CHERRY HILL'S HORSEKEEPING ALMANAC

CHERRY HILL'S HORSEKEEPING ALMANAC

THE ESSENTIAL MONTH-BY-MONTH GUIDE FOR EVERYONE WHO KEEPS OR CARES FOR HORSES

Illustrations by Elayne Sears

Storey Publishing

The mission of Storey Publishing is to serve our customers by publishing practical information that encourages personal independence in harmony with the environment.

Edited by Deborah Burns
Editorial assistance by Melinda Sheehan
Art direction by Cynthia N. McFarland and Alethea Morrison
Cover design by Alethea Morrison and Jon Valk
Text design by Vicky Vaughn Design

Illustrations by Elayne Sears
Maps and image coordination by Ilona Sherratt
Photograph on page 14 by Randy Dunn

Indexed by Susan Olason, Indexes & Knowledge Maps

Printed in the United States by CJK
10 9 8 7 6 5 4 3 2 1

Library of Congress Cataloging-in-Publication Data

Hill, Cherry, 1947-
Horsekeeping almanac / Cherry Hill.
p. cm.
Includes index.
ISBN 978-1-58017-684-2 (pbk. : alk. paper)
1. Horses–Calendars. 2. Horsemanship–Calendars. I. Title.
SF285.H549 2007
636.1–dc22

2007032328

DEDICATION

To my mother, Sally George,
91 years young, who followed her own Almanac
while raising five children.

Thanks, Mom, for passing along your love of nature
and for teaching me how to cook, can, and make soap!

And to Richard,
husband, best friend, and fellow horsekeeper,
who has helped make my dreams come true.
Thank you, Richard, for everything!

CONTENTS

LATE WINTER

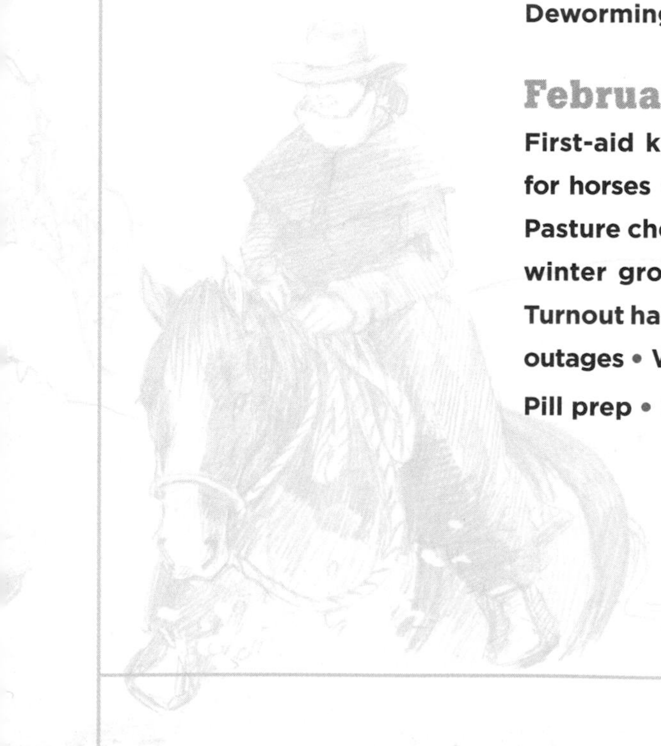

SPRING

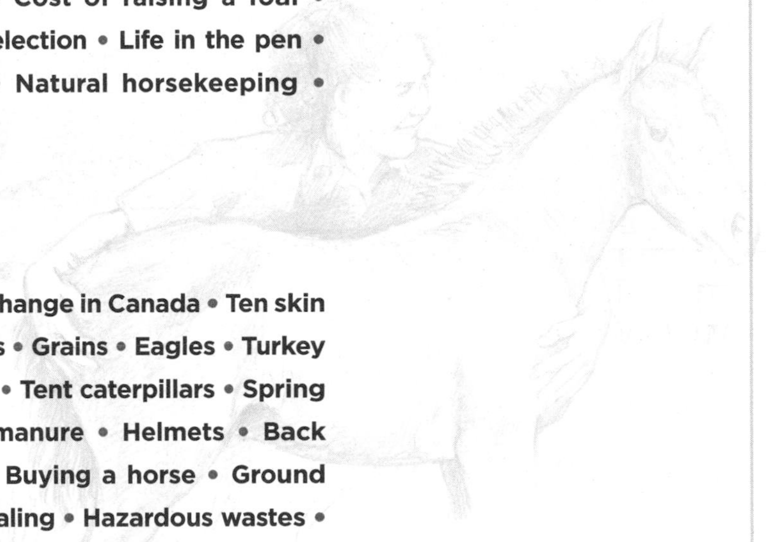

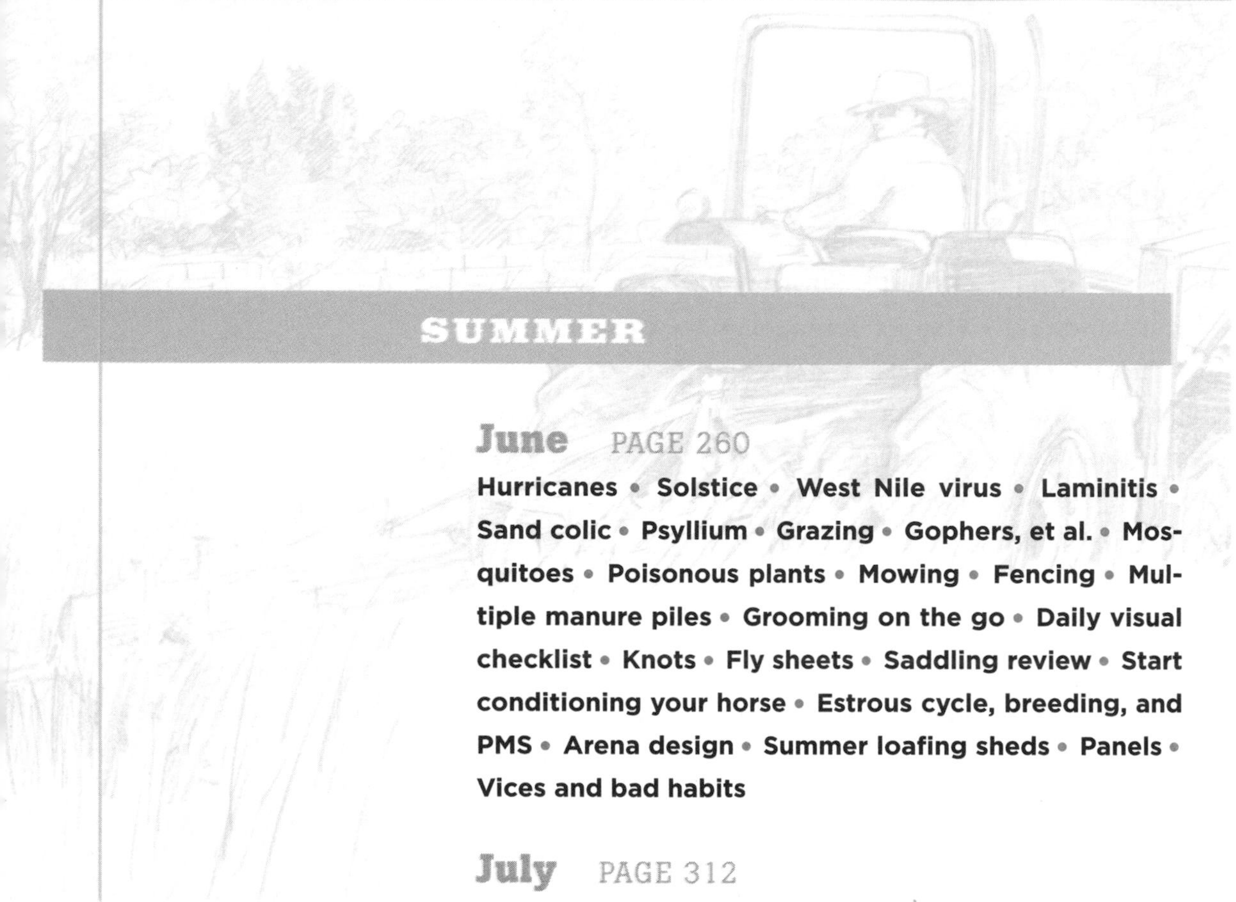

SUMMER

FALL

EARLY WINTER

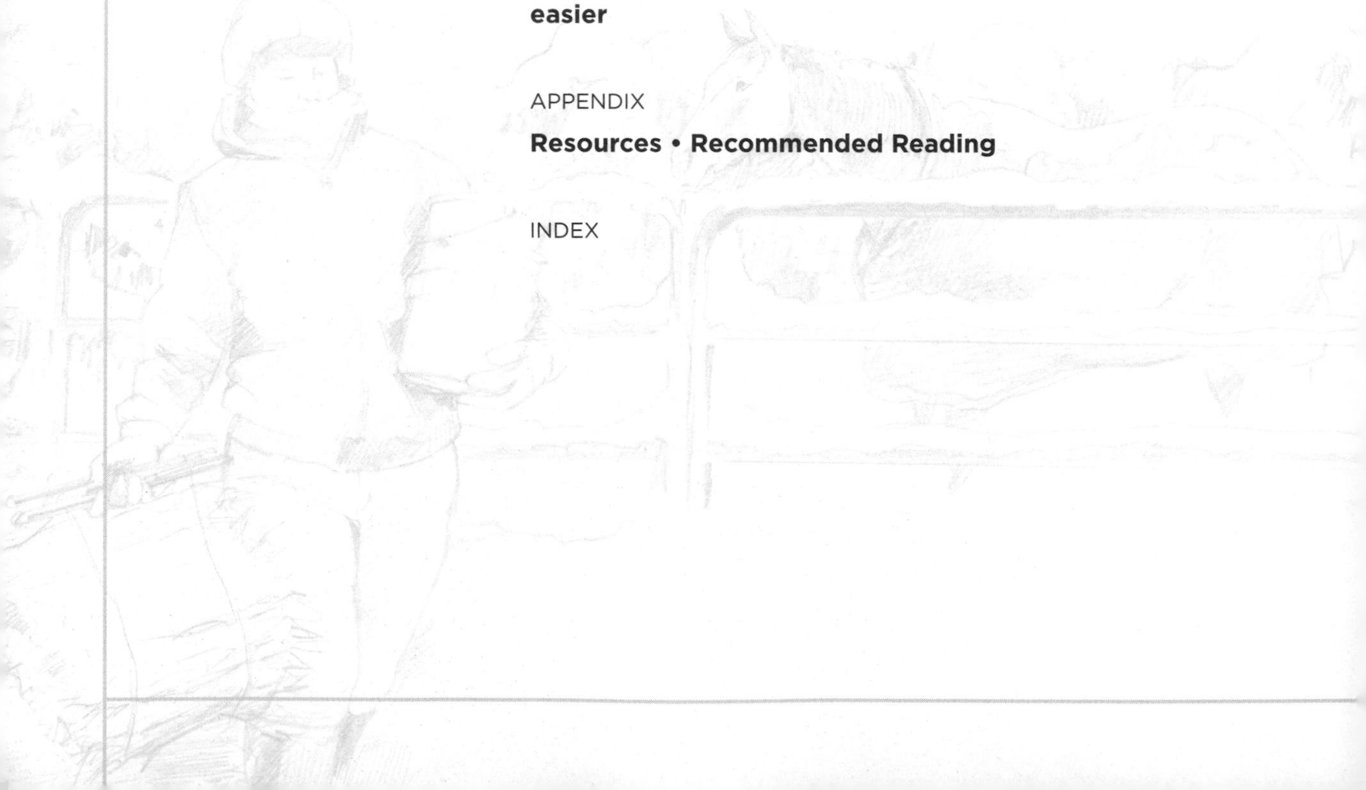

PREFACE

"God forbid that I should go to any heaven where there are no horses."

— Robert Bontine Cunningham-Graham
in a letter to Theodore Roosevelt, 1890

I CAN'T IMAGINE life without horses. They are the thread that ties the stuff of life together. Horse ownership asks us to give, but we receive so much more in return. Although horsekeeping is a year-round task requiring dedication and hard work, the benefits are there for us every day.

We Horsekeepers

We horsekeepers tend to our horses' needs every day at least twice a day, often before our own. We tend to their feeding, grooming, and exercise, as well as buying feed, cleaning and repairing tack, maintaining land and facilities, and much more. Many aspects of horse ownership require hard physical labor: shoveling manure, toting bales, carrying water, training, and riding. Sometimes we have to make trade-offs. We might have to give up something we'd like to do or have in order to ensure that our horses receive proper care. We might have to interrupt our sleep, work schedule, or love life to take care of a foaling mare or an injured or ill horse, or to meet with our veterinarian or farrier. During the winter, when we are least likely to ride, our horses require just as much care as they do during the summer. We also have legal obligations to our horses, our neighbors, and other horse owners in the area, as well as to pedestrians and motorists that pass by our properties.

We horsekeepers are dedicated and hardworking and reap the many benefits that horsekeeping provides. A relationship with a horse can be very fulfilling. A horse doesn't talk back but does tell us, using body language and other nonverbal communication, how he interprets our actions. A horse reveals our tendencies and provides the opportunity for us to become better people. Caring for and interacting with horses can make us more reliable, thorough, trustworthy, honest, and consistent. People who have difficulty working with other people often find that a horse can teach them the meaning of teamwork. When we work closely with a horse, it becomes a partnership. Each of us has certain obligations to the other, and when those are met consistently on both sides, there is the potential for a great relationship.

An honest, trustworthy horse can provide invaluable therapy for us when our life is hectic. Riding can reduce stress and stop unhealthy mental conversations. Few experiences equal a trail ride in the fresh air, especially amid gorgeous scenery. Riding down a road or in an arena can also be enjoyable and beneficial for us and our horses in many ways. A rein-swinging walk can connect us to natural rhythms; a brisk trot with its metronome-like quality is physically invigorating; a rolling cross-country gallop rekindles the sensations of freedom.

We horsekeepers receive regular exercise and daily inspiration. Grooming, cleaning, health care, and riding involve many muscle groups and types of activities. Horsekeeping can help us establish good habits and routines and bring order to a chaotic life. Horses are a feast for the eyes. But then, you already know that if you are a horsekeeper. They are beautiful to watch resting, grazing, playing, and moving with energy and grace. They provide a valuable opportunity for learning about animal behavior. Their reactions and interactions are fascinating and provide us with stories to tell our family and friends. Horses are such treasures. They encourage us to live passionately. Our work becomes our play.

"The master in the art of living makes little distinction between his work and his play, his labor and his leisure, his mind and his body, his information and his recreation, his love and his religion. He hardly knows which is which. He simply pursues his vision of excellence at whatever he does, leaving others to decide whether he is working or playing. To him he's always doing both."

— Zen text

Long Tail Ranch

TO GIVE YOU AN IDEA of where my horsekeeping advice comes from, I thought I'd describe our facilities, climate, horses, and horse activities. We have 70 acres of nonirrigated semiarid pasture in the foothills of the Colorado Rocky Mountains in northern Colorado. There is a year-round creek running through the three largest pastures. A seasonal spring runs through two other pastures. Natural shelter includes trees, ravines, and large rock outcroppings. The pastures are fenced and cross-fenced as indicated on the accompanying map and result in 12 pastures that range in size from approximately ½ acre to 10 acres.

The climate is semiarid; we average 15 to 17 inches of precipitation per year. It is a mild climate for its 7,000-foot elevation. During the summer the temperature rarely rises above 90°F, and during the winter, we have only short patches of days below freezing. Occasionally there is a string of days below zero and snow over 3 feet.

We average between five and nine horses, ranging in age from newborn foals to seniors. We have Quarter Horses and Warmblood/Quarter Horse crosses, which we use for arena western horsemanship, dressage, and trail riding, as well as for photos and videos.

My husband, Richard Klimesh, and I do it all: training, riding, grooming, feeding, health care, shoeing, and facilities maintenance. We are like a well-oiled machine

Our Facilities

Buildings and improvements include:

- 52′ x 33′ four-stall horse barn with sheltered runs; 1′ overhang on west; 15′ overhang on east; 26′ roof extension on the south end.
- 40′ x 80′ enclosed hay and equipment barn with additional 20′ roof overhang on the east end where the senior center is located.
- 24′ x 40′ shop and farm-office building
- Three large metal pens
- 66′ diameter round pen
- 100′ x 200′ arena.

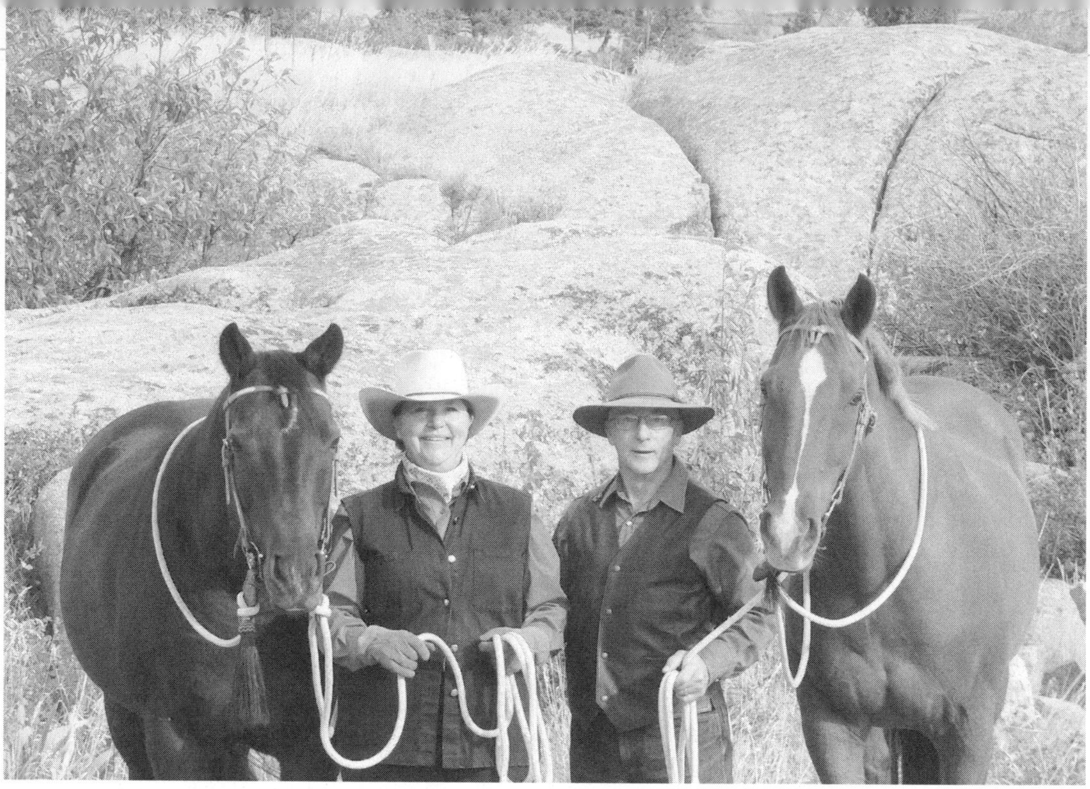

CHERRY HILL AND RICHARD KLIMESH

when it comes to doing chores. As we head out the back door one of us might say something like “What a great day,” or “Gosh, it’s bitter . . . brrr,” but we rarely have to discuss what we are going to do. It is like a well-rehearsed play that runs every day. The script changes from season to season, but the natural division of duties always seems to fall into place.

For example, in midwinter, when our six horses are out on five different pastures, here is how we proceed. I head to the main horse barn to mix up mashes and grain rations while Richard is off to the hay barn to make up big hay suitcases to carry to four of the pasture horses. I take the grain buckets and single servings of hay to the other two horses. While I am in their pastures, I check their water troughs, breaking ice if necessary and making note of when the troughs will need refilling. Richard checks the creek while he is out feeding his four, breaking ice and noting whether there is enough flowing water to meet their needs.

Even though we are working across 70 acres, I sense where Richard is at all times by either seeing him, seeing the horse’s reactions, or seeing a light on or off in the hay barn. I’ll bet he has his own ways of keeping track of me too. It isn’t unusual for us both to finish with our portion of chores at the same time and be walking in the back door together.

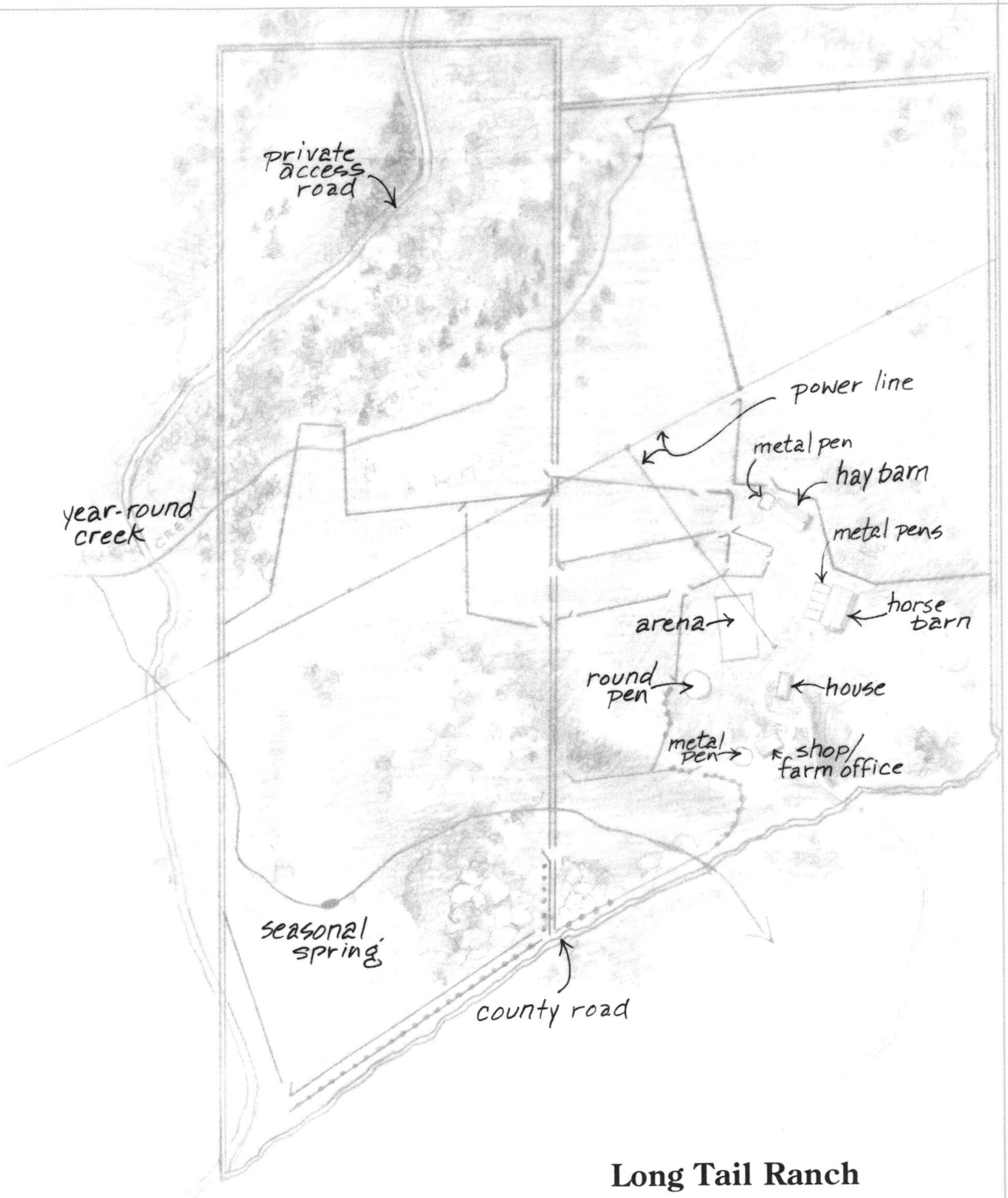
private access road
power line
metal pen
hay barn
year-round creek
metal pens
horse barn
arena
round pen
house
metal pen
shop/ farm office
seasonal spring
county road

Long Tail Ranch

Using This Book

Whether you have one horse or a hundred, horsekeeping tasks are many and varied. To help you organize what needs to be done when, I've set up this book as an almanac tracking a year of activities for horsekeepers in temperate climates (the majority of the United States). Although I now live in Colorado and have included many of my personal schedules, lists, and ideas, I have kept horses everywhere from Alaska to Arizona and as far east as Michigan, so I kept climate-specific issues in mind as I wrote.

Horsekeepers in Canada and the extreme northern United States and those in the South will need to adjust the timetable a bit to fit your locale. For example, while Southern horsekeepers enjoy beautiful riding weather, those in North Dakota might be in the deep freeze, so your horsekeeping concerns and tasks will be different. Each month, I've included topics that are specific to certain areas in North America to target some of these regional issues.

Besides the topics you'd expect me to cover in this book (feed, health care, hoof care, and facilities maintenance), I've included some other departments that I hope you enjoy as much as I do.

Horse Movie of the Month. Richard and I are great movie fans so I thought I'd tell you about some of my favorites. It was hard to pare my list down to twelve!

Wacky Wonderful Weather. I'm also a weather enthusiast, having reported data from the station on our ranch for more than 20 years, so you'll be reading a bit every month about wind and precipitation and other atmospheric issues.

Ranch Recipes. I love to cook and make concoctions so I'll share some of my ideas, mostly for horse stuff.

Wild Life. Each region has its own rich flora and fauna, and wildlife plays a huge role here in Colorado. I'll include some facts and stories that you might find interesting.

En español. Here I'll give recognition to some of our many horse words that have their origin in Spanish. Some scholars say that Spanish has contributed more than 10,000 words to the English language. Each month I'll present a word or two that arises from the rich equestrian history of Spain, Mexico, Latin America, South America, and other Spanish-speaking regions of the world.

Historical Horsekeeping. Under this heading I'll share tips and techniques I've gleaned from my collection of very old horse books. In some instances, the advice is still gold; in others, I was tempted to retitle the box "Hysterical Horsekeeping" because the information is truly from the Dark Ages.

It was great fun putting this book together. I hope you read it, write in it, tuck feed tags and receipts in it, take it to the barn, and use it to design your own Horsekeeping Master Plan.

My warmest regards,
Cherry Hill

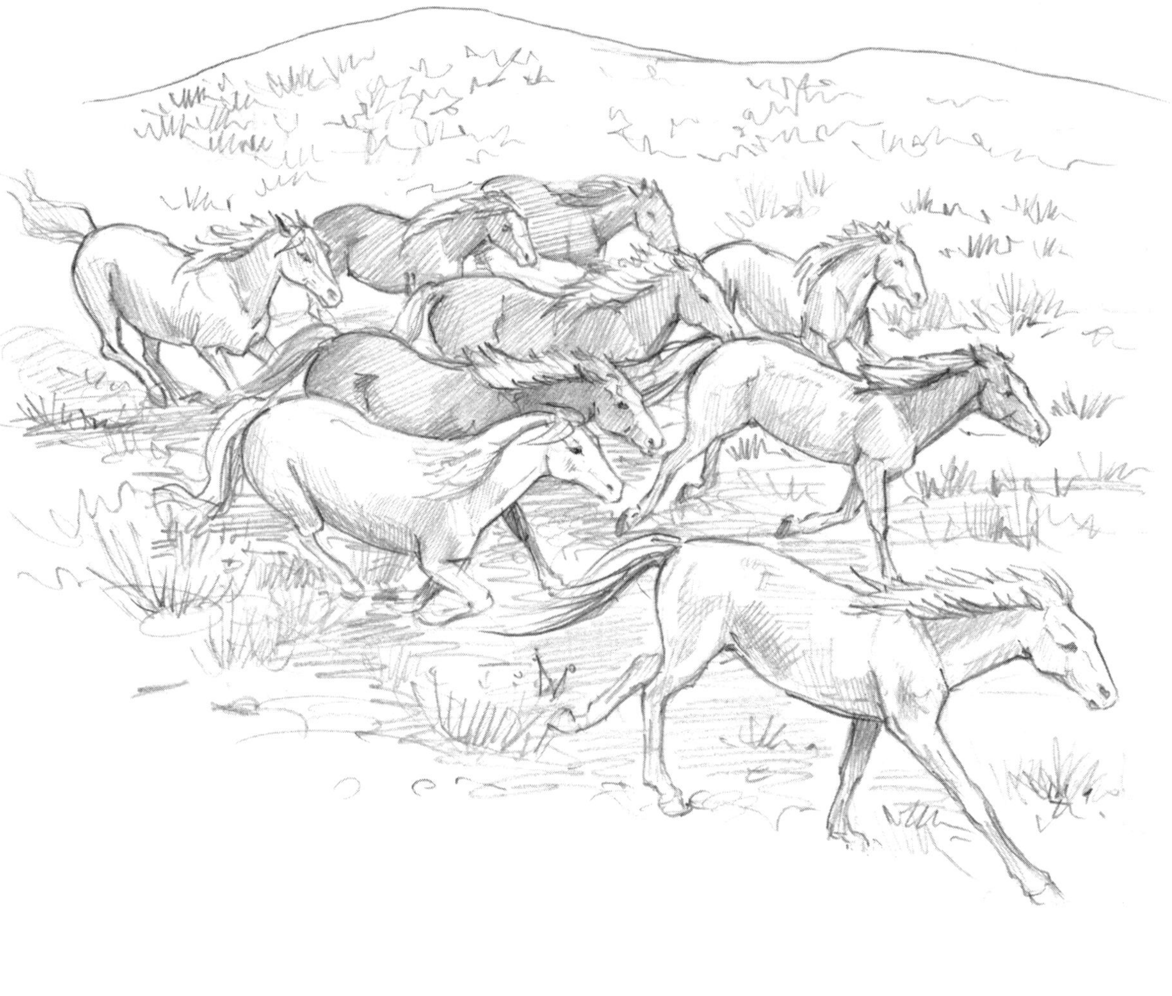

LATE WINTER

JANUARY AND FEBRUARY

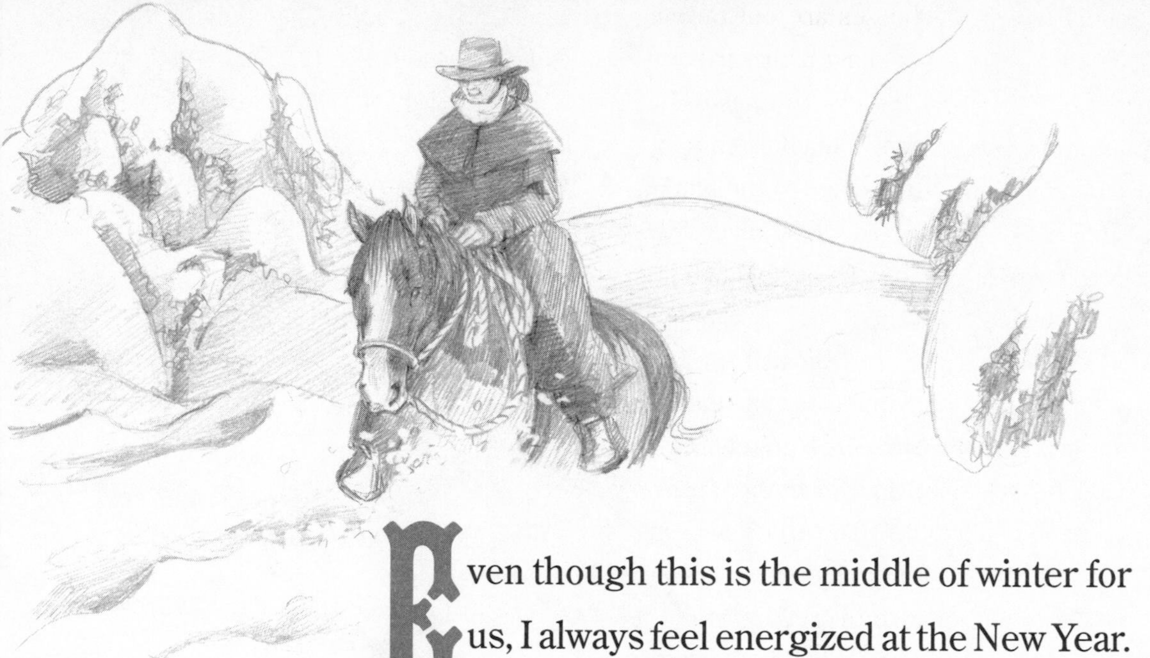

Even though this is the middle of winter for us, I always feel energized at the New Year. January is an opportunity for a fresh start, setting new goals, making plans, and preparing for the next busy horse season. From April 1 through November 15, the days are packed, and we spend a lot of time outdoors. From mid-November to the end of March, we hibernate a bit, writing the books and video scripts that are the basis of our work.

That's why January is a good time to make lists and set up calendars and notebooks. They help me stay organized and keep track of all the things that a horsekeeper must do.

The horses kick back at this time of year. It is usually too windy and cold for much training and riding, so if there is sufficient snow cover, the horses are out on winter pasture — unless we have a blizzard or very strong winds. As long as the pastures are protected with a snowy blanket, the horses don't do too much damage to the land, and the snow makes a nice clean place to feed them; plus, they get free-choice exercise and a soft place to lie down.

Some winters, I let some of the horses grow a full-length winter coat. In other years and with certain horses, I blanket all winter. (See July, October, and November for everything about blankets.) I do little grooming of pasture horses this time of year, because I don't want to disturb the natural protective sebum that lies next to the skin and acts as a windproof and waterproof layer. One or two horses are usually shod with winter shoes and pads for days when the weather allows training or riding, but the rest are barefoot.

The horses are fed at 7:00 a.m. and 6:00 p.m. Only the seniors get concentrates at this time of year; the rest do quite well on just hay. The horses are carrying a little bit more weight at this time of year than usual. The extra layer of fat helps to keep them warmer. Their full-time turnout keeps them in good shape physically, because they have to walk down to the creek several times each day to drink and they mosey around between feedings.

In addition to the exercise from doing chores, I find it essential to go for a walk every day. As an added benefit, a healthy dose of sunlight helps prevent those winter blues. I am usually champing at the bit to begin working with the horses full time, so I pacify myself with pre-riding exercises to stretch and strengthen those muscles that might have become slack over the winter.

Late Winter Visual Exam

OVERALL STANCE AND ATTITUDE. As I approach with feed, does the horse have his head up, are his eyes bright, and is he eager

Weekly Tasks

- ❑ Restock the hay supply in horse barns
- ❑ Check grain supply
- ❑ Dump and scrub all waterers, troughs, tanks, tubs, and buckets
- ❑ Scrub feed dishes
- ❑ Check veterinary supply needs
- ❑ Check upcoming farrier and veterinarian appointments and get ready for them
- ❑ Keep winter feeding areas clean of old feed that might have become wet from snow

Seasonal Tasks

- ❑ Spread manure
- ❑ Clean tack
- ❑ Get ready for spring!

for feed, or is he lethargic, inattentive, or anxious?

LEGS. I look at the horse from both sides so I will quickly spot any wounds, swelling, or puffiness. If the horse is shod, I look for four shoes, tightly nailed.

APPETITE. Have the horses finished all of the hay from the previous feeding? Are they all anxious to get the new ration?

WATER. Is there evidence that the horses have taken in a sufficient amount of water?

MANURE. Although difficult to assess on pasture, I try to observe whether the fecal material is well formed or if it is hard and dry, loose and sloppy, covered with mucus or parasites, or filled with whole grains.

MOVEMENT. Does the horse move comfortably and soundly as he approaches?

✳	My Day	A Horse's Day
6:00 AM	Rise.	Stand near feed spots.
7:00 AM	Chores and visual exam of the horses (see above).	Eat.
8:00 AM	Breakfast.	
9:00 AM	Work in office with a mid-morning exercise break.	
10:00 AM		Walk down to the creek for a drink.
10:15 AM		Mosey around the pasture.
12:30 PM	Lunch.	Lie down for a nap.
1:30 PM	Work in office or barn.	
3:30 PM	Walk down to the creek.	
4:30 PM		Stand near feed spots.
5:00 PM	Chores and visual exam.	Eat.
6:00 PM	Supper.	
7:00 PM	Domestic duties.	Head back down to the creek for a drink.
7:15 PM		Mosey until dawn, keeping an eye and ear ever vigilant for coyotes, stray dogs, mountain lions, and blowing objects.
8:00 PM	Nightly movie.	
10:30 PM	Bedtime.	

JANUARY

Short days and long nights provide plenty of time for well-deserved and necessary R&R (that's Research and Reading, of course!). The number of daylight hours has a great effect on biological functions in plants and animals, and it can affect moods and emotions in humans, too. It is a good idea to be aware of the day length in your area so you can plan and adjust chore schedules, set up lights for shedding or breeding, and implement other management decisions.

Day Length in Hours

Latitude	Jan 1	Jan 16	Feb 1
60°N	5.66	6.35	7.51
55°N	7	7.5	8.37
50°N	7.93	8.32	9.01
45°N	8.64	8.95	9.51
40°N	9.21	9.46	9.92
35°N	9.69	9.89	10.27
30°N	10.1	10.27	10.58

See page 22 to find your latitude.

WACKY WONDERFUL WEATHER

To Do

- ❑ Set up records
- ❑ Establish baseline vitals
- ❑ Prepare foaling kit
- ❑ Tractor maintenance
- ❑ Hoof trim and shoe
- ❑ Deworm
- ❑ Rhino #2 for broodmares
- ❑ Repair barn brooms
- ❑ Scrub feed tubs and buckets
- ❑ Move hay to barns
- ❑ Annual barn cleaning

To Buy

- ❑ Beet pulp pellets
- ❑ Senior feed
- ❑ Corn oil
- ❑ Hoof supplement

TRACKING YOUR WEATHER

Keeping a log of the weather at your farm or ranch is not only interesting, but it will also help you calculate cold-weather rations, manage pastures, and know when there is a livestock alert. Livestock alerts are issued by the National Weather Service when temperatures, precipitation, and/or wind are severe enough to be harmful to the safety of animals. Perhaps you could become a weather spotter or station for your regional weather service or university. If so, you might be able to obtain some of the equipment for providing data, free of charge.

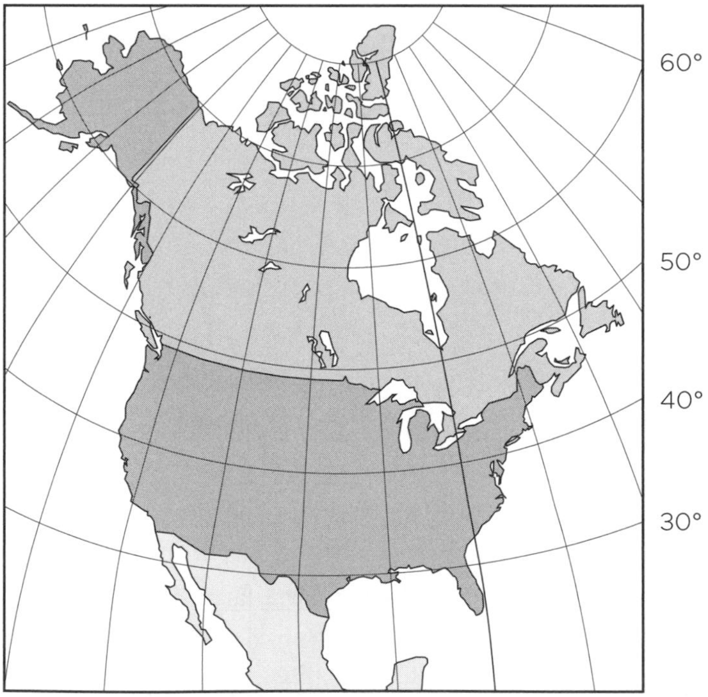

Latitude and season determine the length of your days and nights.

Horses and the Weather

Horses are in tune with the weather. Perhaps it is due to changes in barometric pressure or shifts in wind direction. Whatever the connection, horses often signal an impending storm by becoming restless and somewhat anxious.

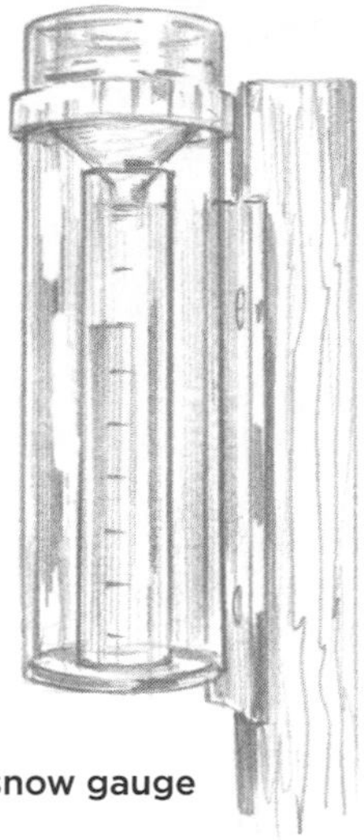

Rain-snow gauge

Weather Equipment

The first and most essential piece of weather-station equipment is a precipitation gauge. My favorite kind is a large, clear tube that is a combination rain and snow gauge. It consists of four parts: a mounting bracket that is screwed onto a post, a large snow-collection tube, a small rain-collection tube that fits inside the large tube, and a receiving funnel that collects rain and sends it into the rain tube. You can also purchase and install an all-purpose digital weather station, which will record and save daily highs, lows, highest wind, lowest wind chill, and more.

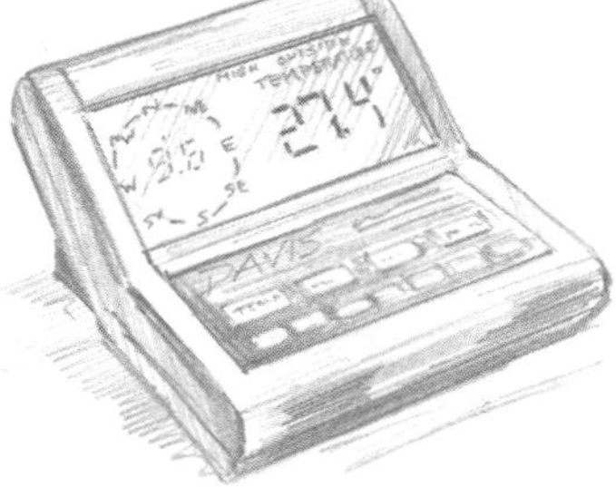

All-purpose digital weather station

SETTING UP RECORDS

January 1 is the traditional time to set up new calendars, notebooks, and other record files for the upcoming year. In my tack room I have a hanging calendar where I write all upcoming veterinary and farrier appointments, plus when I need to deworm or vaccinate. I check the calendar every week so I can get ready for upcoming sessions. On my tack room desk I have a 4x6 recipe-card box with a divider tab with each horse's name. I record vet, farrier, breeding, and other information on individual horse cards. In addition, I have a two-drawer file cabinet where I store all registration papers, equipment instructions, and warranties as well as old veterinary and breeding records.

Ranch Notes

Jan. 1 Gopher explosion. I see Yoda eat a gopher at 7 AM, Noon, and 6 PM. There are gopher holes everywhere in the pastures but very few mice in the fields or buildings.

In a general horse journal I write any unusual events related to the horses or horsekeeping. From November to April, the journal is usually near one of my favorite chairs in our home, but at other times, it is handier in the tack room. I bring out a brand-new blank journal in January and when it is filled, I file it away for reference.

On my home-office computer, I have a calendar that makes the sound of a cracking whip when something related to the horses needs to be done. That way I will receive a reminder of an upcoming deworming or "psyllium week" when I am at a computer and near a phone, so I can order necessary supplies or make an appointment.

In the barn aisle, I have a board that lists each horse and his or her current age, height, weight, blanket size, and any other useful data. I update this on January 1, as all horses become a year older on that date no matter what date they were born.

In the feed room, I have an erasable feed board with each horse's name and his morning and evening feeding amounts. Although I keep this board updated regularly throughout the year, during the first week of January I wipe the entire board clean and start fresh, redrawing all the lines and squares. (See page 33 for more on feed boards.)

An old horse **does not forget his path.**

— Japanese proverb

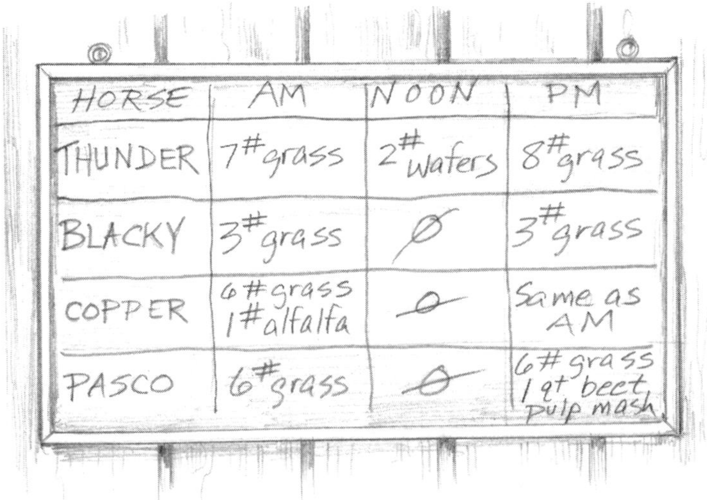
HORSE
AM
NOON
PM
THUNDER
7# grass
2# wafers
8# grass
BLACKY
3# grass
Ø
3# grass
COPPER
6# grass 1# alfalfa
Ø
Same as AM
PASCO
6# grass
Ø
6# grass 1 qt beet pulp mash

An erasable feed board helps keep track of feed changes.

VET CLINIC

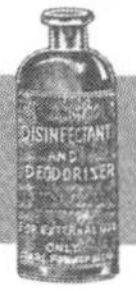

MONITORING VITAL SIGNS

A basic task of horsekeeping is to monitor your horse's health by regularly taking his vital signs, beginning with temperature, pulse, and respiration.

Every horse is different, so learn what is normal for each of your horses in order to recognize immediately when there is a problem.

TEMPERATURE. To take a horse's temperature I use a glass-mercury animal thermometer (digital thermometers require a battery). First check the thermometer to be sure it is reading below 96°F. If it is still registering a temperature from the previous use, hold the thermometer securely at the top and shake it sharply, which forces the mercury to the bulb of the thermometer. Then apply a small amount of petroleum jelly to the business end of the thermometer. The lubricating jelly should be at least at room temperature, somewhere around 65°F.

Baseline Vital Signs

January 1 is a good time to establish baseline vital signs for each horse. Vital signs measure a horse's body functions and are a good indication of his overall state of health. I record the normal stats for each horse, because every horse is an individual, and like us, horses change as they grow up, mature, and then age. When I suspect something is wrong, I can refer to that horse's normal stats. This is valuable information to have on hand if I need to call my veterinarian.

To establish a current set of normals, I perform the following procedure each year. I take each horse's temperature, pulse, respiration, and capillary refill time; perform the pinch test; and listen to his heart, lungs, and intestines with a stethoscope. I take the vital signs twice a day for three days and average the readings. I choose various times of day, but always when the horse is at rest, not when he has just been working or is excited. I write the average in each horse's record.

An assistant should hold your horse, or you can tie him if he is used to having his temperature taken. Move his tail off to one side. This tends to cause less tension in the horse than lifting the tail up.

Insert the thermometer into the anus at a very slight upward angle, gently easing it inward and upward until about 2 inches remains outside the anus. Do not insert the thermometer all the way. If you do, it has a greater chance of contacting warm fecal material, which will give you an inaccurate temperature reading.

Move the tail back into position. After two minutes, take a reading.

Using a Mercury Thermometer Safely

If you use a glass mercury thermometer to take your horse's temperature, it is smart to protect it with a case and a string clip. You'll need a 24-inch length of nylon string (builder's cord works great), an alligator clip (available at hardware and electronic stores), and a drill of some sort.

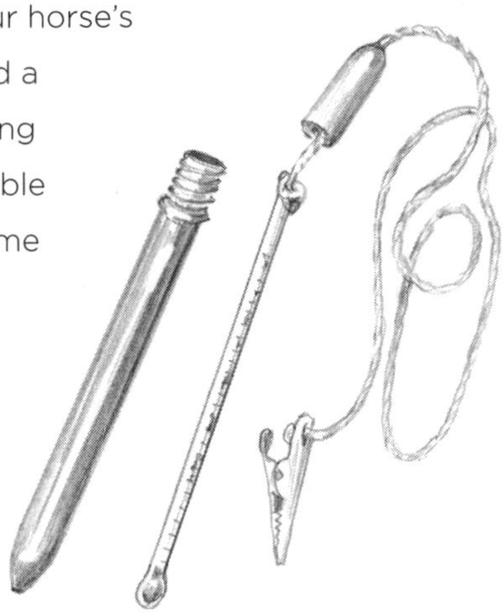

1 Tie the alligator clip to one end of the string. To prevent fraying, melt the end of the string with a flame.
2 Drill a hole in the cap of the thermometer case and thread the string through the cap from the pointed end of the cap.
3 Tie the end of the string to the eyehole at the end of the thermometer.

When you take your horse's temperature, clip the string to his tail. If he defecates, the thermometer will not fall to the ground and break; instead, it will hang from his tail. The case protects the thermometer from breakage between uses.

PULSE. Pulse rates can be taken anywhere an artery lies close to the surface of the skin. (Arteries carry blood from the heart to the tissues.) Two convenient places are at the digital artery of the fetlock and at the maxillary artery under the horse's jaw.

Hold your index and middle finger over the artery. The artery will feel like a thin cord. Press until you feel it throb. Your thumb has its own artery and pulse, so although you can use your thumb to anchor your hand, don't use it over the artery to take the pulse, or you might be counting your own pulse instead of your horse's.

Once you can feel the pulse distinctly, count the beats in one minute. If your horse is restless, you can count for 15 seconds and multiply by four.

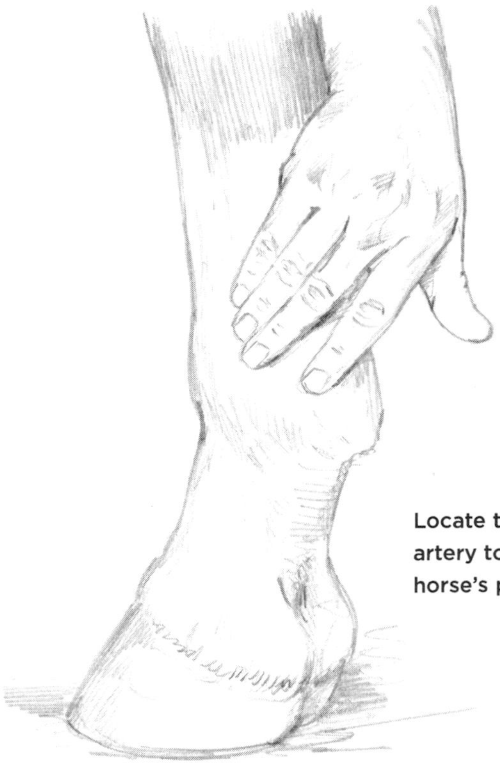

Locate the digital artery to take a horse's pulse.

What's Normal?

Temperature

The average resting temperature of an adult horse ranges from 99° to 100°F. Temperature increases with exertion, excitement, illness, and hot, humid weather. Temperature decreases with shock, and a horse's temperature can be a few degrees lower in very cold weather.

Pulse

Normal resting pulse for an adult horse is 30 to 40 beats per minute. Pulse rates are higher with excitement, pain, nervousness, elevated body temperature, shock, infectious disease, and exercise. Pulse rates are lower on fit horses and in cooler weather.

RESPIRATION. Respiration is a little harder to measure, and it is one vital sign that you will want to pay attention to as a horse rests, eats, works, and recovers from exercise. A horse's normal resting respiration rate is usually between 12 and 25 breaths per minute. One breath is measured as one inhalation and one exhalation. The ratio of the pulse to the respiration rate is often a more significant measure of stress than each of the actual figures is.

When a horse is exercising heavily, it is easy to measure his respiration rate by watching his nostrils dilate and relax (each cycle counts as one breath) or by watching his ribs move in and out. This is very hard to detect in a resting horse, however, so the best way to determine a respiration rate is to use a stethoscope on the trachea.

Standing near your horse's shoulder, face forward with the earpieces of the stethoscope in your ears and your right hand resting on the horse's withers. With your left hand, press the bell firmly into the underside of the horse's neck about four inches below the throatlatch. Count the breaths for fifteen seconds and multiply by four.

What's Normal?

Respiration

Depending on the horse's age, his normal resting pulse-to-respiration ratio should range from 4:1 to 2:1. If the ratio becomes 1:1 or 1:2 (called inversion), the horse is suffering from oxygen deprivation, which indicates serious stress.

CRT

One to two seconds is normal. If the CRT is prolonged, the horse is showing signs of circulatory impairment and could be suffering from colic or shock.

CRT. Capillary refill time (CRT) measures how long it takes blood to return to blanched tissues. It is used as a general indicator of circulation. To determine the CRT, exert light thumb pressure on your horse's gums above the upper incisors for two seconds to temporarily push the blood in the capillaries out of the tissues. (Capillaries are the smallest blood vessels.) When you remove your thumb, you will see a white spot the size and shape of your thumbprint. Note how long it takes for normal color to return to the spot. That is the CRT.

Also inspect the mucous membranes around his eyes and gums for a bright pink color and appropriate moisture. If the mucous membranes are very pale or white, the horse is suffering from blood loss or circulatory impairment.

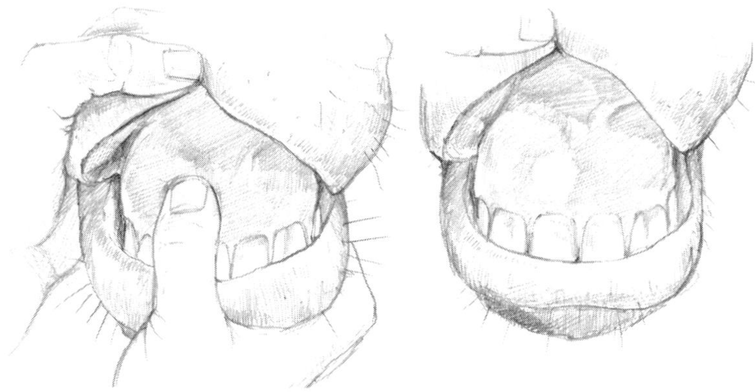

Normal CRT is one to two seconds.

Bright red gums indicate a toxic condition (poison). If the gums are grayish blue, the horse is probably in shock.

PINCH TEST. The pliability and resiliency of a horse's skin is a good indicator of his level of hydration, or the amount of water in his tissues. To determine if your horse is dehydrated, use the pinch test. Pick up a fold of skin in the shoulder or neck region and then release it. It should return to its flat position almost instantaneously, or at least within a second or two. If the skin remains peaked for more than two seconds, this is termed a "standing tent," and indicates some degree of body fluid loss. A standing tent lasting five to 10 seconds or longer indicates moderate to severe dehydration and requires immediate veterinary attention.

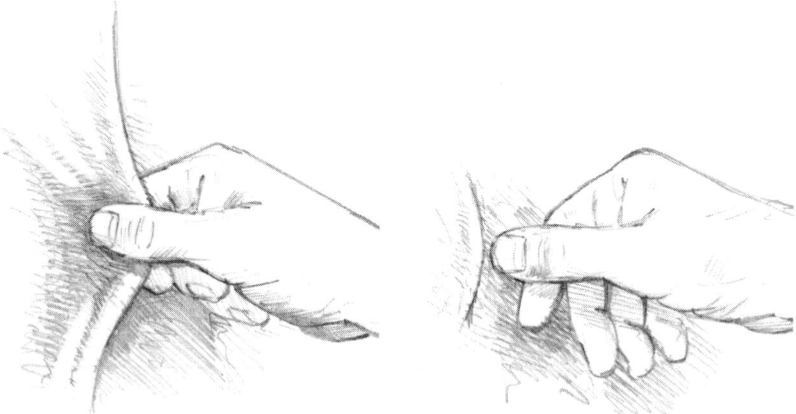

A normal pinch test is flat within two seconds.

Ranch Notes

Jan. 4 Turned out all horses and put new 3/8" minus pea gravel in their pens; ordered another load.

PERFORM A DAILY VISUAL EXAM

Make a New Year's resolution to assess the overall health and well being of your horse with a daily visual exam. You will develop your own daily visual exam depending on where your horse lives (in a stall, pen, or pasture) and if he is in a group, wears a blanket, is shod, and so on. But here are some basics to get you started. (See the seasonal notes for guidelines according to the time of year. See June for my pasture check routine and what I carry in my pasture kit.)

A visual exam is a quick but methodical once-over that you conduct with your eyes as you feed your horse. If you see something abnormal, take the time to touch your horse and if necessary, take his vital signs. As you feed, try to view your horse from both sides and from the front and the rear.

If you see something abnormal, take the time to touch your horse and if necessary, take his vital signs.

- ❑ Is his head up? Are his eyes bright? Is he eager for his feed?
- ❑ Is he lethargic, inattentive, or anxious?
- ❑ Are his legs free of wounds, swelling, or puffiness?
- ❑ If he is shod, does he have all four shoes and are they well fitted?
- ❑ Did he finish all of his feed from the previous feeding?
- ❑ Has he taken in a sufficient amount of water?
- ❑ Is his manure well formed or loose and sloppy? (Take a closer look to detect the presence of mucus, parasites, or undigested whole grains.)
- ❑ If he lives in a stall, do you see signs of pawing, rubbing, rolling, or thrashing?
- ❑ Are there signs of wood-chewing in stalls, on fence posts, or on rails?
- ❑ Watch your horse move. Is there any irregularity in his gait or does he lag behind the other horses?

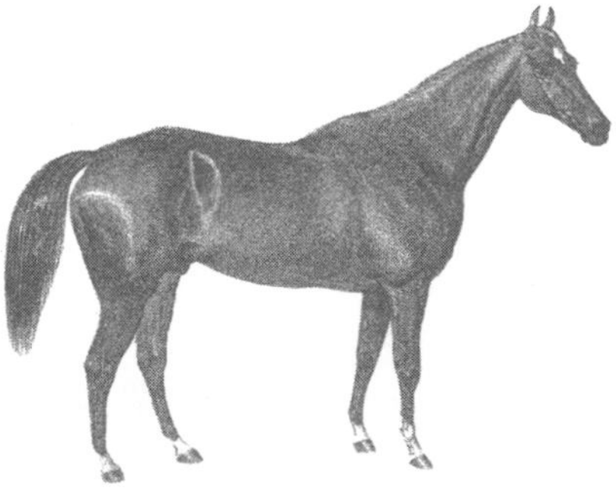

FOOT NOTES

GOOD MANNERS FOR FARRIER VISITS

A horse should pick up his hoof readily when asked and be able to stand on three legs in balance while your farrier works on the fourth. The inactive time in January is a perfect time to review manners for trimming and shoeing. It is my job, not my farrier's, to train my horses for farrier care.

THINK LIKE A HORSE. First I try to see things from a horse's perspective. A horse doesn't reason things out, he reacts. He has deeply ingrained reflexes. And he is very socially connected to other horses. Some don't like being separated from buddies. Although a temporary fix might be to bring a buddy in the barn when a horse is being shod, ultimately each horse should be secure alone. One way I do this is to routinely separate each horse from other horses in an isolated pen or stall or tied to a hitching post so every horse sees that he can survive in a variety of situations away from his buddy, his stall or pen, the barn, and the herd.

I also remind myself that horses are nomads and don't naturally choose to stand still. They are also fearful of restraint, which is one of their means of survival. Horses must be trained to accept being tied and to stand still. Understandably, a "fresh" horse (one that has not been turned out recently) is likely to get antsy when asked to stand still for shoeing.

I try to make sure my horses are well acquainted with tying and standing for periods of time, and that they are regularly exercised. Bringing an untrained, insecure, under-exercised horse into the barn, confining him in crossties, and asking a farrier to shoe him is inconsiderate and just plain foolish.

TIPS & TECHNIQUES

Comfort Zone

Many horses are reluctant to defecate or urinate if they are standing on a surface that will splash back. So if one of my normally quiet horses becomes extremely restless, I might let him urinate in a pen or deeply bedded stall while the farrier is shaping a shoe.

It is my job, not my farrier's, to train my horses for farrier care.

TIPS & TECHNIQUES

Hoof-Lifting Tips

Don't pull the leg out to the side. Hold the hoof so that the knee is bent at about a 90-degree angle and the cannon is parallel to the ground. If he likes to snatch his leg away, tip the toe upward so that the fetlock joint is bent. It will be more difficult for the horse to jerk his foot out of your hand.

LIFTING A HOOF PROPERLY. I do not want a horse to pick up his hooves every time I touch a leg. Sometimes I want his legs to stay put for grooming, clipping, and bathing. But when I do want him to lift his foot so I can clean his hooves, I am not strong enough to actually lift his leg, so I will ask him to lift his leg for me.

I do this by running my hand down his leg to just above the fetlock where I give a light pinch to his tendon. An alternative signal is to squeeze the chestnut. (Chestnuts are horny growths above the knees and below the hocks.) When you are training your horse to pick up his foot, hold the foot up for only a few seconds to begin with, and gradually hold it for longer periods of time as his training progresses.

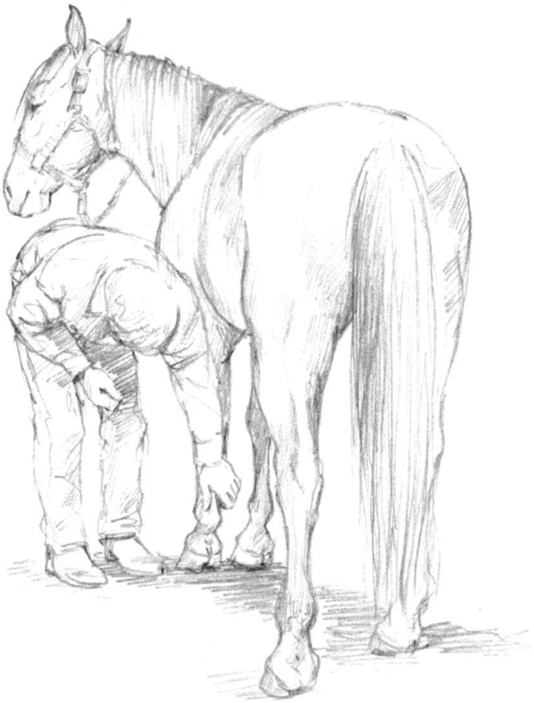

Signal your horse to pick up his foot with a light pinch to the tendon.

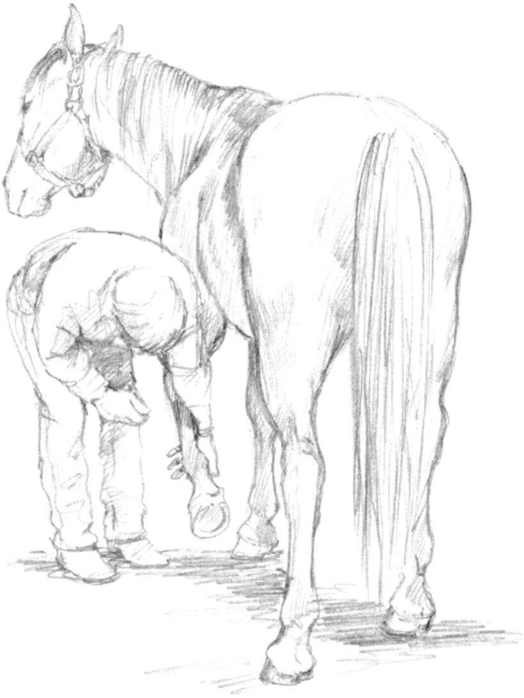

Be ready to catch and hold the foot when he lifts it.

FEED BAG

COLD WEATHER FEED RULE

Here in Colorado, I have to adjust the horses' rations on a daily basis according to the weather. The safest and most sensible way to increase a ration suddenly is to increase the hay.

Human nature makes us think when the weather is cold, we need to give our horses more grain to keep them warm, but if you heap up the grain bucket every time the temperature drops, your horse could suffer colic, become overweight, and be too full of energy, but still not really be warmer. Grain is digested relatively quickly and the heat from its digestion is soon gone. On the other hand, hay generates heat over a longer period of time and is safer to increase suddenly.

For every 10°F below freezing, increase your horses' roughage by 10 percent. If your 1,100-pound horse normally receives 16 pounds of hay per day (in two 8-pound feedings), when the temperature dips to 22°F, increase his hay ration by 10 percent, or 1.6 extra pounds, for a total of 17.6 pounds of hay per day. When the temperature is at 0°F, he should be receiving 30 percent more hay per day:

(16 x 0.30) = 4.8

4.8 + 16 = 20.8

So the horse should receive a total of 20.8 pounds of hay per day at 0°F.

CALCULATING YOUR HORSE'S WEIGHT

The first step in properly feeding a horse is to determine how much he weighs, so that he can be fed according to his weight. Knowing his weight will also help you administer the proper dosage of medication. There is an easy and fairly accurate way to measure your horse's weight using a

Labeling Feed: The 3 Bs

In my feed room I have an erasable **board** with feeding instructions. That way, if someone else needs to do chores, I know my horses will receive the correct rations. I list each horse, the type and amount of each feed the horse gets, and at what time. I keep the board current as I make changes to my horses' rations.

Each feed **barrel** in the feed room is labeled. I label the barrel, not the lid, since lids can be switched accidentally.

Each horse has a feed **bucket** with his or her name on it.

All of these details help prevent feeding errors.

specially designed equine weight tape that's available from tack shops and vet supply catalogs. Measure weight by running the tape snugly around the horse's heart girth.

The approximate weight of your horse can also be determined by using a livestock scale or a heart girth table, or by calculation. To use a heart girth table, first measure the horse's heart girth in inches. With the horse standing square, place a tape measure around the horse's body just behind the withers and about 4 inches behind the front legs. Pull it tight enough to slightly depress the flesh, and take the measurement just after expiration. Refer to the chart below.

Odd Words

heart girth. The circumference of a horse's barrel measured over the withers and just behind the front legs.

withers. The prominent area of the horse's spine where the neck joins the back.

MEASURING HEIGHT

Horses are measured in hands. One hand equals 4 inches. It is easiest to measure a horse's height with a specially

Formula for Weight

You can also calculate an estimate of weight using a formula. Measure the heart girth as above. Measure the body length in a straight line from the point of shoulder to the point of buttocks. Then use this formula:

Heart Girth (in) ×
Heart Girth (in) ×
Body Length ÷ 330 =
Body Weight (lbs)

Estimating Horse Weight by Heart Girth

Heart Girth		Weight	
(inches)	(cm)	(lbs)	(kg)
30.	76	100	45.5
40.	102	200	91.
45.5	116	300	136.5
50.5	128	400	182.
55.	140	500	227.
58.5	148	600	273.
61.5	156	700	318.
64.5	164	800	364.
67.5	171	900	409.
70.5	178	1000	455.
73.	185	1100	500.
75.5	192	1200	545.
77.5	197	1300	591.

designed horse-measuring stick or a height/weight tape. Be sure the horse is standing with weight on all four feet, with his legs set squarely under his body. He should be standing on a flat, level surface such as concrete or a rubber mat. Place the toe of your boot on the designated line of the tape. Hold the measuring tape vertically in one hand and the stick horizontally, resting on the highest point of the horse's withers, in the other hand. Be sure to keep the stick level. If you angle it up, the result will be too high. If you angle it down, the result will be too low. When the bottom of the level stick lines up with the tape, that reading is the horse's height.

If you use a standard tape measure instead, divide by 4 to convert inches to hands. [60 inches ÷ 4 = 15 hands.] If your horse were to measure 63 inches, you would figure it this way: [63 inches ÷ 4 = 15 hands and 3 inches, which is written 15•3 or 15-3 but not 15.3].

TIPS & TECHNIQUES

Scrub That Tub

Before I fill a water tub, I always scrub it and rinse it thoroughly. Even in cold temperatures, hay or grain that is dropped into the tub can deteriorate and foul the water. Buy several inexpensive toilet brushes and hang them near your water troughs. They make great tub scrubbers.

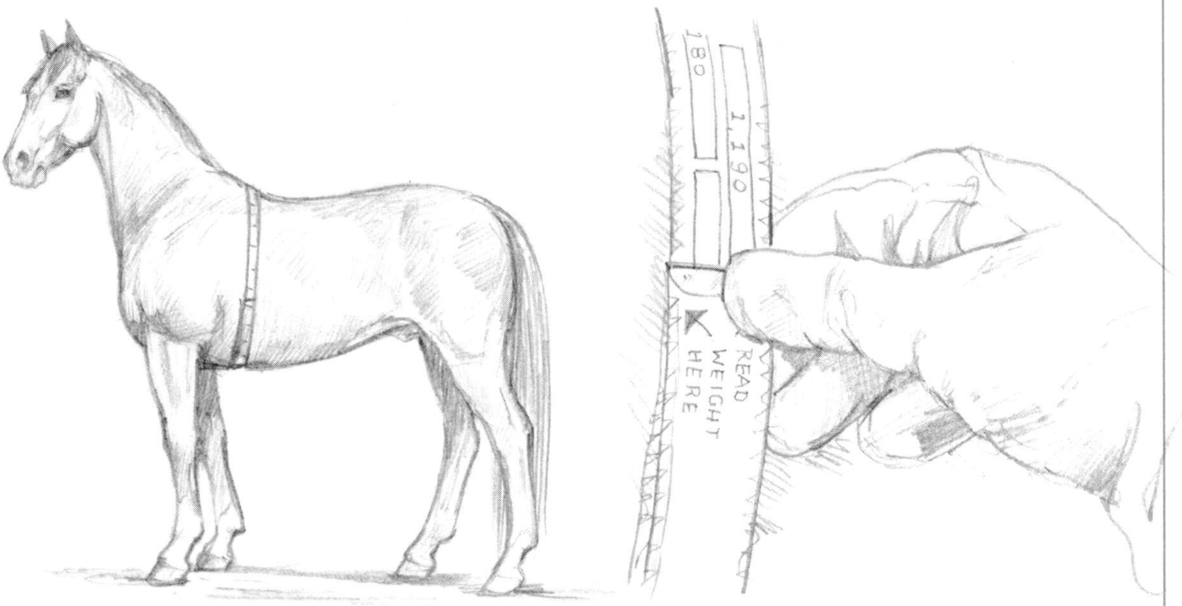

A weight tape is a simple way to estimate your horse's weight.

WILD LIFE

MOUNTAIN LIONS

The only wide-ranging, long-tailed wild cat in North America, mountain lions roam throughout the western United States, in the Rocky Mountains, and in parts of Canada, Texas, northern New England, and Florida. Also referred to as pumas, cougars, panthers, and catamounts, they are officially known as *Puma concolor* or *Felis concolor*, which means "cat all of one color."

Ranging from a tawny brown to a light cinnamon, mountain lions have many similar characteristics to housecats: a cat face, the ability to purr, a long tail for balance, retractable claws, and the ability to leap and climb. Adult males can weigh up to 160 pounds, and females weigh an average of 25 pounds less than males. From nose to tip of tail, they can measure up to 8 feet.

Mountain lions are solitary and come together to mate every two years. Breeding can take place during any season, and gestation is about three months. Kittens are usually born from April to July in litters of two to three. At two months of age, the spotted kittens leave the den, usually in late summer or early fall; at six months they lose their spots. The young remain with the mother until 18 months of age, at which time they must find their own territory.

Mountain lions live to about 12 years of age and subsist on deer, elk, mice, rabbits, squirrels, porcupines, raccoons, coyotes, moose, bison, and grasshoppers, but they generally will not eat carrion. When

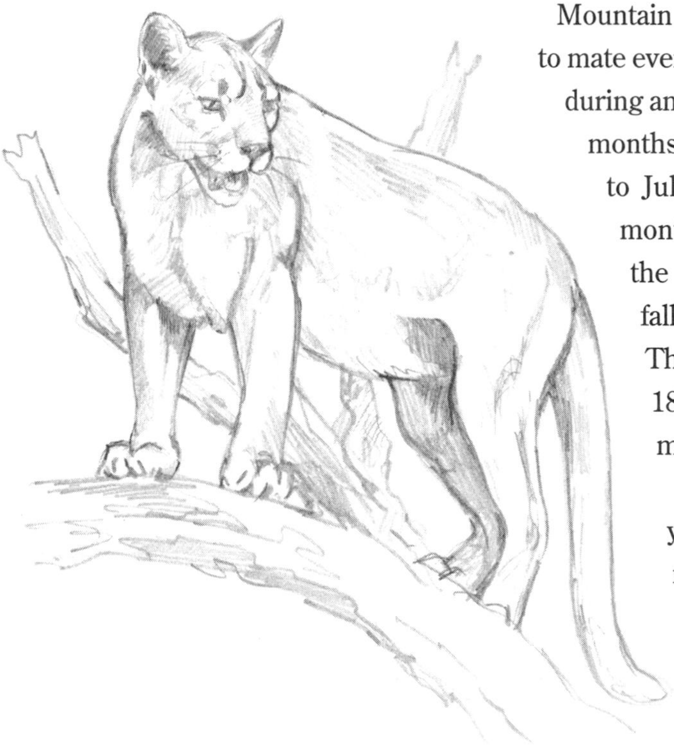

Mountain lions are predators and an important part of the ecosystem.

natural food is scarce, lions might prey on domestic livestock such as foals, ponies, calves, sheep, and goats.

Although they might use a promontory to spot prey, mountain lions stalk their victims from the ground. They leap onto the back of larger prey, using their canine teeth to break the neck or puncture the jugular. The remains of a carcass might be cached (covered with pine needles, leaves, and other debris) for later feeding. Adult mountain lions have few natural enemies (and none in some areas); bears, wolves, and other lions are their predators.

PROTECT AND PRESERVE. Lions play an important role in the ecosystem, helping to control overpopulation of deer herds. When a predator has taken pets or livestock in an area, permits are often issued for killing the animal, which is a shame. If you take steps to protect your animals, therefore, you not only keep them alive, but you help mountain lions to survive as well.

FYI

A Lion's Share

Although a mountain lion's territory may cover 100 miles, the individuals encountered by humans have a much smaller range, due to a more concentrated food source and less available habitat.

How Did the Egg Cross the Road?

Richard and I were finishing up chores yesterday and he asked me if I wanted to see something strange that he found in the pasture while feeding our horse Seeker. Absolutely!

To my surprise, it was a 4-inch by 6-inch forest green egg. Though it looked prehistoric and out of place, I immediately recognized it as an emu egg. We have neighbors who raise emus, but they live a half mile away from us, with several hills, fences, and buildings in between. How, then, did this egg arrive in Seeker's pasture?

Subsequent phone calls to neighbors revealed that a mountain lion had recently been in the valley, taking a dog and a pony. Could he have carried this large egg in his mouth all the way to our place, only to drop it when something startled him? We're sticking with that story.

Here are some ways to protect pets, foals, and ponies from possible mountain lion attack.

- Keep animals in or near buildings from dusk to dawn, lions' most active hunting time.
- Clear brush from around buildings.
- Keep yards lit if necessary.
- Bring all pet food in at dusk.

Bobcats rarely pose a threat and provide rodent control.

Finally, consider acquiring a guard dog to alert you to the presence of a predator. This is an age-old practice used around the world. Breeds of guard dogs used for livestock protection in the United States include Akbash (from Turkey), Great Pyrenees (from France and Spain), Komondor (from Hungary), Shar Planinetz (from Yugoslavia), Maremma (Italy), Kuvasz (Hungary), Anatolian Shepherd (Turkey), Tatra (Poland), and Mastiff (Tibet).

These measures, according to the Department of Fish & Game, help protect livestock from lions, domestic dogs gone wild, and coyotes.

BOBCATS AND LYNX

Bobcats and lynx are small, short-tailed ("bob-tailed") cats. The lynx *(Lynx canadensis)* is 3 feet long and weighs 20 to 30 pounds, with a short, black-tipped tail, huge hind feet, and ear tufts. Its coat is usually grayish, with obscure spots.

The more common and widespread bobcat *(Lynx rufus)* is slightly smaller (13 to 30 pounds) and reddish with less prominent ear tufts and smaller hind feet. It can have spotted or lined markings in brown or black.

Both species prey on rabbits, ground birds, squirrels, and rodents, and they occasionally eat carrion. Breeding season is December to April and the gestation period lasts 50 to 70 days. Although they hunt during both night and day, they are not generally a threat to horses or pets.

Another member of the rodent patrol, the lynx has characteristic ear tufts.

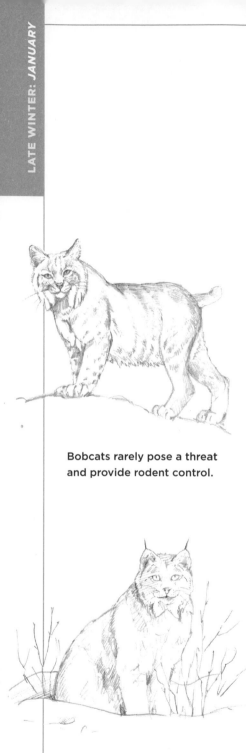

PEST PATROL

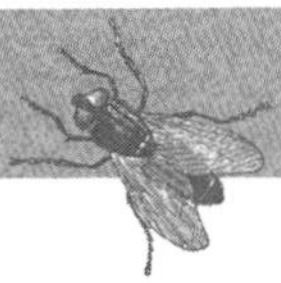

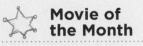

INTERNAL PARASITES

All horses have internal parasites. Worm eggs in manure hatch into larvae that the horse eats as he grazes. Once inside the horse they subsist on the horse's blood while they mature, lay eggs, and continue the cycle. Excessive worm populations can cause a horse to become dull coated, pot bellied, and lethargic. To prevent these problems, deworm him regularly, and remove manure from his living quarters daily.

Bots, another type of internal parasite, live inside the horse until the pupae drop to the ground with manure and hatch into bot flies. Although bot flies look like bees, they don't sting but lay eggs on the horse's hair. Nose bots try to fly up the horse's nose, which causes most horses to strike viciously with their front legs and run frantically. This is a very dangerous situation. Bots can also be treated with regular deworming.

Movie of the Month

***THE HORSEMAN ON THE ROOF* (1995)**

During the second European cholera pandemic, in 1932 as southern France is ravaged by the disease, we meet Angelo (Olivier Martinez) and Pauline (Juliette Binoche). Both actors show great equestrian skills on their exceptional horses as they race for life across gorgeous Provence, all the while chatting flirtatiously.

DEWORMING DOS AND DON'TS

To most effectively break the reproductive and developmental cycle of common internal parasites, most horses should be dewormed every eight weeks, year round. There are four exceptions to this rule:

1. **Horses in crowded turnout areas with continually changing population.** This environment, prevailing at many boarding stables, is usually host to a high parasite concentration. In this case, consider deworming every six weeks or possibly daily with a pelleted dewormer. This decision should be made in conjunction with post-treatment fecal exams and veterinary consultation. A fecal exam is a laboratory test performed on a fresh manure sample to determine what parasites are present.

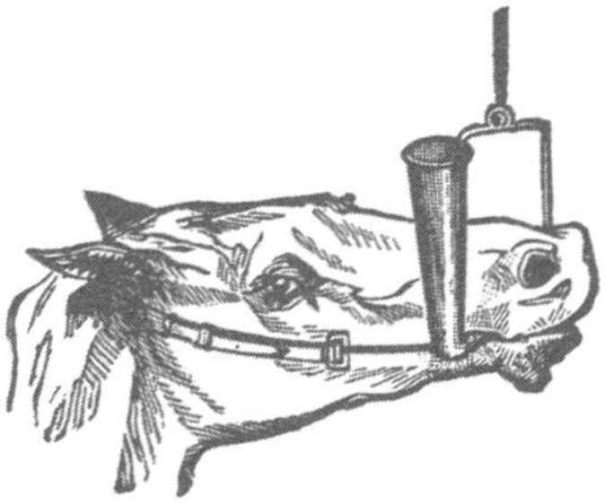

See this month's More in Depth for more on deworming.

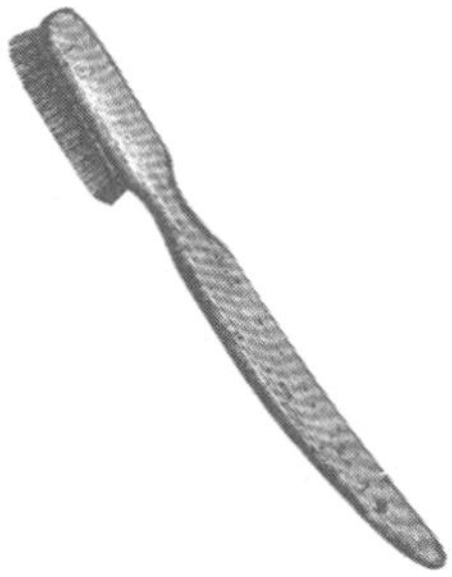

2. **Foals less than one year of age.** Foals under one year of age are susceptible to heavy parasite infestation. The usual recommendation is deworming at one month of age, and then every month until weaning. After weaning, deworm every six weeks until 12 months of age, then every eight weeks thereafter. Threadworms can also be a problem for foals under six months of age. They are not common in the older horse. Ivermectin and oxibendazole (a benzimidazole) are effective on threadworms.

3. **Older horses.** From the late teens on, older horses often have a weaker immune system than adult horses in their prime, so they are more susceptible to parasites. They may require deworming every six weeks, especially if they experience any of the digestive tract problems that often accompany old age.

4. **Horses that share a large pasture** with a relatively unchanging population. If a small, unchanging herd is on a large pasture and has been on an eight-week-cycle deworming program for a year or two, and fecal egg counts are low, it may be practical to decrease the deworming frequency to four times per year. Confer with your vet.

Your Horse's Toothbrush

Before giving your horse an oral medication, such as dewormer, bute, or oral antibiotics, it is best if his mouth is clean. If he has leftover feed in his mouth when you medicate him, he could spit out the feed and the dewormer. Use an old toothbrush to get your horse to release his hidden feed wads prior to medication.

Insert the toothbrush in the interdental space at the corners of his mouth and stroke the roof of his mouth and his tongue with the bristles. Then insert the toothbrush between his molars and cheek and move it back and forth, on both sides. Your goal is to get major tongue and mouth action.

Now when you deworm him, the medication will go to the worms, not the wads.

Winter Grooming

During the winter, if a horse is not in work, I do very little grooming. The horse's sebaceous glands produce waxy exudates that create a waterproof coating next to the skin. Vigorous grooming would remove this protective material. I usually use a pair of grooming gloves with rubber bumps on them to regularly give my pasture horses a once-over, mainly looking for any problem areas with the coat. I also straighten out the mane with my gloved fingers, removing any burrs or hay or other material from the long hair. If a horse has a long mane, I apply a leave-in detangler to keep the wind from whipping it into "witches' curls." Since the tails have been put up in the fall (see October Beauty Shop), there is no tail care this time of year.

PASTURE PERFECT

PROVIDE WINDBREAKS

This time of year, I sure am glad we have windbreaks in the pasture for feeding, and so are the horses. Windbreaks can be natural, they can be made from downed trees or railroad ties, or they can be three-sided sheds. In addition to windbreaks, pastured horses should have easy, safe access to shelter from precipitation – either natural (trees, rocks, or terrain) or man-made (sheds).

Trees out in the open can act as a windbreak, but during the winter the bare branches of deciduous trees don't offer much protection from precipitation. Thickly wooded areas, on the other hand, may provide shelter, especially if they include evergreens, but the undergrowth can be hazardous for a horse's legs, especially if there is a snow cover.

Odd Word

chamois (usually pronounced "shammy"). A soft under-split of a sheepskin (without wool) that has been oil-tanned and suede-finished.

LOCATION AND ORIENTATION. A man-made pasture shelter is typically a rectangle with one of the long sides

TIPS & TECHNIQUES

A Portable Facility

You might consider a portable shed built on skids that can be relocated with a tractor. You can routinely move the shed to a different location or a different pasture depending on the season or when the area around it becomes damaged and needs renovation. (See more on sheds in June Fine Facilities.)

open. The shelter is oriented so the prevailing winds (usually from the north, west, or northwest in North America) hit the back wall, and the open front faces the east or south. Although a south or southeast opening usually provides winter sun and protection from the cold north winds, each locale and each spot on your land may have different wind patterns that you must take into consideration before building.

Locate the shelter on well-drained high ground so it doesn't become a quagmire during wet seasons. Select one of the highest points in the pasture, unless it is the windiest spot. The shed should not be located so remotely that you rarely visit it.

DESIGN AND CONSTRUCTION. Figure a 12-foot by 12-foot space for each horse, so if you plan to pasture three horses, a 12-foot by 36-foot shed should give them enough room to cohabit comfortably.

The shelter should be constructed of materials that are safe for horses. Wood is usually safe but would need to be treated periodically to prevent chewing. In addition, nails tend to creep out of wood, so they need regular checking. Steel is lower maintenance, but sharp edges must be covered.

As with stalls in a barn, line the shelter on the inside with a material (such as 2-inch-thick lumber) durable enough to prevent a horse from kicking through the walls.

FOOTING. Inside the shed, the footing should be a clean, comfortable material that drains well. A deep bed of pea gravel (3⁄8″ minus round gravel) works well. Horses readily lie down in pea gravel, stay clean, and don't develop hock sores the way they do on bare ground. Avoid using sand if you plan to feed inside the shed during stormy weather, as it can lead to sand colic.

Ideally a shed should be large enough to have a feeding area with a smooth surface, like rubber mats, and a soft loafing area, where a horse can stand comfortably out of the sun or wind or lie down if the pasture is wet or muddy. Don't bed the shed unless you are using it for foals or if you produce bedding on your farm and cost is not a factor. Bedding will invite horses to urinate and defecate in the shed, so unless you are looking for a daily job of cleaning, skip the bedding. In fact, you might want to devise a way to lock horses out of the shed during nice weather to discourage them from using the shed as a toilet.

Ranch Notes

Jan. 8. 50 mph winds all night. The wind caved in Sherlock's pen because of the wind screens fastened to the panels. Richard pried it back into position with a long bar.

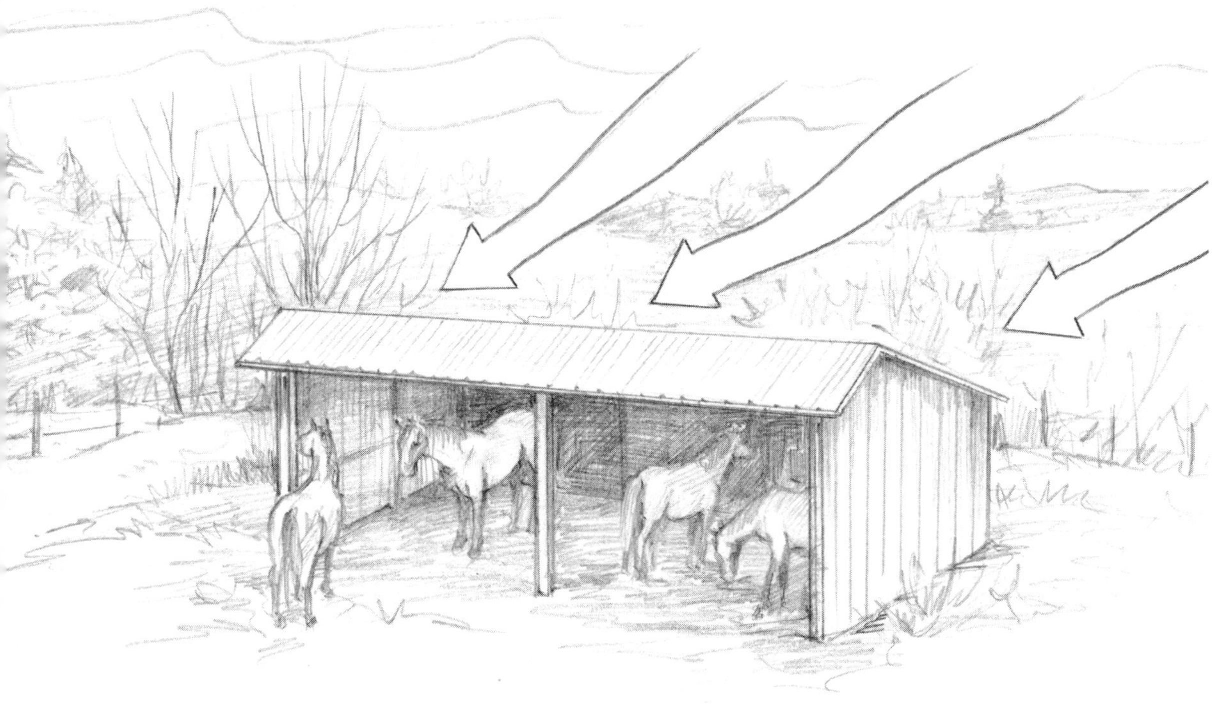

Pasture shelters typically have shed roofs (a single slope) that are higher at the front than the back. The height should be a minimum of 8 feet at the rear of the shed and 10 feet at the front. A 4- to 6-foot overhang along the front makes a shed roof into an offset gable or "salt box" to keep wind and precipitation from blowing in and to provide more shade for loafing.

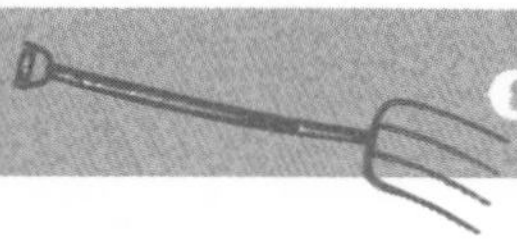

CLEAN-UP CREW

SANITATION

Keeping your horse and his living quarters clean will minimize parasite reinfestation, cut down on grooming time, and help him look great. This includes cleaning up manure, keeping the area around the barn and pens dry, and keeping flies and other pests to a minimum.

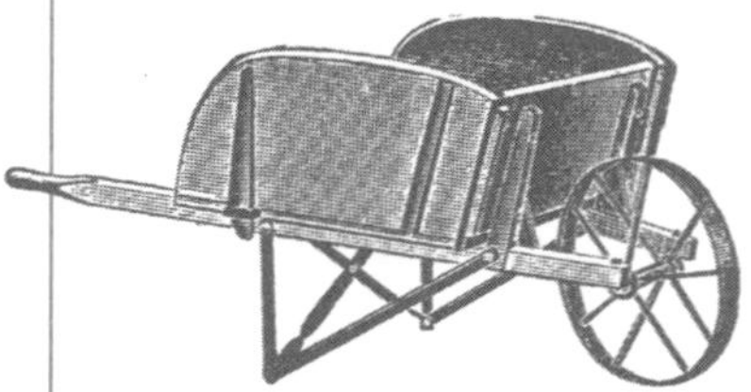

To give you an idea of how much manure you might expect a group of horses to generate, here's how it stacks up at our place. Our annual manure pile usually makes 12 to 16 spreader loads. We have an International 540 PTO-driven spreader with a capacity of 5.5 cubic yards (120 bushels). We pull it with a 60 hp Massey Ferguson 1190 diesel 4WD tractor. We have between five and nine horses. Two to four are usually on pasture, and the others are in stall/pen in-and-out setups with a short daily pasture turnout. We go through minimal bedding because most of the manure is deposited in the pens or on the pastures.

Pens are cleaned twice a day and the manure is composted until it is spread during the winter. We spread our manure on the pastures that we won't be using until mid to late summer. For us, January or February is usually the ideal month to spread because it is often dry, and thus we

Space Needed for Manure Compost Piles

Number of Horses	Space Needed (in feet)
One horse	12 x 12 x 12
Up to five horses	Two or three compost bins, 8 x 8 x 4 (hand turned)
More than five horses	One 30 x 30 pad for three piles (turned by tractor)

do minimal damage to the pastures by driving on them. Pasture is fragile here, and tire tracks can remain as visible scars of poor timing.

Our winter snows usually fall from February through May, here at 7,000 feet in the foothills of the Rockies. As the snow cover melts throughout the spring, it carries the decomposed manure's nutrients into the soil. (Read all about composting in May.)

JANUARY
Manure Pile Maintenance

It is ideal to have at least three compost piles going at all times: one to which fresh manure is being added daily (A), one that is in the process of decomposing (B), and one that is fully composted and ready to spread (C). Each month will have a monthly manure task associated with each of the piles.

PILE A
Sell, store, or spread

PILE B
Turn once, water as needed

PILE C
Turn twice, water as needed

Manure Statistics

A 1,000-pound horse produces approximately 50 pounds of manure per day, or a little more than 9 tons per year. In addition, a horse produces 6 to 10 quarts of urine per day, which, when soaked up by bedding, can constitute another 50 pounds daily.

If you have five average-sized horses living in pens, therefore, they will produce more than 45 tons of manure per year. If you keep them in bedded stalls, you will have 90 tons of manure and used bedding to manage yearly.

Spending that many hours in the saddle gave a man plenty of time to think. That's why so many cowboys fancied themselves Philosophers.

— Charles M. Russell

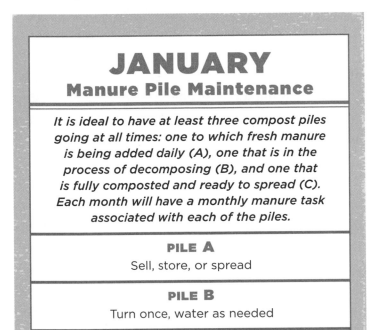

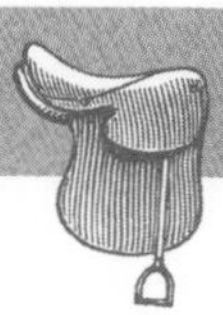

TACK ROOM

Tack Tactics

For routine leather care, follow these three steps to protect your tack:

1. Clean it
2. Feed it
3. Seal it

TIME FOR A SADDLE CHECK

Each winter, I prepare my tack for its spring, summer, and fall use, starting with the saddles in January. English saddles are pretty easy: they need a thorough cleaning and conditioning, and in addition, I check all billet straps and corresponding girth straps for signs of fatigue or wear. This is the time of year to have a part repaired or replaced.

If your tack is well cared for, however, it will last a very long time, and you will rarely have to replace items. On an English saddle the stirrup leathers may need to be replaced soonest, since they come in contact with sweat, dirt, and hair and they endure the repetitive stress of a rider posting.

Western saddles require a little more time for cleaning and conditioning, due to their larger size and heavily tooled leather. Brush the sheepskin on the underside of the saddle. Inspect the latigos or half-breeds (the leather straps that attach the cinch to the saddle) for cracking, fatigue, and worn spots, especially where they attach to the saddle itself. These are the items that most frequently need replacement. Also inspect the cinches, and if using a string mohair cinch, wash it and then hang it to dry with a weight on one end to prevent it from shrinking to pony size. When not in use, leather articles can be covered with fabric for protection from dust and dirt. Allow adequate ventilation.

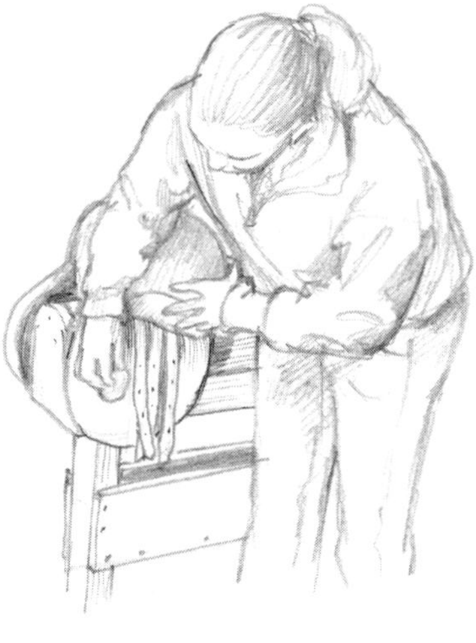

Routine leather care will ensure that your tack will last longer, be safer, and look first-rate.

Leather Tack Care and Cleaning

Leather's greatest enemies are water, heat, dirt, and salt from sweat. Store fine leather articles at room temperature and out of direct sun and light. Keep humidity moderate and the room well ventilated and as dirt free as possible. If a dehumidifier is impractical, discourage mold and mildew by wiping leather articles periodically with a mild acid solution, such as white vinegar and water (2 tablespoons to 1 cup) or a 1:1 ratio of denatured or rubbing alcohol and water. If mildew persists, wash with a specialized leather wash or a thick suds of a germicidal or fungicidal soap. Follow by exposure to air and sunlight.

Here are the three steps of rountine leather care.

CLEAN IT. First, brush or vacuum all dirt and dust from tack. This is especially important for tooled Western tack, on which dirt can get into the crevices of the tooling. Then use warm water and Turkish toweling to remove dirt, hair, sweat, and previous applications of saddle soap and oil. Tooled saddles may benefit from the use of a soft bristled brush, such as an old toothbrush, and neglected saddles will require the addition of a cleaning agent to the water.

Specially designed leather-cleaning products get leather very clean, and do so safely without stripping oils.

FEED IT. Once the leather is thoroughly cleaned and rinsed of soap residue, allow it to partially dry. While it is still damp, nourish the flesh side of the leather with oil. Damp leather absorbs oil more readily by drawing it into the pores as the water evaporates.

Leather loses some of its fat every day and needs to be fed. Overfeeding, however, can create a limp, flabby, greasy article with deteriorated threads and weakened leather fibers. Routine light conditioning is far superior to a one-time saturation. Choose a compound specifically designed for fine leather.

SEAL IT. Once the conditioned leather has dried, seal the conditioner into the leather. This final coat not only locks in the conditioner, but it also makes daily removal of sweat and mud much easier. You can finish large leather surfaces easily with a finish spray.

Sealing: Choose Your Method

For articles such as bridles, use the hard wax method. Apply a good-quality soft saddle soap directly from the can using a sponge or small piece of sheepskin. Let it dry thoroughly and then buff and polish the piece with a barely damp chamois or a soft lint-free cloth.

For stirrup fenders and leathers, back cinches, and skirts, use a finish spray or the hard wax method. Apply the lather liberally to areas that especially need protection from sweat and mud and to areas that come in contact with the rider's clothes.

See May Horsekeeping Across America for more on mold and mildew.

Clothes Horse

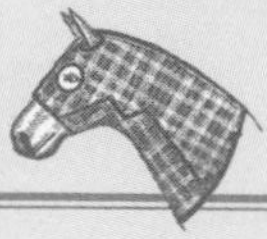

Field-Washing a Blanket

Blankets and sheets get very dirty keeping your horse clean. Dirt and mud on the outer shell can prevent a blanket from breathing, while sweat and dirt buildup on the lining can cause hair loss and skin problems. When you can't find a Laundromat that allows horse gear and your home washing machine isn't large enough, you can field-wash blankets and sheets.

You'll need: a brush or vacuum, a bucket of warm water, mild soap or blanket wash, a push broom with medium bristles, a stiff hand brush, a hose with a spray nozzle, a clean, flat surface, and a fence or rail.

1. Wet hairs are almost impossible to remove, so before you wet the blanket, use a brush or vacuum to remove as much hair as possible from the blanket lining.
2. Presoak extremely dirty areas, such as the trim around the neck, with a spray stain remover or a concentrated soap solution. Spread the blanket out flat on a clean concrete pad or rubber-matted surface such as a wash rack or driveway and wet it thoroughly with warm water. Let it soak for a few minutes to loosen the dirt.
3. Add a small amount of mild soap or blanket wash to a bucket of warm water. Pour some of the soapy water on the blanket and scrub it with a push broom.
4. Flip the blanket over and scrub the other side.
5. Lay the straps on top of the blanket and scrub both sides with a stiff hand brush. Place removable straps in the wash bucket to soak first.
6. Scrub the trim. Don't forget the shoulder and tail areas where body oils and manure stains concentrate.
7. Hang the blanket over a fence or rail and rinse it thoroughly. Flip it over and rinse again to remove all soap residues, which could cause skin irritation. Continue flipping the blanket and rinsing until no trace of soap remains.
8. Hang the blanket in an airy place to dry.

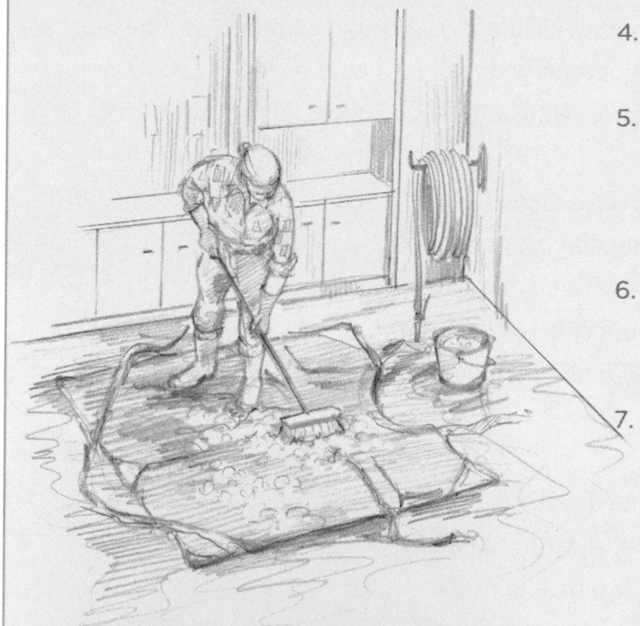

Stand on the blanket to hold it in place while brooming.

FARM OFFICE

AN INCOME TAX OVERVIEW

January signals the beginning of income tax time. If you run your horse farm or ranch as a business with profit intent, you probably already have a tax counselor or advisor who has experience with farm accounts. Even if you don't, it is a good idea to keep track of expenses as a matter of economy and budget planning, using formal income and expense records.

PROFIT INTENT. A horse business needs to show profit intent in order to retain its business or farm status.

In case of an audit, the IRS will note whether you have sought advice from experts, such as marketing and financial counselors, and will evaluate the time and effort you expend in your business. Keep a log of the hours you actually work in your business. You should have a projected profit plan available, which you update each year.

INCOME. You must report all income related to your horse business. This includes horses bought for immediate resale, horses raised and sold, and assets acquired for the business and then sold (such as a truck, tractor, trailer, saddle, or breeding stock). It also includes prizes and awards, show and track winnings, boarding fees, training fees, lesson fees, proceeds from hosting events and clinics, and income from the sale of farm-raised grain, hay, and straw.

If you engage in bartering, the services or goods you receive are considered income and must be recorded at the fair market value of the item or service. For your half of the trade in bartering, what you gave will be considered an expense if it would have been a deduction in the normal course of business.

TIPS & TECHNIQUES

Separate Is Best

It is best if you keep your horse operation transactions separate from monies used for domestic matters, other farm ventures, hobbies, and your other work. One of the best ways to do this is to maintain a separate checking account for your farm. All equine-related expenses and income and no others should be handled through this account.

TIPS & TECHNIQUES

1099 for Services

Whenever you pay $600 or more to an individual or a non-incorporated business in one year for services, you are required by law to fill out a Form 1099 and send it to the IRS and to the person or business for them to report as income.

For example, if your bills for veterinary work totaled $600 or more and your veterinarian's business is not incorporated, you should issue a 1099 to your veterinarian. The same goes for your farrier, farm laborers, and so on.

Expenses

Horse business expenses generally fall into one of three categories:

- Operating expenses that are entirely horse related and fully deducted in the year they are incurred;
- Expenses shared with domestic or other businesses that must be pro-rated, with the horse portion deducted in the year incurred;
- Major expenses that are spread out (depreciated) over several years.

OPERATING EXPENSES. The operating expenses are fairly straightforward and include feed, vet supplies and services, farrier services, and so on. Either your expenditures are "ordinary and necessary" for your particular business (deductible) or they are not (not deductible). Be sure you fully understand the definitions and requirements for an expense to qualify for a particular category so you don't claim something you shouldn't that might invite an audit. Some expenses are only partially deductible (such as business meals) and others are deductible only if your horse operation is showing a profit (such as an office in the home).

PRO-RATED EXPENSES. Expenses that need to be prorated include vehicles, taxes, and utilities. In each situation, you must determine, to the best of your ability, what percentage of the expense is directly attributable to the horse operation.

For example, if a vehicle is shared between domestic and farm purposes, keep a log book with the starting and ending mileage each time you use the vehicle for business-related activities, along with the business purpose of the trip. At the end of the year, determine what percentage the business miles are of the total miles traveled by that vehicle during the year. Keep all receipts concerning vehicle operation and maintenance.

The portion of property taxes that are deductible is usually determined by consulting the itemized breakdown on your property valuation and tax statement. The tax resulting from the assessed value of horse-related buildings is deductible, as is the tax assigned to the portion of the land you use for the horse operation. If you have ten acres, you may be using two for house, yard, and other domestic uses and eight for the horse operation. The tax related to the eight acres and farm improvements on them is deductible.

Utilities may be a little tougher to divide up as a pro-rated expense. With electricity, for example, unless you have separate meters for your barn and your house, you will have to estimate what percentage is farm related. If you have just added horse facilities to your residential acreage, you can compare utility bills before and after the additions to help you calculate business-related kilowatt-hours and dollars.

LARGE ASSETS. Large assets purchased for the business (such as a truck, trailer, buildings, or tractor) or those converted to business use are often depreciated. Your tax counselor will either advise you to take a full expense in the year incurred for an item (depending on the cost of the item and the status of your profit or loss) or will determine what depreciation schedule each item will follow. Then each year of the depreciation schedule, a certain percentage of the cost of a tractor, for example, will be available to use as a deductible expense. It must be remembered, however, that during the year you sell a business asset, its expense potential will have to be recaptured and treated as income.

This summary is meant just as an overview of the financial records you need to keep if you have a business. Your tax advisor will cover all the details with you as they relate to your specific circumstances.

Estimating Utility Usage

To help you determine your utility business percentage, you may be able to get hourly rate estimates from your utility company on the kilowatts required to operate various electrical devices. Note that what you determine as a percentage for electricity may be totally different than the business percentage for gas, water, or other utilities. Most small horse operations located on a residence use between 20 to 60 percent of the total utilities.

TRAINING PEN

KNOW YOUR KNOTS

Some years I spend more time working with my horses inside the barn in January than I do training or riding outdoors. Therefore, it is essential that they are very comfortable being tied for farrier work, body clipping, or clothing changes. It is a good time of the year to review tying.

Whenever I tie a horse, I make sure he is wearing a strong rope or nylon web halter and that the lead rope and hardware are heavy duty. If I am tying to a hitch rail or tie ring, I use a quick-release knot. (See June for Knots.)

Even when in a hurry, I never tie a horse with bridle reins. It would be far too easy for the reins to snap, which may cause damage to the horse's mouth and increase the potential for the horse to develop the bad habit of pulling when tied. The only exception to this is if a Western horse's headgear has a tie rope incorporated into the bridle, such as with a mecate or get-down rope.

A bad-tempered man will never make a good-tempered horse.
— Anna Sewell, *Black Beauty*

Cross-tie horses in the aisle of the barn for grooming, vacuuming, clipping, farrier work, and tacking up, and in the wash rack for bathing.

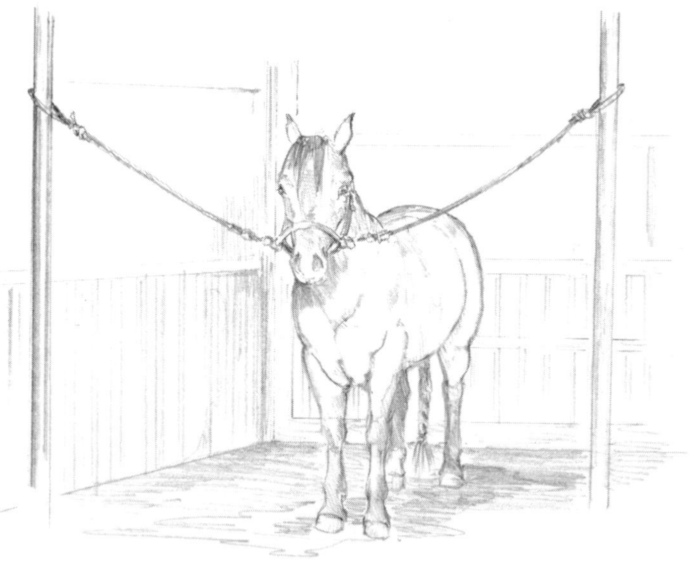

CROSS-TIES. Cross-tying is a means of tying a horse in which a chain or rope from each side of an aisle is attached to the side rings of the horse's halter. Be sure your horse is well accustomed to being tied in other ways before you attempt to tie him in a cross-tie. If I have more than one horse in the barn, I tie them a safe distance from each other.

Tying Tips

When I tie a horse, here are some things I keep in mind.

★ I make sure the point of attachment of the lead rope to the hitch rail or ring is at the level of the horse's withers or higher. This will discourage him from pulling back, because he will not be able to get very good leverage.

★ I leave about an arm's length of rope (24 to 30 inches) between the snap on the horse's halter and the post, rail, or ring he is tied to. If tied shorter than this, some horses will panic and pull back. Tying too short creates an uncomfortable position for the horse's neck, as he cannot relax. But if you tie too long, the horse can easily get into trouble. He can move around too much or get his head wrapped in the rope.

★ If I straight-tie, I use a strong post, a tie ring, or a specially designed hitch rail. It is very dangerous to tie to any object that would move or be pulled loose if a horse pulled back, as it would frighten the horse and likely cause him to panic and run with the object following him.

★ Never tie to:
- a board fence
- a wire fence
- the mirror on your truck
- a bird bath
- a door handle
- a lawn chair
- a lawnmower
- a porch railing
- a barbecue grill
- a tire
- a bicycle
- a bird feeder
- a wheelbarrow
- a motorcycle
- a swing set
- a water hydrant
- or anything other than an object specifically designed for tying horses

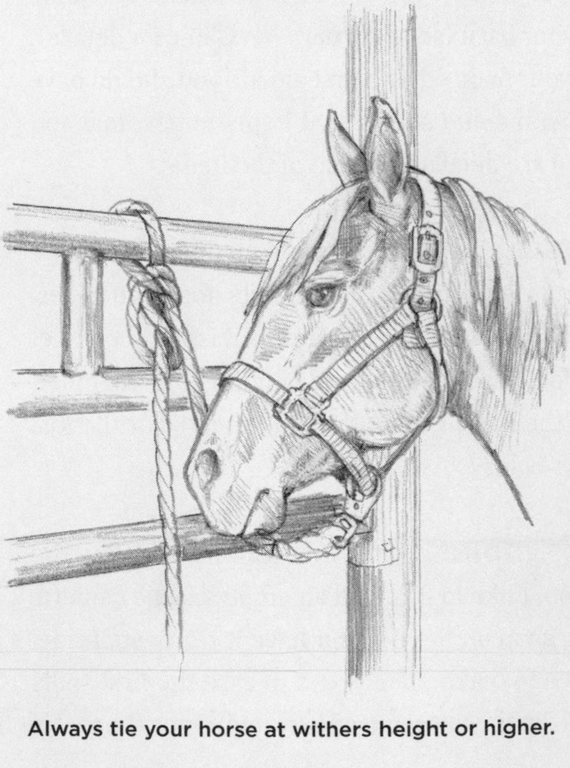

Always tie your horse at withers height or higher.

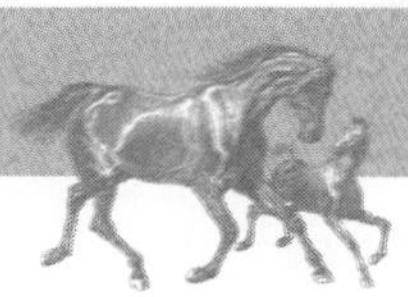

REPRODUCTION ROUNDUP

RHINO #2 FOR YOUR MARE

Depending on when you bred your mare, January might be time to give her the second rhinopneumonitis shot. Pregnant mares should receive vaccinations against rhinopneumonitis virus (equine herpes virus 1p and 1b) to help prevent abortion due to infection by the virus. Vaccinations are usually given at the fifth, seventh, and ninth month of pregnancy. Other horses on your premises might also require rhinopneumonitis vaccines. Ask your veterinarian to recommend which type of rhino vaccine to use for your situation.

ASSEMBLE A FOALING KIT

Foaling season is quickly approaching, so make sure you have your supplies ready. You should have a general equine first-aid kit in your barn (see February Vet Clinic for details). In addition to your main equine first-aid kit, you should have a Foaling Kit with some specialized items for the foal and the mare. Here are details on some of the items.

CLEAN TOWELS. For many uses, including to dry the foal, stimulate circulation, and clean out its nostrils if necessary. But don't do too much of this unless it is very cold. Let the mare and foal have their natural bonding time together. Step in only if the mare is not attending the foal or the foal is very weak or cold.

TINCTURE OF IODINE (7%). You can dip or spray the umbilical stump. I like to dip. I fill an empty plastic camera-film container, snap on the lid, and have it ready stall-side. It is a good idea to make up an extra in case the first spills while trying to dip the navel on a frisky foal. Once the foal is

TIPS & TECHNIQUES

IM Injections

Administer injections only if you are fully capable of giving an aseptic intramuscular (IM) injection. The rhinopneumonitis vaccine must be administered IM, deep into heavy muscle. Be sure your horse is able to exercise following the injection to promote absorption and to prevent muscle soreness.

Foaling Kit

- ❑ Vet's phone number(s)
- ❑ Cell phone (if no phone in barn)
- ❑ Camera (a digital camera takes great pictures without a flash so as not to disturb mare and foal)
- ❑ Flashlight and batteries
- ❑ Clock or watch to keep track of intervals
- ❑ Notebook and pen to take notes
- ❑ Book (see Recommended Reading)
- ❑ Lots of clean towels in various sizes
- ❑ Ivory liquid soap
- ❑ Iodine navel dip
- ❑ String
- ❑ Tail wrap
- ❑ Fleet enema
- ❑ K-Y Jelly
- ❑ Obstetrical sleeves
- ❑ Clean buckets
- ❑ Muck bucket and/or garbage bag

up and the umbilical cord has broken, have someone hold the foal around the chest and hindquarters. Raise the film container of iodine up and press it over the navel cord and surrounding area. Hold for five seconds. Be sure to always use 7% iodine. "Gentle" 1% iodine is not strong enough to sterilize the navel area fast enough.

FLEET READY-TO-USE ENEMA. This is a convenient method of relieving constipation caused by difficulty passing the meconium (hard dark feces) that is present at birth. The adult, green-label Fleet works well and is available in most drug stores for a few dollars. Have two on hand.

K-Y JELLY. This water-soluble lubricating jelly, made by Johnson & Johnson, is available in any drug store for a couple of dollars for a 4-ounce tube. It might come in handy for lubricating the foal's enema tip or lubricating an obstetrical sleeve during a vaginal exam of the mare prior to foaling. During foaling, artificial lubricants are not necessary; the mare's natural secretions provide enough lubrication.

Fleet Enema

Ask your vet if he or she recommends that you give your newborn foal an enema as a matter of course shortly after birth or if you should wait to see if the foal has difficulty with his bowels. There are differing opinions on this and you should follow your vet's advice.

TIPS & TECHNIQUES

It's a Wrap

If you want to use a cotton bandage to wrap your mare's tail, here's how.

1. First wrap the top of the tail and then put the rest of the tail inside a tube sock.

2. Bring the tube sock up to the tail wrap.

3. Using several rounds of sticky adhesive tape, tape the top of the tube sock to about the middle of the tail wrap.

4. Alternatively, you can braid the mare's entire tail, fold it up on top of the top portion of the tail, and then wrap it all up in one thick bundle.

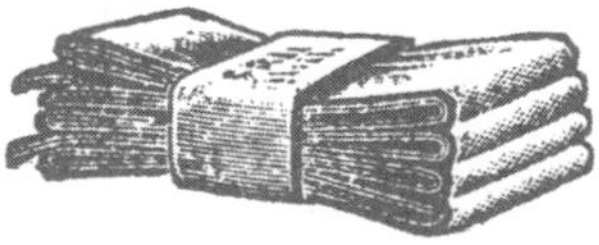

MILD SOAP AND CLEAN CLOTHS. I prefer Ivory liquid soap for washing the mare's perineal area and udder prior to foaling. But take care you don't use too much soap on the udder, and be sure to rinse it thoroughly. Otherwise the soap residue could cause the foal to reject the mare's udder, or if he ingests soap, it could cause him to have diarrhea.

TAIL WRAP. Prior to foaling, wrap your mare's tail completely with either a bandage or Vetrap. Be sure to wrap not only the top, but also the entire length of tail, to keep the long hairs out of the way during foaling. Since the wrap will get pretty dirty during foaling, I prefer to use Vetrap, which is conveniently disposable, rather than a bandage.

OBSTETRICAL SLEEVE. You can purchase a box of 100 sleeves from a vet supply or just get a few from your vet. These disposable, shoulder-length, thin plastic gloves come in handy in case the foal does not present in the proper position for delivery and a vaginal assist is required. The sleeves are not for the protection of the attendant; they are for the protection of the mare. No matter how well-scrubbed your hands are, they are not as clean as the sleeves.

STRING. Have several 2- to 3-foot lengths of thick string or baling twine available to tie up the placenta. Some mares release their placenta right away, so tying it up isn't necessary. But for those mares who take an hour or more to shed their placenta after foaling, you'll want to bundle it up and tie it to itself to keep the mare from stepping on it.

CLEAN PLASTIC MUCK BUCKET OR GARBAGE BAG. In case your vet wants to examine the placenta, you can temporarily store it in a clean plastic muck bucket (lay an old plastic bag on top of it to keep it from drying out) or you can put it in a garbage bag for disposal.

FINE FACILITIES

A CLEAN BARN FOR THE NEW YEAR

January is the time for our annual barn cleaning. A healthy horse barn is a well-ventilated barn, which means windows and doors are often open. This can result in the breezes carrying in fine dirt, which settles on almost everything in the barn. And if you store even a small amount of hay in your barn, as we do, you'll find that even the cleanest hay brings in some field dirt and dust, which becomes airborne as you feed. Bedding may also contribute to the particulate matter in the air. A main contributing factor to heaves is unhealthy air in a closed building.

What this all means is that once a year we do a really thorough barn cleaning to remove dust and dirt. This will protect our horses' respiratory systems, and ours too.

You may laugh when you read "vacuum" in the list, but it is a great way to remove the fine silt that would just become airborne again if you tried to sweep it up or if a gust of wind came in a door or window and stirred things up again. I use an industrial vacuum with a cloth bag. Every hour or so, I remove and empty the bag, which gets quite heavy with fine silt that looks like black talcum powder. Many heavy-duty vacuums have a place to attach an exhaust hose, so I attach a 20-foot hose, which I bought at a second-hand store, to the exhaust pipe with hose clamps and poke the end of the hose out a door so the exhaust doesn't stir up the air inside the barn as we work.

When we are finished, the barn actually sparkles! So if we have a severe spring blizzard and my horses are forced to spend time inside, they will have healthy air to breathe.

Barn-Cleaning Tasks

- ❑ Sweep down all cobwebs
- ❑ Vacuum all dust and webs from electrical receptacles and light fixtures
- ❑ Remove all bedding from stalls
- ❑ Sweep stall floors
- ❑ Vacuum stall mats
- ❑ Vacuum stall walls
- ❑ Sweep barn aisles
- ❑ Vacuum barn aisles
- ❑ Clean feed room
- ❑ Tidy and vacuum tack room
- ❑ Tidy tool room
- ❑ Wipe down all stall grills and blanket bars
- ❑ Scrub all hay and grain feeders and water buckets
- ❑ Lubricate all door latches and hinges

Honey Do Oatmeal Cookies

Since January is the time for a fresh start, I usually start making my "honey do" list for summer projects that I hope Richard has time to do, such as new fencing or a remodeling job on one of the buildings. I know that my mixed-nut oatmeal cookies will help me persuade him.
Yield: 4–6 dozen

Mix together A:
6 cups old-fashioned oats
5 cups flour (see note below)
6 cups salted mixed nuts
3 cups dark chocolate chips (optional)
1 cup ground flax
3 Tablespoons baking powder

Mix together B:
4 eggs
1½ cups milk (I use unsweetened soy)
1 cup peanut oil (or golden sesame oil)
4 teaspoons vanilla
1 cup honey or stevia equivalent

1. Mix A and B together. Refrigerate 4–10 hours.
2. Preheat oven to 350°. Form dough into 3-inch-diameter cookies. For crispy, brown cookies use an ungreased, dark, heavy, commercial-grade steel cookie sheet; for lighter, softer cookies, use an ungreased light-colored aluminum pan.
3. Bake 20 minutes.
4. Cool overnight on raised racks.
5. Store extras in unmarked paper bags in the very back of the refrigerator where *honey* can't find them until you want him *to do*.

Flour note: With each batch, I use varying combinations of spelt, barley, oat, corn, brown rice, and garbanzo flours, each with its own flavor, texture, and character.

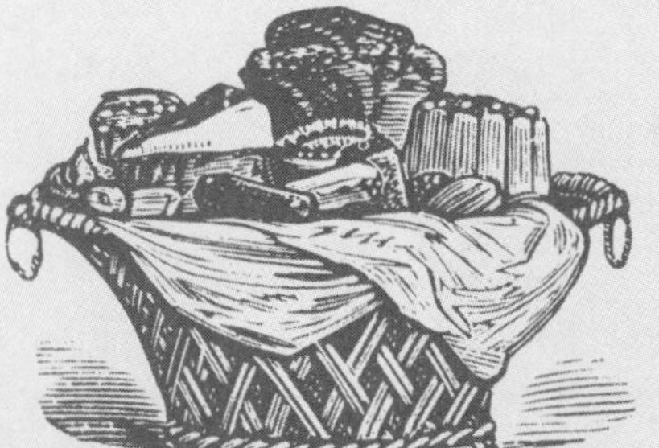

RPMS & PTOS

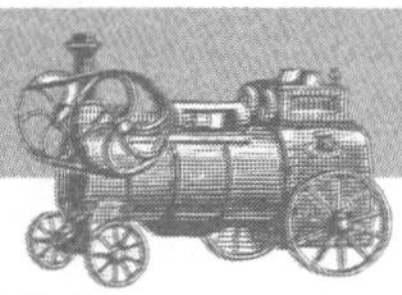

MAINTAINING YOUR TRACTOR

Especially if you have a place indoors to service your tractor and implements, January is a good time to do maintenance work when you might not be using the tractor so much. Alternatively, you might schedule the maintenance with your dealer during this slow time of year. Refer to your owner's manual for the service schedule. Annual maintenance for your tractor may include the following:

- Change the engine oil and filter according to the schedule in your owner's manual.
- Check the transmission oil, power steering oil, and filters, and change if necessary. If you have a 4WD tractor, check the front axle oil.
- Grease the fittings. Your operator's manual will have a diagram of the fittings. Check all hoses, belts, and clamps.
- Drain and flush the radiator.
- Clean the screen and grill in front of the radiator.
- Check fuel hoses for rubbing and leaking. Check the fuel filter sediment bowl to be sure it has no particles in it.
- Remove and clean air filters and replace as needed.
- Check and adjust the brakes regularly and ensure they are evenly adjusted.
- Look over tires closely for checks, cuts, bulges, or incorrect pressure. Service or replace tires as needed.
- Check the battery and service as required and recommended in your owner's manual.

en español

savvy. Comes from *sabe*, meaning 'you know'. Pronounced SAH-veh.

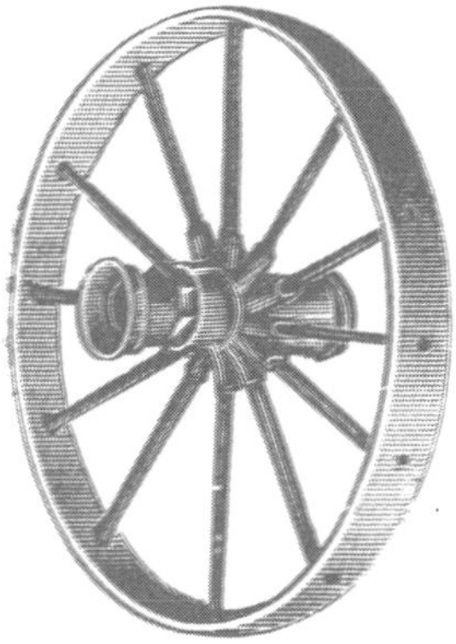

RANCH RECIPES

A WINTER TREAT: BEET PULP MASH

I use beet pulp pellets, not shreds (shreds are more expensive and not as absorbent) and mix each horse's ration individually in a bucket marked by name. I mix only what I will offer for the next feeding.

See page 125 for more on beet pulp.

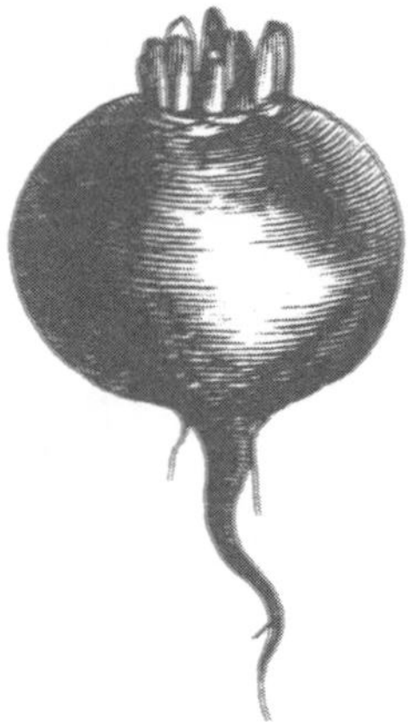

Start out with one part pellets to five parts warm or cold (not hot) water and let it sit from two to 12 hours. During temperatures of 40° to 70°F, you can let the mixture sit for as long as 12 hours. When it is warmer than that, I mix up the beets only a few hours before I feed to avoid spoilage by fermentation. When it is below freezing, I keep the soaking beets in a heated area (my tack room) so they don't freeze.

To the beet pulp mash, I add various of the following enhancements, depending on the horse's needs.

HOOF SUPPLEMENT. All horses receive a maintenance portion of this nutrient supplement, which contains amino acids, vitamins, and other nutrients for healthy hooves.

GROUND LINSEED (FLAX) MEAL. All horses receive an appropriate (according to their weight, condition, and work) amount of linseed meal, a great source of soluble fiber and Omega-3 fatty acids, including alpha-linolenic acid. Omega-3 fatty acids are essential because the horse can't produce them in his body; he must receive them in his feed.

VEGETABLE OIL. For horses over 20 years of age, I use ¼ to ½ cup of corn oil. Oil is a good source of calories for energy or weight gain and has the added benefit of contributing to a healthy skin and hair coat.

ANTIOXIDANT SUPPLEMENT. All horses over age 20 receive this complex because their ability to produce some of these vitamins is reduced with age.

LARGE COMPLETE FEED WAFERS OR PELLETS. I add between a few wafers and several cups. The addition of these large, treat-sized wafers slows down horses that gobble. They could be difficult for seniors to chew, so to their ration I add senior pellets instead.

PSYLLIUM. Once a month for five days, I add psyllium husks to the ration of all horses. I add all other additives on top of the soaked beet pulp, and then put the psyllium on top. I mix the psyllium in just before I feed the ration to the horse so that the psyllium doesn't absorb too much water before it gets inside the horse. (See June Feed Bag for more on psyllium.)

TIPS & TECHNIQUES

Wet, Dry, or Moist?

The beet pulp pellets in your area might be different than mine, so you will have to experiment to end up with a consistency that your horses like. I have found that a moist but fluffy consistency works best. The horses like that better than a wet sloppy mess, and it is easy to mix supplements with a moist mash. (See March Feed Bag for more information on beet pulp.)

STILL TRUE TODAY

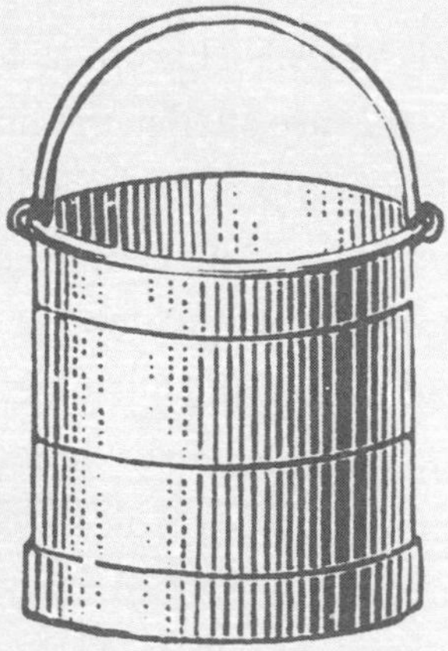

Historical Horsekeeping

"If a large quantity of cold water is taken into the stomach while the system is agitated, by the circulation being so increased as to open the pores of the skin freely, it is liable to chill the stomach and close the pores of the skin, and thus excite some one of the common alimentary derangements, as colic or inflammation of the bowels, etc."

— Magner's Standard Horse and Stock Book, *by D. Magner, 1916*

MORE IN DEPTH

TIPS & TECHNIQUES

Parasite Prevention

★ Remove manure daily from stalls and pens and weekly from pastures.

★ Ensure that pastures and paddocks are well drained and not crowded.

★ Compost manure to kill parasite eggs. Keep manure pile at 145°F for two weeks.

★ Don't spread fresh manure on fields where horses graze.

★ Feed on the ground only if snow-covered or if covered with mats that are kept clean.

★ Use feeders for hay and grain when necessary.

CHEMICAL CLASSES OF DEWORMERS

The decision on which dewormer to use involves knowing what parasites you want to destroy at what particular time and what chemical is effective against those parasites. Routinely you will be concerned with strongyles, roundworms, and pinworms, and at least once a year you should target tapeworms. Additionally, in the early spring and late fall, you'll need to use a boticide.

Ivermectin is the drug of choice against bots and it will also kill all other worms except tapeworms and encysted small strongyles. Both praziquantel and double-dose pyrantel pamoate will kill tapeworms. Moxidectin will kill encysted small strongyles and provides 84-day suppression of strongyle eggs.

TREATING INTERNAL PARASITES

Although we treat many of the internal parasites as a group, it helps to know more details about each parasite for the most effective control.

STRONGYLES. Large strongyles are also known as bloodworms or red worms. The eggs that are shed in the horse's manure hatch into larvae that crawl up onto grass blades and are consumed by a grazing horse. The larvae mature in the horse's intestinal tract, burrow out into blood vessels, and migrate through organs and back to the intestine. During the migration, the larvae can cause extensive blood vessel damage. Large strongyle infestations result in weight loss, anemia, or colic, sometimes fatal.

Small strongyles don't migrate but they do become encysted (burrow into the intestinal wall). While they are encysted, only a certain dewormer can eradicate them. Small strongyle infestation can result in colic, diarrhea, weight loss, poor condition, and stunted growth in young horses.

ASCARIDS. Also called ascarids, roundworms are more often a problem in young horses than in mature horses. Since ascarids are from 6 to 12 inches long, it doesn't take many of them to steal a horse's nutrients and give him a pot belly. Symptoms include colic, coughing, and diarrhea. Impaction colic could result from blockage by large masses of worms, especially after deworming a badly infested foal.

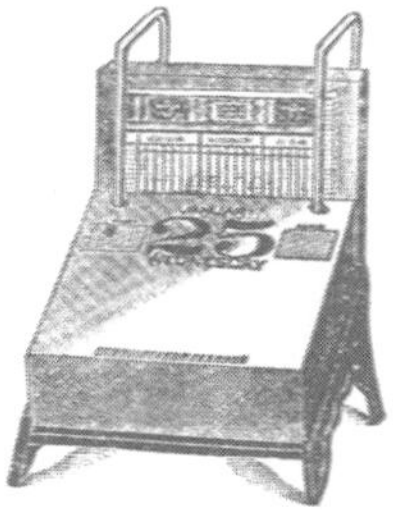

Ascarid eggs are picked up where feces have contaminated feed, pasture, or water. The eggs hatch in the intestines, and the worms bore through the intestinal wall and head to the lungs. Ascarids migrate through lung tissue and can cause pneumonia. The young worms travel up the trachea to the mouth where they are coughed up and

Deworming Plan

January is a good time of year to make up a deworming plan based on the following recommendations:

- ★ Deworm six times per year (every eight weeks).
- ★ Twice a year, use an ivermectin product against bots.
- ★ In the summer, treat your horse for tapeworms using praziquantel.
- ★ The other three times, alternate dewormers according to your veterinarian's recommendations. Consider using moxidectin once or twice a year for encysted larvae following ivermectin treatment.

Here is the schedule I follow in Colorado, at 7,000 feet and with few other horses in the valley.

January/February: Variable (usually pyrantel pamoate or fenbendazole)

March/April: Ivermectin

May/June: Moxidectin

July/August: Praziquantel

September/October: Ivermectin

November/December: Moxidectin or pyrantel pamoate or a benzimidazole

Odd Word

deworming vs. worming. When someone tells me that they are going to worm their horse, I wonder, “Hmm, doesn’t your horse already have enough worms?” The proper term is *deworm* and the product we use is a *dewormer.*

swallowed, arriving in the intestines for a second time. This time they stay for two to three months until mature enough to lay eggs, which are shed with feces, thereby continuing the cycle. One female ascarid can lay up to 200,000 eggs per day.

PINWORMS. More of an annoyance than a severe health threat, pinworms cause anal itching, which can result in bald patches on the tail and hindquarters.

Horses pick up the immature worms from consuming contaminated water, grain, hay, or grass. The young worms mature in the large intestine in three to four months, then crawl part way out of the anus to deposit their sticky eggs, which cause the itching. When the eggs hatch, they drop to the ground.

TAPEWORMS. Horses that live on pasture can ingest tapeworm eggs by eating pasture mites that have eaten the eggs. Tapeworms can cause colic, and they require a specialized deworming product. Confer with your veterinarian for the most effective treatment plan for your horse.

Tapeworms are a bigger problem in some regions of the United States than in others.

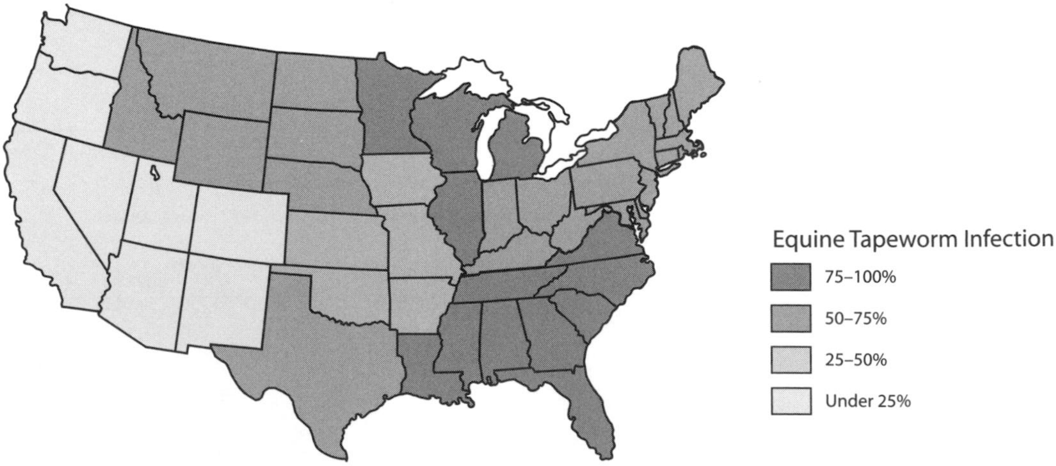

BOTS. During late summer and early fall, a stingless, bee-like fly, called the bot fly, lays eggs on the hair of your horse's forelegs, flank, chest, nose, and throat. When the horse licks the area, the eggs hatch and the larvae enter the mouth and settle in the gums, cheek, and tongue. A month later, the larvae migrate to the stomach and attach to the lining, which causes a host of problems including obstruction to the small intestine. The bot larvae live in the stomach for eight to 10 months and are shed with the feces, from where they burrow into the ground. When the time is right, the bots mature into adult bot flies and the cycle begins again. Customarily, boticides are used one month after the first hard frost to break the cycle.

How to Administer a Dewormer

Dewormers are available as paste, pellets, powder, and liquid suspension.

Paste in a syringe-type tube is the most common form available to horse owners. Some dewormers are low-volume and thus more convenient to administer. Larger-volume dewormers can be messy in paste form, and significant amounts can end up on the ground if the horse is uncooperative or has food in his mouth when the paste is given. For best results, insert a toothbrush in the corner of a horse's mouth to stimulate him to spit out feed wads, or rinse his mouth with several large syringes of water. Wait until all water has dripped out and then administer paste.

Pellets are designed to be fed mixed with grain. Some horses, however, will not eat grain with dewormer pellets in it. This is a major drawback to purge dewormer pellets, those that are fed once every eight weeks to rid a horse of parasites. You can't count on all of your horses eating all of the dewormer at once. The other type of pelleted dewormer is designed to be fed at a low level every day to prevent parasite infestation.

Consult Your Vet

As a final note, deworming your horse is usually routine and does not require veterinary help. However, if you have questions, or are concerned about particular parasites or about a deworming drug, consult your veterinarian. These are, after all, medications used to eliminate potentially harmful parasites. (See the AAEP Web site in the appendix.)

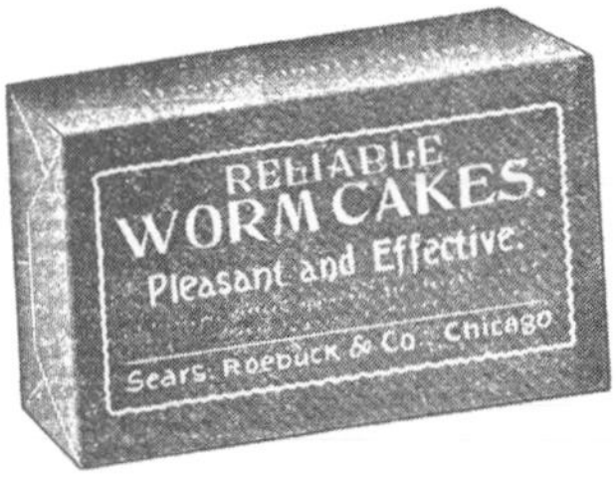

Following Up

If you want to do a post-treatment fecal check to see if the dewormers you are using are doing their job, do it two weeks after treatment. You can purchase a kit or have your vet perform the test.

The wagon rests in winter, the sleigh in summer, the horse never.

— Yiddish Proverb

Powder and liquids are usually available only to veterinarians and used as a drench through a stomach tube — a long, flexible, plastic tube passed through the horse's nose and into the stomach — for a "direct hit." Tubing is not commonly used today, due to the ease and effectiveness of paste dewormers.

A BIT MORE ABOUT BOTS

If you use the daily dewormer Strongid C, realize that it does not kill bots. Therefore, you'll need to administer an ivermectin paste in the spring and fall to control bot infestations.

The most effective times of year to treat against bot flies are usually during early spring (approximately April or May here in Colorado) just before bot larvae leave the stomach, and in late fall after a killing frost and after all bot eggs have been removed from the horse's coat (approximately October or November here).

Keep on the lookout for the presence of bot flies or eggs on your horses' legs or flanks. If you are in a heavy bot fly-way (for instance, your neighbors deworm their horses every other year whether they need it or not) you may have to step up your bot control program to three or four times per year — two spring and two fall treatments.

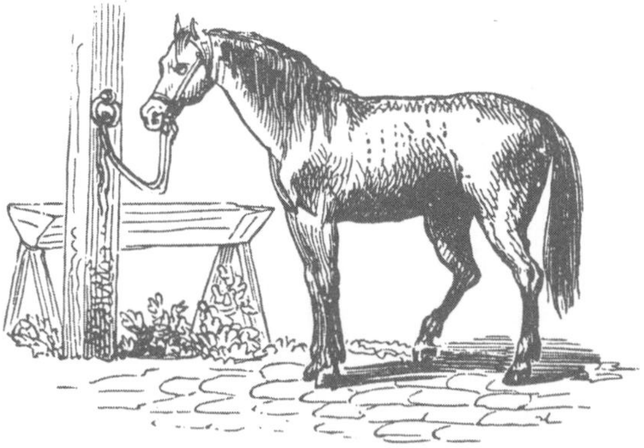

WINTER WEATHER PATTERNS

In our part of the country, January is notorious for blizzards. However, in every geographical area, winter weather has different components, characteristics, and names. The Federal Emergency Management Agency (FEMA) is a good source for information on natural disasters. (See the FEMA Web site in the appendix.)

In the mid-Atlantic and New England states, the classic winter storm is called a "Nor'easter." Since the Atlantic region has an ample supply of moisture, these storms

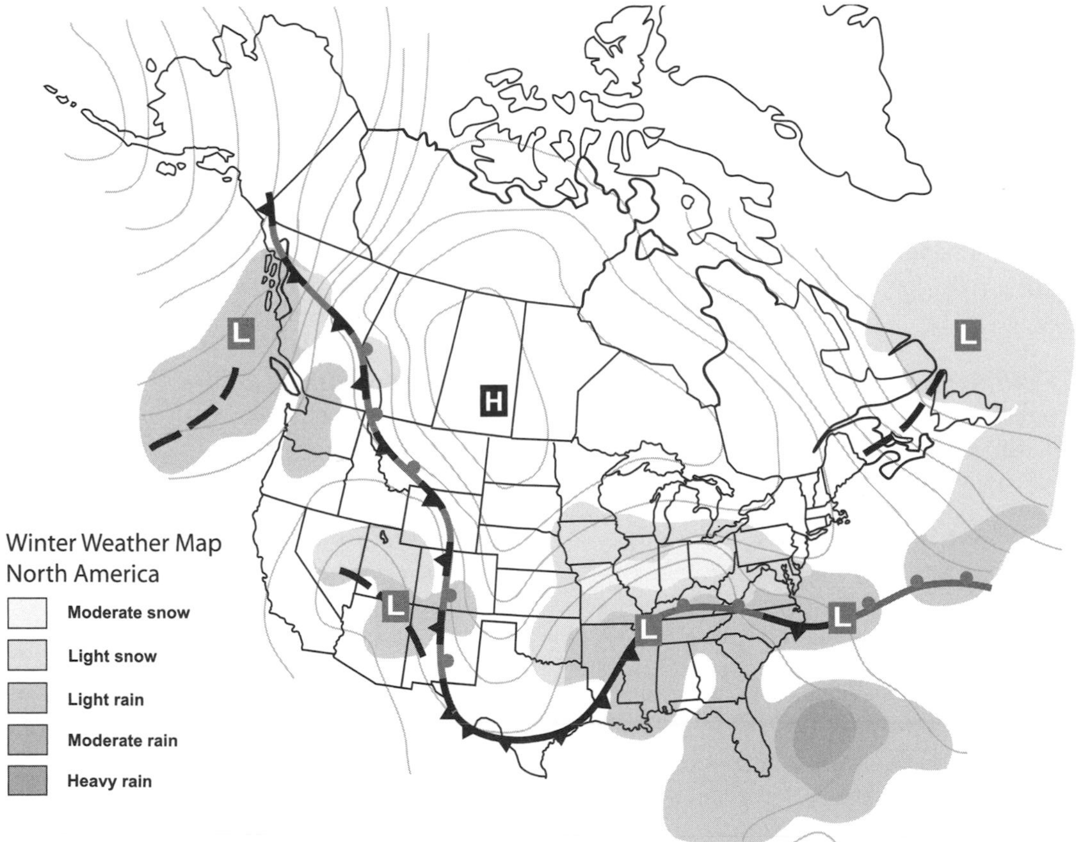

It's useful and rewarding to learn to read a typical weather map. This one shows storms off both coasts and mild weather in the High Plains and Northeast.

often result in very heavy snow. When the wind kicks in, blowing and drifting can shut down some areas. That's why it is recommended to have emergency supplies on hand at all times. Ice storms can also complicate travel and everyday farm management.

The southeastern United States doesn't usually get snow, but when it does, it can be an inconvenient surprise, freezing water lines, plants, and trees, and resulting in traffic accidents due to drivers' lack of practice maneuvering on ice and snow.

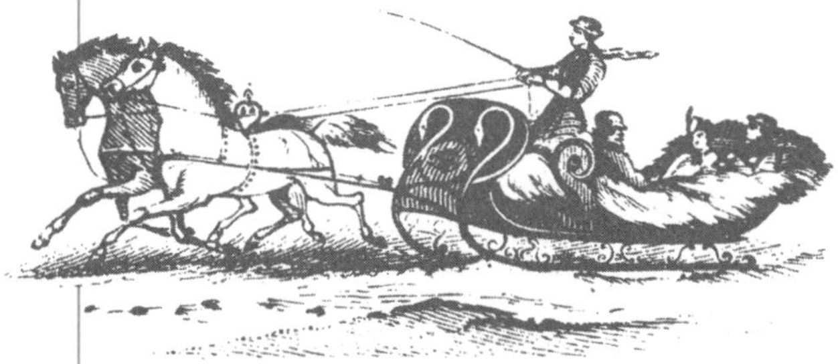

The midwestern United States is famous for its blizzards. When storms that develop over the Colorado Rocky Mountains are hit by a blast of cold Canadian (called "arctic" or Siberian) air and the moist air flow from the Gulf of Mexico, conditions

Winter Weather Warning Terms

See the appendix for the Web sites of the National Oceanic and Atmospheric Administration (NOAA) and the National Weather Service.

★ **Winter Storm Watch.** Severe winter weather conditions may affect your area. (Freezing rain, sleet, and heavy snow may occur separately or in combination).

★ **Winter Storm Warning.** Severe winter weather conditions are imminent or occurring, and are expected to meet or exceed selected criteria.

★ **Heavy Snow Warning.** A snowfall of at least 6 inches in 12 hours or 8 inches in 24 hours is expected. (Under certain conditions, heavy snow may be included in Winter Storm Warnings.)

★ **Blizzard Warning.** Considerable falling and/or blowing snow and winds of at least 35 miles per hour are expected for several hours.

★ **High Wind Warning.** Sustained winds of at least 40 miles per hour or gusts of at least 58 miles per hour or greater are expected to last for at least one hour. (In some areas, this means strong gusty winds occurring in shorter time periods.)

★ **Wind Chill Warning.** Used with wind chills of 25°F below zero or colder due to brisk winds and very cold temperatures.

are ripe for a blizzard. Accompanying strong winds create extremely low wind chill and blowing and drifting snow. Livestock can be stranded and farms have to dig themselves out. Often a series of blizzards can pile up snow so deeply and densely that it becomes very difficult to plow with an average farm tractor or get to livestock feed. Inadequately engineered farm roofs can collapse from the weight of the snow.

In the Pacific Northwest, storms that enter the United States from the ocean can bring snow to Washington, Oregon, and northern California. As the storms move into the Rocky Mountains, road closures are common and avalanches are possible. As the cold air works its way over the contours in mountainous areas, the terms "air funnels" and "wind tunnels" are used to describe windstorms that can reach sustained speeds of 100 miles per hour with higher gusts. Such winds can peel off roofing and injure livestock.

In Alaska, the intense wind-driven storms coming across the Bering Sea can result in coastal flooding, including the dashing of large chunks of ice onto shoreline buildings. The Arctic coast is infamous for its record breaking "white-outs" (blinding snow) and wind-chill temperatures as cold as 90°F below zero. Other characteristic Alaskan winter weather includes ice fog that might last a week and extremely heavy snow in the interior. That snow builds Alaskan glaciers, but it also can cause drifting that collapses buildings and suffocates trapped animals and humans.

Alaskan winters are not for the faint of heart. However, a "warmer-upper" in the form of a foehn wind is a frequent visitor to Alaska. Called a Chinook, this is a warm, dry wind that descends off a slope. It occurs not only in Alaska but all along the Canadian and U.S. Rocky Mountain areas as well. The wind, blowing usually from the southwest or the west, can be quite strong and drying.

en español

cinch. Comes from *la cincha*, meaning 'a girth for a saddle'.

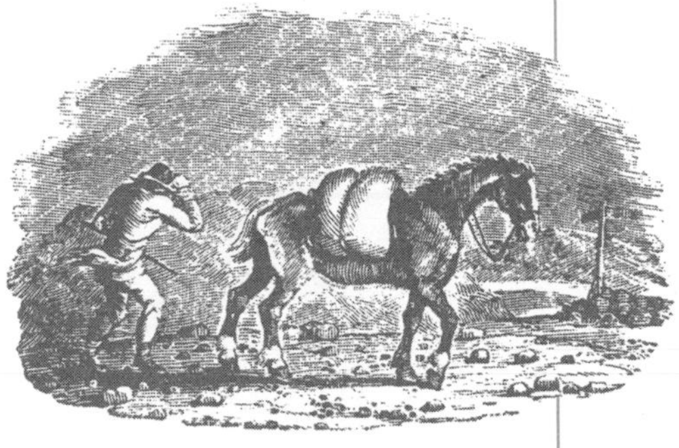

Horse Sense and Safety

Approaching a Horse

★ Always speak to a horse as you are approaching him. Move toward a horse at an angle, aiming for his shoulder.

★ Never approach a horse by aiming directly at his head or his tail. Remember his "blind" spots. Touch a horse first by placing a hand on his shoulder or neck.

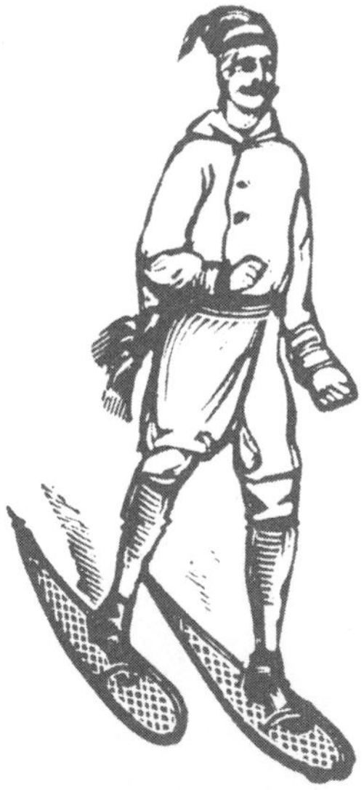

CANADIAN WINTER WEATHER PATTERNS

Canada's weather can be similar to that of the United States, in general from west to east, but it also has its unique weather patterns. In British Columbia, the low-pressure systems that develop over the Pacific Ocean are usually one of two types: powerful lows that remain well offshore, and those that approach the coast and then develop rapidly, sometimes in as little as nine hours (called "bombs"). Combination storms that spread, weaken, then drift and reorganize are also common in this area.

High pressure forms in the cold air over Alaska and the Yukon and moves southeast to the Canadian prairies (northern Saskatchewan, Manitoba, and Alberta). The prairies also suffer destructive blizzards from low-pressure systems that originate in Colorado.

A winter storm particular to Alberta is a cold air dam, which occurs when cold air is trapped against the Canadian Rockies and prevents warmer air from coming in from the west. The warm (British Columbia) air is forced to rise over the cold air dam in Alberta, so the Canadian prairies often miss the benefit of a midwinter warm-up.

The Yukon can have long and severe winters with very short days. Anyone that has ever driven the AlCan (Alaska Canadian) Highway knows that there are only a few weeks in the middle of summer when you can be positive that you won't encounter snow!

Low-pressure systems also carry winter storms to Ontario and Quebec, but their severity varies greatly depending on the location in these provinces. Winter storms in eastern Canada usually have broad cloud cover, both snow and rain, high winds, and freezing precipitation.

The Atlantic Canadian provinces of New Brunswick, Nova Scotia, Newfoundland, and Prince Edward Island are in some ways microclimates, with a wide variety of winter weather with one thing in common: cold.

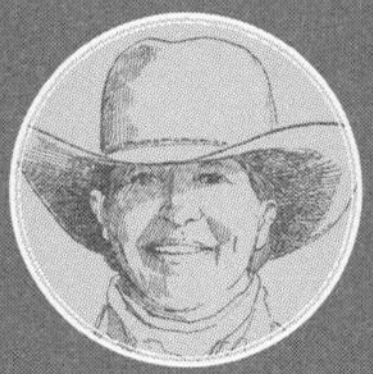

Ask Cherry

Post-Foaling Care

Q

Our mare is due on Feb 9. This is our first foal — is there a list of things that I should have (and do)? Thank you very much.

A

See page 55 for a Foaling Kit. But first, be sure you talk with your veterinarian about medical treatment your mare and foal should have prior to and after foaling. Your veterinarian might recommend:

- ★ tetanus antitoxin for foal
- ★ penicillin for mare and/or foal
- ★ immunity testing of foal
- ★ deworming of mare right after foaling with ivermectin
- ★ probiotics for foal (vitamins, minerals, enzymes, and live organisms in a paste to "jump start" the foal's digestion)
- ★ other tests or medical procedures

Water Trough Heater Safety

Q

How do you stop a horse from playing with the tank heater cord and ripping it out of the plug, and how do you prevent a horse from standing and playing in her water trough? The trough is filled with mud, urine, and manure, and very undrinkable when she is done.

A

A water trough should be about 30 inches tall so a horse can't put a hoof in it. Try placing large rocks around the base so she can't back up close enough to poop, but still can drink.

All tank heaters must be inaccessible to horses. This is customarily done by partitioning off the area where the tank heater will reside, using a wooden cover and a heavy mesh containment area for the heater. If the cord is accessible to a horse, she could be electrocuted. Locate the tank half in and half out of a paddock, pen, or pasture, so the heater cage and cord are well on the outside and the horse has access only to the safe half of the tank for drinking. To keep a horse from getting at it, run the cord through a steel or heavy plastic pipe that is buried or firmly attached to a pen or wall.

FEBRUARY

We've rounded the corner and are heading toward warmer weather, so I'm champing at the bit and getting things ready for spring. When it's too blustery to ride, I work in my tack room, giving bridles an inspection and cleaning. It's also a good time to bring some of the younger horses into the barn for some bridling practice sessions. When there is a still, sunny day, I'll grab my clipboard, walk the property, and do a pasture and fence check.

Day Length in Hours

		Date		
		Feb 1	Feb 16	March 1
Latitude	60°N	7.51	8.78	9.96
	55°N	8.37	9.37	10.32
	50°N	9.01	9.82	10.61
	45°N	9.51	10.18	10.83
	40°N	9.92	10.48	11.02
	35°N	10.27	10.73	11.18
	30°N	10.58	10.96	11.33

See page 22 to find your latitude.

Wind Chill

Wind (mph)	Temperature (°F)																	
Calm	40	35	30	25	20	15	10	5	0	-5	-10	-15	-20	-25	-30	-35	-40	-45
5	36	31	25	19	13	7	1	-5	-11	-16	-22	-28	-34	-40	-46	-52	-57	-63
10	34	27	21	15	9	3	-4	-10	-16	-22	-28	-35	-41	-47	-53	-59	-66	-72
15	32	25	19	13	6	0	-7	-13	-19	-26	-32	-39	-45	-51	-58	-64	-71	-77
20	30	24	17	11	4	-2	-9	-15	-22	-29	-35	-42	-48	-55	-61	-68	-74	-81
25	29	23	16	9	3	-4	-11	-17	-24	-31	-37	-44	-51	-58	-64	-71	-78	-84
30	28	22	15	8	1	-5	-12	-19	-26	-33	-39	-46	-53	-60	-67	-73	-80	-87
35	28	21	14	7	0	-7	-14	-21	-27	-34	-41	-48	-55	-62	-69	-76	-82	-89
40	27	20	13	6	-1	-8	-15	-22	-29	-36	-43	-50	-57	-64	-71	-78	-84	-91
45	26	19	12	5	-2	-9	-16	-23	-30	-37	-44	-51	-58	-65	-72	-79	-86	-93
50	26	19	12	4	-3	-10	-17	-24	-31	-38	-45	-52	-60	-67	-74	-81	-88	-95
55	25	18	11	4	-3	-11	-18	-25	-32	-39	-46	-54	-61	-68	-75	-82	-89	-97
60	25	17	10	3	-4	-11	-19	-26	-33	-40	-48	-55	-62	-69	-76	-84	-91	-98

Frostbite Times: 30 minutes | 10 minutes | 5 minutes

You will hear the term *wind chill* only in the winter. It is a calculation that combines the air temperature and the wind speed to represent the perceived loss of body heat.

VET CLINIC

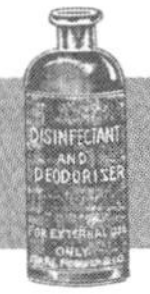

FIRST-AID KIT

The purpose of a first-aid kit is to provide the tools and supplies you need to give immediate care to your horse. I have three barn first-aid kits. One is next to the cross-ties and holds frequently used items for both horses and people. The other two are in the tack room: a comprehensive commercial human first-aid kit by the door, and my custom equine trauma kit, both at room temperature.

I keep all of the essential tools and supplies for dealing with a wound in a large plastic container with a snap lid. When an emergency strikes, I know that when I open my kit, all of the necessary items will be there, ready to use.

Remember, this is a first-aid kit, with all that you need as a first responder. Your tack-room medicine chest will contain many more supplies as needed by your specific horses and your level of experience.

To Do

- ❑ Hoof trim and shoe
- ❑ Fill in pathways with gravel
- ❑ Restock first-aid kits
- ❑ Clean out bluebird houses
- ❑ Scrub feed tubs and buckets
- ❑ Move hay to barns

To Buy

- ❑ Broodmare feed
- ❑ Antioxidants for seniors
- ❑ Complete feed wafers
- ❑ Anti-chew product
- ❑ Grain
- ❑ Dewormer

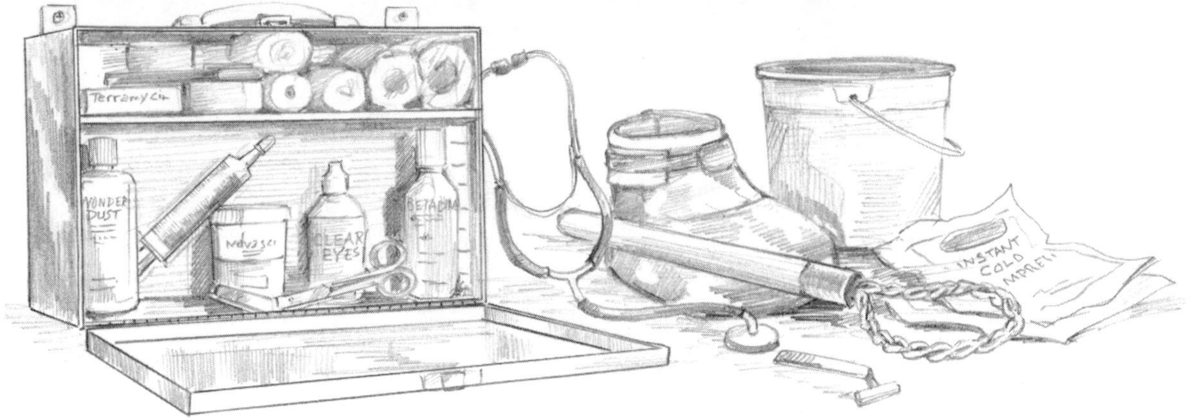

Locate your first-aid kit in a handy place, stock it well, and update products as needed.

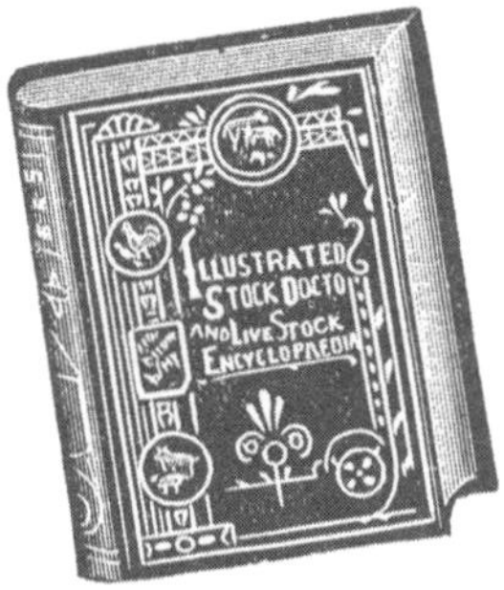

WOUND WIPES. Once you've opened a bulk package of 4x4 gauze squares, it is difficult to keep them clean in the paper bag they came in. I have a few square plastic kitchen containers that are the perfect size for the gauze squares. As you might know, tending a wound uses a good number of gauze squares soaked in a Betadine solution. Put a tall stack of 4x4 squares into one of these containers, pour in enough Betadine solution to saturate the pads, and snap on the well-sealing lid. There should be just enough room around the edges of the squares for you to be able to easily grab them.

Store the full container out of the sunlight. When you no longer need it for daily wound care, store it clean and dry, or use it to store a stack of dry pads.

Round-hoof'd, short-jointed, fetlocks shag and long,
Broad breast, full eye, small head, and nostril wide,
High crest, short ears, straight legs and passing strong,
Thin mane, thick tail, broad buttock, tender hide:
Look, what a horse should have he did not lack,
Save a proud rider on so proud a back.

— William Shakespeare, *Venus and Adonis*

INSIDE YOUR FIRST AID KIT

- ★ First-aid book (see Recommended Reading)
- ★ Veterinarian's phone number
- ★ Flashlight and batteries
- ★ Latex gloves
- ★ Thermometer
- ★ Lubricating jelly (K-Y Jelly)
- ★ Betadine solution
- ★ Betadine ointment (povidone-iodine, 10%)
- ★ Triple antibiotic ointment
- ★ Furacin ointment (nitrofurazone)
- ★ Saline solution for eye and wound wash
- ★ Phenylbutazone (Butazolidine)
- ★ Banamine (flunixin meglumine)
- ★ Wooden applicator sticks
- ★ Nonstick gauze pads (4" x 4")
- ★ Padding (leg quilts or disposable diapers)
- ★ Rolls of gauze bandage (preferably conforming)
- ★ Self-adhering stretch bandage (Vetrap)
- ★ Elastic adhesive tape
- ★ Scissors (blunt-tipped surgical type)
- ★ Pocket knife
- ★ Tweezers and/or forceps
- ★ Stethoscope
- ★ Watch with second hand
- ★ Disposable syringes and needles for injections
- ★ Large-dose syringe for flushing wounds
- ★ Alcohol and cotton balls or premoistened alcohol wipes for site prep
- ★ Instant cold compress

In Refrigerator

- ★ Antibiotics
- ★ Epinephrine

Readily Accessible

- ★ Chain twitch
- ★ Protective hoof boot
- ★ Hoof pick
- ★ Weight tape
- ★ Clean buckets
- ★ Clean cloths
- ★ Clean spray bottle
- ★ Portable lights (clamp or stand)
- ★ Extension cords

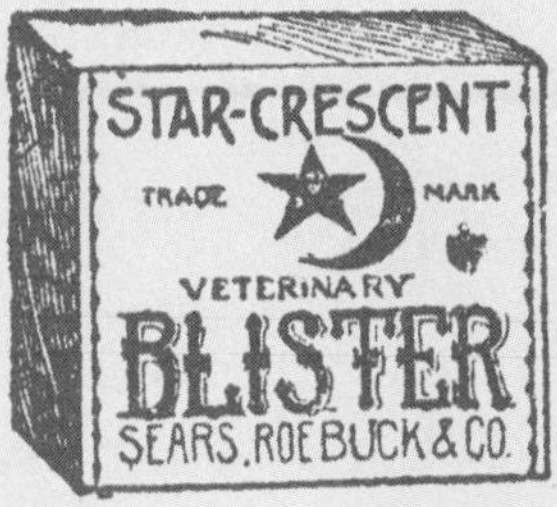

FOOT NOTES

RECOGNIZING A GOOD FARRIER

You depend on your farrier to keep your horse well trimmed and shod, so choose a good one, treat him or her well, and be a conscientious horsekeeper and trainer. What makes a good farrier?

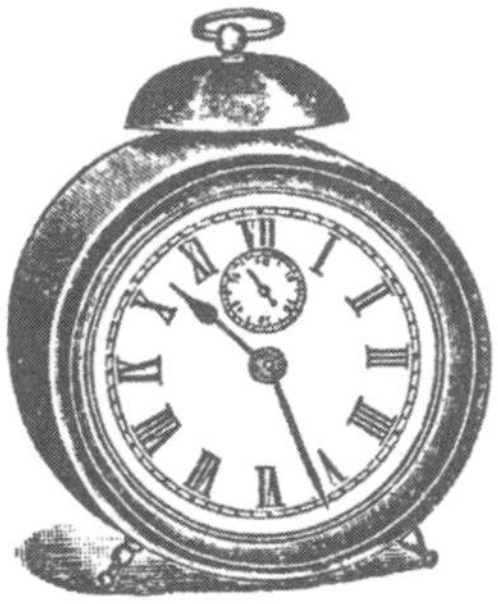

INTEREST AND PRIDE. A farrier should be a true craftsman with genuine interest and pride in his work. He should look at each hoof that he prepares and shoes as one that will bear his trademark and demonstrate the quality of his work. A keen farrier wants to keep informed of the latest research and developments in hoof care technology. A farrier that does not stay updated is outdated.

GOOD TIME MANAGEMENT. Because a farrier must usually be the secretary, accountant, and chief laborer in his small operation, he must be a good business manager. Time is one of his most valuable assets and it must be properly managed. In order to be successful, a farrier must be organized when making and keeping appointments. A farrier who is not dependable or punctual can cause unnecessary inconveniences and frustrations for horse owners, and his negligence can result in irregular care for his client's horses. A horseshoer must be careful to not pack his schedule so full that he becomes hurried, because then he will not do his best work. If he jams the entire week with appointments or falls behind schedule, he may have no time left for emergencies such as replacing lost shoes or working with your veterinarian on an emergency lameness.

GOOD HORSE-HANDLING SKILLS. In order to get along with the variety of horses belonging to clients, a farrier must

Horse Sense and Safety

Moving Around Horses

★ Don't pet the end of a horse's nose. Doing so might cause him to move away, or it might encourage him to nibble.

★ Either walk around a horse well out of kicking range or move around the horse by staying close, with your hand on his hindquarters to let him know you are there. Never walk under or step over the tie rope.

understand and be comfortable using standard methods of horse handling. Although a farrier needs to remain flexible to the different ways of doing things at various barns, he should never consent to work in unsafe conditions or on an untrained or unmannerly horse. A big part of being a good horseman is knowing when to say no when a client presents an unruly horse for him to shoe. (More on this later for you, the horseowner.)

GOOD COMMUNICATION. Storytelling is not a prerequisite to being a good horseshoer, but being able to explain hoof care principles and management to owners is important. You should be able to ask your farrier what thrush is and get a thorough, intelligent, and accurate answer. After all, the health and care of hooves is his area of expertise. If the answer to "What is thrush?" is "Black gook, and you don't want it," then you haven't really learned anything. Although your farrier doesn't have the time to teach you everything he has learned, he should be able to give you a good answer and then refer you to books or articles that deal with the topics that concern or interest you.

Ranch Notes

Feb. 1 Made a pasture check with notebook and map.

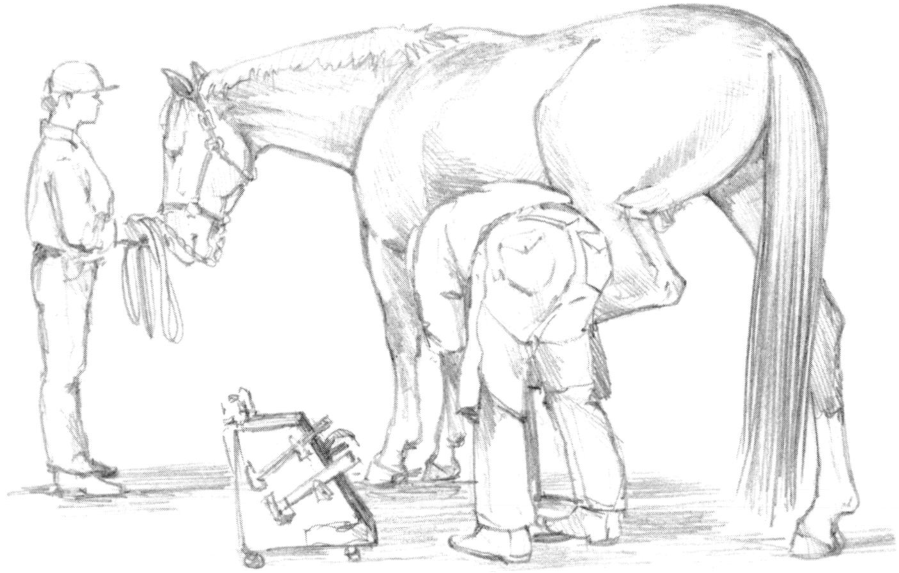

If your farrier prefers that you hold your horse for shoeing, learn safe handling practices.

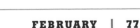

APPROPRIATE SKILL LEVEL. Just as there are all levels of horsemen, there are all levels of practicing horse shoers as well, from very basic, self-taught individuals to thoroughly educated, high-tech farriers. Horses with abnormal hoof problems require the experience and skill of an upper-echelon farrier. When an inexperienced horseshoer

NO WAY!

Historical Horsekeeping

I collect antique horse books. One day I opened a book I had just purchased and found a clipping from a 1910 edition of the Sunday Boston Post *inside. The "Sunday Post Veterinary" column was sponsored by the Massachusetts Society for the Prevention of Cruelty to Animals to promote the welfare of horses. Questions were answered weekly by Harvard graduate Dr. D. L. Bolger. These two examples give us an idea of what horsekeeping was like a hundred years ago:*

QUESTION: I have a valuable horse 18 years old. I don't use her a great deal; she has been out to grass all summer. Her right forward shoulder is all swollen up in the muscle. It extends in the inside of her leg to her body. It runs down the inside of the leg to her ankle. It is stiff and she cannot pick up her foot; she seems to drag it. We have been bathing it in warm water and sal. soda. — C. A. J.

ANSWER: *Feed the mare on bran for one day with no hay, and give one quart of raw linseed oil on empty stomach in the morning. Bathe the shoulder and leg at least five times a day, half an hour each time with a pail of hot mustard water, no hotter than you can bear with your hand in it, one tablespoon of mustard to a pailful of water. Write us again in about two weeks.*

QUESTION: Will you kindly tell me whether or not there is any help for cocked ankle? Have tried several liniments, but they do not seem to straighten my mare's ankle so that she will stand erect, though it does not make her lame. — J. E. W.

ANSWER: *Have her shod with a good long shoe. Rub her ankles well twice a day with skunk's oil. Persist in this and I am sure it will help her some.*

is faced with quarter cracks, underrun heels, laminitis, or navicular syndrome, he may not know what to do and could make the situation worse.

The greater the performance demands are on a horse, the more precise the shoeing needs to be. The backyard pleasure horse with normal hooves may get along very well being trimmed and shod by a farrier who has only very basic (but acceptable) skills. However, when that horse is headed into the reining pen, over a hunter course, or on an endurance ride, his shoeing requirements may become much more specialized and the margin for error becomes smaller.

PRICE. With farriery, as with many other things, you usually get what you pay for. Although the price of a standard shoeing (four keg shoes) can vary by as much as $100 among farriers, the range will be based on level of experience, education, skill, demand, and location. Prices also vary regionally, with West Coast farrier fees generally being the highest, followed by the Southeast, the East Coast, the Midwest, the West, and the Southwest.

Ads Aren't Adequate

Do not rely solely on printed advertisements in your search for a farrier, because some of the best ones don't need to advertise. Their reputation is spread by word of mouth. While some farriers that advertise may be new to the area and very qualified, others might be desperately seeking business and end up creating long-term problems for your horse.

Finding and Choosing a Farrier

There are several ways you can go about finding a good farrier: certification, recommendations, and interview. I recommend that you use a combination of methods to find the individual best suited to your needs.

Start your list by jotting down the names and phone numbers of farriers who advertise in newspapers and local horse publications or on bulletin boards in feed stores, tack shops, and stables. Keep a notebook so that you can modify your list and take notes as you go.

The greater the performance demands are on a horse, the more precise the shoeing needs to be.

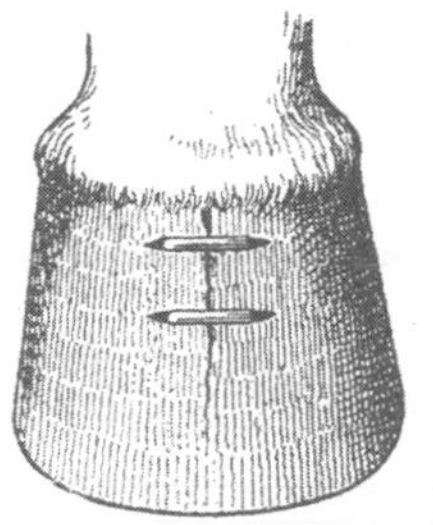

CERTIFICATION. There are many horseshoeing schools in the United States, with courses ranging from one week to one year. Some will issue a certificate or diploma after a

Ranch Notes

Feb. 16 Musical pens and pastures. Plan for March:

- ❑ Move Zipper between Aria and Seeker on east side of horse barn.
- ❑ Return Dickens to his SW horse barn pen.
- ❑ Put Sassy in pen by lower red barn.
- ❑ Leave others where they are (Zinger in senior center, Sherlock in pen by lower red barn)

student has completed the course. Some farriers who have attended these schools will list "certified farrier" or "graduate farrier" after their names to indicate that they have been to school and have received a certificate. To help standardize the skill level ratings of farriers (no matter what school they attended) the American Farriers' Association (AFA; see its Web site in the appendix) has developed a means of testing and certifying farriers by using standardized exams and testing procedures across the country.

Although AFA membership and testing are open to any farrier, only a small fraction of the farriers in the United States belong to the AFA. Applicants are required to pass written shoeing and veterinary-related exams as well as demonstrate shoeing skills in practical exams. In addition, at most levels, the applicants are required to present a display of various types of shoes that the applicant has made or modified. As the applicant rises through the levels, the testing becomes more difficult and thorough. The AFA maintains an updated directory on its Web site of farriers' names, addresses, phone numbers, and level of certification.

However, if you rely solely on the AFA farrier list, you may miss finding a very talented and capable farrier who lives just down the road from you. So take the list you began compiling from advertisements, cross-reference the AFA farriers with it, and start asking for recommendations.

Certification

A farrier can be certified at the following levels from more basic to advanced:

- ★ AFA Intern Classification (IC)
- ★ AFA Certified Farrier (CF)
- ★ AFA Certified Journeyman Farrier (CJF)

RECOMMENDATIONS. When you ask people who their farrier is, you'll likely either get an overwhelmingly enthusiastic recommendation, a reluctance to "share," or blatant dissatisfaction. Try to talk with about 10 people, drawing from the following groups: your vet, other vets, professional horsemen, and horse owners.

Beginning with your own veterinarian, ask him or her which farriers are capable and open-minded in solving hoof problems, and which work well with owners in developing a hoof care program. Ask your veterinarian to name both the farriers he recommends and those he does not recommend. Then ask the same of two other equine veterinarians in your area. Ask some local professional horsemen (trainers, instructors, stable managers, and breeders) which farriers they've used and which ones they currently employ.

But don't take one person's opinion so strongly that you either cross a farrier off your list or put five stars by his name. Just keep adding data to your list, including details such as: "never on time," "great with young horses," or "he's hard to get along with." Ask how long it takes for various farriers to replace lost shoes; if a horse has ever been lame right after shoeing and what the farrier did about it; if the farrier works well with the farm veterinarian; if the farrier gets along well with horses.

Then choose three horseowners who are very similar to the type of horse person you are or aspire to be. If you are a casual trail rider, for example, it would be inappropriate to ask a gaited show-ring rider for his or her farrier recommendations. Find three people who follow the same level of management that you do and ride as frequently as you do in similar activities, and ask them the same sorts of questions that you asked of the professional horsemen.

By now, you should have a notebook bursting with valuable personal recommendations. Look for three or four names that kept coming up in a positive way. Also, if there are names that consistently brought negative comments, make a "don't go there" list. And while everything is fresh in your mind, rank those that are left in a middle group. This will be particularly useful if you call your top three and none of them are taking on new customers. Good farriers are busy.

INTERVIEW. Next you will need to speak either in person or on the phone to your top choices. Hiring a farrier to work on your horse requires a good measure of trust, so you

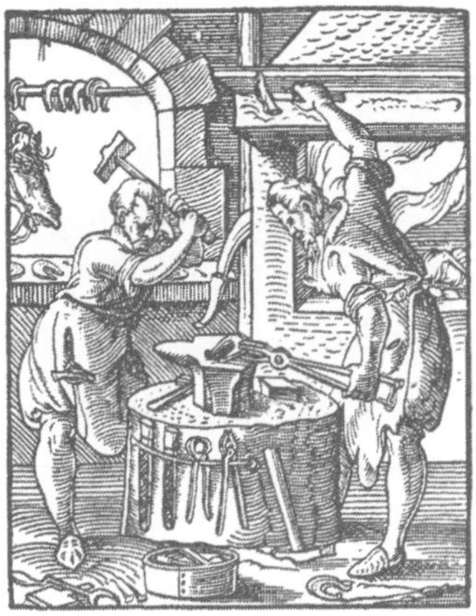

"*For the want* of a nail, the shoe was lost; for the want of a shoe, the horse was lost; and for the want of a horse, the rider was lost; being overtaken and slain by the enemy, all for the want of care about a horseshoe nail."

— Benjamin Franklin, in the Preface of *Courteous Reader*, 1758

> *en español*
>
> **hackamore.** Comes from *la jáquima*, meaning 'a headstall or a halter for a horse'. Pronounced HA-kee-ma.
>
> Note: A hackamore consists of a *bosal* (braided rawhide noseband), a *mecate* (horse hair rope and reins), and a *fiador* (rope throatlatch). All three are Spanish words.

have every right to request background information. Some farriers have a biographical sheet that they give to prospective clients, listing their education, experience, and rates. If you present your questions in a courteous, respectful manner, no farrier should take such inquiries as an affront. If he does, it may tell you something about how the two of you will get along.

Besides giving you a sense of a farrier's level of expertise and his manner, a brief telephone or personal interview will also help you find out his rates and scheduling procedures, two very important business details that must be clearly discussed to prevent misunderstandings.

Once you have found the farrier that suits your needs, here's how to keep him.

KEEPING YOUR FARRIER

Since scheduling is the most common problem in obtaining continuous farrier service, find out if your farrier likes to schedule a definite appointment seven weeks in advance or if he'd rather you make an appointment the week before

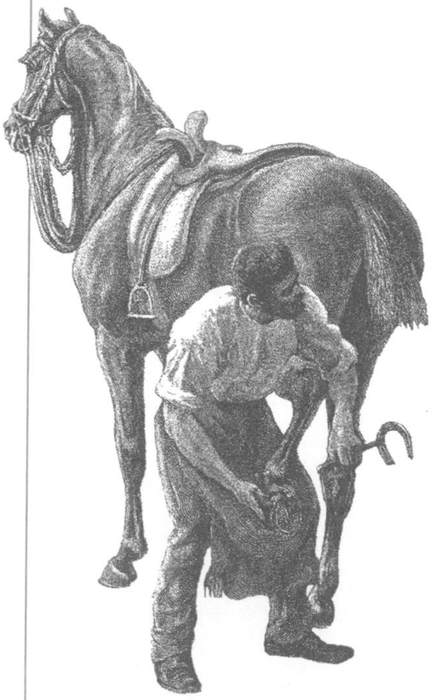

> ### Questions to Ask a Farrier
>
> It's appropriate to ask a prospective farrier about the school he or she attended, how long he or she has been shoeing, and his or her areas of specialty. Make sure he or she has had experience in the activities you are likely to pursue. If you are interested in riding reining horses, for example, you'd better be sure your farrier knows about sliding plates; if you will be raising foals, he must understand the developmental process of the young horse's limbs.

you need him. Ask if you need to call to verify the appointment the day before.

Also, make sure you know if the farrier requires someone to be present when he is working. If you have a large number of horses, or if your horses' shoeing schedules differ greatly, it may be best to arrange for your farrier to come to your farm on a particular morning each week unless otherwise notified.

PREPARING THE WORK AREA. All horses scheduled for work should be ready when the farrier arrives, tied or cross-tied in the barn or in nearby stalls or small pens conveniently located to the working area. The shoeing area should have a secure place to tie horses safely at a height above their withers, or a competent person should hold the horse.

The area should be well lit, uncluttered, and level. Some shoers like to work on a concrete slab, others on a rubber mat. A rocky paddock or a barn aisle full of potholes isn't comfortable or productive.

Although direct sunlight might help your farrier see what he is doing, hot summer sun can be extremely fatiguing. Provide shade and shelter, and perhaps a fan, for summer as well as for winter work. Besides making your farrier happy, you will be making your horses more comfortable and cooperative as well.

The farrier's work area should not be Grand Central Station. Shoeing in the cross-ties in a barn aisle can be a real nightmare if traffic in and out of stalls requires the farrier to constantly move the horse he is working on. A place where the farrier can concentrate without interruptions will enable him to do his best work. Children and dogs have no place in the farrier's area. The nearby operation of noisy machines such as motorcycles, snow machines, snow blowers, weed eaters, tractors, and chain saws should be scheduled at a time other than when the farrier is working.

Making an Appointment

When you make an appointment, have an accurate list of what you need done, such as two horses to shoe all around, and three broodmares and one yearling to trim. Also mention any problems that might require special supplies. Discuss payment arrangements, because some farriers require payment at time of service, while others prefer to send a bill.

Most Essential

Finally, one of the best ways to keep a good farrier is to be genuinely interested in the health of your horse's hooves. Be a conscientious manager and rider and learn all you can about hoof care and shoeing.

Farrier Etiquette

- ★ **Do** offer to hold your horse if it is his first time for trimming or shoeing, but
- ★ **Don't** object if your farrier prefers to work alone with the horse tied.
- ★ **Do** have plenty of fly repellent on hand, but
- ★ **Don't** wait until your farrier's visit to acquaint your horse with a spray bottle.
- ★ **Do** introduce your dogs to your farrier when he first arrives, but
- ★ **Don't** let your dogs loose while the farrier is working.
- ★ **Do** tell your horseshoer the name, age, and use of each horse and any problems he might have, but
- ★ **Don't** expect him to listen to long stories or carry on a conversation. He is there to shoe your horse.
- ★ **Do** pay attention to your horse's behavior, but
- ★ **Don't** take your nervous horse for a hike down the gravel driveway on freshly trimmed feet while the farrier is shaping a shoe.
- ★ **Do** discuss stable management and hoof care with your farrier. Ask him about the symptoms of problems he may see in your horse's feet and listen to his recommendations to remedy them, but
- ★ **Don't** expect miracles from your farrier. If you bought a horse that had been neglected for two years, or if you have a horse with crooked legs, or if you board at a stable that only cleans stalls once a week, don't think that your farrier has a magic rasp that can cure cracks, founder, conformation flaws, or thrush. You must work together toward gradual, permanent results.
- ★ **Do** have your payment in full ready before he leaves (if that is what he prefers), and
- ★ **Don't** make him ask.
- ★ **Do** offer him a place to wash up and a glass of water.
- ★ **Do** make an appointment for the next shoeing.

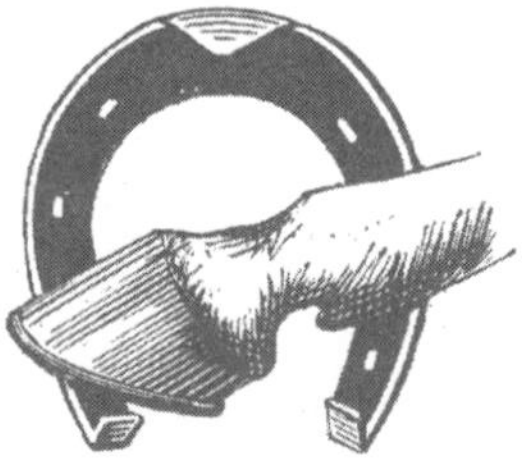

PREPARING THE HORSES. If your horses have come out of muddy lots, be sure to clean them, especially their shoulders, hindquarters, and legs, the areas that will be in direct contact with the farrier. Scrape and then wipe the mud off the hooves, rather than hosing them off. Clean, dry hooves are much better for the farrier to work on than slippery, wet hooves.

If your horse is trained to be cooperative about having his legs handled and his hooves worked on, your farrier will be safer and can do his best work. (See January.)

Make things nice for your farrier. He will appreciate it a lot more than cookies, I'll guarantee it.

FEED BAG

HAY IS FOR HORSES

A horse's digestive system is designed to handle a high amount of bulk (roughage, like hay or pasture, which is high in fiber) and a low amount of concentrate (grain). Feeding too much grain or rich hay is not good for a horse. It can lead to excess body weight, excess energy, colic, laminitis, or possibly a calcium-to-phosphorus imbalance. I feed a grass-mix hay (brome, orchard grass, and timothy) or a grass/alfalfa mix (alfalfa is a legume with purple flowers) that contains no more than 15 percent alfalfa. Both hays are ideal for horses.

> **Go Natural**
>
> Natural feeding can be summed up pretty simply:
>
> ★ Feed at ground level.
>
> ★ Maximize roughage, minimize grain.
>
> ★ Feed little or no alfalfa hay.
>
> ★ Give your horse many little meals.
>
> ★ Provide free-choice water, trace minerals, and salt.

Hay Amount

To maintain my horses' optimal weight and to minimize my feed costs, I feed hay at the rate of 1.5 to 1.75 pounds of hay per 100 pounds of body weight. That way, the horses get filled up but not filled out. Using my rule of thumb, Zipper, my 1,100-pound gelding, eats between 16.5 and 19.25 pounds of hay per day:

1,100 ÷ 100 = 11 cwt (cwt [hundredweight] = 100 pounds)
11 cwt × 1.5 = 16.5 pounds of hay per day, or two feedings of 8.25 pounds each
11 cwt × 1.75 = 19.25 pounds of hay per day, or two feedings of 9.5 pounds each

A horse's digestive system is designed to handle a high amount of bulk (roughage, like hay or pasture, which is high in fiber) and a low amount of concentrate (grain).

Some horses require less bulk and more concentrate, so I feed them less than 1.5 pounds of hay per 100 pounds of body weight. These include horses in heavy work, mares in late pregnancy, and weanlings. However, lactating mares usually require both more concentrate and more than 1.5 pounds of hay per 100 pounds of body weight.

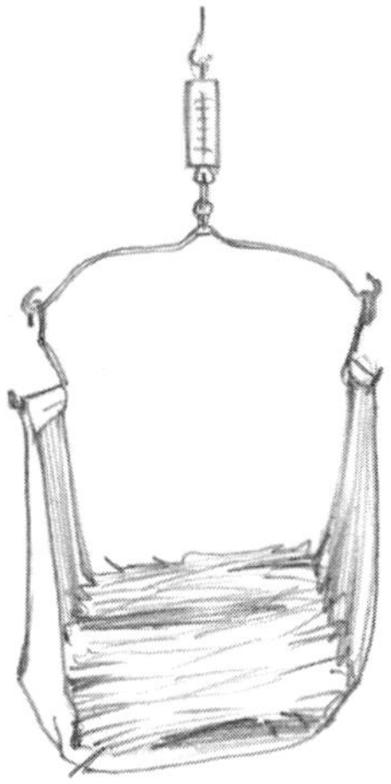

A simple hanging hay scale will tell you exactly what you are feeding your horse.

WEIGH YOUR HAY. Depending on where you live, the sections of a bale of hay are called by various names such as flakes, flecks, leaves, slabs, sections, biscuits, and slices. Flakes of hay will vary greatly in weight depending on the type of hay, moisture content, how tightly the hay was baled, and the adjustment on the baler for flake thickness. One flake might weigh 3 pounds while another could weigh 9 pounds.

That is why it's important to feed hay by weight, not by flakes. If you weigh your horse's hay daily, he will get the ration he needs and you will save feed costs by not overfeeding.

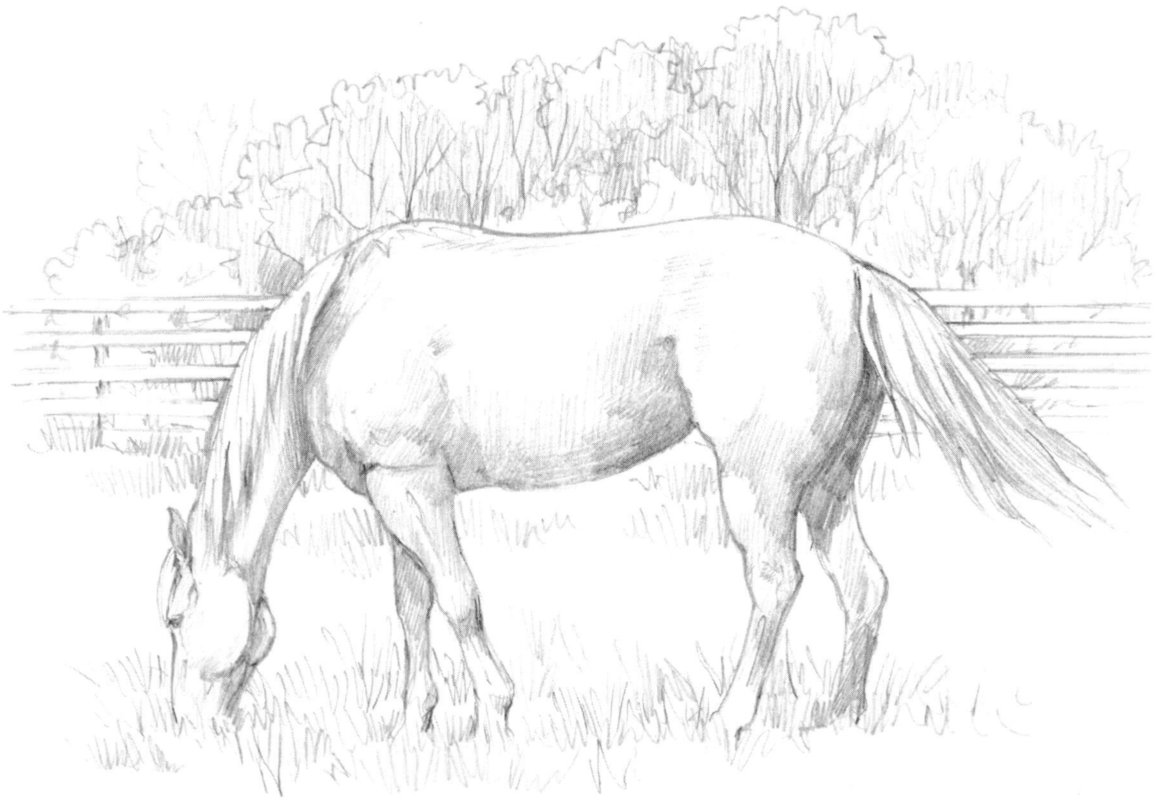

Pasture grass is the most natural horse feed.

Natural Feeding

There is nothing as gratifying as opening up a bale of hay to feed your horse in February and seeing clean, green grass hay that stills holds the sweet smell of summer. Pasture grass is the mainstay of a wild horse's diet, so the most natural way for a horse to eat is on a good grass pasture. If you don't have adequate pasture for grazing and for the winter months when pastures are resting, good quality grass hay is the next best thing. (See Health Food for Horses in More In Depth, page 108.)

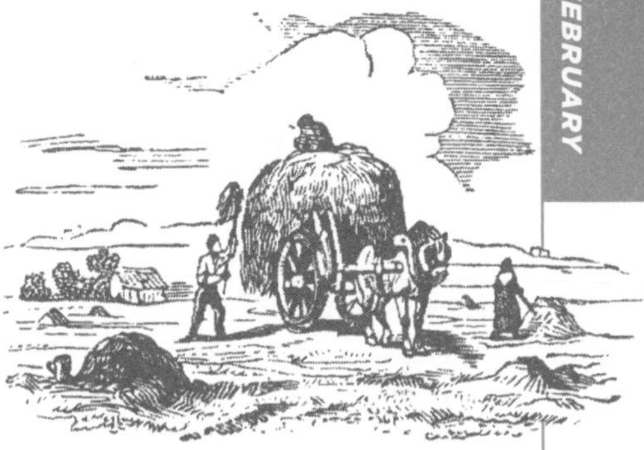

WILD LIFE

PREDATORS

Predators are beautiful, natural members of the ecosystem, but in some situations they can become dangerous killers of people and livestock. Some of the predators that might threaten you or your animals are bears, mountain lions, wolves, coyotes, and wild dogs. Depending on how big of a problem they are in your area, how much loss or damage has occurred on your farm or ranch, and the laws in your state, your method of control will be either nonlethal or lethal. Each situation is very different and will require a unique solution.

Some *nonlethal* means of predator control include:

- **Fencing.** Erecting barrier wire or electrical fences to keep predators out of pastures.
- **Guard dogs.** Using certain breeds of dogs to guard livestock and alert the manager when predators approach. Such breeds as the Great Pyrenees, Akbash, and Komondor are noted livestock guard dogs. (See January Wild Life).

WOLVES

Twice the size of coyotes, wolves (*Canis lupus*) rarely cause problems for horse owners. Once abundant in the Lower 48, the gray wolf (a.k.a. timber wolf) and its subspecies are now found only in the northernmost United States and throughout Canada and Alaska. Males weigh more than 100 pounds and increase with latitude, reaching more than 150 pounds in Alaska.

Last Resort

Lethal means of predator control include hunting, trapping, snaring, and poisoning, all of which must first be checked for legality and considered only as a last resort.

- **Herders.** Employing people to live out with a herd of livestock.
- **Scare devices.** Using devices (such as lights, radios, sirens, and cannons) to frighten predators away from livestock. This is only a temporary measure, because predators become accustomed to the devices and are no longer frightened away.
- **Relocation.** Capturing offending predators and moving them to a more remote area; this task is usually performed by local or state wildlife agents.

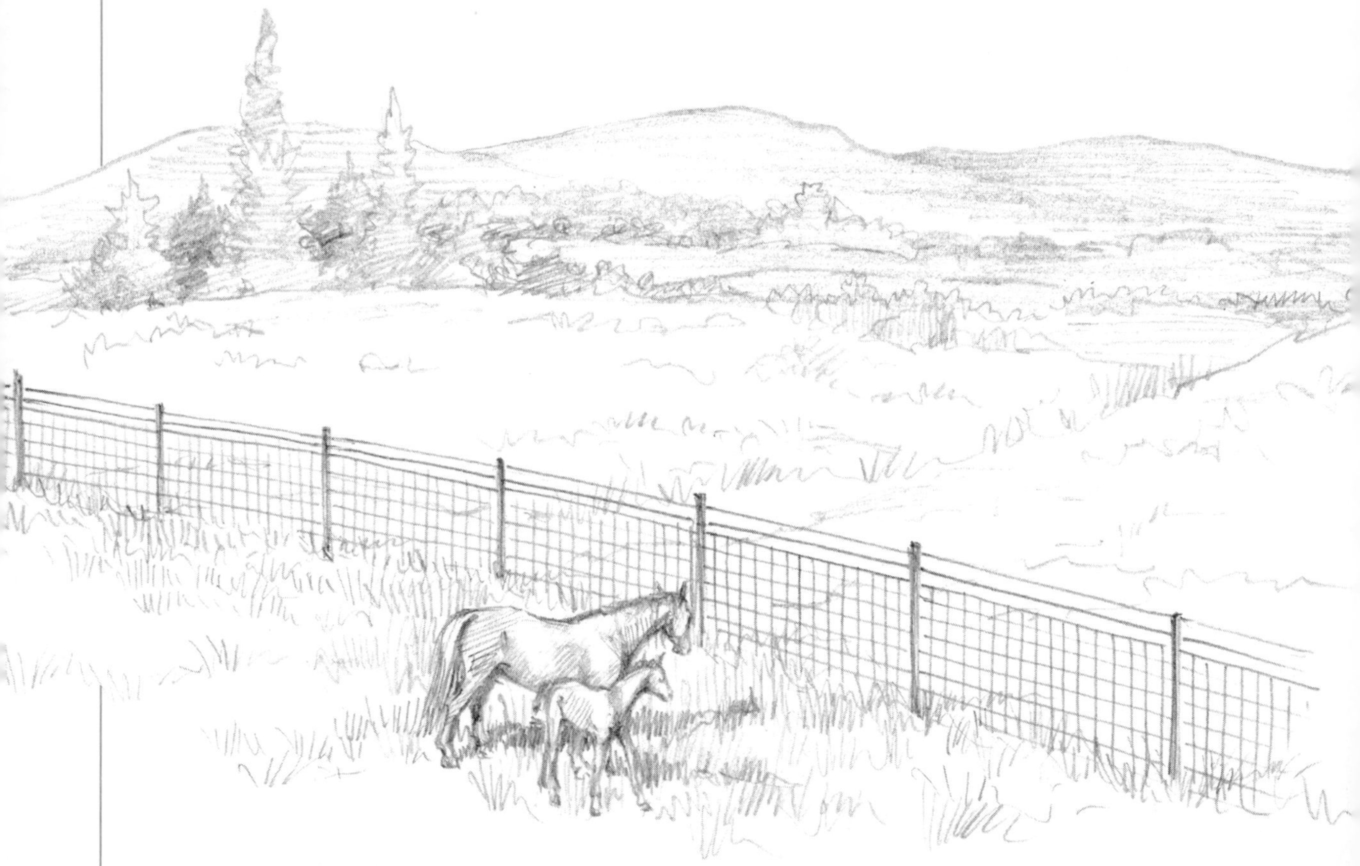

To keep loose or wild dogs off your property, you may need to install a predator fence.

Pest Patrol

Coyotes and Wild Dogs

Because coyotes (*Canis latrans*) and wild dogs hunt both solo and in packs, they could be a risk to your pets and to small or old horses. It is odd that on one hand, certain dogs are a deterrent to predators while others become predators. In my experience, more problems occur on horse farms and ranches due to wild dogs or loose domestic dogs than to coyotes.

A neighbor of ours, years back, routinely used to shoot any dog that came on his property. Some of his llamas had been maimed or killed by loose domestic dogs that got into very bad company and developed a dangerous game. Legally, our neighbor was within his rights. Unfortunately, many people move out to the country and believe they can just turn their dogs loose to roam free. Once a dog experiences the taste of blood and the excitement of a chase and kill, he often reverts to his instincts and behavior patterns and changes from a loose domestic dog to a wild dog. In addition to chasing livestock, wild dogs also form packs and chase wildlife.

We've had great success in catching wild dogs, some still wearing collars and tags from their previous domestic situation. We are ever-vigilant, as are our horses and neighbors, for predators on the loose. Keeping one another informed is an excellent way to avoid problems.

You'll see and hear coyotes, but most likely you will not have a horse problem with them. Although their main diet is rabbits, mice, and gophers, they could prey on domestic pets, chickens, young foals, calves, and sheep. They are also capable of breeding with and "stealing" domestic dogs. Pups are usually born in April and May.

Coyotes weigh 20 to 50 pounds. Their scat is 2 to 5 inches long, round, and approximately an inch in diameter. In the winter, scat will contain some seeds, but mostly hair and bone fragments.

Coyote tracks are 2 to 3 inches long, with four toes and round pads. A coyote's front feet, which he uses for digging, are larger than his back feet. Coyote tracks are more elongated than dog tracks.

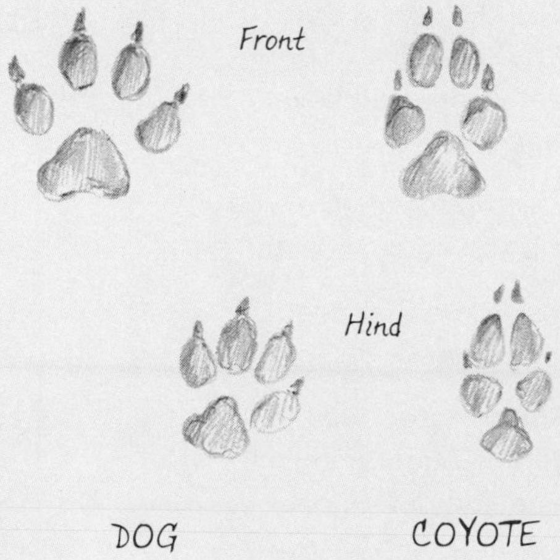

PASTURE PERFECT

PASTURE CHECK

This time of year, we bring all of our horses in off pasture to let the grass grow and to protect the land from hoof damage during the muddy spring months. During this period, I turn off the electric fence controllers and, with a map of our property (which has twelve pastures), walk around each pasture, making note of needed repairs.

I make notes and symbols on the map showing the exact location of these repair jobs and get ready to bake yet another batch of those cookies for Richard.

Annual Fence Walk

Here are some things to look for as you check your fences in February.

★ Posts or support braces that might need replacement

★ Gates that require a tune-up to counteract the sag of soil shifting or old age

★ Wooden posts that need a new coat of preservative or anti-chew compound

★ Electric fence wire that is frayed or broken

★ Insulators that need replacement

★ Smooth steel wire that needs tightening or refastening due to deer damage

ELECTRIC FENCES

Electric fencing can be used as temporary or permanent fence, either by itself or with other fencing. Electric fences can train horses not to chew, lean over, push, or rub on other

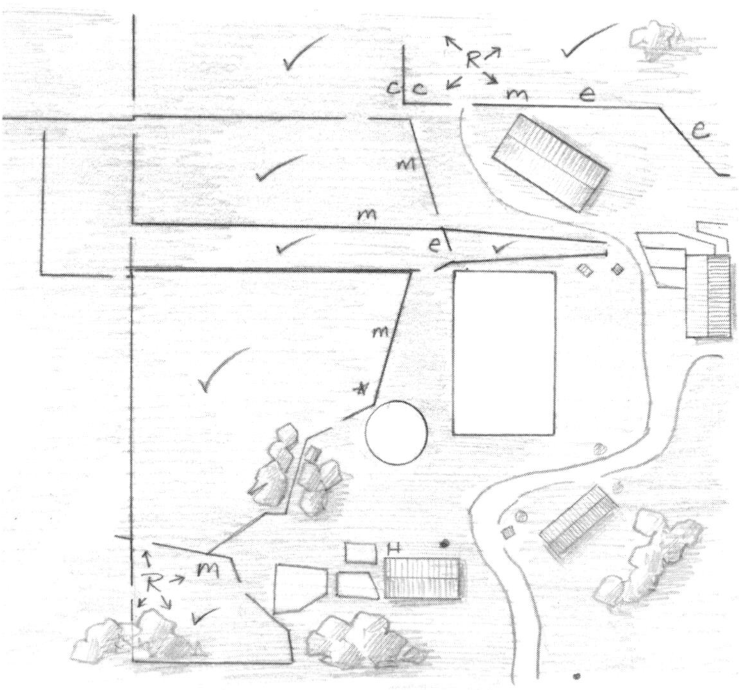

types of fences. An electric fence system consists of wire, insulators, posts, and a grounded power source.

There are a variety of electric fencing options. You can use solid steel wire, either galvanized 12-gauge smooth or barbless twisted galvanized cable. More popular is ⅛-inch to ⅜-inch polymer rope or cord with woven-in stainless steel or copper. Another option is ½-inch- to 2-inch-wide poly tape or ribbon.

The power source for an electric fence is called a controller, charger, fencer, transformer, or energizer. It is usually one of three types: plug-in, battery, or solar.

Plug-in electric transformers (also called "mains") that run off 110/120-volt household current are effective and economical, but not convenient for pastures away from buildings and electricity.

Battery-powered transformers are handy for temporary or remote situations, but the need to replace or recharge the batteries every two to six weeks adds more cost and time.

Plastic vs. Steel

For both my horses and me, plastic (poly) has great advantages over steel, such as:

- ★ The color of the plastic makes it more visible than steel wire.
- ★ If a horse becomes tangled, plastic will break more easily, while steel will often cut the horse.
- ★ Plastic fence can be put up or repaired with just a pair of scissors and a simple knot.
- ★ It is light and flexible and does not need to be stretched tightly, as steel wire does.

With plastic electric fence, you use plastic insulators that snap onto fiberglass or steel T-posts or are nailed or screwed onto wooden posts.

Looking at Horses

Head Proportions

For the brain to coordinate the horse's movements, adequate cranial space is necessary. Here are some pointers on how to judge head proportions.

- ★ The length from the base of the ear to the eye should be at least one-third of the distance from ear to nostril.
- ★ The width between the eyes should be the same distance as that from the base of the ear to the eye.
- ★ A wide poll with ears far apart allows the atlas to connect behind the skull rather than below it.
- ★ A wide, open throatlatch permits proper breathing during flexion.

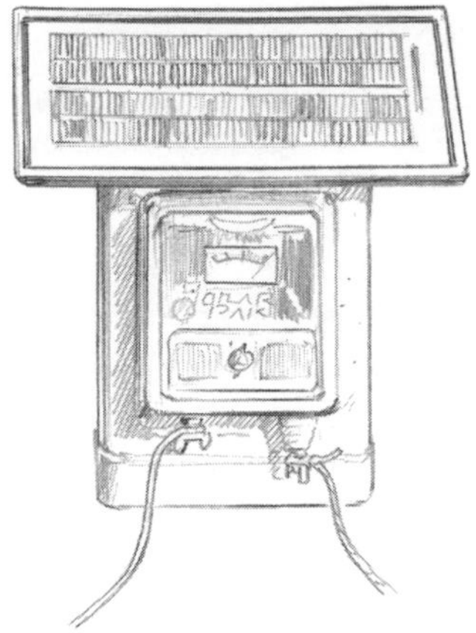

Solar fence charger

And as a battery begins to wane, it no longer has enough charge to do its job, so often leaves the fence insecure.

Solar-powered chargers have photovoltaic cells that convert sunlight into electricity to charge the battery continuously. It takes only three to four hours of sunlight per day to maintain a charge, and a fully charged battery can last three weeks without a sunny day. Mount the solar charger facing south in a place where horses can't reach it.

INSTALLING THE CHARGER. The charger converts electricity (from a battery or a 110-volt service) into shock pulses that are transmitted to the fence wire. The charger must be properly installed according to the directions for the specific model.

Some models require a clean, dry location where moisture cannot drip or blow onto the unit. Others are designed to be weather resistant and can be mounted right on a fencepost; however, it is still advisable to protect them with a weatherproof box. The exception to this is the solar fence charger, which must be open to the sun.

If your power unit is inside a building, as most plug-in types will be, install a tube insulator through the wall so you can run a "hot" wire from the unit to your fence outside without it being grounded by the wall. A piece of small-diameter plastic pipe or rubber tubing works well.

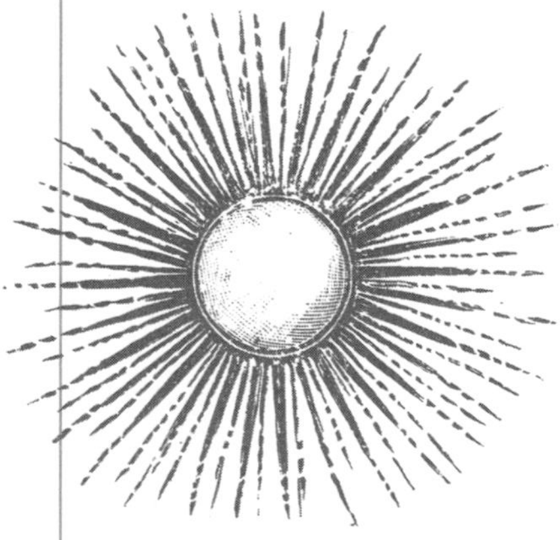

GROUNDING. The controller unit itself must be grounded. In order for a horse to feel a shock, the current must travel from the controller to the wire to the horse to the ground (earth) and back to the controller. (That's why a bird can sit on an electric fence and not be shocked. The current hasn't completed the circuit by touching the ground.) Improper grounding causes many fence problems. The ground rod or tube should be of copper, steel, or galvanized pipe and should be driven 6 to 8 feet into the ground, where it reaches permanently moist earth. If you are in a very dry climate, you may need three or more ground rods driven deeper than 8 feet. This will help the controller work steadily and efficiently.

Connect the ground rod to the controller using 14-gauge copper wire. A hose clamp works well to attach the wire to the rod. You can solder the attachment for a positive connection. In semiarid climates with dry soil conditions, to maintain a difficult ground, use a wide-impedance charger that increases the amount of power.

CAPACITY. You should be able to power from 3 to 25 miles of electric fence with your controller, depending on the rating of your model and the type of fencing you are charging. The rating indicates capacity for a single strand of steel wire and is based on using quality insulators with no weeds touching the wire. If your model is rated for 20 miles and you run two strands of steel wire, the charger will power 10 miles of fence.

Poly wires and tapes add resistance to the flow of electricity; they decrease the distance capacity to about 10 percent. So a charger rated for 25 miles would power 2½ miles of one strand poly rope. Low-impedance chargers are specially designed to maintain high power when poly rope or tape is used or where weeds are a problem. They are also less likely to cause a fire.

If a transformer is making a clicking sound, it does not necessarily mean the fence is working.

TESTING THE FLOW. Although horses seem to be able to sense when a fence is working and when it is not without actually touching it, few humans have that ability. Purchase a fence tester so you can check to be sure that ample current is flowing through the fence without having to touch it. A

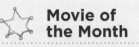

Movie of the Month

***THE MAN FROM SNOWY RIVER* (1982)**

The thrill of riding one of my horses down our steep Colorado slopes pales in comparison to Jim Craig's downhill gallop while on a solo muster. The hardy Australian Brumbies and their tough riders are at their finest in spectacular outback scenery. No foo-foo horsemen here. A great glimpse into harsh country, intense people, and an Australian style of horse handling.

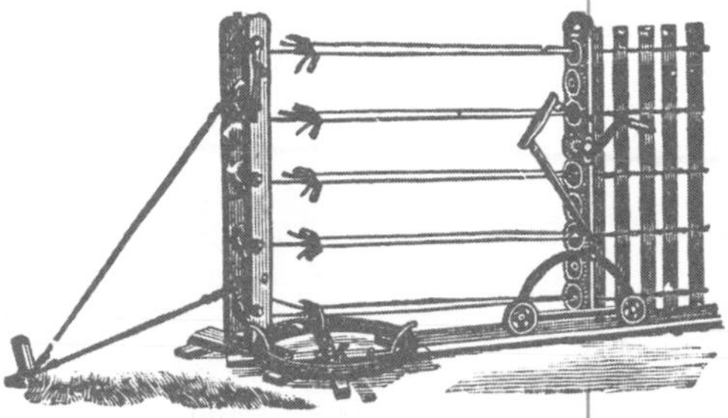

Your Horse and the Fence

Train your horse to respect an electric fence by putting feed on the other side of it, to tempt him to touch it. Once he realizes what this new fence means, he will be less likely to run through it. You may wish to — or be legally required to — post warning signs for people so they will be aware that a fence is live.

hand-held voltmeter provides a specific reading and is easier to read in bright sunlight than a tester that lights a bulb. Some newer controllers have a current meter built in.

SHORT CIRCUITS. A short circuit can significantly weaken the shock of an electric fence or ground it out, making it totally "dead." A short occurs when the electric fence wire touches a stationary object, most frequently a metal post or steel fence wire, which carries the electricity to the ground. Weeds and grass can also ground out an electric fence, especially when they are wet or snow covered. If the wire comes close to a grounding object without touching it, the electricity can arc and spark across the gap. Arcing can also occur between the ends of a broken metal wire strand in poly wire or ribbon. This arcing can melt and weaken the plastic, causing it to break, and can even cause a fire if highly combustible material is close by.

CLEAN-UP CREW

SPREAD COMPOST

For us, February is the best time to spread humus on our pastures. We select one or two vacant, dormant pastures that have not received fertilization recently, and then we

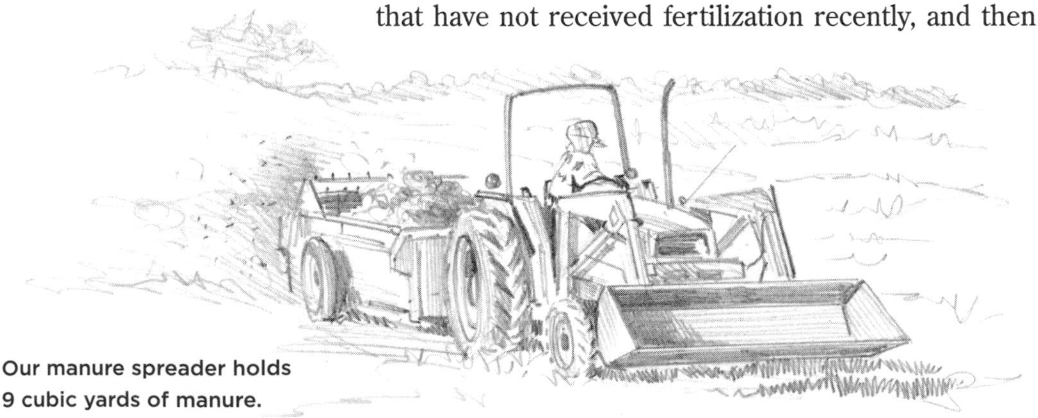

Our manure spreader holds 9 cubic yards of manure.

spread the humus at a rate suitable for our soil. We usually receive the majority of our winter snow in March and April, which helps to carry the nutrients from the humus into the soil. This year we had eight and a half loads of humus, which we spread on the fields indicated on the map.

Afterwards, we blow the debris off the tractor's radiator and screen with a high-pressure air hose. If the temperatures are mild, we wash the tractor and manure spreader right away. If not, we wait until the next decent day.

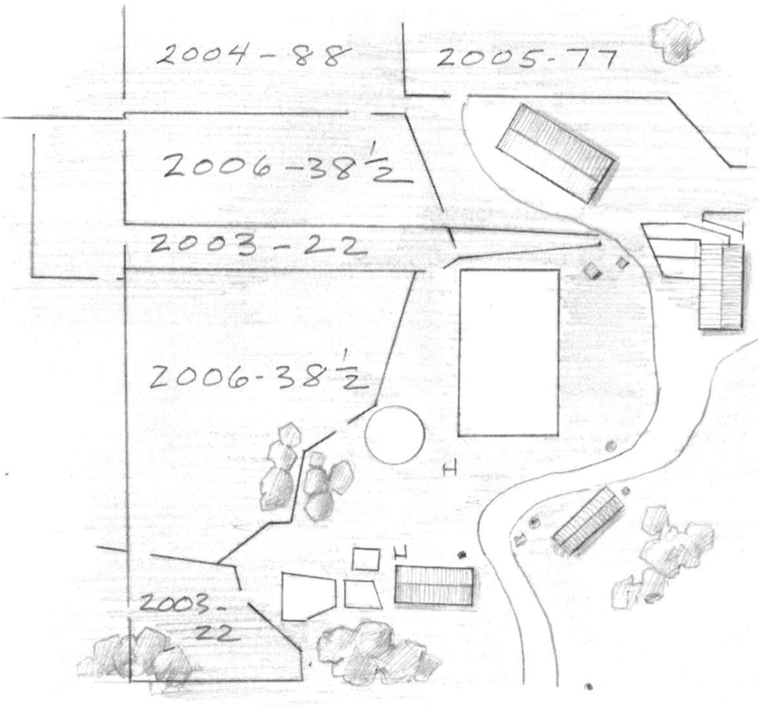

I make note of where I spread humus each year and how many cubic yards are spread.

FEBRUARY Manure Pile Maintenance

It is ideal to have at least three compost piles going at all times: one to which fresh manure is being added daily (A), one that is in the process of decomposing (B), and one that is fully composted and ready to spread (C). Each month will have a monthly manure task associated with each of the piles.

PILE A
Sell, store, or spread

PILE B
Turn once, water as needed

PILE C
Turn once, water as needed

A Horseman should know neither fear nor anger.

— James Rarey

BEAUTY SHOP

LATE WINTER GROOMING ROUTINE

Depending on the year, February might mark the shift from low-key winter grooming to the accelerated spring grooming routine. Most of the horses have started responding to the increasing daylight and are shedding. For the seniors who hold onto their long winter coat, I've found that a grooming rake, which is like a comb with a handle set perpendicular to the teeth, works the best this time of year. If a horse received a body clip in the fall, I might do one last touch-up clip in early February.

When a horse begins shedding in earnest, however, it is too late to body-clip because the summer coat is growing in at this time. If you clipped, you would nip off the tips of the summer hairs and the summer coat would never achieve its deep color and rich luster. (See December Beauty Shop for the whole scoop on body clips.)

A well-groomed horse is less apt to develop skin problems and is a feast for the eyes. Daily grooming is required when a horse is worked, is shedding, or rolls frequently. I keep a separate set of grooming tools for each horse and wash them regularly. If any horse is having a skin problem, wash all grooming tools with a disinfectant.

Why Groom?

Grooming serves many purposes, such as:

- It removes dirt, dried sweat, and dead skin cells.
- It helps the shedding process and it brings body oils to the surface, which makes a horse shine.
- It gives me a chance to make a close inspection of my horse's skin, head, mane, tail, legs, and hooves.
- It accustoms a horse to being handled, helps desensitize ticklish areas, and is a great workout for you and a warm-up for your horse.
- It results in cleaner tack and less tack maintenance.

SHEDDING

Shedding is triggered by longer daylight hours, not increased temperatures, even though both might occur at the same time. Most horses in the United States begin shedding their winter coats between January and March and finish shedding by mid- to late May. Older horses tend to shed late, and some retain a thick coat all summer. Horses can be encouraged to shed earlier by increasing their exposure to light to 16 hours per day. A 200-watt light bulb per stall is adequate. (See November Reproduction Roundup for more on using lights.)

Feeding 3 ounces of corn, soybean, or canola oil per day often hastens shedding and results in more pliable skin and a more lustrous coat. Biotin and lysine are also thought to have a beneficial effect on the quality of the hair and the skin.

A soft rubber curry is better for shedding hair than a sharp metal blade or hard plastic curry, which tends to scratch the skin and can create an entry site for undesirable dermal organisms. (See March Beauty Shop and April Vet Clinic.) Soft rubber "grabs" the long winter hair and is gentler than a shedding blade for removing it from the sensitive areas: face, flanks, and legs. Most horses act as if they enjoy being groomed with a soft rubber curry, but not a shedding blade.

Shedding is triggered by longer daylight hours, not increased temperatures, even though both might occur at the same time.

It's a lot like nuts and bolts – if the rider's nuts, the horse bolts!

— Nicholas Evans

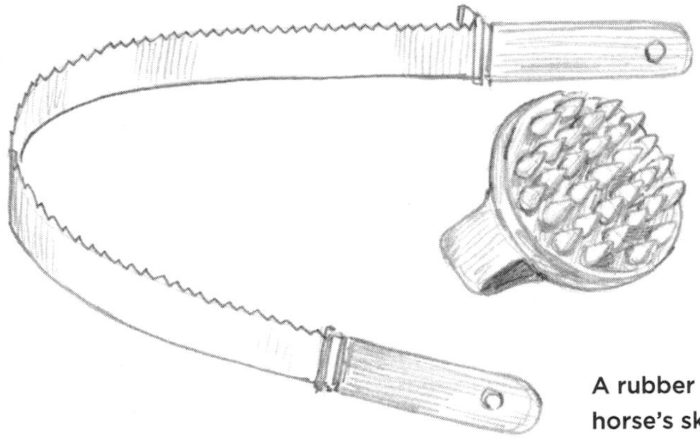

A rubber curry is safer and kinder to your horse's skin and coat than a shedding blade.

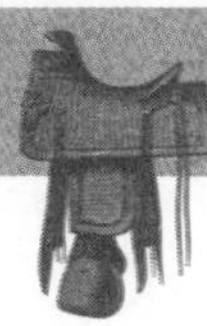

TACK ROOM

BRIDLE CHECK

A good bridle is a substantial investment and an important piece of tack. To keep my bridles in safe working order, maintain their good looks, and extend their useful life, I keep them clean and store them on a contoured bridle rack.

Here in semiarid Colorado (annual precipitation at Long Tail Ranch is 17.5 inches), wooden bridle racks work great. If you live in a very humid climate, on the other hand, an open-style bridle rack will allow the crownpiece to dry more thoroughly.

Just as with my saddles, during the slow months I give my bridles a once-over to make sure all leather and hardware is in good working order. I pay particular attention to folds in the leather where there might be hidden dirt or the beginnings of a crack. I use the same leather-cleaning regimen as I do for saddle leather. (See January Tack Room.)

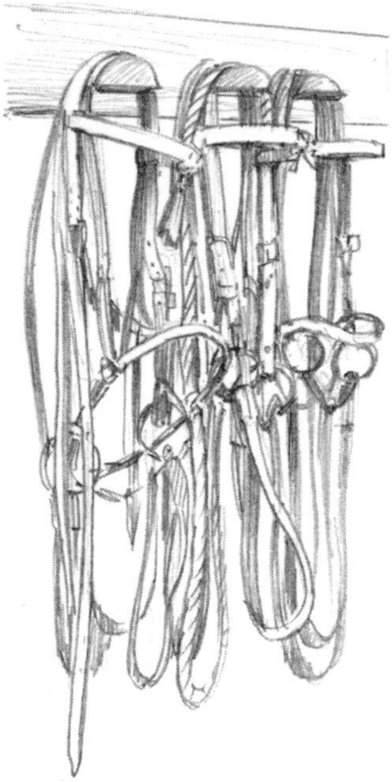

If you hang a bridle on a nail, the crown will take the shape of the nail and could crack at the sharp bend in the leather. If you store bridles on contoured bridle racks, they'll tend to keep the shape of your horse's poll.

Looking at Horses

Arm's Length

The length of the horse's "arm" or humerus (from the point of shoulder to the point of elbow) affects his stride length. A long humerus is associated with a long, reaching stride and good lateral ability; a short humerus with a short, choppy stride and poor lateral ability.

The steeper the angle of the humerus, generally, the higher the action; the more toward horizontal, the lower the action.

CLOTHES HORSE

TURNOUT HALTER

Exercise is essential for the health and well-being of any horse, and turnout is an ideal way to achieve it naturally. Although it is tempting to leave a halter on a horse on pasture to make him easier to catch, it is just too dangerous, as he could get the halter caught on a fence, a tree, or his own horseshoe when scratching. It is best to teach a horse to be caught and haltered (see December Training Pen).

When a halter is absolutely necessary, however — such as when an overweight or foundered horse needs to wear a muzzle to limit grazing — be sure the halter is a safety or breakaway halter. An alternative to a safety halter is buckling a safety strap insert onto a regular halter. This device has a strip of elastic that will break under stress and may prevent serious injury to your horse.

Never use a breakaway halter for tying a horse, because it wouldn't take much for the horse to break or release the halter and learn the bad habit of pulling to get free. In fact, leading an unruly horse with a breakaway halter is also risky, because one sudden pull could release him and teach him a very bad habit.

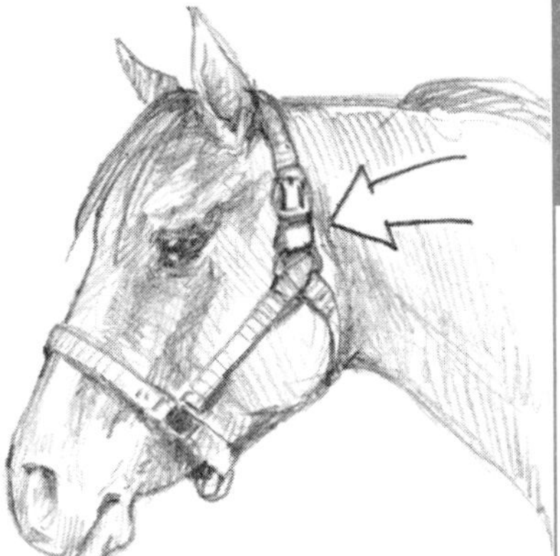

Safety halters are constructed so that one portion will break or release if the horse becomes caught on a post or tree.

STILL TRUE TODAY

Historical Horsekeeping

"The food should be of the quality and quantity to impart strength, vitality, and elasticity; and this requires some discrimination and care, as the food should be harmonized both to the condition of the horse and the severity of the labor to which he is subjected."

— Magner's Standard Horse and Stock Book *by D. Magner, 1916*

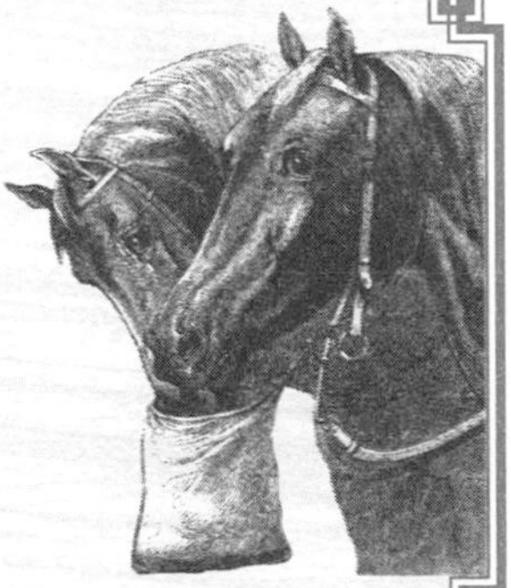

TRAINING PEN

When the fierce winds of February blow, but I still want to make progress with my horses, I'll identify an area that needs improvement and that I can practice indoors.

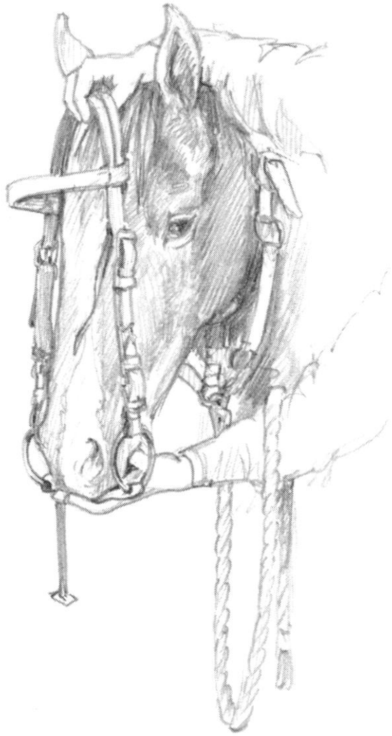

BRIDLING

With young horses, a few thoughtful bridling sessions can set the stage for good manners for years to come.

1. In order to keep control of the horse while bridling, I hold these chilly winter bridling lessons in a stall.
2. I remove the halter from the horse's head, and refasten the halter around his neck.
3. Depending on the horse, I either drop the end of the lead rope on the ground if he is trained to ground-tie, or I drape the lead rope over my left arm as I bridle. If the horse is in cross-ties, I remove the cross-ties from his halter and buckle the halter around his neck. If I feel I need to add a lead rope, I will.
4. I hold the crownpiece of the bridle with my right hand and drape the reins over my left arm. I hold the bit in my left hand and present the bridle to the horse by moving both of my hands from the left side of his face to the front of his face.
5. I position my right hand in the area of his forehead while I move the bit into position between his upper and lower teeth with my left hand.
6. When the horse opens his mouth, I smoothly move the bit up and in between his teeth while raising the bridle's crownpiece upward toward the horse's ears with my right hand.
7. I use my left hand to help put the horse's right ear into the headstall, then his left ear.
8. I step in front of the horse to check for balance and adjustment and then look at each side of the bit to see that it is sitting level.
9. Then I fasten the throatlatch and noseband.

FARM OFFICE

LIABILITY INSURANCE

If you have a hobby (recreational) horse farm, your homeowner's policy will usually cover public liability and property damage. Be sure, however, that you understand what your particular policy means by the difference between "recreational" horse use and a horse business. A business is indicated when you file a Schedule F (Farm) or a Schedule C (Business) with the IRS. Often, however, even if you consider yourself a hobby farmer, the insurance company may treat you as if you were running a horse business. If one of your horses is used for showing, parades, or rental, or if your facilities are used for boarding, training, instructing, or breeding, you may have to obtain additional liability coverage with a supplemental business policy.

It is important that all horsekeepers be covered by a personal or professional liability policy as appropriate for the situation. Homeowner's policies in some states come into play if someone is injured on the property or if a horse escapes onto the road and damages a vehicle or injures a person, depending on who is found negligent. If you run a small lesson or training business at your acreage, you'll need additional liability coverage.

To decide whether additional liability insurance is appropriate for your horse farm or ranch, contact various insurance companies and review their policies. Read the terms carefully and ask the agents how worst-case scenarios would play out. Use examples of situations you would most likely encounter at your farm and ask if you would be covered. Before you invest any money, be sure your insurance agent is experienced, reliable, and qualified.

The Best Policy

The best insurance against losses from accident and illness is conscientious care and employment of safe procedures. If additional protection is required, carefully consider the various forms of equine insurance available today and work with a knowledgeable agent.

Before you invest any money, be sure your insurance agent is experienced, reliable, and qualified.

Taking Inventory

List the major items with a brief description and serial or registration numbers if applicable. List the value and include receipts if possible. Photographs or videotapes of your tack room inventory can also assist with identification and description. Keep one copy of the inventory and visual supports with your insurance policy at home and one in your safety deposit box.

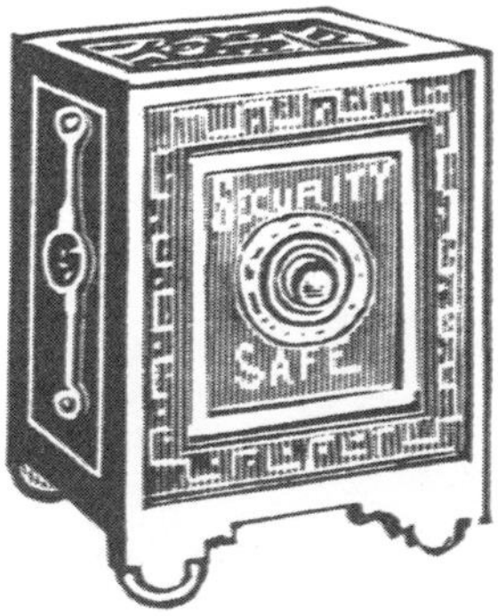

The cost of liability insurance will depend on the type of policy, the amount of coverage, and the terms and exclusions. Various terms are used in naming and describing types of coverage. Some overlap or are very similar, and others use the same words and mean different things. The following is a general guideline to types of policies.

PERSONAL OR GENERAL LIABILITY. The terms describe liability coverage in homeowners' policies. Such policies may have limitations, because they are not written expressly for the needs of a horse owner. They are designed to cover human bodily injury and property damage claims on home premises, yours or someone else's. Such policies should cover a visitor to your home who gets kicked, or the passengers and vehicle in an accident caused by your loose horse, depending on whether you were found negligent (see July Farm Office). The insurance company should cover the cost of the claim as well as your legal expenses. The choice of coverage might range from $300,000 to $500,000 to $1,000,000.

Most general liability policies do not cover incidents that happen to the horse. They usually specifically exclude coverage for damage to any animal (injury or death) that you have in your care, custody, or control. Renters can purchase horse owner policies in lieu of homeowners' policies.

COMMERCIAL LIABILITY. If you receive money for an equine activity, you would probably not be covered by a personal liability policy. See more about liability releases in July Farm Office, and read on for business insurance.

CARE, CUSTODY, AND CONTROL. This type of insurance covers injury or death of an animal that is in your care when the mishap takes place. For example, it should cover a claim if a horse in your care died.

PROFESSIONAL ERRORS AND OMISSIONS. With this type of policy, coverage is for professional services. If you do something wrong while you are working with or caring for a horse or client, whether or not you are aware of it and whether or not the result is apparent immediately or later, this type of policy should cover you.

PROPERTY INSURANCE

Your horse property insurance should cover your horse facilities, equipment, and tack. If you are a hobbyist, this should be covered on your homeowner's policy, but be sure to check the details. If you use your facility or horses for a business, then you'll need a business property insurance policy.

For either your homeowner's or business property insurance policy, you will need to have an itemized inventory of your tack and equipment. This will help you determine how much coverage you need and will also help you identify items that are stolen or destroyed.

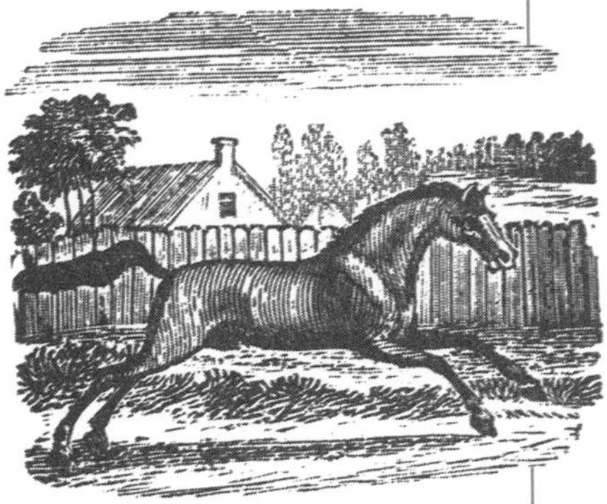

HORSEKEEPING ACROSS AMERICA

SOUTHERN UNITED STATES: BROWNOUTS OR POWER OUTAGES

Sometimes a freak winter storm will hit the southern United States and cause icing of power lines and tree limbs, which can result in a power loss or reduction. When all power is lost, it is called a power outage or blackout. When power is greatly reduced, it is called a brownout. A rolling blackout is a planned event by a power company to alleviate an overloaded system. This can occur when power sources have been damaged or in peak power usage times.

Power Play

Power problems can occur during natural disasters, during intense cold when electric heat is in high demand, and during intense heat when air conditioning is in high demand.

FINE FACILITIES

WOOD CHEWING

Cold, wet winter weather tends to bring out the beaver in any horse. Wood chewing seems to be most common in horses that aren't being fed enough long-stemmed hay or that are otherwise unsatisfied. It seems to be a socially contagious behavior, as you will often see horses standing around chewing a fence rail together. If you use wood for fences or stalls, you will have to protect the edges with heavy metal edging or regularly apply anti-chew deterrents to the wood.

To nip wood chewing in the bud, apply an anti-chew product on the wood as soon as you see a "test nibble." To do this, you need to have your products and applicator at the ready. Anti-chew products are notoriously messy to work with. For tidy application, fill an old ketchup or mustard bottle with the anti-chew product. Store a designated paintbrush in a can alongside the squirt bottle, and keep an old rag and a pair of disposable latex gloves nearby. When you spot a nibble, grab your kit, dribble some product on the brush, and apply it to the wood.

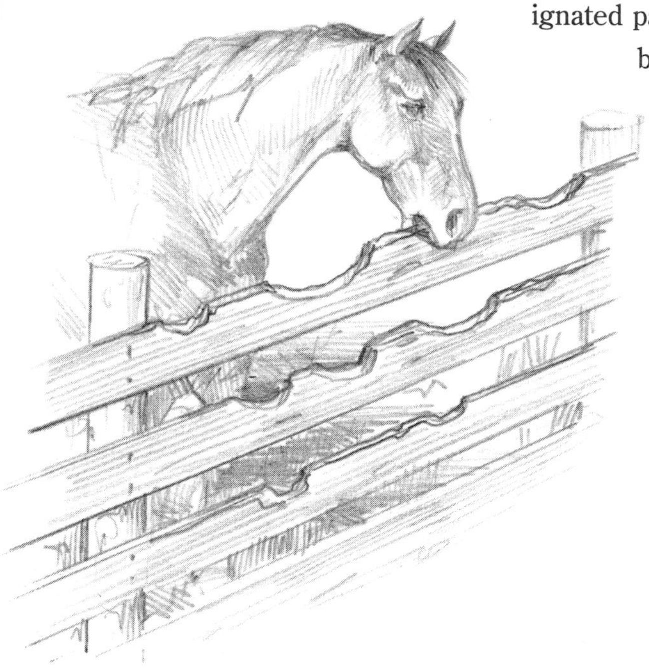

Wood chewing is destructive to facilities but can be prevented with proper management.

RPMS & PTOS

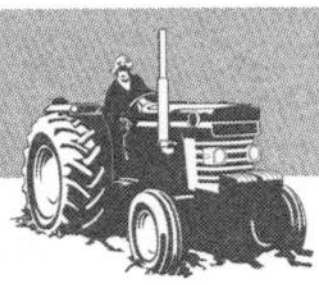

MANURE-HANDLING EQUIPMENT

Because February is the month we spread our humus, it is the ideal time to talk about manure-handling machinery. (See Recommended Reading for more information.)

TRACTORS. First of all, you'll need a tractor that is of a suitable size to operate your spreader. There are trade-offs in relation to tractor size. Small tractors are more affordable and maneuverable but might make your annual manure-spreading task take weeks. Large tractors can be pricey and are sometimes tough to operate in small spaces, but you can use larger spreaders and harrows and get the job done in a matter of hours or days. For a small horse farm of fewer than 10 horses and less than 50 acres, consider a tractor in the 50- to 65-horsepower range or smaller.

Be sure the tractor has a power takeoff (PTO) attachment if you are going to run a PTO spreader. The PTO is a revolving shaft on the back of the tractor that provides power from the tractor's engine to the equipment. If you plan to use a harrow that requires a three-point hitch, be sure your tractor has a PTO. A three-point hitch is the linkage on the back of the tractor that hydraulically raises and lowers attached equipment. Also, the tractor should have a bucket on the front for loading the manure into the spreader; otherwise you'll have to do that job by hand!

I'd rather have a goddam horse. A horse is at least human, for God's sake.

— J.D. Salinger, *The Catcher in the Rye*

It's better to have more tractor and not need it than need more tractor and not have it.

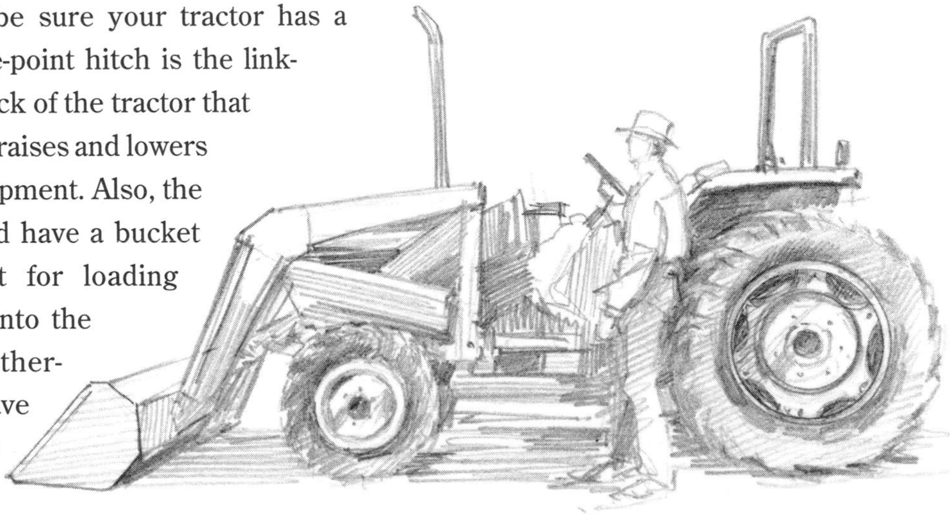

Time to Harrow

I frequently harrow the pastures in February, because it is usually bone-dry here then. The manure breaks up easily and the ground is not damaged. It is a great feeling when I time it right and just as I park the tractor and harrow, the heavy spring snows begin.

MANURE SPREADERS. A manure spreader is a wagon with a mechanical apparatus designed to distribute manure as the tractor pulls the spreader through a pasture or field. Spreaders are either friction-drive or PTO-drive. We use a PTO-driven International Harvester 540 spreader that holds more than 5 tons of manure. (See more about manure spreaders in August RPMs & PTOs.)

PASTURE HARROWS. Harrows are useful for breaking up and spreading manure on pastures. There are three basic types of pasture harrow or drags, as they are sometimes called: the chain (or English), the spike tooth, and the spring tooth. (See more on pasture harrows in October RPMs & PTOs.)

In dry, sunny climates, harrowing is a good practice as it exposes parasite eggs in the manure to the sun, which kills them. In humid climates, however, harrowing the manure in pastures may spread the parasite eggs over a larger area while still allowing them to be viable, so in effect it increases a horse's chances of reinfestation. In such a situation, the manure should either be collected instead of harrowed or the pasture should not be used for horses for a year after harrowing.

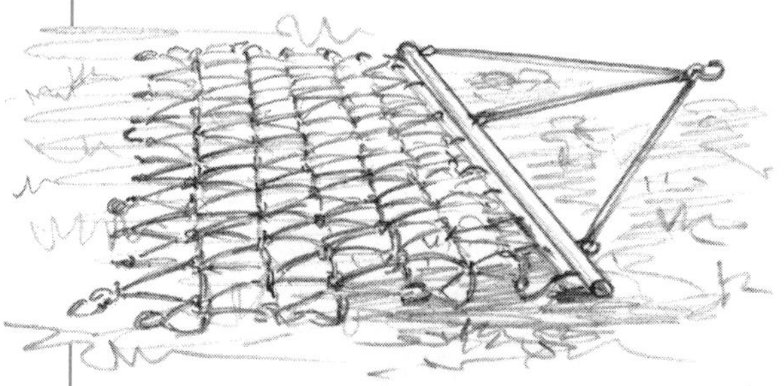

An English harrow is ideal for pasture work.

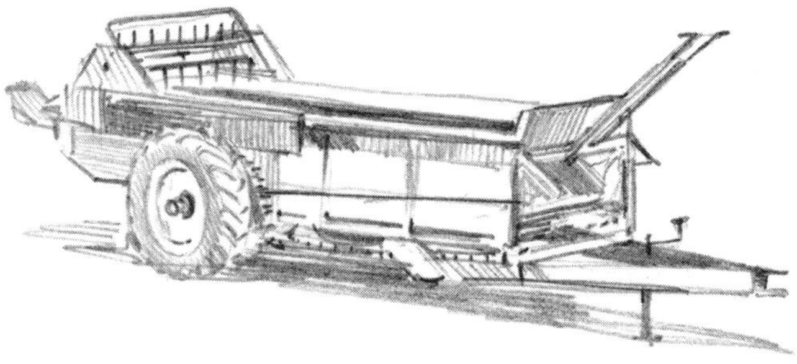

A friction-drive spreader does not require a PTO.

RANCH RECIPES

PILL PREP

When your horse must take oral medications, you need to crush the pills. A mortar and pestle is the traditional way to grind pills. Choose a heavy marble mortar and pestle that won't slide around as you work. You can also use an electric coffee grinder, which is quick and thorough. I keep a coffee grinder in the barn specifically for this purpose.

There are several ways you can feed the crushed pills to the horse. You can mix them with his grain. But, depending on the medication, your horse might either sift out the meds or turn his nose up at the entire grain ration. To be sure to get the medication into the horse, use the syringe method.

EASY SYRINGE METHOD

If your horse is taking a bland or flavored pill, such as grape triple sulfa tablets, try this. Cut the tip off a 35cc syringe. Place the whole pills in the syringe and, holding a finger over the end, fill the syringe with just enough water to cover the pills. These pills dissolve very quickly. Give them a stir with a chopstick, checking consistency. You might need to add just a bit more water. Dose your horse. (Also see April Ranch Recipes for Pill Paste.)

Keep one leg on one side, the other leg on the other side, and your mind in the middle.

— Henry Taylor

Keep your mind in the middle and a leg on each side.

— Cherry Hill

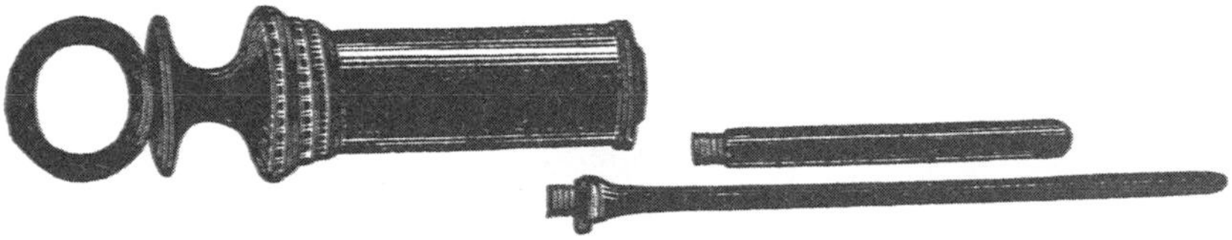

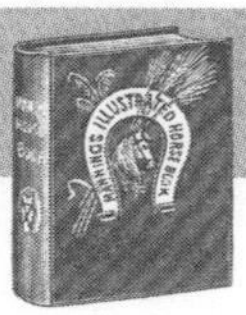

MORE IN DEPTH

HEALTH FOOD FOR HORSES

I am often asked what I feed my horses because they are healthy and good looking, with long tails and manes and mellow dispositions. Part of that comes from genetics, training, and management, but nutrition also plays a big role.

The Feed

I'll describe how I feed my horses without providing exact amounts, which will vary according to age, activity level, quality of feed, and more. This is the art of horse feeding;

Meet the Horses of Long Tail Ranch

Zinger. Thirty-year-old Quarter Horse mare. Retired, lives in a deluxe individual sheltered pen complex off one end of the hay barn (called the "senior center"). An easy keeper who can become overweight. *See Feeding Plan A.*

Zipper. Twenty-one-year-old Quarter Horse gelding. On vacation, barefoot (for the first time since he was two), and turned out for a few months during the winter on 18 acres of pasture with creek. Active, easy keeper. *See Feeding Plan B.*

Dickens. Sixteen-year-old Quarter Horse/Selle Français gelding. Shod, in light work, lives in sheltered pen off main barn. Hardest keeper of the six, can get ribby. *See Feeding Plan A.*

Seeker. Ten-year-old Quarter Horse/Trakehner mare. Barefoot, taking some time off, lives in individual sheltered pen off main barn. Easy keeper. *See Feeding Plan A.*

Aria. Ten-year-old Quarter Horse/Trakehner mare. Shod, in moderate work, lives in individual sheltered pen off main barn. Easy keeper. *See Feeding Plan A.*

Sherlock. Four-year-old Quarter Horse/Akhal Teke gelding. Barefoot, in occasional work, lives in large individual pen. Active, easy keeper, stays trim. *See Feeding Plan C.*

for a more scientific discussion, refer to a nutrition book (see Recommended Reading in the appendix).

Hay. Generally I feed grass hay or a grass/alfalfa mix containing no more than 15 percent alfalfa. Any exception to this is noted in the Feed Plans.

Water. Horses in pens all have free-choice well water in 50-gallon water barrels. Horses on pasture drink out of a creek.

Salt and minerals. All horses have free-choice access to plain white salt blocks and 12% calcium/12% phosphorus trace mineral salt blocks.

Beet pulp and supplements. Supplement options and quantity of beet pulp are individually tailored to fit each horse's needs. (See January Feed Bag.)

Flax. Flax (linseed) has a high concentration of Omega-3 fatty acids. A horse cannot produce these fats, so they are called "essential fats" and need to be part of his diet. Flax is also a good source of soluble fiber rich in lignin, which gels when it contacts water (similar to psyllium) so is thought to help prevent impaction and sand colic. (That's why I add it last to the beet pulp mash.) Flax seed or linseed shouldn't be fed whole to horses because the small, hard seeds would pass through the horse unchewed and undigested. You can grind flax seed fresh daily for your horses, cook or soak the seeds, or buy freshly ground meal. Meal needs to be stored in an airtight container in a very cool place (like a refrigerator). Seeds can be stored longer.

Mature pasture. I am never in a hurry to turn my horses out on spring pasture. First of all, dry-land mountain pasture is fragile, so I like the plants to get a good head start before the horses start eagerly grazing. But mainly, I find that I sleep better at night knowing that when my horses are on pasture, they are eating safe forage. For more information on the current research on and the prevention of pasture-related laminitis in horses, see the appendix.

Odd Word

easy keeper. A horse that requires minimal feed to keep in the proper weight. In fact, many easy keepers must have strict management of their feed to prevent them from becoming overweight.

See more on winter feeding on page 85.

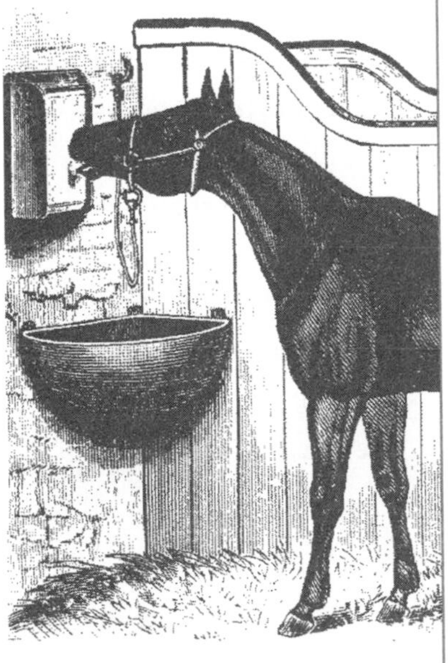

THE FEEDING PLANS

FEEDING PLAN A. In this group are the hardest keepers and some of the easiest keepers. The hard keeper receives a proportionately larger amount of the grass/alfalfa mix hay, and the easy keepers receive a smaller ration of the straight grass hay.

Dawn. Each horse receives one fourth of his daily hay ration. If a horse gets 16 pounds a day, he would get 4 pounds in the morning. I work the horses in the morning so the light feeding allows me to get started earlier.

Noon. Each horse receives one half of his daily hay ration, or 8 pounds per the above example. I measure out beet pulp pellets for all seven horses and soak them in water for the evening feeding.

Evening. Each horse receives the last fourth of his daily hay ration and his individual beet pulp ration. (Additives to soaked beet pulp will be discussed later.)

FEEDING PLAN B. One older gelding is in this group.

Dawn. The horse is on pasture with plenty of grass so at this time, he does not receive hay in the morning. (Pastures are evaluated each day on my morning walk and rides.)

Noon. No hay.

Evening. This horse receives his individual beet pulp ration in the evening.

FEEDING PLAN C. One young gelding is in this group.

Dawn. This horse receives one fourth of his daily hay ration in the morning.

Noon. This horse receives either one half of his daily hay ration and is kept in or one fourth of his daily hay ration and is turned out on pasture for four to five hours.

Evening. This horse receives his individual beet pulp ration and one fourth of his daily hay ration. (See January Ranch Recipes for Beet Pulp.)

Reproduction Roundup

Feeding the Broodmare

During the last trimester, which is after seven months of pregnancy, the fetus is developing rapidly inside the mare. Because 65 percent of fetal growth occurs after the seventh month, the mare's nutritional requirements change.

The mare's protein requirements increase by about 30 percent and her energy requirements increase by about 20 percent. In addition, depending on the type of hay you are feeding, she will likely require calcium and phosphorus supplementation for the formation of the foal's skeleton.

Confer with your veterinarian as to what type of supplementation he or she recommends.

CARBOHYDRATES

At this point you may be asking yourself, "A low-carb diet for horses? No grain?" A horse can't really go on a low-carb diet because carbohydrates are a necessary part of his diet. However, many horses benefit from a low-glycemic diet — one without sugar, molasses, refined grains, or sweet young pasture.

Carbohydrates include simple sugars, starches, and cellulose. Cellulose, the fiber or roughage portion of grass and hay, is a complex carbohydrate. A horse digests cellulose in his cecum, where small microbes break it down over a period of time. Grains, grass, and hay all contain sugars, starches, and fiber. Grains such as corn, oats, and barley are lower in fiber and higher in energy than roughages.

Of the grains, oats are the safest to feed with hay because they are high in fiber and low in energy, and higher in protein than corn. Corn has the highest energy content of any grain and can put weight on a horse quickly. Barley is an intermediate source of energy and protein content.

FATS

Fats are found in grains and roughages at a low level (2 to 4 percent), but horses benefit from and can tolerate a ration that contains as high as 10 percent fat. A ration higher in fat than that can cause runny stools. Fats are necessary for metabolic functions and are associated with healthy, sleek hair coats. Fats produce 2.25 times the amount of energy as an equal weight of carbohydrates and they produce less heat.

ENERGY FOOD

Horses get energy from fats and carbohydrates. Excess fats and carbohydrates lead to excess energy, obesity, and other problems. Although a natural and necessary part of a horse's diet, just as with people, complex carbohydrates are often healthier than simple carbohydrates.

Healthy Feeding in a Nutshell

To state it simply, it is healthier for a horse to eat **oats** than sugar, but better that he eat **beet pulp** than oats; better that he eats **grass hay** than third-cutting alfalfa hay; safer for him to be turned on **mature pasture** than new, vigorous, high-fructose growth; and there might be a place in your horse's ration for **oil**.

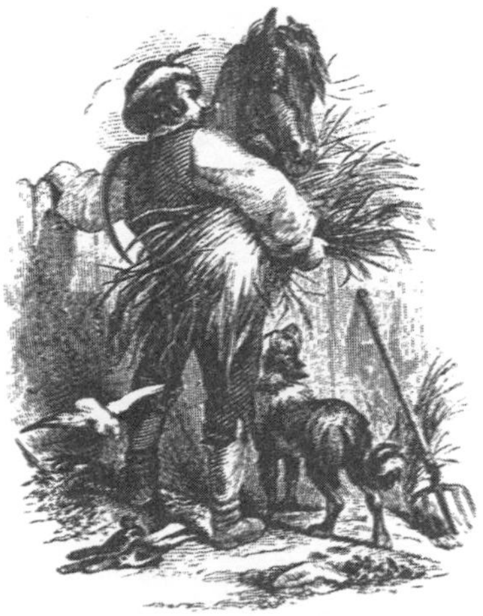

Spreading Manure on Frozen Ground

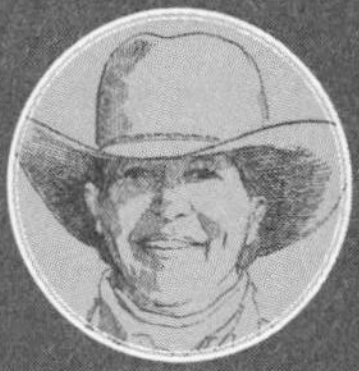

Ask Cherry

Q

You offer a good forum for folks to get credible information for equine management. I don't discredit any of your practical advice but question the recommendation of spreading composted manure on frozen ground. Ag producers on the East Coast are discouraged from applying manure to frozen ground because of the potential for it to leave the site during rain events. Your interest in not tearing up the pasture is admirable relative to preserving vegetation and reducing soil loss. Just curious as to any alternatives such as midsummer spreading.

A

Thanks for your question. Midsummer spreading would be ideal on crop land or on land that will not be grazed by horses for the next 12 months. So, if a landowner could set aside one or two pastures to rest each year, then application could be made in the season that suits the climate the best in that locale. Here in the foothills of Colorado, we spread during January or February when the ground is dry. Our tractor tires do the least damage to the pasture during that time and then when our big snows come in late February, March, and April, the composted manure is sealed in place under a blanket of snow until the spring melt. As the snow slowly melts, it tends to carry the nutrients into the soil and the humus adds cushion and aeration to the soil.

As I think you are suggesting, you are right: it would not be a good idea to apply raw manure or composted manure to land (frozen or not) just before heavy rain periods, especially if the precipitation would cause the manure to run off. With runoff, not only are the nutrients lost to the pastures but lakes, rivers, and streams can be contaminated.

Like so many management tasks, each horsekeeper needs to make responsible decisions by being informed and then using trial and error to see what works best. When to spread manure is one of those questions that can only be answered when considering all of the specifics of the situation: how much land is available for spreading; what will the land be used for during the next 12 months; when does the heaviest precipitation occur; and so on.

SPRING

MARCH TO MAY

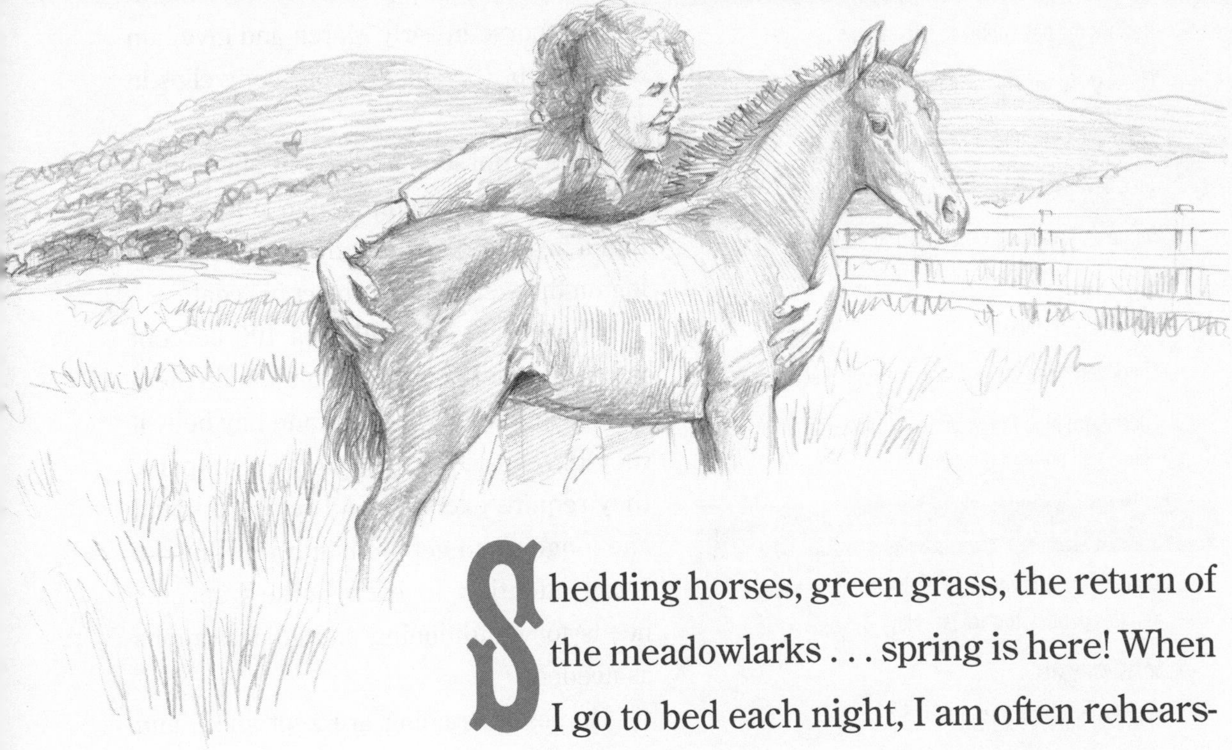

Shedding horses, green grass, the return of the meadowlarks . . . spring is here! When I go to bed each night, I am often rehearsing all the things I want to do the next day as I slip into dreamland, and when my feet hit the floor every morning, they are in high gear. This is the beginning of a new horse season, and it can't start too early for me.

Mother Nature, however, can bring some interesting events to the mix. We usually have our deepest and wettest snowstorms during March, April, and even May. So although I am revved, I always need a backup plan in place if the weather makes it unsafe or impossible to train or ride.

Weekly Tasks

- ❑ Restock the hay supply in horse barns
- ❑ Check grain supply
- ❑ Check bedding supply
- ❑ Take hay inventory
- ❑ Dump and scrub all waterers, troughs, tanks, tubs, buckets
- ❑ Scrub feed dishes
- ❑ Check veterinary and grooming supply needs
- ❑ Check upcoming farrier and veterinarian appointments and prepare for them

Seasonal Tasks

- ❑ Keep horses off pasture or limit grazing to a few minutes per day toward late May
- ❑ Spray early weeds
- ❑ Check all horses for ticks
- ❑ Extensive shedding, grooming, clipping
- ❑ Get fly gear ready
- ❑ Wash winter blankets, repair, and store them
- ❑ Tune up mowing equipment
- ❑ Schedule routine veterinary appointments for dental care and immunizations

The horses are all brought in from winter pastures in March, if not before, to allow the land to rest and the plants to grow. Each horse has his own separate sheltered pen. I bring the horses back into work one at a time, starting with a grooming program. I might vigorously groom a horse daily to remove as much of the shedding hair as possible, or in some cases, I might bathe a horse in early March and give him a body clip. (See more about body clips in December.)

Until a horse is 95 percent shed out, I don't put a sheet on him. Then I either give him a turnout sheet or a fly sheet, depending on the weather, to protect his coat.

The horses are still on a 100 percent hay ration, but I cut back a bit to help them start losing their winter fat and hay belly if they have one. Because they are in pens, they require exercise, so I review in-hand and longeing to get them into work mode. I pay attention to each horse's specific needs for conditioning and adjust rations as needed.

Horses in training are kept shod, and even some that are not in training are kept shod to protect their hooves from our abrasive Rocky Mountain terrain. It is great having a resident farrier!

This time of year, the horses are fed three times per day, at 6:00 a.m., noon, and 7:00 p.m. The seniors are still getting their beet pulp and supplements, and the rest of

✳	My Day	A Horse's Day
5:00 AM		Stand near feed spots.
5:15 AM	Rise.	
6:00 AM	Chores and visual exam (see Chore Sandwich in March Feed Bag).	Eat.
7:00 AM	Breakfast.	
8:00 AM	Work in office, etc.	Walk over to the water tub for a drink.
8:15 AM		Return to the feed area to vacuum up the dregs.
9:00 AM	Head to the barn for grooming, tacking up, training, and riding.	
10:00 AM		Exercise and training (this varies for each horse; some will be exercised in the afternoon), doze, or lie down.
12:00 PM	Noon feeding, then lunch.	Eat.
1:00 PM	Work in office or barn, do domestic duties, or nap in my recliner.	
2:00 PM	Back to the barn.	Drink.
2:15 PM		Doze, lie down, or exercise and train.
5:30 PM		Stand near feed spots.
6:00 PM	Chores and visual exam.	Eat.
7:00 PM	Supper.	
8:00 PM	Nightly movie.	Drink.
8:15 PM		Mosey or doze until dawn, keeping alert for unusual sights or sounds.
10:30 PM	Go to bed.	

the horses receive beet pulp with additives as their level of work dictates.

Spring makes us all feel great. I'm spending lots of time outdoors. I always wear a broad-brimmed hat, a bandanna around my neck, gloves, and a long-sleeved shirt. This is mainly to protect my eyes and skin from sun damage. I often find that from this time of year through fall, I get plenty of varied exercise from chores, grooming, training, riding, mowing, and facilities maintenances tasks, so the indoor exercise equipment gets a little dusty over the summer. The early mornings and late afternoons can still be a bit chilly, so mainly for my horse's sake, I try to do vigorous training and riding either midmorning or midafternoon, giving them plenty of time to cool out thoroughly before chilly evening temperatures.

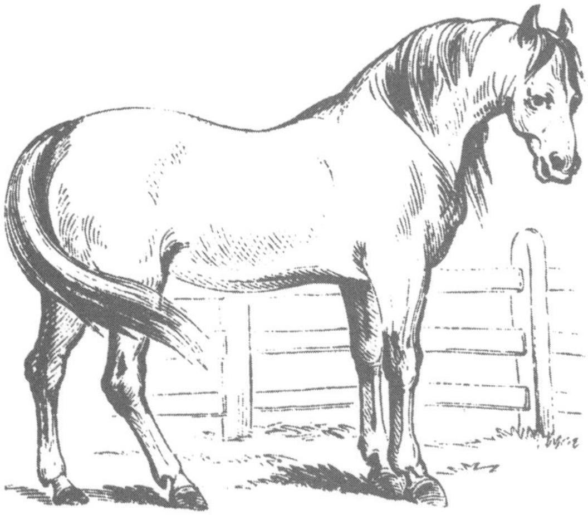

Spring Visual Exam

OVERALL STANCE AND ATTITUDE. As I approach the barn, does the horse have his head up, are his eyes bright, and is he eager for feed or is he lethargic, inattentive, or anxious?

LEGS. I look at the horse from both sides so I will quickly spot any wounds, swelling, or puffiness.

APPETITE. Has the horse finished all of his feed from the previous feeding?

WATER. Is there evidence that he has taken in a sufficient amount of water?

MANURE. Is the fecal material well formed or is it hard and dry, loose and sloppy, covered with mucus or parasites, or filled with whole grains? Are there at least three to four manure piles since I last fed? (Six to eight bowel movements per 24-hour day is normal.)

PEN, SHELTER, OR STALL. Are there signs of pawing, rubbing, rolling, thrashing, or wood-chewing?

MARCH

The spring equinox, also called the vernal equinox, occurs on March 20 or 21 in the Northern Hemisphere. At the equinox, the sun crosses the earth's equator, so night and day are of approximately equal length everywhere. In North America, the days often become wetter and warmer, which brings on mud and emerging insects, two realities we horsekeepers learn to deal with. When I think March, I gear up for immunizations in order to stay ahead of the insect vector season. I also take the necessary steps to minimize mud.

Day Length in Hours

Latitude	Mar 1	Mar 16	April 1
60°N	9.96	11.35	12.84
55°N	10.32	11.46	12.69
50°N	10.61	11.55	12.58
45°N	10.83	11.62	12.48
40°N	11.02	11.68	12.41
35°N	11.18	11.74	12.34
30°N	11.33	11.78	12.28

See page 22 to find your latitude.

FLOOD ALERT

Flooding can occur from many causes and can damage property, destroy utilities, be a health hazard, and cause great inconvenience, at worst becoming life threatening. Common areas of flooding include coastal, river, and low-lying regions. In addition, any area with intense rain or snow and ice melting can experience flooding. If you are in a flood-prone area, devise an emergency evacuation plan. (See more in this month's Horsekeeping Across America.)

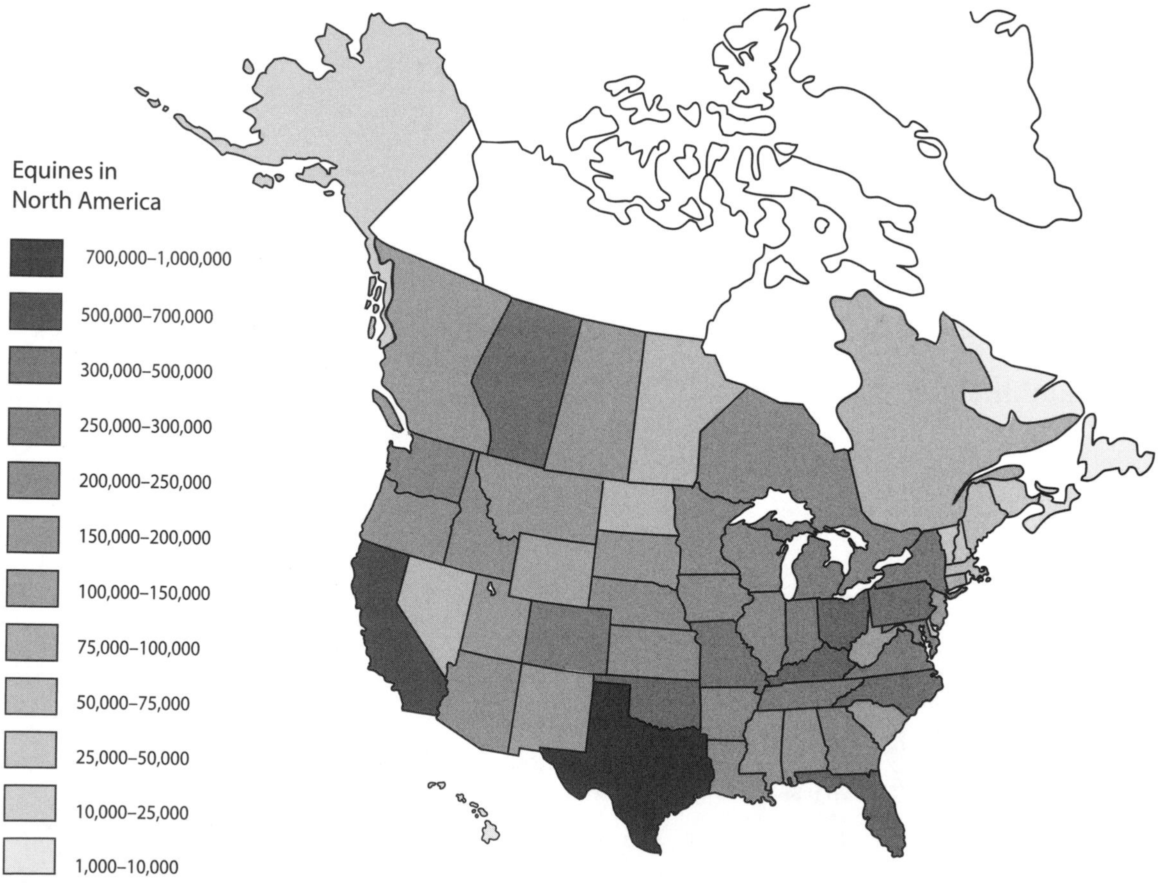

TIME CHANGE

Remember to "spring forward, fall back." During the change to Daylight Saving Time, clocks are turned forward an hour, effectively moving an hour of daylight from the morning to the evening. The names in each time zone change along with Daylight Saving Time. Eastern Standard Time (EST) becomes Eastern Daylight Time (EDT), and so forth. In the United States, clocks change at 2:00 a.m. local time. So, in the spring, clocks spring forward from 1:59 a.m. to 3:00 a.m.

Although we used to change our clocks in April, on August 8, 2005, the Energy Policy Act of 2005 adjusted the time-change dates for Daylight Saving Time in the United States. Beginning in 2007, DST will begin on the second Sunday of March and end the first Sunday of November. The Secretary of Energy will report the impact of this change to Congress. Congress retains the right to continue with the new schedule or revert the Daylight Saving Time back to the 2005 time schedule once the Department of Energy study is complete.

Daylight Saving Time is not observed in Hawaii, American Samoa, Guam, Puerto Rico, the Virgin Islands, and Arizona. Even though the Navajo Nation lies partially in Arizona, it participates in the Daylight Saving Time policy, due to its large size and location in three states. (See April Wacky Wonderful Weather for Canada's DST policy.)

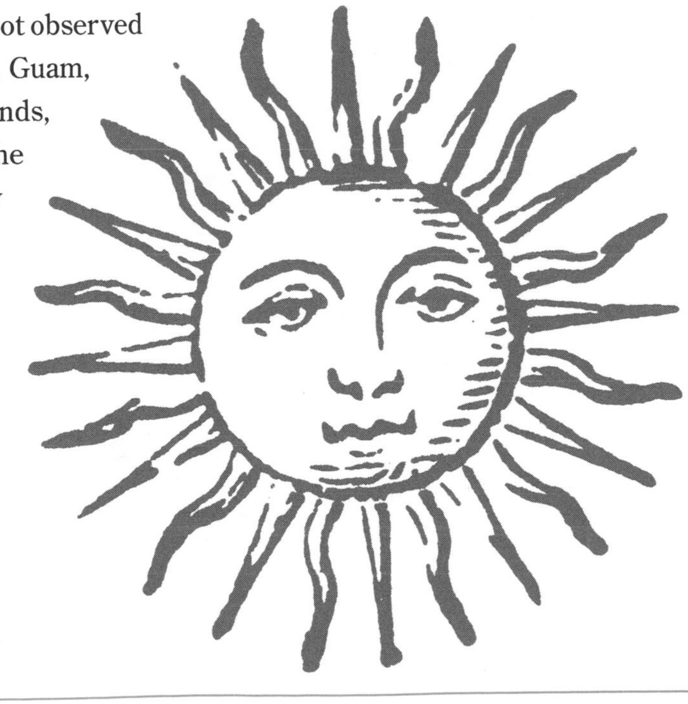

To Do

- ❑ Set clocks ahead
- ❑ Immunize or schedule vet to do so
- ❑ Rhino #3 for broodmares
- ❑ Deworm
- ❑ Scrub feed tubs and buckets
- ❑ Move hay to barns
- ❑ Income tax

To Buy

- ❑ Psyllium
- ❑ Senior feed
- ❑ Antioxidant supplements
- ❑ Beep pulp pellets
- ❑ Corn oil
- ❑ Vaccines
- ❑ Absorbent sweeping compound

VET CLINIC

IMMUNIZATION TIME IS HERE

Spring is the traditional time of year to give spring boosters. Depending on where you live, however, you'll adjust the time to fit the arrival of insect vectors. Here, at 7,000 feet in the foothills of the Rockies, we rarely have mosquitoes and our stable-fly season doesn't start until late summer. But in early spring we have our highest incidence of ticks, and we have a brief but intense horse-fly season. So, to be on the safe side, I usually vaccinate in March or April. Confer with your vet as to which vaccines are necessary for your locale and your horses and when is the best time to immunize them.

Stable flies begin emerging this month in the southern United States. To read about flies, go to July Pest Patrol.

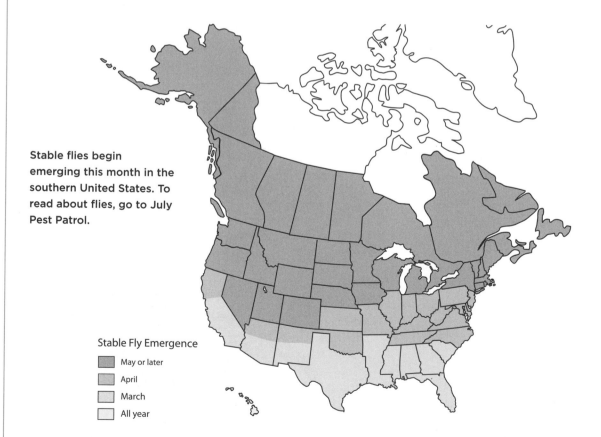

COMMON HORSE DISEASES

Vaccines are available for most of these common diseases.

★ **Equine encephalomyelitis** (sleeping sickness) is caused by a virus, carried by a mosquito from a wild bird or animal to your horse. The brain and spinal cord are affected; symptoms include high fever, weakness, lack of coordination, and stiffness. The mortality rate is 25 percent for WEE (see page 274); 100 percent for EEE. VEE is often fatal; WNV fatalities are rare.

★ **Tetanus** (lockjaw) is an infection of the nervous system caused by bacteria that enter through a wound or a foal's umbilical cord. The muscles stiffen so severely that within a few days the animal dies or must be euthanized.

★ **Influenza** (flu) is caused by a virus. It's a common respiratory disease, spread by coughing, and rarely fatal.

★ **Rhinopneumonitis** (snots) is of two types: a respiratory infection, which usually affects four- to six-month-old foals and can cause pregnant broodmares to abort; and a neurological form, which can cause hind-leg ataxia. Vaccination protects only against the former.

★ **Strangles** (distemper) is a highly contagious bacterial infection from *Streptococcus equi* that causes the glands near the throat to swell. The horse will not eat or drink and has a very high fever, but rarely dies.

★ **Rabies** rarely affects horses, but when it does, it is nearly always fatal. The virus is transmitted from an infected animal to the horse by a bite, usually from a dog, a skunk, a fox, or a bat, and causes severe depression or aggressiveness.

★ **Potomac Horse Fever** can cause diarrhea, laminitis, or abortion.

★ **Equine Protozoal Myeloencephalitis** (EPM) is a disease that affects the central nervous system, and without treatment it can lead to death.

★ **Equine Infectious Anemia** (EIA or swamp fever) is a virus that infects the horse's blood and is spread from one horse to another through a biting insect. There is no vaccine to protect your horse against swamp fever, but the Coggins test identifies carriers.

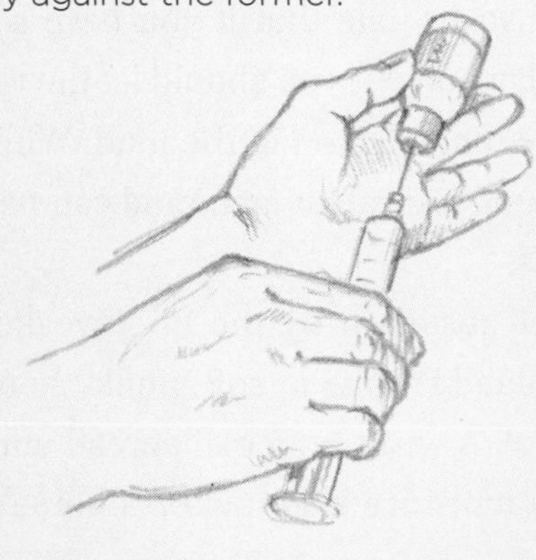

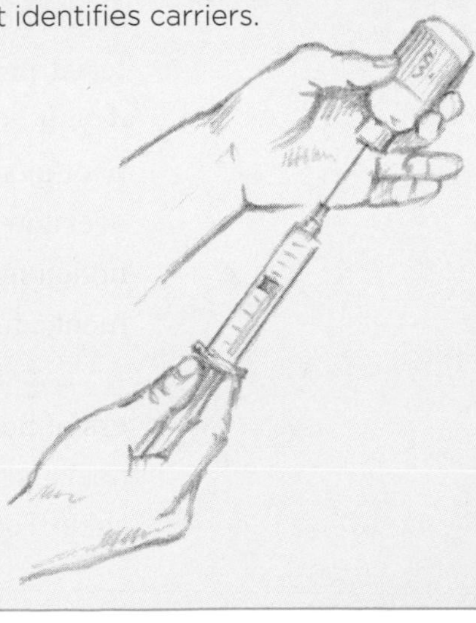

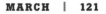

TIPS & TECHNIQUES

Disinfecting

Disinfectants can include bleach, phenol solution, and boiling water or steam. Confer with your vet.

Contamination and Isolation

Diseases are spread either directly from one horse to another, from a contaminated stall or feeder to a horse, between horses eating or drinking from communal areas, or through the air. If a horse is contaminated, use a combination of treatment, disinfection, and isolation to keep the disease from spreading and to eliminate the organism that caused it.

Quarantine is a good idea every time your horse returns from a show, clinic, vet hospital, or group trail ride. An ideal quarantine period is 14 days, because it covers the incubation period of most diseases. Therefore, it is a good idea to have both temporary quarantine and permanent isolation areas separate from the herd and from each other. Horses must not share water, feed, facilities, tack (especially bits), or caretakers (unless the caretakers disinfect themselves).

FOOT NOTES

IT'S MUD SEASON

March and April are usually our wettest, muddiest months, so the horses are off the pastures and in well-drained, sheltered pens. Horse hooves are healthiest when they are dry. It is an old wives' tale that if you have a horse with poor-quality or dry hooves, you should let the water trough overflow to force him to stand in the mud. While the basic notion might sound logical, in fact, mud can be very detrimental to hooves.

Excess water absorbed by the hoof weakens the layers of hoof horn and results in soft, punky hoof walls that peel and separate. A weak hoof can spread out like a pancake. Too much moisture also makes a horse's soles soft and susceptible to sole bruises and abscesses. Hooves subjected to repetitive wet-dry conditions undergo a stressful expansion and contraction, leading to cracks and other problems.

THRUSH

Another common problem among horses that stand in dirty, wet footing is the condition called thrush. Thrush is a decomposition of hoof tissues that usually starts in the clefts of the frog. Anaerobic bacteria, those that survive and flourish without air and are present almost everywhere on the farm, are sealed in the clefts of the frog by mud and manure and kept moist by urine and muddy conditions. The bacteria destroy the hoof tissue and produce a foul-smelling, black residue that you will never forget once you have smelled it. Erosion in the clefts of the frog can become so extreme as to reach sensitive tissue and cause lameness. One of the best ways to preserve your horse's hooves is to keep them clean and dry.

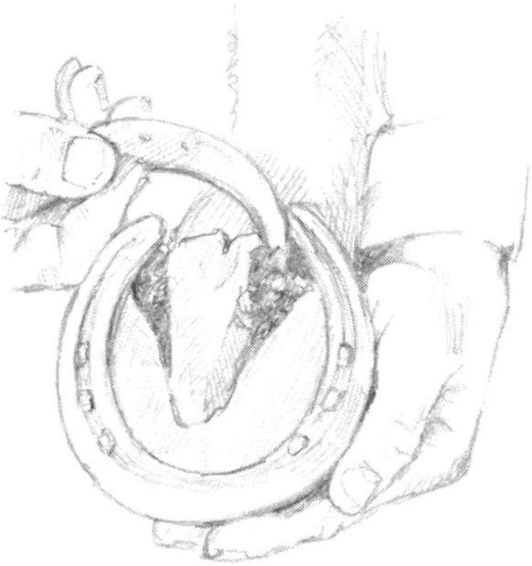

Thrush commonly affects the clefts of the frog.

A Muddy Experiment

If you want a firsthand example of how drying such situations can be, stick your fingers into some fresh mud past your fingernails, and then let them dry. Your "hooves" (fingernails) and "coronary bands" (cuticles) will probably show signs of drying and cracking after just one episode! Mud has the effect of drawing out moisture and oils and tightening pores, as in a poultice or a mud facial.

Wherever man has left his footprint in the long ascent from barbarism to civilization we will find the hoofprint of the horse beside it.

— John Moore

> **Thrush in a Nutshell**
>
> Although thrush most commonly affects the grooves on either side of the frog (collateral sulci) and in the center of the frog (central sulcus), it can invade the white line and even areas of the sole. The bad news is, thrush bacteria are almost always present in the soil, just waiting for the opportunity to move into the warm, dark, moist environment found in the bottom of your horse's hoof.
>
> The good news is, thrush is anaerobic — the bacteria don't survive in the presence of air. So, the best way to avoid thrush is to keep your horse's feet clean and dry so air can reach the tissues.

As every horseowner knows, however, this is easier said than done. Horses, especially those in confinement, often don't have a dry place to stand, and even if they do, they often choose to stand in wet bedding, manure, or mud at least part of the time. One of the consequences of wet footing is thrush. Do not apply bleach or hydrogen peroxide to a horse's feet. These so-called "treatments" can burn the healthy tissues of the frog and actually retard healing.

COMMERCIAL THRUSH REMEDIES. These vary in effectiveness and ease of use, and can cost up to $12 per ounce! Many products in squirt bottles are very messy to apply. Some contain fungicides and bactericides (like gentian violet and copper naphthenate) that are also staining agents. The purple or green color of the liquid lets you see where the product is being applied, but stains everything it touches, including your clothes and hands and your horse's hair, and it is difficult, if not impossible, to remove. Other products smell worse than the thrush itself (which is pretty bad!).

TREATING THRUSH PROPERLY. To treat thrush, first trim loose and overgrown flaps of frog so air and medication can reach the affected tissues. If you're not comfortable doing this, ask your farrier or vet for help. Wash the hoof thoroughly with mild soap, such as Betadine scrub, and plenty of warm water. Pat the hoof dry with a cloth and apply Sugardine (see this month's Ranch Recipes) deep into the clefts of the frog using a small brush, such as an acid brush. An acid brush has short, flat, black bristles and a 6-inch-long tubular metal handle, and is available at hardware stores for about 25 cents. The sugar will settle to the bottom of the container, so you'll need to stir Sugardine thoroughly before each use. Apply Sugardine daily until the thrush is gone, and keep the horse's feet as clean and dry as you can to prevent recurrence.

FEED BAG

BEET PULP

Beet pulp is a byproduct of the sugar beet industry. Once the sugar has been extracted from the beets, the pulp is wet and soft and so would be prone to mold. Dried into shreds or pellets, it is a very fibrous material that makes an excellent source of digestible fiber, which agrees nicely with a horse's digestive system. Since it is a relatively low-protein (8 to 10 percent) and low-energy feed (similar to hay), it does not make a horse hyper the way grain often does. It is also relatively high in calcium, so it makes a good addition to feed with grass hay. It is ideal for senior horses, horses with dental problems, and hard keepers (horses that are difficult to put or keep weight on).

Beet pulp is customarily fed as a mash and nutritionally is a better choice than wheat bran mash (see November Feed Bag). Mashes are ideal to feed in the winter to ensure water intake. I have found pellets to be more economical than shreds, and they soak up much more water.

Some say it is not absolutely necessary to soak beet pulp pellets before feeding. However, I have always added a moderate amount of water because the resulting fluffy mash allows me to mix in supplements, powders, and psyllium, and it gives my horses added moisture (see January Ranch Recipes). It seems to be more palatable, too, and there is less chance of choke.

You can use beet pulp in addition to hay or in place of hay, up to approximately 45 percent of the horse's ration.

Ranch Recipes

Sugardine for Thrush

Costing only around 34 cents per ounce to make, Sugardine is a homemade thrush remedy that's effective, easy to use, and has no bad odor. Used for years in human medicine to treat wounds and burns, it reduces edema (swelling), nourishes surface cells, and speeds healing.

To make Sugardine, mix white table sugar with a povidone-iodine product (such as Betadine scrub, solution, or ointment) to form a thin paste. Generic povidone-iodine is often half the price of Betadine and is basically the same product.

The Spring Diet

Most horses enter spring out of condition and with a hay belly. Adjust the diet to decrease bulk and increase energy in accordance with work.

Try a Chore Sandwich

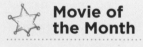

No, it is not a snack that I eat while doing chores! It is a visual image of the way I do chores and take my morning walk.

The bottom slice. Each morning, the first thing I do is go out and feed all of the barn horses their hay.

The filling. While they are munching, I take a brisk walk around some of the pastures and down to the creek. This accomplishes several important tasks:

- I check the perimeter and cross fences (mainly for deer damage)
- I make sure the creek is running freely
- I give the pasture horses their daily visual check
- I enjoy the magic of nature — the transformation of the pasture grasses and trees through the seasons, the majesty of our resident bucks and their herds of does, and the morning light changing on the rock cliffs
- I get my morning warm-up exercise

The top slice. After my walk, I feed the barn horses their grain ration, which usually consists of beet pulp and supplements. In the time it takes me to cruise around the property, they have eaten almost half of their hay ration. This has taken the edge off their appetites so they are less likely to bolt their grain. They thoroughly chew their grain, resulting in more efficient feed utilization and better digestion (less colic). I'm all for that.

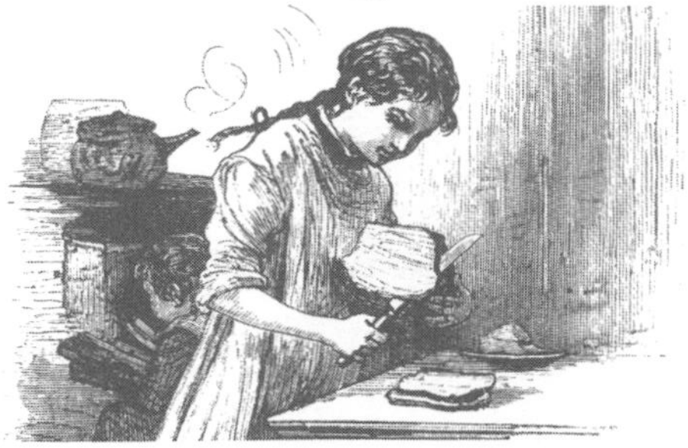

Movie of the Month

LADYHAWKE **(1985)**

This film has beautiful dream-like horse scenes in the woods. But it is worth the whole movie to see Rutger Hauer trot his powerful Friesian into the medieval church and battle with the knight of the evil bishop, all the while with their horses charging and rearing on the brick floor.

SPRING: *MARCH*

WILD LIFE

BIRDS

Because bluebirds are making their way back to breed here in the mountains, early in March I clean out the houses from last year's broods. And my very favorite bird, the Western meadowlark, arrives on or around our wedding anniversary in March. When the sweet melody of the meadowlark wakes me, I know it is spring!

Build a bluebird house of wood, preferably cedar.

1. Mount it on a pole, fence post, utility pole, or tree, with the bottom of the house 4 to 5 feet above ground.
2. Face the entrance to the house away from prevailing winds. In hot climates, face the house north or east to avoid direct midday sun.
3. Space multiple houses at least 100 yards apart.

Clean bluebird houses before nesting season. Here, we clean them out in March.

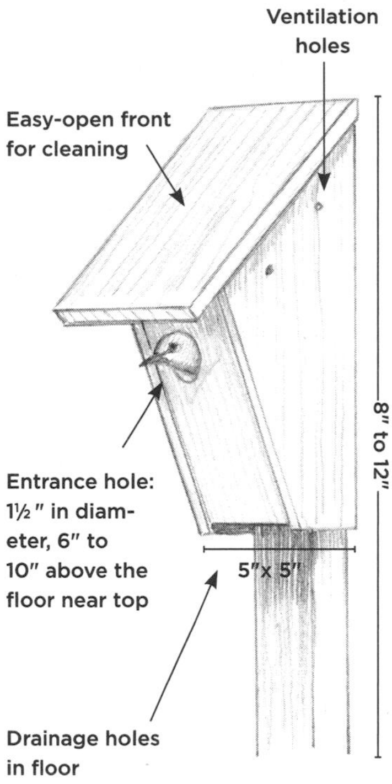

Bluebirds will raise their families in a well-designed bird house.

Bears Are Awake

In March I have frequently seen a black bear or its tracks in the snow down at the creek. I expect there is a den nearby, and hibernation ends in March. See more about bears in September Wild Life.

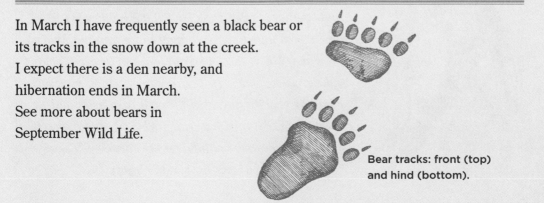

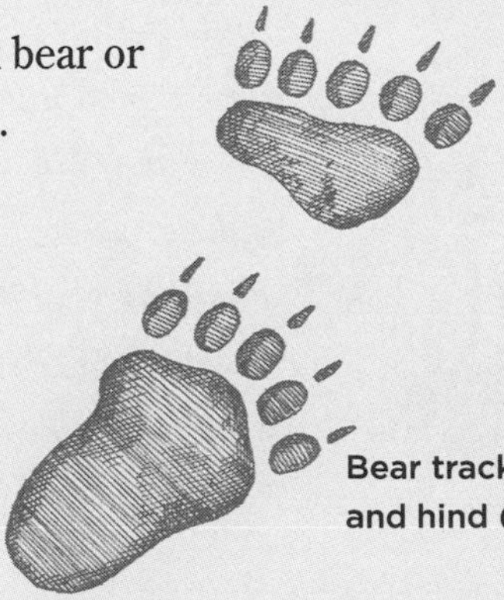

Bear tracks: front (top) and hind (bottom).

PASTURE PERFECT

. . . *daffodils,*
That come before
the swallow dares,
and take
The winds of March
with beauty. . . .
William Shakespeare,
The Winter's Tale

TIME TO LET YOUR LAND REST

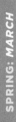

Although I hate to take away their freedom to roam, March 1 usually marks the time when I bring all horses in from pasture. Since March and April are our muddiest months, this is when horses would do the most damage to the earth, so despite their longing to be out, all the horses are in stalls or pens near the barns while the pastures rest for two to three months. This allows the emerging plants a chance to grow without eager nibbling and damage from hooves.

No matter how good a pasture is, it needs to lie dormant for some months each year, especially during the muddy months. Mud plus hooves equals lost shoes, pasture damage, and weed invasion. Mud is also an excellent breeding site for insects and harbors bacteria and fungi that lead to thrush, rain rot, and scratches.

NOT ALWAYS TRUE

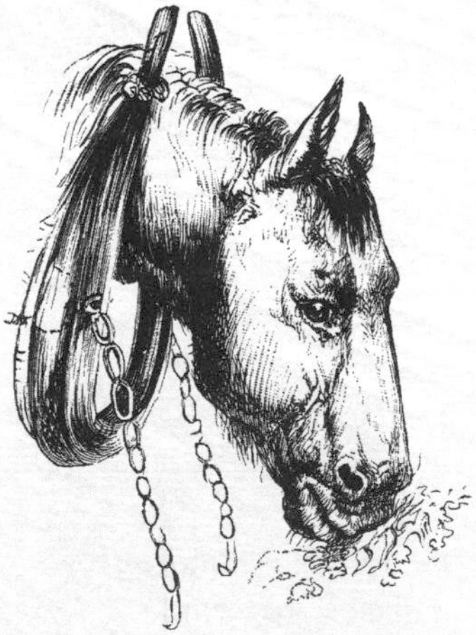

Historical Horsekeeping

"Hay is most perfect when it is about a year old. Horses would perhaps prefer it earlier, but it is neither so wholesome nor so nutritious, and may cause purging. When it is a year old, it should retain much of its green color and agreeable smell. In packing or stacking hay, salt should be slightly sprinkled through it so as to destroy insects. It also aids in preserving it bright, and makes it more palatable and healthful for the horse." — Magner's Standard Horse and Stock Book *by D. Magner, 1916*

Pest Patrol

Skunks, Opossums, Squirrels, and Raccoons

Some wild animals may be darling members of the natural world but a nuisance or a hazard to your horse's health. Skunks, members of the weasel family, can carry rabies, yet they are an important part of rodent control since they eat mice, moles, and shrews. Opossums carry and shed the protozoan that causes EPM (see page 121), so contact between horses and opossums or hay from opossum country should be eliminated. Squirrels can wreak havoc in your barn loft or feed room. Raccoons are nocturnal rummagers that can make a mess in your barn and carry rabies.

The best way to keep your horse farm unattractive to these varmints is to keep things tidy: secure garbage containers, put away pet food and water bowls, and close barn doors during cold weather and at night. Screen windows, vents, and chimneys that could become entry points. Don't be tempted to make pets of these critters. It is unwise, and in many states it is illegal to possess most species of wildlife, including birds and snakes.

Raccoons, which can reach 40 pounds, breed in February or March and have two to five kits in April or May. Although their native diet consists of berries, nuts, grains, frogs, insects, and bird and turtle eggs, they adapt to forage on garbage and pet food.

If you have a nuisance raccoon, contact your local Division of Wildlife. They may suggest that you use a live trap baited with sardines and relocate the animal. Take care when handling the cage, as raccoons can transmit distemper, parvovirus, and roundworms to humans.

Relocation is not a perfect answer, though, and it is illegal in some states. The relocated animal could be leaving young behind, and usually another animal will soon fill its vacant territory anyway. And if you live-trap certain animals (like skunks) you might be required by law (depending on your state) to destroy them because health laws don't permit relocation. That's why, taking everything into consideration, it is best if you can learn to coexist with wildlife and just develop good management practices that don't attract animals to your buildings.

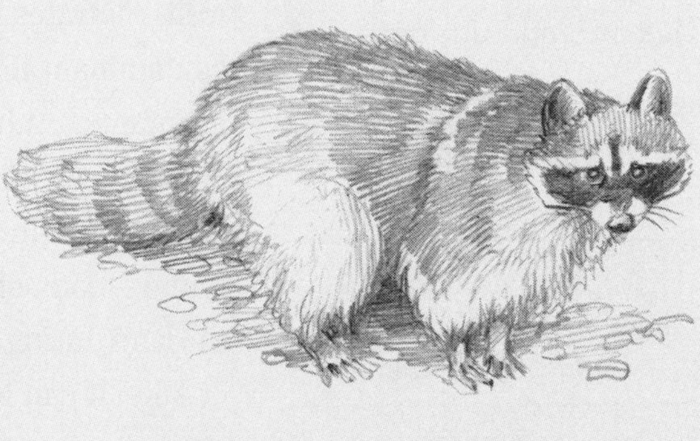

It's best to make your buildings unattractive to these masked marauders.

CLEAN-UP CREW

MARCH
Manure Pile Maintenance

It is ideal to have at least three compost piles going at all times: one to which fresh manure is being added daily (A), one that is in the process of decomposing (B), and one that is fully composted and ready to spread (C). Each month will have a monthly manure task associated with each of the piles.

PILE A
Start pile.

PILE B
Sell, store, or spread.

PILE C
Quit adding, turn once.

See April and May for more on handling manure and composting.

MANURE MANAGEMENT

Horse manure can be a valuable commodity. About one-fifth of the nutrients a horse eats are passed out in the manure and urine. Manure is composed of undigested food, digestive juices, and microorganisms. The bacteria make up as much as 30 percent of its mass! Because urine (usually in the form of soaked bedding) is a liquid, it contains more readily available dissolved nutrients than do feces. If the manure is properly handled, about half of those excreted nutrients can be utilized by pasture or crop plants in one growing season, with the balance being used in subsequent years.

Horse manure is valuable because it is "hot," or capable of breakdown by composting. A ton of horse manure will supply the equivalent of a 100-pound sack of fertilizer (the exact nitrogen-phosphorus-potash ratio will vary) and provide valuable organic matter and trace elements.

Even if manure is not to be used as a fertilizer, it must be properly managed to control odor, remove insect breeding areas, kill parasite eggs and larvae, and prevent nitrogen and phosphorus in the manure from contaminating water.

Locate your manure piles away from all water sources. Nitrates entering the groundwater can affect streams and wells. Nitrates in drinking water above the EPA maximum contaminant level can cause health problems, particularly in infants. Although horses tolerate elevated nitrate levels somewhat better than humans do, they are more susceptible to nitrate poisoning than most other monogastric (single-stomach) animals. If excess phosphorus runs off the land during rainfall or snowmelt and settles in your pond or lake, it can lead to eutrophication, the process whereby excess nutrients in water cause excessive and unhealthy aquatic plant growth, particularly of algae.

BEAUTY SHOP

GROOMING TOOLS FOR EARLY SPRING

Although a shedding blade is handy for removing thick pads of hair from a long winter coat, it can be hazardous to your horse's health! Shedding blades with very sharp pointed teeth can easily scrape or scratch his skin. Breaks in the skin then open the door for bacterial, fungal, and other skin problems. Be aware of how sharp the teeth on your shedding blade are, and how hard you are pressing down as you stroke. Do not use a shedding blade on a short coat. A soft rubber curry is safer for your horse's skin, and kinder to your horse's coat.

Basically, there are four types of curries: soft rubber, soft bristled, hard plastic, and metal.

Soft rubber curries come in many colors in round, rectangular, and oval shapes with various types of "nubs." Soft rubber is safest for the head and for bony areas like legs, and it is effective for giving your horse a good rub down, provided you add that elbow grease!

Soft-bristled curries are ideal for combing through a clean, long winter coat.

Hard plastic curries don't conform to your hand or the horse's body as well as rubber curries but they are good at breaking up mud clumps on thickly muscled parts.

Metal curries are not designed to be used on the horse at all. Rather, they are for cleaning the stiff bristles of a mud brush or dandy brush as you groom your horse. I hold the metal curry in one hand and the mud brush in the other. When I want to clean the bristles of the mud brush, I run them over the metal curry.

en español

ranch. Comes from *el rancho*, meaning 'farm', especially in the West.

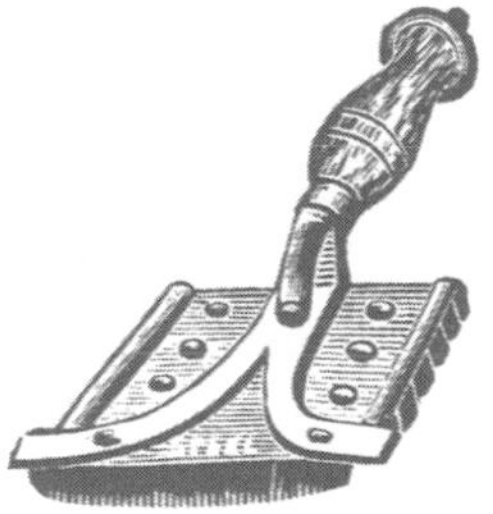

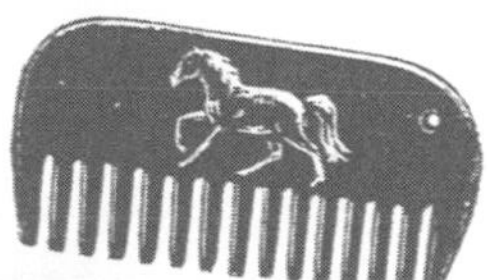

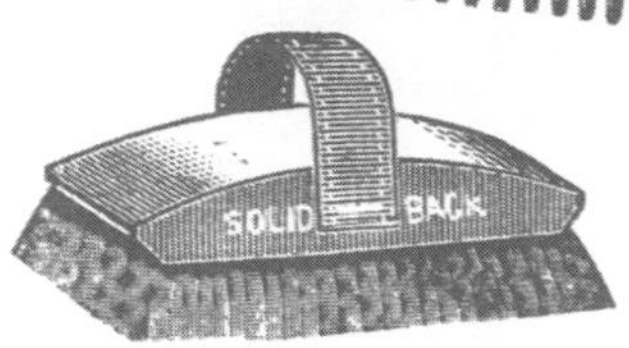

Grooming Tools: How and Where to Use Them

Metal curry. Not to be used on the horse at all; is designed to clean other brushes.

Shedding blade. Use only on heavily muscled portions (neck, shoulder, hindquarters) with long strokes and light to moderate pressure to remove a long, thick winter coat.

Sweat scraper. Use on heavily muscled portions (neck, shoulder, hindquarters) with long strokes and light to moderate pressure to remove water from coat after bath.

Very soft rubber curry. Use on face, lower legs, belly, and flank with appropriate pressure and circular motion.

Rubber curry. Use on all other areas with moderate pressure and circular motion.

Stiff-bristled mud brush. Use on heavily muscles portions (neck, shoulder, hindquarters) with short, flicking motions.

Medium brush. Use on ribs and upper legs, and possibly on mane and tail.

Soft brush. Sometimes made of fine horse hair. Use on face, lower legs, belly, and flank with smooth, soothing strokes and flicks.

Cloth or sponge. Use on face, under tail, in the flank area, and to clean udder and sheath (wiping, not scrubbing.)

Grooming glove. Use on face, ears, and muzzle. Use hands to strip water off lower legs.

Hoof pick. Use to remove mud and foreign objects from clefts and sole.

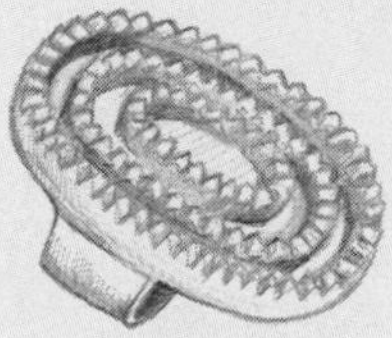

Rubber curry

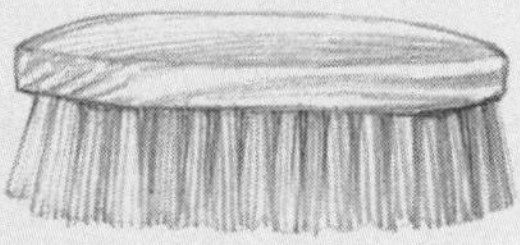

Stiff-bristled mud brush

Medium brush

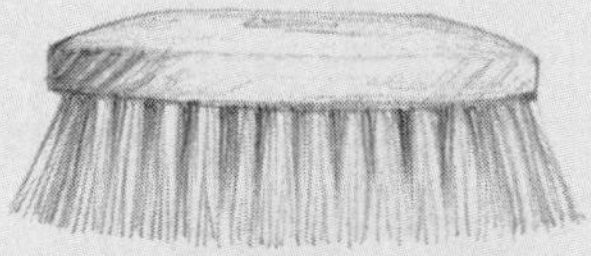

Soft brush

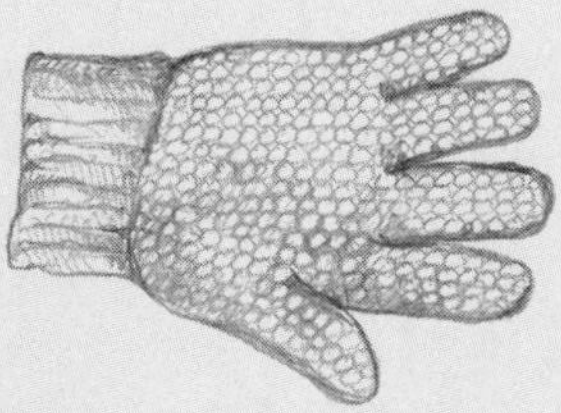

Grooming glove

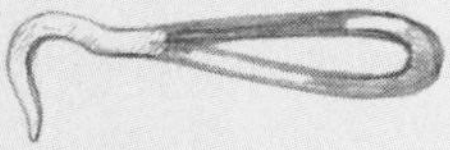

Hoof pick

TACK ROOM

FITTING A STRAP HALTER

It is easier to fit a strap halter properly if you start with the right size. Depending on the manufacturer, halters are usually available in suckling, weanling, yearling, cob (Arab), horse, Warmblood, and draft sizes.

When fitting a web halter, try to buckle it on the middle hole to allow the halter to be the most balanced on your horse's head. If a halter has buckles on both cheekpieces, as leather halters usually do, try to buckle them on the same hole on each side to balance the halter.

Also bear in mind that the crownpiece of the halter should be located at the poll, where it will give a clear signal to your horse when leading. If you let the crownpiece slide back on the horse's neck, which happens if the halter is too big or is adjusted too low, you won't be able to give the horse a very good signal.

A horse is a thing of such beauty – none will tire of looking at him as long as he displays himself in his splendor.

— Xenophon, 400 B.C.

FITTING A ROPE HALTER

Rope halters come in a variety of sizes, from weanling to draft. Once you have found the right size halter for your horse, you can adjust it in a couple of simple ways, using two knots. One is the fiador knot, which is located below the jaw of the horse (*fiador* is Spanish for 'guarantor, one

STILL TRUE TODAY

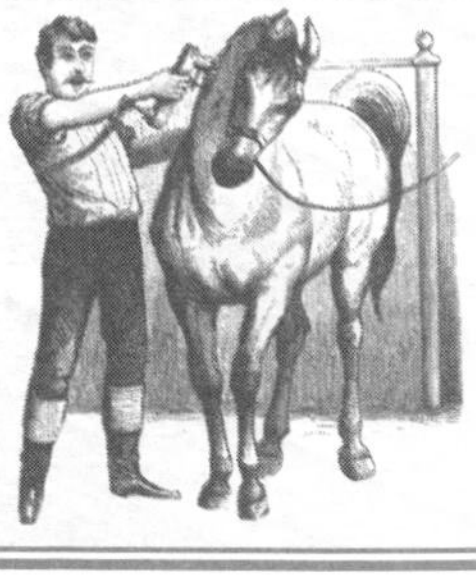

Historical Horsekeeping

"As a rule, any horse may be properly cleaned with a scraper, a curry comb, a brush, a sponge, a comb, a wisp of straw and a rubbing cloth."

— Gleason's Horse Book *by Prof. Oscar R. Gleason, 1892*

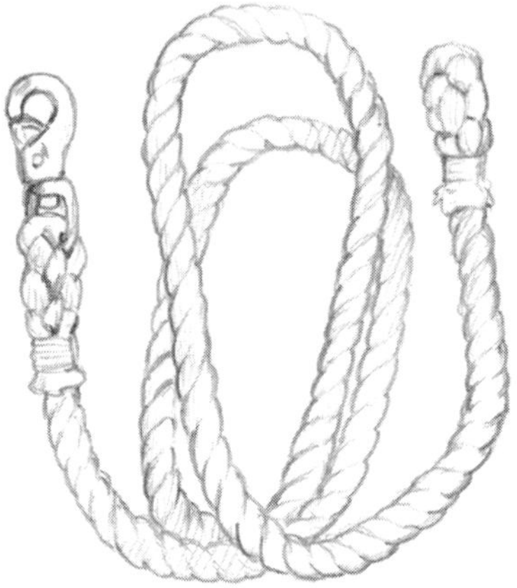

A cotton lead rope with bull snap.

who provides security'). The other is the sheet bend knot, which is used to fasten the halter onto the horse.

To raise or lower the noseband, adjust the sheet bend knot. Loosen the knot, raise or lower the noseband, and then refasten the knot.

If the noseband is too loose or too tight, you can adjust the fiador knot. First take the halter off the horse. Then grasp the rope above and below the fiador knot and push together, loosening the knot to allow you to work the rope through it. Move the fiador knot down if you want to make the noseband larger, or move it up to make the noseband smaller. Then tighten the knot and put the halter back on the horse.

Two-Finger Rule

When checking halter fit, use the two-finger rule in three places:

- ★ Two fingers below the prominent cheekbone
- ★ Two fingers under the noseband
- ★ Two fingers under the throatlatch

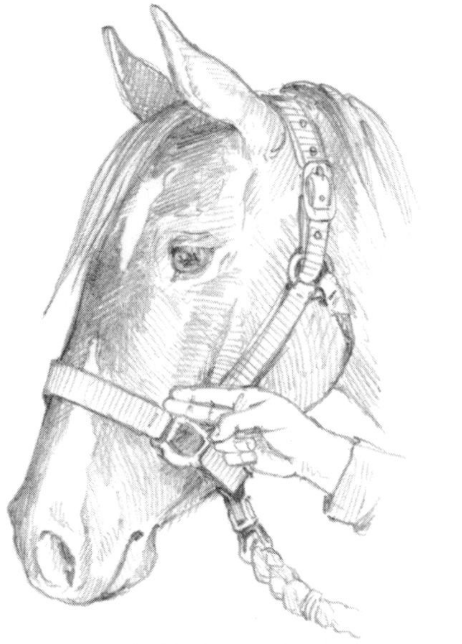

CHOOSING AND USING A LEAD ROPE

I like a lead rope that is ⅝- to ¾-inch thick and 10 to 12 feet long. Cotton is a natural fiber that is soft and nice to handle, so it makes an ideal in-hand rope; however, cotton is difficult to untie when it's wet or has been pulled tight. In addition, it can fray and rot, making the rope no longer safe to use.

Nylon lead ropes resist moisture and rot, and they are about four times as strong as cotton ropes of the same diameter. Due to their slick surface, however, they can be difficult to grip, so they are not my choice for an in-hand rope. Nevertheless, when I want a weatherproof rope for tying outside, I usually choose nylon.

Never wrap or loop a rope around your hand, arm, or other part of your body, thinking it will help you hold onto your horse better. I have seen children seriously hurt because they wrapped the rope around themselves and couldn't let go.

Never wrap or loop a rope around your hand, arm, or other part of your body, thinking it will help you hold onto your horse better.

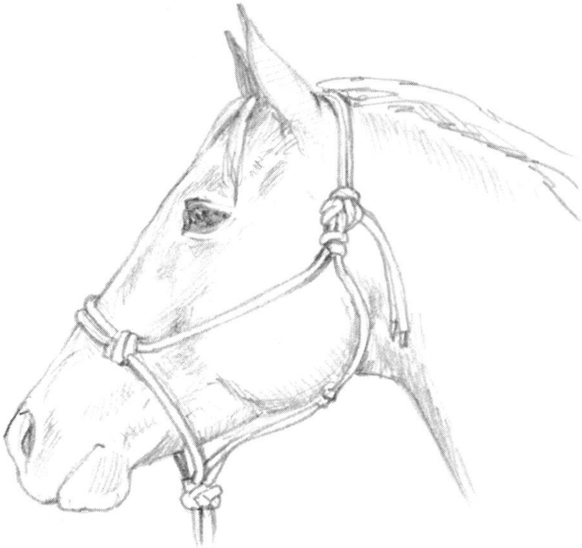

A properly fitted rope halter.

Horse Sense and Safety

Handling a Horse

★ Know your horse and his habits.

★ Protect your head by wearing protective headgear.

CLOTHES HORSE

Ranch Notes

Mar. 14. 5'— long icicles (the longest ever) on horse barn scared horses when they crashed down (scared me too!)

SELECTING TRAILER (SHIPPING) BOOTS

If you plan on trailering to some spring trail rides or shows, you'll want to round up your horse's trailer boots by March. I pay special attention to my horse's legs, both for his welfare and because they are one of the essentials for a peak performance. There is nothing more disappointing and unnecessary than opening the trailer door to find a horse with a wound. A well-designed trailer, safe driving habits, proper training in trailer loading and unloading, and familiarization with traveling all help to prevent injury. Even the most seasoned equine traveler, however, will occasionally scramble or take a misstep while en route. That's when a good pair of shipping boots helps.

Because shipping boots are used where there is a lot of activity, dirt, moisture, and manure, they must be well designed and tough. They should cover the hocks and the knees and be cut so that when they are positioned over the point of the fetlock, the bottom of the boots reaches the ground. I prefer shipping boots with durable scuff plates at the base of the boots to further protect the horse's bulbs and coronary band, as well as to shield the bottom of the boots from urine, manure, and shredding by the horse's hooves.

See December Clothes Horse for more on hook-and-loop closures.

Shipping boots should provide a cushion and be comfortable for the horse. Although fleece lining is easy on a horse's legs, the extra care needed to pick or brush shavings, sawdust, hay, hair, manure, or dirt out of the fleece between and before washings is time consuming. Travel boots lined with a smooth, soft, conforming, stretchable fabric that can easily be brushed off are best. The exterior fabric should be made of a tough, waterproof, breathable fabric. The most common fastener type is hook-and-loop (such as Velcro).

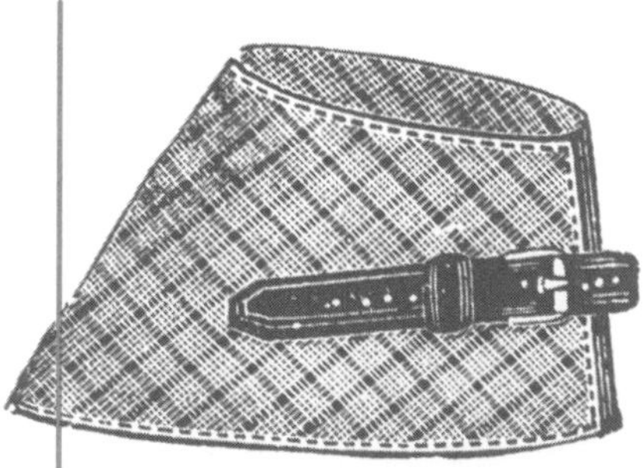

BUDGET

About the time I have finished my income taxes, I have a pretty good idea of what the farm's expenses have been and what I need to plan for the next year. Hay is my single biggest expenditure. Although I take my official hay inventory in May (see May Farm Office), I have a pretty good idea in March of how much hay I have left and what I will need to buy. When I budget, I group things into three categories: normal operating expenses, repairs, and large purchases. I also try to project the farm income for the year.

When your expenses exceed your income, you need to decrease your expenses or increase your income. It is best, of course, if you can justify your budget each year, not carrying over any debts to a new year.

Cost of Raising a Foal

One place where many people spend more money than they anticipated is in the raising of a foal. It is often much less expensive to buy a foal from a breeder who is set up to raise large numbers of foals and has a stallion and breeding farm facilities, and often even a veterinarian on staff. Although it is quite gratifying to raise your own foal, here is an idea of what it might cost you to do so.

THE MARE. She needs to be of the quality to breed. Her price can range from $1,000 to $100,000, with an average, for the sake of discussion, at about $5,000.

THE STUD FEE. The cost to have a stallion breed your mare can range from free to $20,000 or more. But in this category, I include not only the stud fee but any of the fees that would be applicable in your situation, such as board at

Expenses Examined

Normal operating expenses include feed; veterinary supplies and services; farrier supplies and services; labor; materials such as footing and bedding; supplies for the tack room and farm office; real estate and income taxes; horse, property, and liability insurance; loan interest; fuel; utilities; and rent.

Repairs generally are to facilities (such as a new roof, stall mats, or fencing) or vehicles (such as the truck, trailer, tractor, or implements).

Large purchases, which might be depreciated or taken as a one-time Section 179 deduction, might include a new truck, trailer, implement, piece of tack, or building.

Income Breakdown

Budgeting basically boils down to comparing what you anticipate taking in against your expected expenses. Projected income might include sale of horses, stud fees, lesson charges, boarding fees, crops, winnings, and so on.

If you have your heart set on a foal by that special stallion, then do your homework (see this month's Reproduction Roundup) and have a good breeding contract.

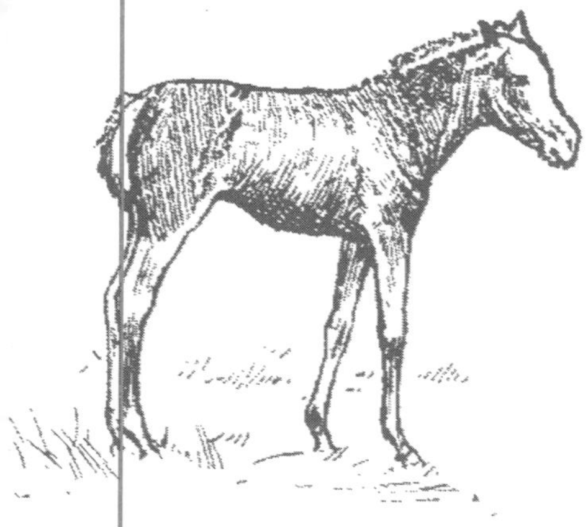

the stud (usually ranging from one month to six months, averaging two months); veterinary fees including palpations, ultrasound, collection, artificial insemination (AI) services, and drugs; and AI transport and shipping. A very conservative total is $7,500.

MARE CARE. During the16-month period from conception to weaning, the mare will either be boarded or cared for at your facility and her expenses will include hay, grain, water, salt, veterinarian supplies and fees, and farrier care. This can range anywhere from $1,600 to $6,000 annually, so for 16 months, figure approximately $5,000.

Note: So far, we are up to $17,500 and it is just now foaling time.

FOALING EXPENSES. If you are experienced, these can be minimal, but could go skyward in a hurry if there are complications. This category includes veterinary supplies and fees or a foaling-out service, and could run from $100 to $1,000 ; I'll use $300 here.

FOAL CARE. From birth to weaning, you'll need to buy more feed, vaccine, and dewormer for the foal than for an adult horse, and you'll have vet and farrier fees too. For the four months until weaning, figure $400 to $1,500 with an average of about $600. Now we are at $18,400.

If we sell the mare for $5,000 or still own her and are using her for the next foal, we can subtract what we received for the mare ($5,000) or transfer the value of the mare ($5,000) from this foal to the next, resulting in a net cost of the foal at weaning of about $13,400. If a mare dies as a result of her role as the dam to the current foal, then the $5,000 remains as a cost of this foal and the mare's value ($5,000) would not be subtracted; the net cost of an orphan foal at weaning would be $18,400.

RAISING THE FOAL TO RIDING AGE. Now you need to get the foal to two-and-a-half years of age to begin training, so figure another two years of feed and care costs, then training costs. . . .

As you can see, the cost of raising a foal to weaning age, or a horse to the age of five with training, is considerable. Think about that when you are horse shopping. If you have your heart set on a foal by that special stallion, then do your homework (see this month's Reproduction Roundup) and have a good breeding contract.

BREEDING CONTRACT

If you are the mare's owner, you must become very familiar with the terms of the stallion owner's breeding contract. Most contracts list the booking fee, a nonrefundable portion (usually about one quarter) of the stud fee that assures the mare a place in the stallion's schedule. The balance of the stud fee is customarily due upon determination that the mare is pregnant.

There are generally two types of contracts — live foal guarantee and one-time breeding — but neither of the types is standard in terms. Live foal can be defined as one who "stands and nurses" or "stands and nurses and is physically

Contractual Requirements

Usually some prebreeding veterinary requirements are stated in the contract, which the owner should attend to before the mare leaves home. These may include but are not limited to:

- ★ Current vaccinations
- ★ Negative Coggins test
- ★ Uterine culture
- ★ Uterine biopsy

Breeding Safety

If breeding is to be live rather than AI, another requirement may be that the mare's hind shoes be pulled before arrival at the stud, as a precaution for the stallion's safety during breeding.

A horse is **worth more than riches.**
— Spanish proverb

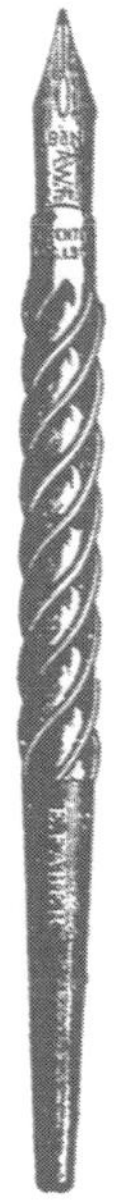

healthy." In the event a mare aborts, a foal is born dead, or a foal dies within the covered terms of the contract, the mare owner is usually allowed return breeding privileges. This will be specifically stipulated as another chance for the same mare, the substitution of a different mare for the one that had the difficulty, or a refund of the nonbooking portion of the stud fee. The mare owner needs to realize that although it is better to have some guarantee than none at all, there will be additional veterinary, mare care, and traveling expenses incurred if it is necessary to return the mare for rebreeding.

No Second Chance

One-time breeding contracts are just that. There are no return breeding privileges.

Most contracts state the mare care fee per day and some quote an adjusted monthly rate. Many stipulate that the farm promises good care but is not held responsible for accidents, injury, or sickness. Most require that all financial obligations be satisfied before the mare leaves the stud. Two copies of each contract are usually sent to the interested breeder. The mare owner provides the information required, signs both copies, and sends a check for the booking fee to the farm. A copy countersigned by the stallion manager is returned to the mare owner.

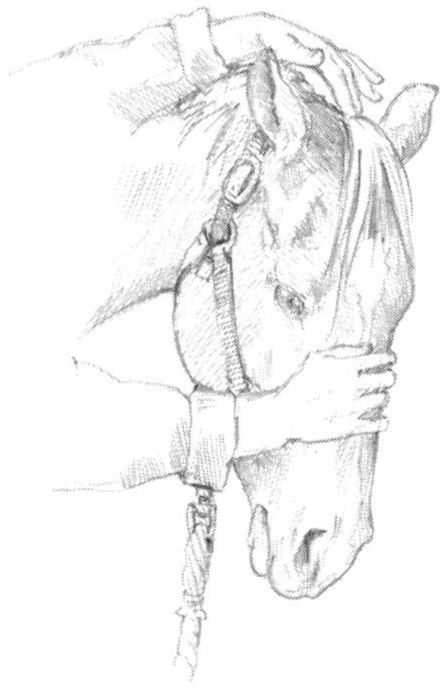

Manners for Deworming

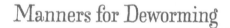

Whether you deworm your animals or your vet does, you should work with your horse so he is cooperative for the procedure and has good manners.

Here are some of the goals:

- ★ Your horse must stand still
- ★ He must lower his head
- ★ He must allow handling all over his head and mouth
- ★ He must allow insertion of a tube into his mouth without raising his head or pulling away

Training Pen

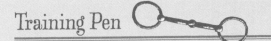

Safe Haltering Procedure

Use proper haltering procedures to develop good habits in your horse and to avoid accidents. Here's how to halter safely.

As you approach the horse from the near (left) side, hold the unbuckled halter and rope in your left hand. With your right hand, scratch the horse on the withers and move your right hand across the top of the neck to the right side.

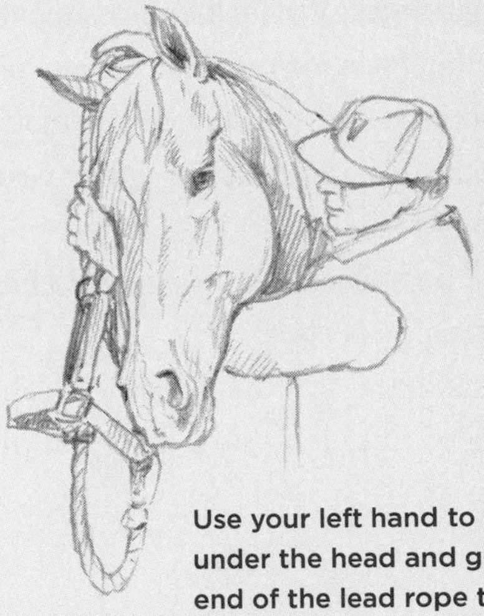

Use your left hand to go under the head and give the end of the lead rope to your right hand.

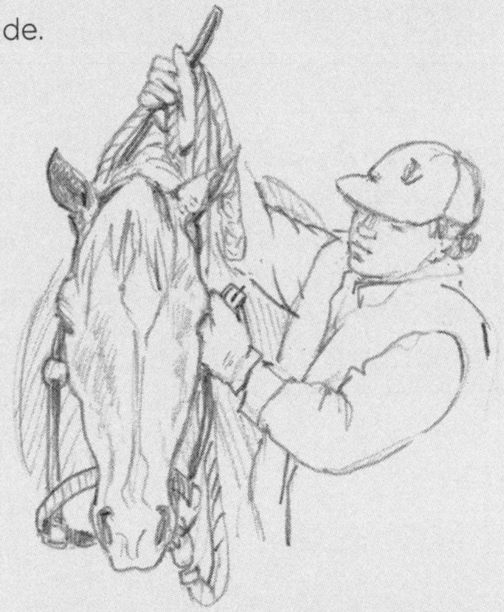

Make a loop of rope around the horse's throatlatch and hold the loop with your right hand. If the horse tries to move away at this stage, you can pull his head toward you with the loop of the rope. Next, hand the halter strap with the holes in it under the horse's neck to your right hand.

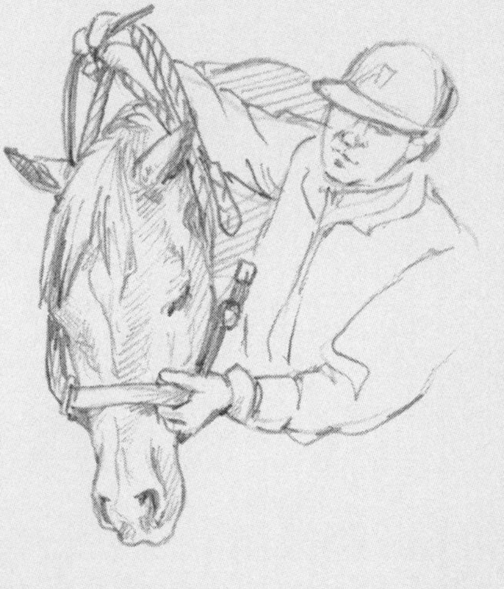

With your left hand, position the noseband of the halter on the horse's face.

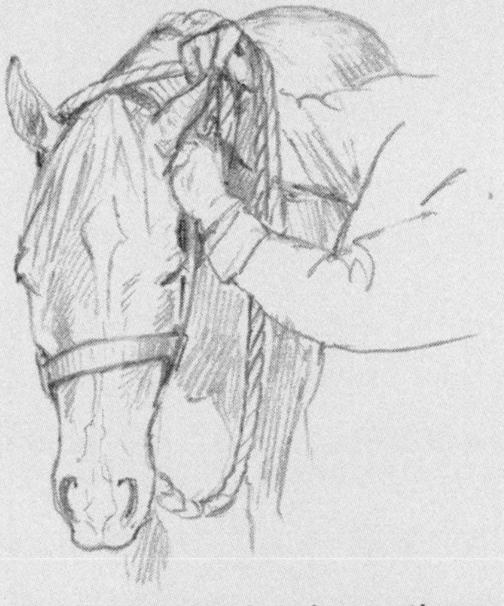

Then bring your hands together on the near side to buckle the halter.

REPRODUCTION ROUNDUP

Breeding value depends on the mare's conformational quality, performance ability, performance record, and prior reproductive performance.

STALLION SELECTION

If you plan to rebreed your mare, you should choose the stallion and make necessary business arrangements. (See this month's Farm Office). Start by providing specific, objective answers to the following questions:

- First of all, is your mare worthy of further investment?
- What are your specific goals for the foal? Is your primary motive profit-oriented or to produce a personal horse? (Although quality is essential in either case, financial strategies differ slightly.)
- What stallions would be suitable for your mare? Limit the field to about three prospects.
- Which of the finalists is the best financial bet? (The word "financial" refers to much more than just the stud fee.)

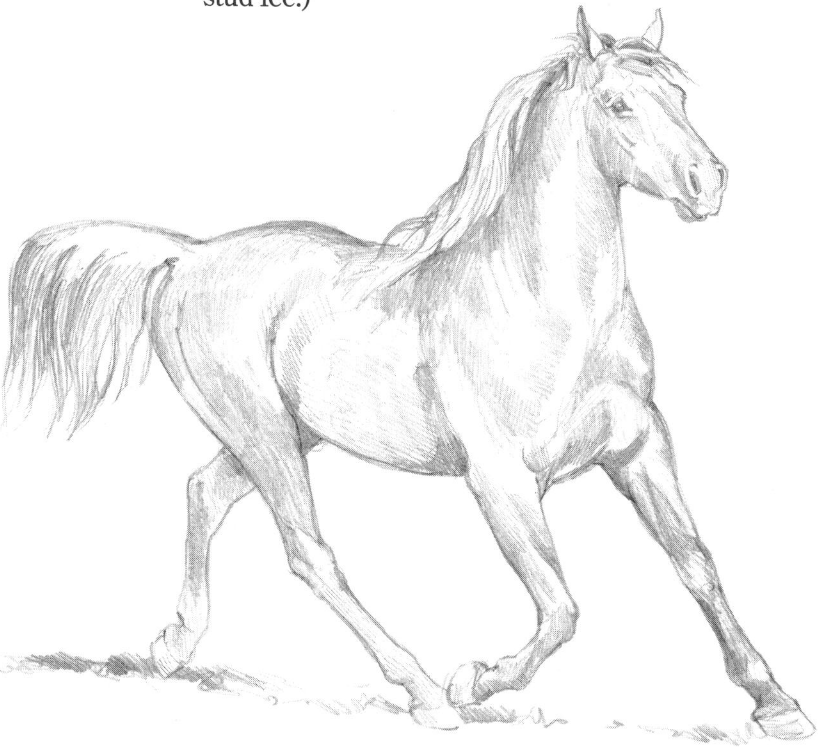

OBJECTIVELY EVALUATE YOUR MARE. Appraising your mare's breeding value might be difficult if you have a strong emotional attachment that prevents you from making objective observations. Breeding value depends on the mare's conformational quality, performance ability, performance record, and prior reproductive performance. A mare that has a heritable unsoundness or is untrainable should never be chosen as a broodmare in a last ditch attempt at recouping the investment cost of her purchase price. Rarely does such a mare magically produce a foal that is exempt from the behavioral or conformation defects that rendered her unusable.

Refer to the standard of perfection of your mare's breed as baseline criteria to evaluate her conformation. Using a numerical system, rate her strong and weak conformation points. While the pencil and paper are still in your hand, compile a separate list of traits that you hope the foal will possess. This will make the selection process more efficient when you are narrowing the field of stallions.

In most situations, after calculating and adding the appropriate costs, you'll find that a stud fee of about one fourth to one half the value of your mare is usually a financially appropriate investment. Therefore, if your mare's actual cash value is $10,000, a suitable stud fee would be in the $2,500 to $5,000 range. Although in some situations an exceptional mare may warrant a gamble on a stud fee above her "price range," in no instance would it make sense to breed a mare to an inferior stallion.

THE STALLION: REGISTERED OR CROSSBRED? First you must decide whether you want a purebred or crossbred foal. Breeding within a breed may give you a better chance of attaining a specific look or type if those traits are predominant in a particular breed. This is especially true with inbreeding or linebreeding, where family lines

Rhino #3

Your broodmares need their third Rhinopneumonitis vaccination in the ninth month of pregnancy, which is often March. For mares heavy in foal, hand-walking 15 to 30 minutes per day for three or four days following the vaccination is a good idea to promote absorption.

A horse gallops with his lungs, perseveres with his heart, and wins with his character.

— Frederico Tesio

Estimating Your Mare's Cash Value

Determining a realistic market value on your mare will help you to establish the stud fee amount that would represent an appropriate investment. Use the real cash value for your mare, not what you have invested in her emotionally or financially through the years. You may need to solicit the aid of an objective professional to help you make this determination.

The strict business approach dictates that the cost of producing a horse up to weaning should never exceed the value of the mare. This means that the total of the following costs should be less than or equal to the value of the mare: stud fee + mare care + veterinary breeding expenses + transportation to and from the stud + cost of maintaining the mare during gestation + cost of raising the foal to weaning. In the case of breeding with shipped semen, semen charges and insemination fees will be a substituted cost for mare care and transportation costs.

are concentrated in an effort to strengthen certain characteristics. Inbreeding can backfire, however, as undesirable characteristics and even lethal traits are also concentrated when closely related horses are mated.

If your emphasis is on performance and registration papers are not important, crossbreeding may work for you. Many crossbred horses have earned well-respected reputations in a variety of horse sports and uses. When you crossbreed, you are combining gene pools from two very different sources. This can result, due to hybrid vigor, in the offspring being a better individual than either one of the parents. Unfortunately, crossbreeding can also produce an individual with such a diverse mix of genes that no characteristics are accentuated, resulting in a mediocre individual. One thing is for sure, with crossbreeding, there tend to be less uniformity and more surprises on foaling day.

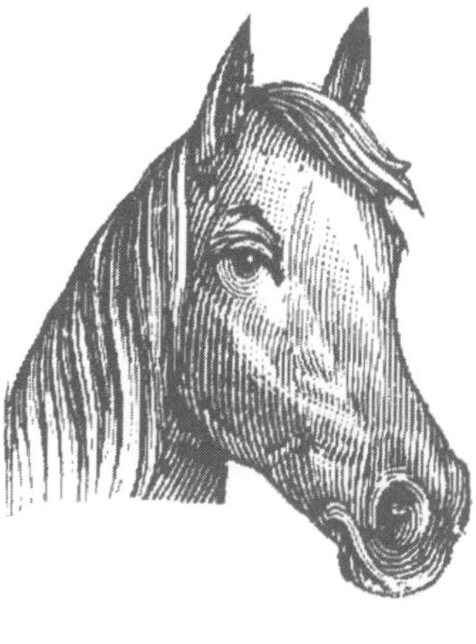

MAKE A CHECKLIST. Before visiting the stallion, make a checklist itemizing important traits that he should possess to complement the mare. The key is to select a stallion capable of enhancing her qualities as they're passed on to the foal. Give each trait a numerical score indicating relative importance. General categories such as balance, symmetry, and proportion can be included on the score sheet as well as such specifics as correctness of angles (shoulder, hip, pastern), substance of bone and muscle, height, weight, and quality and soundness of legs and hooves.

Having a checklist in your hand might prevent you from being overwhelmed by the presence of a stallion, and it can provide you with a written reference for later objective comparison. It is not necessary to make a big deal out of your checklist evaluation. It can be an inconspicuous 3" x 5" card, previously prepared with categories that you can use for quick notations, checkmarks, or numbers.

EVALUATE THE STALLION IN PERSON. Visit the stallions and their offspring in person, if possible. Do not rely solely on advertisements, testimonials over the phone, or videotapes. Seeing the horse in the flesh, watching him (and hopefully his offspring) move, and observing him perform will give you a clear, firsthand view of the stallion's abilities. If distance precludes your visiting the stud farm, videotapes can help you in your assessment. Be aware, however, that a well-produced videotape is essentially advertising, which showcases the horse's positive attributes and fails to mention any drawbacks.

The inspection of the stallion should include a thorough in-hand evaluation, at which time you can employ your checklist. Depending on the breed, type, and use of the horse, you will place different emphasis on some of his structural components. However, all horses should have functionally sound conformation.

Looking at Horses

Quality and Substance

Quality is defined as "flat" bone (indicated by the cannon bone), clean joints, sharply defined (refined) features, smooth muscling, overall blending of parts, and a fine, smooth hair coat.

Substance refers to thickness, depth, and breadth of bone, muscle, and other tissues; overall weight and height; hoof size; depth of heart girth and flank; and spring of rib.

Best viewed from the rear, spring of rib refers to the curve of the ribs. Besides providing room for the heart, lungs, and digestive tract, a well-sprung rib cage provides a natural, comfortable place for a rider's legs. A flat-ribbed or "slab-sided" horse is difficult to sit properly, whereas a wide-barreled horse can be stressful to the rider's legs.

A stallion's own competition history should be studied as well as that of his offspring. Fastest times, dollars or ribbons won, weight pulled, and heights jumped are some possible indicators of excellence. Agility and trainability are important gauges as well, but are harder to measure in specific terms. Here is where knowledgeable observation pays off. For example, a horse's natural ability to move well in the three gaits is essential for a pleasure riding horse. If a young stallion has no show record, perhaps you can assess the quality of his movement and level of cooperation by watching an at-home training session.

> You can tell a gelding, ask a mare, but you must discuss it with a stallion.
> — Anonymous

Even if a stallion is an exceptional performer, however, he may not possess the prepotency to pass his abilities on to his offspring. Look at several sons or daughters, and if possible their dams, to get an idea of which type of mare produces a better "nick" with a particular stallion.

STILL TRUE TODAY

Historical Horsekeeping

"The law of like producing like is inexorable; consequently, to raise good horses, good horses must be bred from. Many farmers, who are keenly alive to other interests, are singularly thoughtless and imprudent in this. If a mare is broken down, and unfit for labor, no matter how coarse or badly formed she is, or what the evidence of constitutional unsoundness, she is usually reserved to breed from. On the same principle, no matter how coarse the stallion, if he is fat and sleek, and if his use can be obtained cheap, he is selected for the same purpose. It costs just as much to raise a poor, coarse-blooded colt as a fine-blooded one."— Magner's Standard Horse and Stock Book *by D. Magner, 1916*

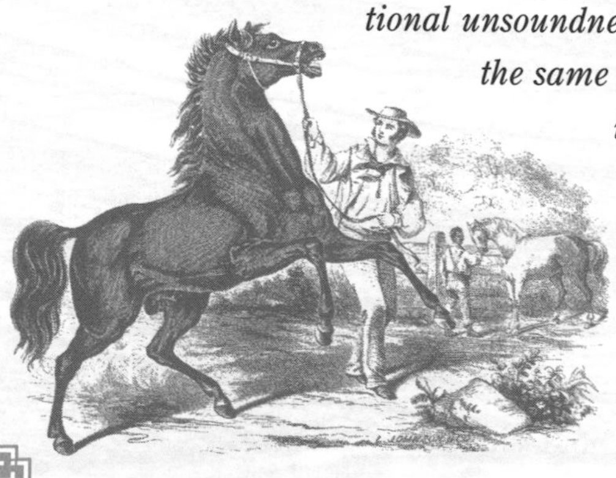

Judging Character

Some traits are more difficult to assess in a one-time visit to a stallion. Since temperament can help or hinder a horse in the expression of his physical abilities, it needs to be near the top of your list of breeding criteria. The trouble is, a horse's general patterns of behavior are difficult to estimate accurately, especially during a brief view, so plan to visit several times. No matter what the use of a horse, it is certain that an honest and intelligent individual has an advantage to succeed in the world of training.

You can get a fairly good sense of the overall attitude of a stallion toward humans by observing him at the farm and at competitions. Whether you place more emphasis on patience or bravery, calmness or aggressiveness, is largely a matter of personal taste and intended use. Nevertheless, any stallion should be tractable, cooperative, and have a high level of self-preservation, evidenced by his adaptability.

INCENTIVE PROGRAMS. Once your mare has passed her critique and the field of stallions has been limited to a few top contenders, look at other factors that can influence your final choice. If you are interested in showing the resulting foal, it is in your best interest if the farm has solid, long-range plans for promoting the stallion and his offspring. This may be evidenced by the partnership of the stallion with a competent trainer who has developed a goal-oriented competition schedule for the horse. Or promotion may be in the form of an awards incentive program for the owners of the stallion's offspring.

STUD FARM MANAGEMENT. Take a careful look at the management of the stud farm. It should not be assumed that a stallion with a fantastic physique and impressive lineage has necessarily landed in the hands of a competent horseman. Although the stallion provides the genes, the overall professionalism at the stud farm can have a large affect on whether or not your mare becomes pregnant.

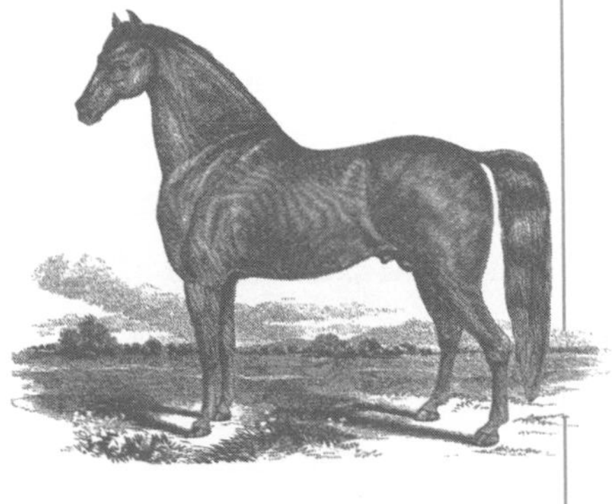

Horse breeding involves a significant investment of time, money, and other resources. If you devise a plan and carefully consider the options, you reduce the risks and increase your chances of ending up with the foal you desire.

Code of the West

- ★ Live each day with courage.
- ★ Take pride in your work.
- ★ Always finish what you start.
- ★ Do what has to be done.
- ★ Be tough but fair.
- ★ When you make a promise, keep it.
- ★ Ride for the brand.
- ★ Talk less and say more.
- ★ Remember that some things aren't for sale.
- ★ Know where to draw the line.

(from *Cowboy Ethics: What Wall Street Can Learn from the Code of the West* by James P. Owen)

QUESTIONS TO ASK AT A STUD FARM. Are the mares exercised daily? Are the stalls and pens safe? Will the mares be mixed in with other horses? Are the farm workers competent, and do they appear to enjoy their work? Are the stalls clean? Do the horses have good feed and clean water? Are the mares fatter or thinner than your mare should be? Is the feeding program flexible? Is the farm's veterinarian a reputable equine specialist? Do you notice any stable vices that you do not want your mare to acquire during her stay? Are the horses handled with respect? Are the visitors and clients handled with professionalism?

Does the farm use natural service or artificial insemination, or does it ship semen to the mare owner? What percentage of mares are settled on the first breeding? This depends on a variety of factors, one of which is viability and quantity of semen. However, even a stallion with low volume, poor-quality semen, if properly managed, can adequately settle mares. The competence of the staff in mare teasing and preparation, stallion handling, and laboratory procedures will greatly affect conception rates.

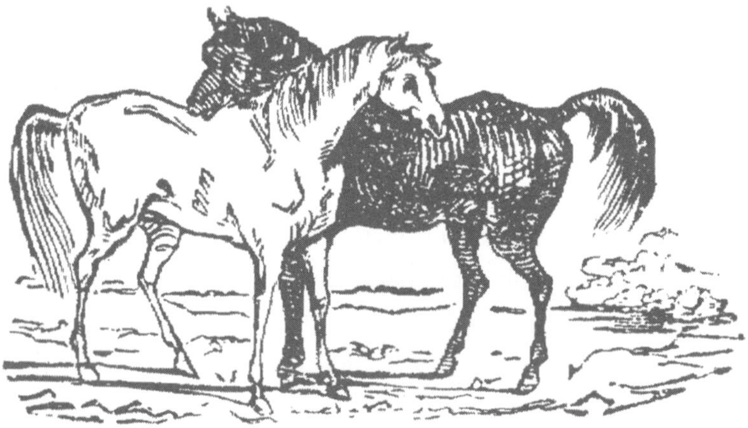

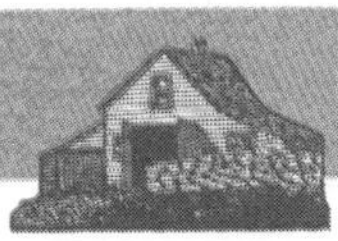

LIFE IN THE PEN

Before we bring the horses in from pasture to their individual pens for the spring, we give all the pens a once-over. This includes checking all panel connections, gates, wooden posts, or other wooden areas that need a new coating of anti-chew product, and laying down a fresh layer of ⅜" minus pea gravel.

Our pens are located adjacent to a barn that provides covered shelter. Pens can vary in size from a bare minimum of a 16-foot by 60-foot individual run attached to a stall to a 60-foot by 100-foot or larger pen off the end of a barn or loafing shed for a group of horses.

A sheltered feeding area with rubber mats allows a horse to eat at ground level without ingesting sand or wasting feed. In the loafing area of the pen, bedding can be used to encourage a horse to lie down, but it usually invites a horse to defecate and urinate there also. This behavior can be minimized or eliminated by locking the horse out of the loafing or eating areas except during specific times.

Pen fencing can be made from metal panels or continuous fencing. Panels don't require setting posts, so they are more adaptable to changing pen size or shape. Whatever pen fencing is used, it needs to be tall enough (5 feet is adequate, 6 feet is better) and strong enough to withstand roughhousing, rubbing, and playing across the fence. Panel connections should be tight and safe.

PANEL GAPS. When choosing panels for horse pens, look for panels with tight-fitting connections. Avoid panels that have gaps that could trap a hoof or jaw. If you already have panels with dangerous gaps, you can use panel caps to close

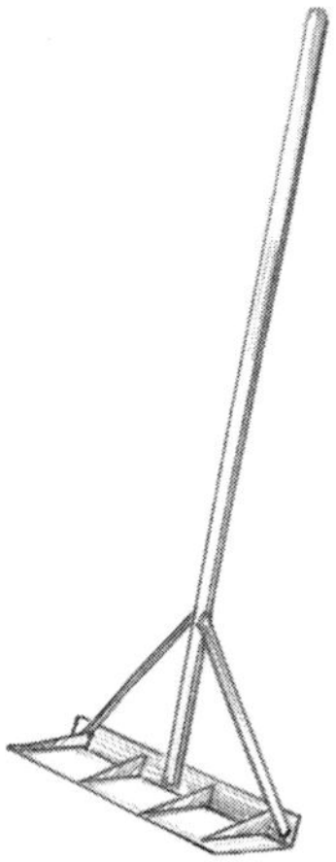

A landscape rake is useful for leveling pen gravel.

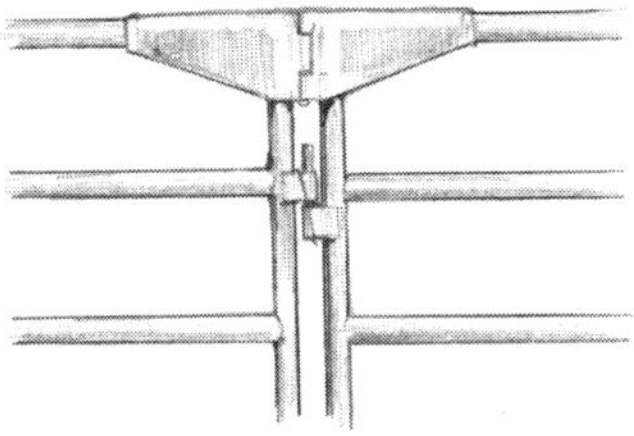

Panel caps close dangerously wide gaps.

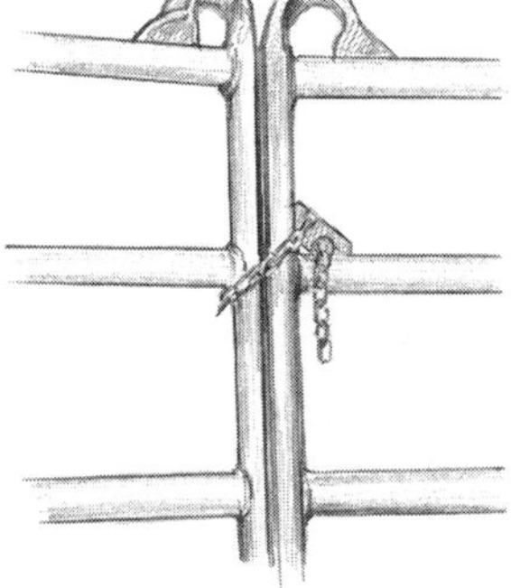

Panels with tight-fitting connections are safest.

A Good Pen

A horse pen should be located on high ground and situated so that the horses can take shelter from cold wind, wet weather, hot sun, and insects as needed. There should be a clean place to feed and a comfortable place for horses to lie down. To prevent feed from blowing away, windscreens can be attached to the outside of the panels. The land in pens and runs is considered "sacrifice" because no vegetation is expected to survive the constant traffic.

If the natural lay of the land doesn't slope away from the barn or shed, then excavation should remedy this so that the shelter under the building is high and dry, and the pen or run gradually slopes, at a grade of about 2 degrees, away from the building. Depending on the native soil, footing can be added to provide cushion and minimize mud. Some choices are decomposed granite, road base, and pea gravel.

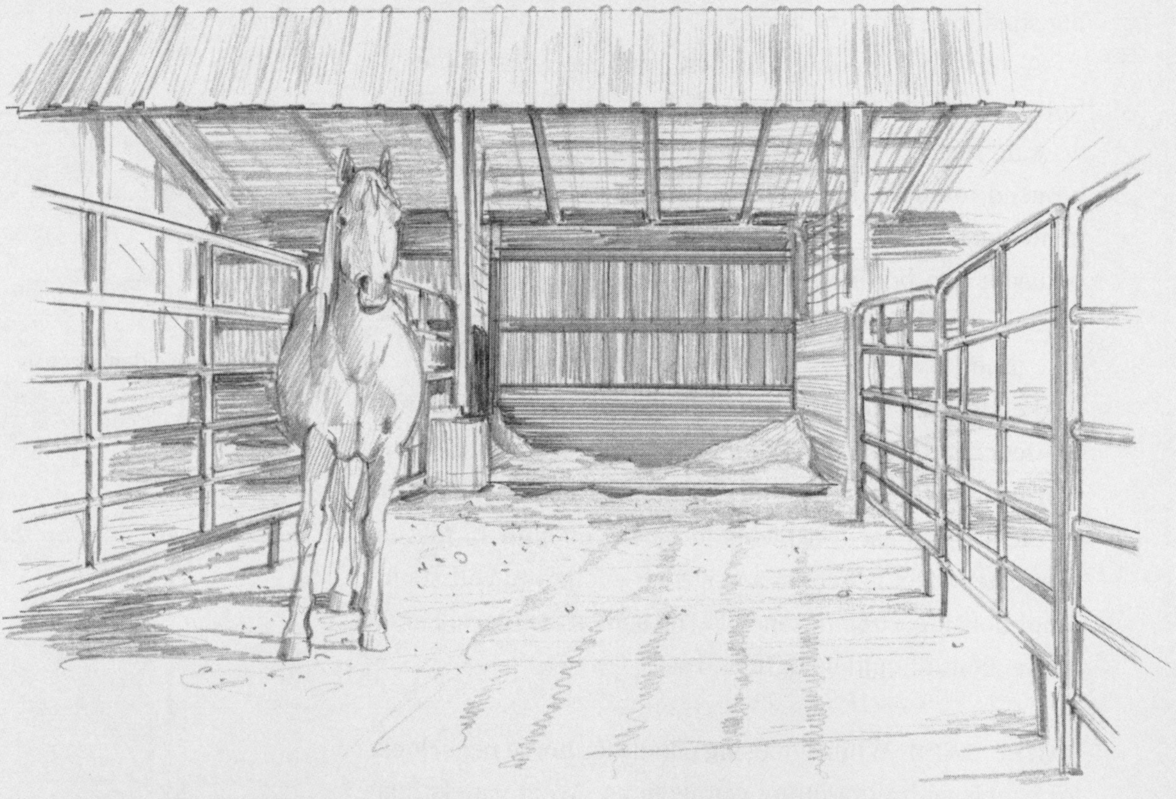

A good pen has shelter, safe, durable fencing, and comfortable, well-drained footing.

the gaps and make the panels safer for horses. A simple, easy-to-install, and tidy way to block the gap on unsafe panels, they are tough, durable plastic connectors with hinges allowing them to conform to various angles. They are adaptable to fit various sizes and styles of panels and gates and quickly attach to the panels with nylon zip ties. (See the Resource Guide at *www.horsekeeping.com.*)

PANEL GATES. Some horses can open gate and panel latches that are supposed to be horseproof. When I want to be sure a horse stays put, I add extra security — a 3⁄16-inch zinc-plated (galvanized) general utility chain and horseproof snap. A short piece of chain and a double-ended snap ensure that a horse will not get loose even if the latch does come open.

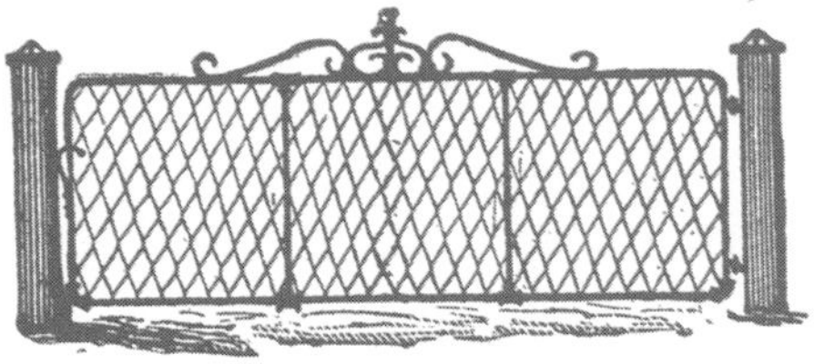

RPMS & PTOS

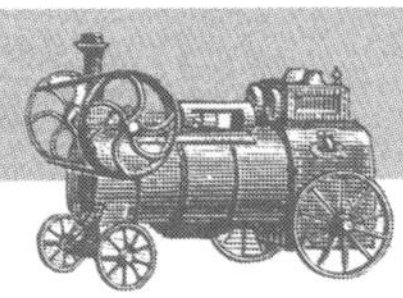

TYPES OF MOWERS

It won't be long before we will need to fire up the mowers, so this is a good time to discuss them. Mowers come in various styles and are designed to cut hay, weeds, or brush. Rotary, sickle bar, and disc are the most commonly used on horse farms.

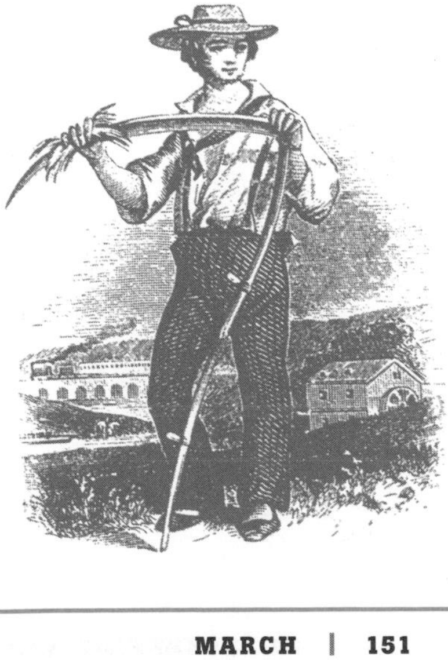

ROTARY MOWER. The most popular choice, rotary mowers are available as either pull-type with self-contained engines, pull-type powered by a PTO (power takeoff), or three-point hitch/PTO models. Engine-driven mowers are small and designed to be pulled behind a small tractor or utility vehicle. Rotary mowers can be found in widths from 3 to 20 feet and can be raised and lowered to the desired mowing height (approximately 1 to 13 inches). Pull-type

Ranking Mowers

Mowers are ranked according to the diameter of material they can cut, from approximately 1 to 4 inches. Those at the low end are turf and pasture mowers; those at the high end are "brush hogs," which are designed to chop and shred brush and small bushes.

mowers are raised or lowered with a manual crank or a hydraulic-assist cylinder. Three-point hitch mowers are raised and lowered using the three-point hitch.

Rotary mowers have from one to four tail wheels to help support and balance the mower in order to minimize scalping (cutting into the earth) on uneven terrain. Most have rubber or metal deflector shields or optional chain guards to keep rocks or other debris from flying out when mowing.

SICKLE BAR MOWER. Sickle bar mowers use a bar of cutting blades pulled back and forth with a pitman arm, which slides across a fixed-position bar of cutting blades to cut

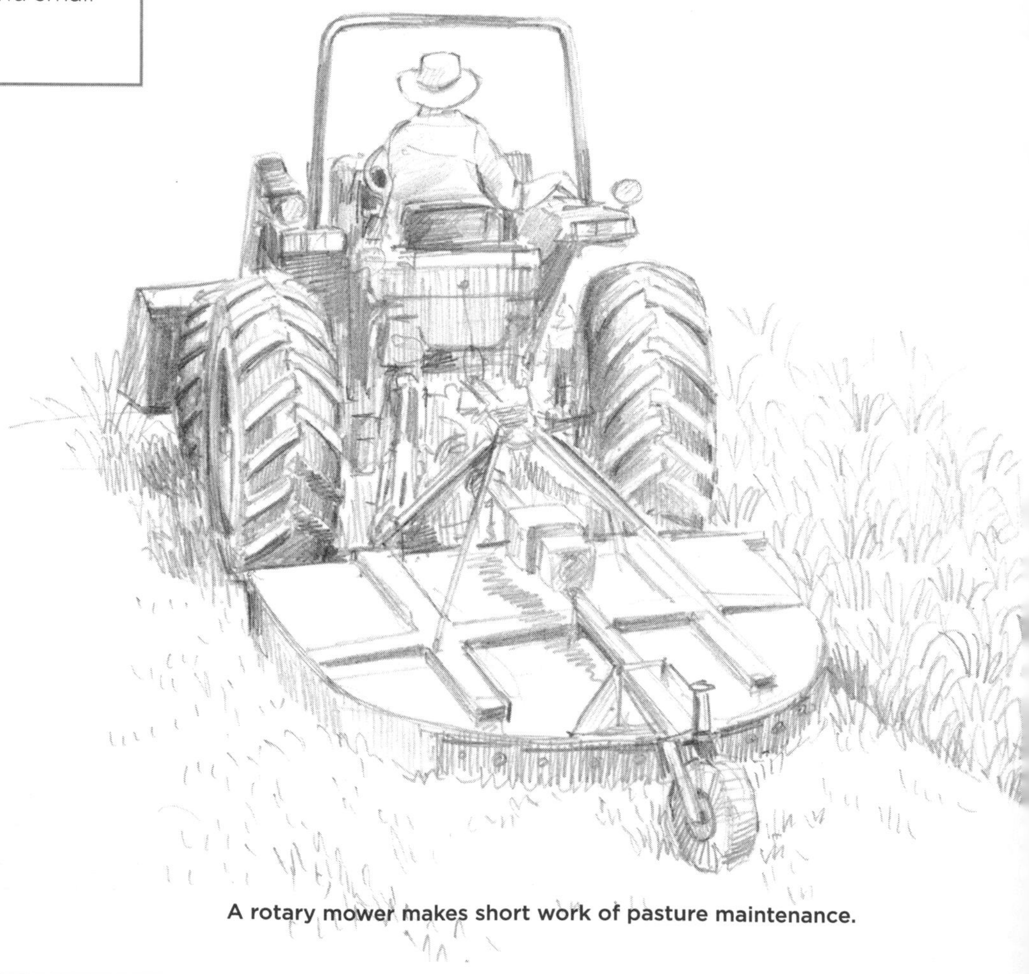

A rotary mower makes short work of pasture maintenance.

grass crops on relatively smooth surfaces. The sickle bars range in width from 6 to 8 feet and can be used for trimming banks as well as mowing fields. Although they cut more cleanly than a rotary mower, they are more costly, they don't have as wide a mowing height range as rotary mowers, and they tend to clog. They are best suited for flat ground.

DISC MOWER. A cross between a sickle bar and rotary mower, disc mowers result in less plugging than sickle bar and higher ground speed than rotary. They have similar height adjustment to a sickle mower.

FLAIL MOWER. A flail mower knocks down high growth with its heavy-duty cutting blades, so it is suitable for coarse growth along roads, field edges, or heavily weeded areas.

Choosing the Right Mower

If your pasture is uneven, a rotary mower would probably be most appropriate. For cutting hay, a sickle bar or disc mower would be best. If you have brush or heavy weed areas that need to be removed, consider a brush hog, which is a heavy-duty rotary cutter/shredder.

Blade Options

Most blades can be sharpened or replaced. Some mowers have a choice of blades depending on the type of soil and vegetation you have.

★ **Low lift.** Aerodynamic design of blade creates minimal updraft so is good in sandy or loose soil.

★ **Medium lift.** The average blade for normal use.

★ **High lift.** Creates high suction to make plants stand up, but requires greater horsepower to operate in dense stands. Not to be used in sandy soil.

★ **Mulching blade.** Irregular edges chop and shred materials rather than just cutting them.

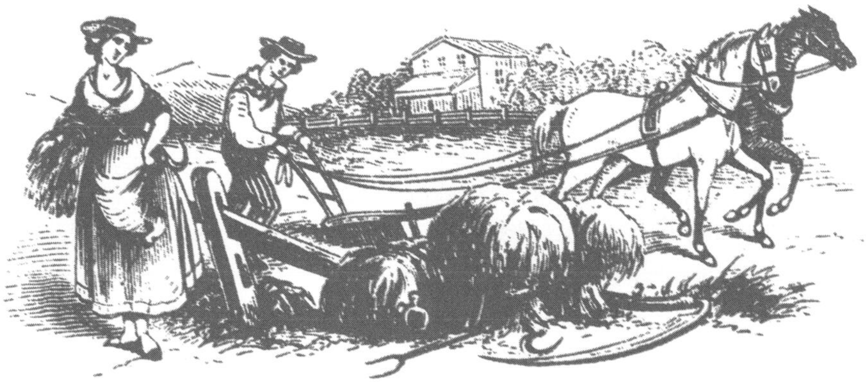

MORE IN DEPTH

NATURAL HORSEKEEPING

Confining horses is inherently unnatural. Yet we can all design our facilities and management routines to give horses as natural a life as our situation allows. The best way to prevent vices is to house and care for your horse using principles of natural horsekeeping. These include:

- Main nutrition from grass pastures or grass hay.
- As much turnout as practical in an area where cantering is possible.
- Living with companions or living near companions.
- Large pen with sheltered loafing and eating areas when pasture is not available.
- When pasture is not available, free-choice grass hay or minimum of three feedings per day of grass hay.
- Minimal or no grain.
- Free-choice salt, minerals, and freshly drawn or naturally aerated water.

Odd Word

sulcus. Cleft. On the bottom of the horse's hoof there is a V-shaped cushion called the frog. On both sides of the frog, there are clefts, referred to as the collateral sulci.

HORSEKEEPING ACROSS AMERICA

FLOODING IN THE SOUTH

The United States federal government prepares floodplain maps based on records of flooding and the integrity of levees, effects of dams, and other factors such as topography. (See the Federal Emergency Management Agency [FEMA] Web site listed in the appendix.) These maps give landowners an idea of how likely their property is to flood. They also provide insurance companies with risk estimates, and inform developers where they can't build.

For horsekeepers, flooding can present a series of problems including:

- Need to evacuate
- Loss of feed
- Loss of drinking water
- Loss of property (such as buildings, tack, or vehicles)
- Loss of utilities

When real-estate shopping, pay very close attention to areas at high risk for natural disasters. Often, risky areas aren't even insurable, so choose another location.

Detailed emergency management guidelines are given throughout this book.

Purchasing a Horse Farm

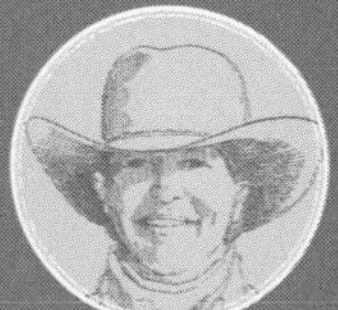

Ask Cherry

Q My husband and I are looking to purchase a small horse farm, mostly for our own use. We have no experience in owning or operating a barn. We were hoping you could recommend 10 of the most important things to look for, a checklist of sorts, as we begin researching and planning to purchase something. Do you have any advice you could give us?

A Ten important things to consider when buying a horse acreage:

1. Location
2. Zoning
3. Size of acreage
4. Homeowner's Association covenants
5. Water
6. Neighbors
7. Existing facilities
8. Soil
9. Native insects and local diseases
10. Price

APRIL

April is always full of hope that we will have a great grazing year. I know that the better I care for our pastures, the better they will care for our horses. My goal is to have well-managed pastures, because part of the dream of having a horse is the satisfaction of seeing him peacefully grazing and knowing that he is getting good nutrition. This time of year, I have either already harrowed or will do so before the grass begins to grow.

Day Length in Hours

		Date		
		April 1	April 15	May 1
Latitude	60°N	12.84	14.22	15.57
	55°N	12.69	13.82	14.91
	50°N	12.58	13.52	14.41
	45°N	12.48	13.27	14.01
	40°N	21.41	13.07	13.68
	35°N	12.34	12.89	13.4
	30°N	12.28	12.73	13.15

See page 22 to find your latitude.

LIGHTNING PRECAUTIONS

During the spring and summer, when you and your horses are leading your active lives, be aware of the potential danger of lightning. In the United States, approximately 300 human injuries and 65 deaths are attributed to lightning strikes each year. There are no statistics on horses or livestock, but the casualties can be quite high when lightning hits a herd.

Lightning is associated with developing summer thunderstorms. As air heats and causes cumulus clouds to grow upward, the stage is set for lightning. When lightning strikes, it can be a direct hit from the cloud-to-ground flash or it can erupt from the charge traveling along the ground.

When a storm is 10 miles away, you can usually hear the thunder, and if you can hear thunder, you are considered within striking range of lighting. The National Weather Service suggests using the 30-30 Rule (see box on page 158) to determine how far you are from the danger of a storm. If you are within 6 miles of the storm, you should seek shelter for you and your horse. It is recommended to stay in the shelter until 30 minutes after you hear the last clap of thunder.

SHELTER FROM THE STORM. What is safe shelter? A large, enclosed building or an enclosed metal vehicle. A fully enclosed building with a roof, walls, and floor is usually safe because it has wiring and plumbing and if lightning struck, the current would travel through the utilities to the ground. Knowing this, you will understand why you should stay away from plumbing and electronics during a storm. Although a picnic shelter, lean-to, carport, shed, or barn overhang might keep you dry, they really aren't a safeguard against lightning strikes.

To Do

- ❑ Hoof trim and shoe
- ❑ Vaccinate (see Immunizations in March Vet Clinic)
- ❑ Scrub feed tubs and buckets
- ❑ Move hay to barns
- ❑ Skin check
- ❑ Pasture tune-up
- ❑ Spring clean-up
- ❑ Review in-hand work
- ❑ Truck/trailer maintenance

To Buy

- ❑ Complete feed wafers
- ❑ Grain
- ❑ Dewormer

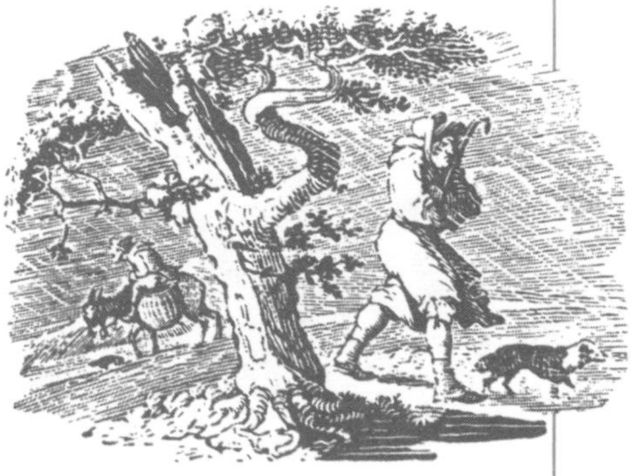

The 30-30 Rule

If you have a clear line of sight to the storm, watch for lightning, then count (or look at your watch) until you hear thunder. If the time elapsed between the lightning and thunder is 30 seconds or less, the thunderstorm is within 6 miles of you and is considered dangerous. You and your horse should seek shelter immediately. Remain there until 30 minutes after you hear the last thunderclap.

— *National Weather Service*

A hard-topped vehicle (such as a car, SUV, minivan, truck, bus, or tractor with a cab) can also be safe. Keep all doors closed and all windows rolled up. Do not touch any metal surfaces while you are riding out the storm. If you are hauling a horse in a trailer and you can't find shelter, pull off the roadway until the storm passes. Do not use electronic devices such as HAM radios or cell phones during a thunderstorm.

TIME CHANGE IN CANADA

Although we used to change our clocks in the United States at 2:00 a.m. on the first Sunday of April, this has been changed to March as of 2007. Read the entry in March Wacky Wonderful Weather. In Canada (except for Saskatchewan) and Mexico, however, the DST change still takes place at 2:00 a.m. local time on the first Sunday in April.

Play It Safe in a Thunderstorm

There is no safe place outside, but if you have no alternative, there are some things that can slightly reduce your chances of being struck by lightning.

★ Seeking shelter under tall, isolated trees actually increases your risk of being struck by lightning.

★ If you are in a heavily wooded area, wait out the storm near a low stand of trees.

★ Stay away from metal objects such as fences. The current from lightning can travel a long distance along a fence.

★ If you are caught riding in the open, and lightning is within 5 miles of you, stop, dismount, and go to a ditch or a low spot and sit down on the ground.

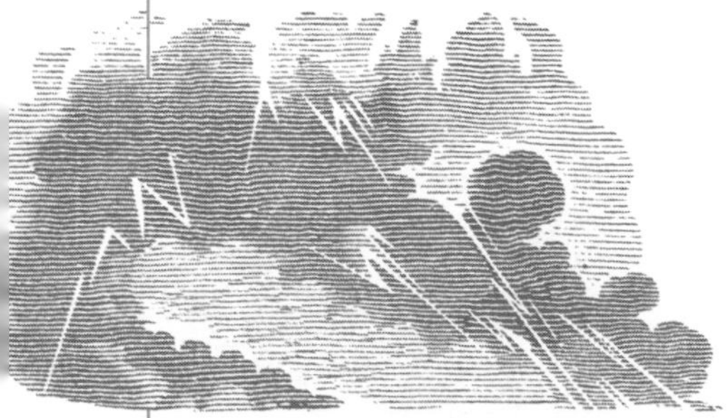

On the last Sunday in October, Canadian areas on Daylight Saving Time return to Standard Time at 2:00 a.m. Some areas of Canada not using Daylight Saving Time include Fort St. John, Charlie Lake, Taylor and Dawson Creek in British Columbia, Creston in the East Kootenays, and most of Saskatchewan (except Denare Beach and Creighton). Canada uses six primary time zones, the last four of which are the same time zones as the United States. From east to west they are Newfoundland Time Zone, Atlantic Time Zone, Eastern Time Zone, Central Time Zone, Mountain Time Zone, and Pacific Time Zone.

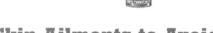

VET CLINIC

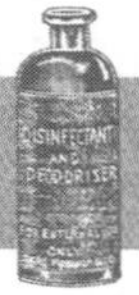

Ten Skin Ailments to Avoid

Here is a brief primer on some of the most common skin problems that might plague a horse.

1. **Rain rot** is caused by *Dermatophilus*, an infectious microorganism from the soil that eagerly becomes established in skin cracks under a dirty hair coat during rainy weather. The painful, tight scabs that form on the horse's neck, shoulders, back, and rump make him uncomfortable and unusable, and require medication and bathing.

2. **Seborrhea** is a skin disease caused by a malfunction in sebum production and function, resulting in flaky skin.

3. **Ringworm** is a fungal infection affecting the skin and hair, characterized by round, crusty patches with hair loss. It is easily spread between horses via tack and grooming tools.

Sweet Itch

Some horses seem to be hypersensitive or allergic to insect bites and, once bitten, go into a rubbing frenzy. This invites other complications sometimes referred to as sweet itch or Queensland itch. Consult a veterinarian, and prevent bites to susceptible animals. Remedies include soothing witch hazel or vinegar rinses, and possibly a corticosteroid prescription from your veterinarian.

4. **Photosensitivity** of the skin (usually under white hair) can result from components of certain plants (ingested). The skin becomes red, then sloughs off.

5. **Warts,** most commonly on the muzzle of a young horse, are caused by the equine papillomavirus. As a horse matures, he develops immunity to the virus and the warts disappear. The same virus also causes aural plaque, a scaly condition inside the ear, which can become painful if flies are allowed to bite and feed inside the ears.

6. **Sarcoids** are common skin tumors with unknown cause. There are several types, mostly occurring around the head or the site of an old injury.

7. **Thrush** is a fungal infection of the hoof that thrives in moist, dirty environments. (See March Foot Notes for more details.)

Skin Check

As your horse is shedding and being bathed and clipped throughout the spring, check his skin closely for signs of bacterial or fungal infections, ticks, or lice. Dermatitis is a general term for inflammation of the skin. There are many skin conditions, including rain rot, seborrhea, ringworm, photosensitization, warts, aural plaques, sarcoids, thrush, scratches, and external parasites including ticks and mange mites.

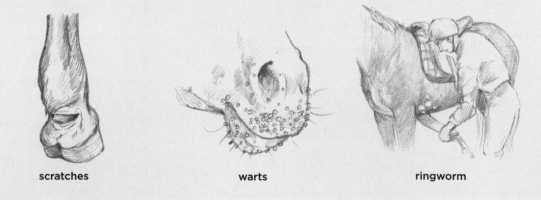

scratches

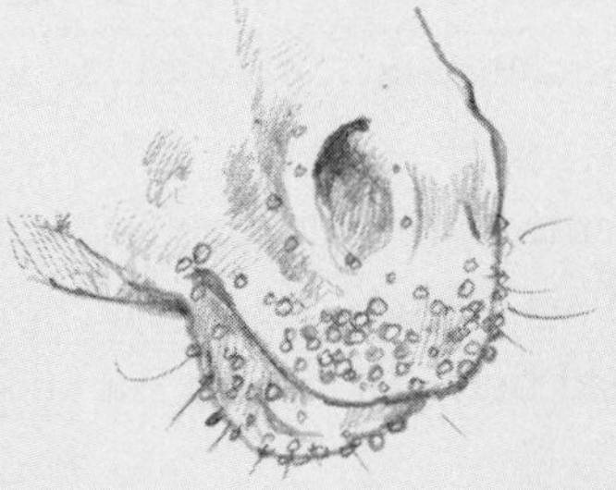

warts

ringworm

8. **Scratches** is a common term that refers to a general localized skin inflammation found on the lower legs of horses. The thick, chronic sores at the heels and rear of the pastern can be quite painful. Scratches are linked to an opportunistic fungus, but can be complicated by bacterial infection.

In a case of scratches, also called grease heel, the pasterns, fetlocks, and cannons become crusty and covered with oozing scabs. In advanced cases, the legs swell and the horse becomes lame. The condition is more common on horses with white legs. Treatment usually includes a topical preparation including a fungicide. Prevention includes good sanitation, minimizing mud, and keeping the legs clean and clipped if necessary.

9. **Ticks** cause crusty scabs and can be disease carriers. Check the mane and tail carefully throughout spring and summer. Use rubber gloves or tweezers to remove ticks, which can carry Lyme disease that can also affect humans (see July Vet Clinic). Be sure to remove the entire tick. If the head is left in, it can cause a painful infection. (See this month's Pest Patrol.)

10. **Lice** are not common in horses unless they are poorly kept and crowded. Then lice can spread rapidly through a group. You'd find the nits (eggs) or the lice themselves along the midline of the horse, such as in the mane and tail head.

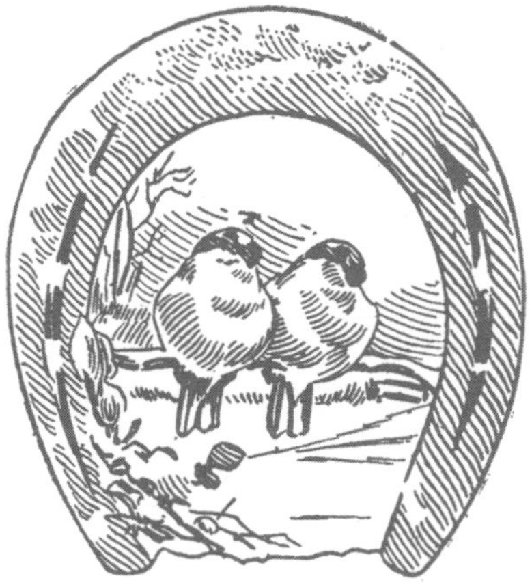

Which Itch Is Which?

Biting gnats, lice, ticks, fungus, and allergies can all cause itching. If your horse rubs bald spots in his mane or tail, check him thoroughly for external parasites such as lice or ticks, parasites (such as pinworms), or fungus, and treat according to your veterinarian's instructions.

Itching can also be caused by ringworm, which is contagious to you and other horses. If a horse has ringworm, you will need not only to treat the horse but also to disinfect grooming tools, halters, blankets, stalls, feeders, and anything else he may have rubbed on.

Ranch Notes

April 2 Bathe Aria
April 3 Bathe Seeker
April 4 Bathe Zipper
April 5 Bathe Dickens

Odd Word

floating a hoof. Trimming that portion of the hoof behind the crack about a quarter inch shorter so it will not contact the shoe.

Cracks do not "heal" back together. The hoof wall must be replaced by new growth from the coronary band, just as a damaged fingernail must grow out, taking nine to 12 months.

CRACKS IN THE HOOF

Cracks are separations or breaks in the hoof wall. Vertical cracks between the hoof horn tubules are referred to by their location, such as toe cracks, quarter cracks, and heel cracks. Sand cracks originate at the coronet, while grass cracks start at the ground surface.

A horizontal crack in the hoof wall is called a blow-out. Blow-outs are caused either by an injury to the coronary band or by a blow to the hoof wall. A blow-out usually will not result in lameness, and many times will go unnoticed until your farrier spots it. Once they occur, these cracks seldom increase in size horizontally and usually require no treatment. However, a blow-out can set the stage for a vertical crack if the hoof is weakened by excess moisture or is not in balance.

Cracks do not "heal" back together. The hoof wall must be replaced by new growth from the coronary band, just as a damaged fingernail must grow out, taking nine to 12 months. For optimal hoof growth, the horse's ration must contain nutrients necessary for healthy hoof horn.

SAND CRACKS. These cracks can result from an imbalanced hoof, an injury to the coronet, or a foot infection that breaks out at the coronet. Sometimes a horse will bump the coronet when loading or unloading from a trailer, or the horse might strike his coronet during fast work or an uncoordinated movement.

A wet environment containing sand or gravel can soften a horse's hooves and force particles up into the white line. If infection results, it can travel upward through the laminae and break out at the coronet, possibly forming a crack.

The first step in dealing with sand cracks is to determine the cause and remove it. This, plus a good shoeing, may be all that is necessary to stabilize the hoof as it replaces the damaged horn. Severe cracks can be held immobile by a variety of methods until the hoof grows out. These may include nailing or screwing across the crack, drilling holes on either side and lacing the crack up like a boot, fastening a metal or plastic plate across the crack with screws or glue, and patching the crack with specially designed epoxy.

Before the crack can be stabilized, it must be thoroughly cleansed of dirt, loose hoof horn, and bacteria. If there is any evidence of moist (live) tissue, the crack must be treated by a veterinarian until it is completely dry. Applying any type of patching material over a moist crack would seal in bacteria, inviting an infection to develop or escalate.

GRASS CRACKS. These cracks most often appear in unshod hooves that have been allowed to grow too long, and often all they need is a good trimming. More severe cracks may require shoes for several months until new hoof tissue can grow down to replace the cracked horn. To help toe cracks grow out, the hoof angle must be kept correct and a square-toed or rocker-toed shoe should be applied to minimize the prying effect of breakover.

SURFACE CRACKS. These tiny fissures, which cover varying portions of the hoof wall, are most often caused by a change in hoof moisture, such as when a horse on wet pasture is put in a stall with dry bedding, or a horse that has been standing in mud then stands in the sun. Surface cracks are remedied by stabilizing the horse's moisture balance, minimizing his exposure to wetness, and using a hoof sealer. Thick hoof dressings may fill the cracks and improve the exterior appearance of a hoof, but a hoof sealer is more beneficial to long-term hoof health.

TIPS & TECHNIQUES

Severe Hoof Cracks

Chronic or very severe cracks toward the heel of the hoof are sometimes dealt with by removing the section of the hoof wall behind the crack. The hoof is then supported by a full support shoe until new hoof grows down.

A simpler approach is to apply a full support shoe and "float" the portion of the hoof behind the crack. By eliminating weight-bearing behind the crack, movement of the two halves of the crack is minimized and the hoof will often grow down intact. A horse that is very active or in work, however, will likely need to have the crack more securely stabilized.

FEED BAG

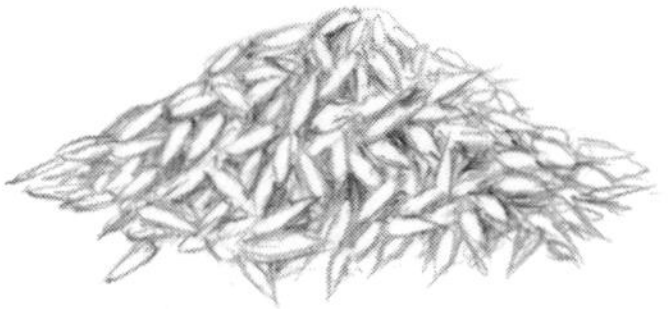

oats

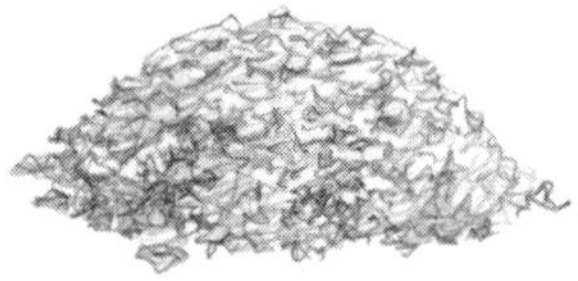

bran

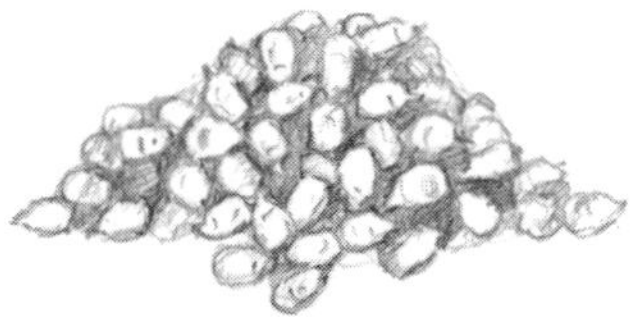

corn

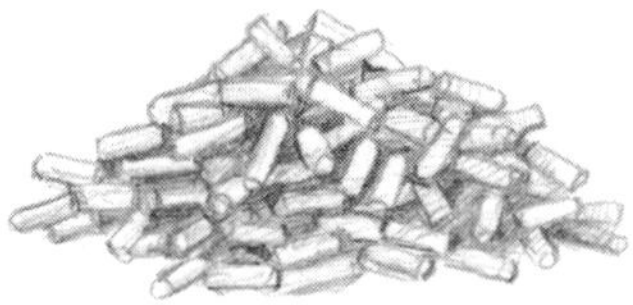

beet pellets

GRAINS IN THE SPRING DIET

This time of year, I might gradually introduce or increase grain in proportion to a horse's workload. Many horses do not need to be fed grain, but young horses, horses in hard work, pregnant mares, and mares with foals usually need grain and supplements.

Oats are the traditional horse grain. They provide fiber from their hulls and energy from the kernels. Oats are the safest grain to feed a horse, because they are a good balance between concentrate and roughage.

Corn has a very thin covering that does not have much fiber, but the kernel does provide a great deal of energy. Because corn is so quickly and easily digested, it is too concentrated for some horses. A can of corn has twice the energy content as the same-sized can of oats.

Commercially prepared horse feeds are available as pellets or grain mixes. Pellets might have both hay and grain in them. "Sweet feed" grain mixes are usually made up of oats or barley and corn, molasses, and a protein pellet. Feed companies create different products for different horse groups — you can find special feed for foals, yearlings, performance horses, broodmares, and even senior horses.

When you feed commercial grain mixtures, be sure to carefully weigh each horse's amount on a scale; do not carelessly give your horse a scoop of feed without knowing how much the grain weighs. Because grains vary so much in their density and feed value, they should always be fed by weight, not volume. For example, a small bucket that holds 2 pounds of bran would hold 5 pounds of sweet feed, 6.25 pounds of oats, and, 8 pounds of corn. Once you have figured how many pounds of what type of grain your horse should be fed, use a scale to weigh his ration. That way, your horse will get the same amount each feeding, which will minimize the likelihood of overfeeding, underfeeding, or colic.

FEEDING HORSES INDIVIDUALLY

Especially when feeding grain, it is important to feed individually. I feed each of my horses separately according to his or her specific needs. I formulate each ration according to the season and the horse's age, weight, and activity level.

I used to be in charge of feeding large groups of horses at colleges and universities, sometimes as many as 100 head. I saw firsthand how feeding in groups can lead to competition, fighting, and injury. The dominant horses would get most of the feed, and the timid horses would get little or none. So we'd end up with one group of fat and feisty horses, and one group of skinny, timid horses. And that is not a good thing. Feeding individually assures me that each of my horses gets his specific ration and can eat in peace.

Preventing Bolting

Bolting is gobbling food without chewing thoroughly. If a horse bolts his feed, he can choke, colic, and lose the nutritional benefits of thoroughly chewing his grain. Instead of using deep feed buckets, which seems to encourage a horse to dive in and gulp, I use large, shallow grain feeders that allow the grain to spread out so that the horse has to nibble smaller amounts of grain with his lips. I also add a handful of complete feed wafers in with the grain, which further encourages a horse to sort and sift.

STILL TRUE TODAY

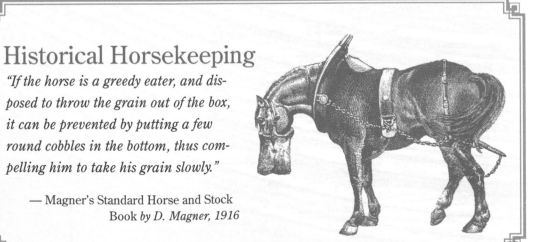

Historical Horsekeeping

"If the horse is a greedy eater, and disposed to throw the grain out of the box, it can be prevented by putting a few round cobbles in the bottom, thus compelling him to take his grain slowly."

— Magner's Standard Horse and Stock Book *by D. Magner, 1916*

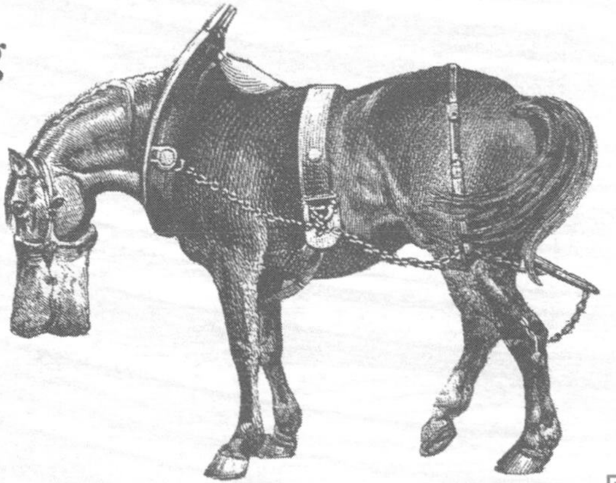

WILD LIFE

EAGLES

We are glad that proud and majestic golden and bald eagles share our mountain home. In fact, a group of four greeted me when I pulled up to our new home with the first load of our domestic possessions. I took it to be a powerful omen of a great place to live, and that has proven to be true.

Thou shall fly without wings, and conquer without any sword. O, horse!

— Bedouin Legend

Eagles, however, can also add unwanted drama, and even tragedy. One spring day when we were outdoors, Richard and I noticed a giant golden eagle on the hill behind our house. He didn't fly away when we approached, which seemed odd. Then he began hopping. We quickly ran through the possibilities: "Is he injured? No, he probably has a rabbit . . ."

Then, to our horror, we saw that he had our beloved cat Yoda, who had spent many years with us on the ranch. In the mountains, cats cheat death every day, and Yoda had lived a full, long life, a good portion of it hunting mice, gophers, and rabbits on the very hillside where he was taken. (See another eagle story in December Wild Life.)

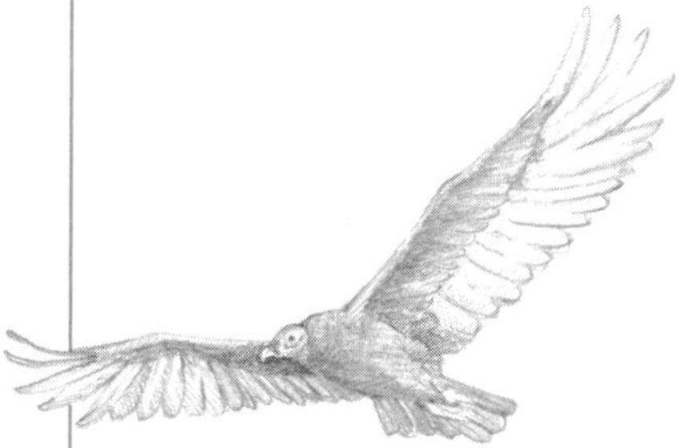

TURKEY VULTURES

About this time of year, we know summer is just around the corner when we see the first turkey vultures, also called turkey buzzards, soaring overhead. I first noticed that they circled our ranch every day about noon when I started taking my lunch on the front porch. Large dark brown birds that from far away could be mistaken for golden eagles, turkey buzzards are the bareheaded "cleaners" of the environment. What the eagles, mountain lions, bears, bobcats, and coyotes leave behind, the turkey buzzards will feast on.

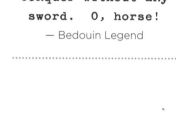

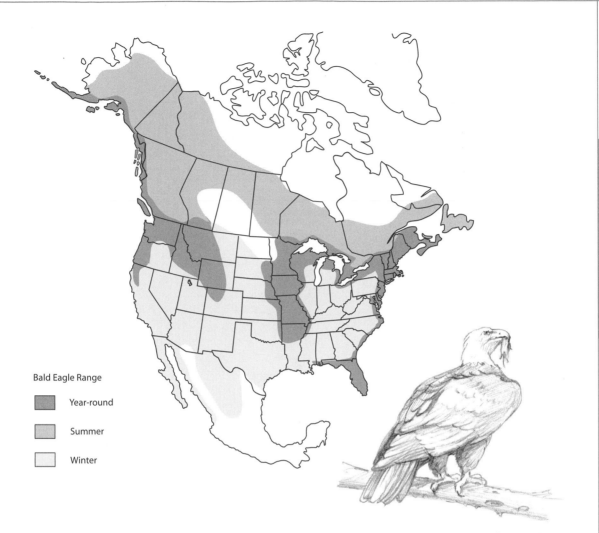

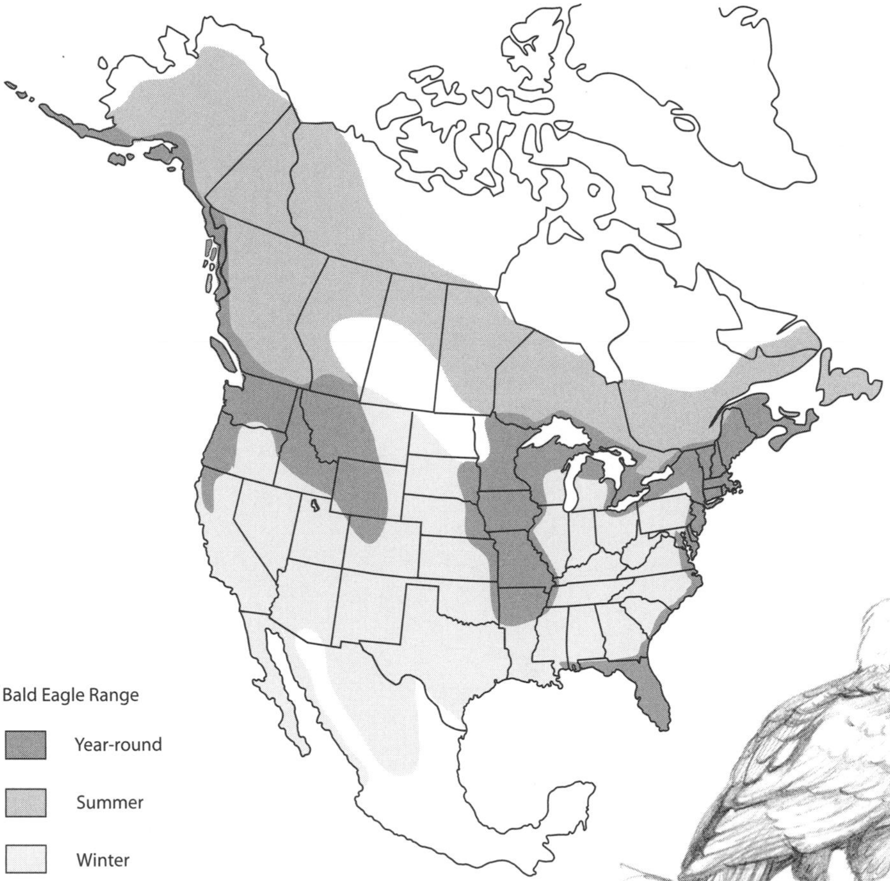

Bald Eagles at a Glance	
Location	Near water in most of North America
Status	Has been protected in United States since 1963
Color	Adopted as U.S. symbol of independence and strength in 1782; DDT banned in 1972 due to thin shells and infertile eggs Brown body, white head and tail, bright yellow bill, and exposed leg
Size	30 in. long; 72–84-in. wingspan; 8–14 lb
Lifespan	30 years or more; adult at 4–5 years
Diet	Fish, mammals, waterfowl, carrion
Breeding	Mates for life; returns to area where fledged; nests near water, in tree; nest often weighs hundreds of pounds

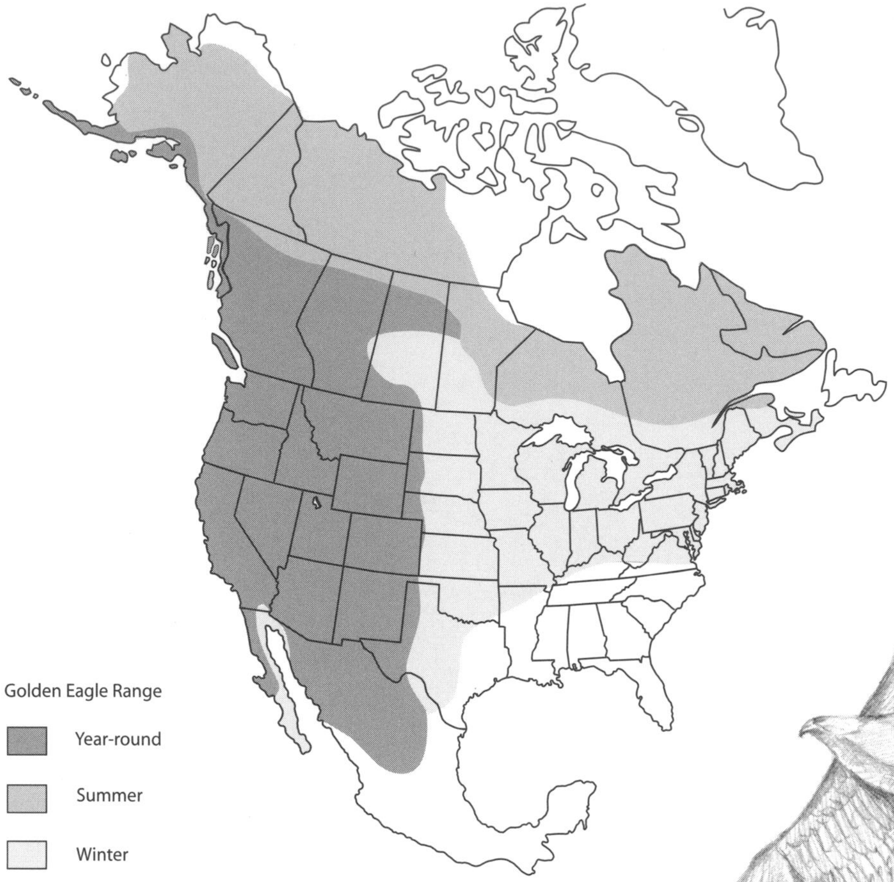

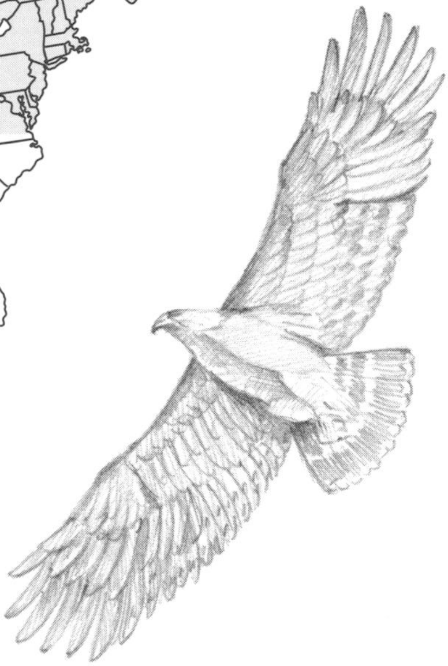

Golden Eagles at a Glance	
Location	Mostly in western states; some in eastern United States and eastern Canada.
Status	Protected in United States since 1963.
Color	Golden brown with light gold head and nape; white patches on underside of wing; broad white tail with dark band; leg feathers all the way down to the toes.
Size	27–33 in. long; 78-in. wingspan; 7–14 lbs
Lifespan	30 years or more; adult at 5 years
Diet	Rodents, rabbits, birds, reptiles, carrion
Breeding	Mates for life; nest of sticks on tree or cliff ledge; 1–2 eggs, rarely 3

PEST PATROL

TICKS: YOU AND YOUR HORSE

Rodents are the reservoir of Lyme disease (see July Vet Clinic), and black-legged ticks are the vehicles that transmit the disease from rodents to horses and humans. Currently there is no USDA-approved vaccine against Lyme disease for horses. The chances of you or your horse becoming infected with Lyme disease in the Northeast and certain parts of the Midwest can be 25 times that in other parts of the United States.

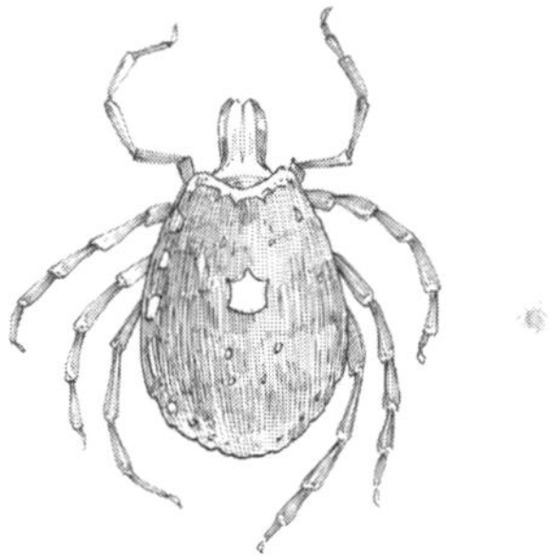

Deer tick shown at actual size and magnified.

Rocky Mountain spotted fever (RMSF) is the most severe tick-borne rickettsial illness of humans in the United States. It is caused by infection with the *Rickettsia rickettsii* bacteria via a bite by an infected tick, usually the American dog tick or Rocky Mountain wood tick. Initial symptoms are sudden onset of fever, headache, and muscle pain, followed by the development of a characteristic black rash. Without prompt and appropriate treatment it can be fatal.

RMSF was first recognized in 1896 in the Snake River Valley of Idaho and was originally called "black measles" because of the characteristic rash. But the name Rocky Mountain spotted fever is a misnomer. The disease is broadly distributed throughout the continental United States, as well as southern Canada, Central America, Mexico, and parts of South America. To date, RMSF has been reported in every U.S. state except Hawaii, Vermont, Maine, and Alaska.

MILLER MOTHS

"Miller" is a general term for moths around the home and stable. Here in Colorado we have the army cutworm. Your local miller moth might come from a different caterpillar. They emerge as flying adults in the spring and sometimes

Tick Talk

Keep your horses out of tick-infested areas, and carefully examine each one at least once a day for presence of ticks, especially during tick season in your area. Remove nymphs (immature ticks usually seen in spring) and adult ticks (usually seen during summer and fall) immediately. Ticks can attach anywhere on a horse, but common areas are on the chest, near the rectum, and along the base of the mane.

The Anti-Tick Attack

Especially if you ride in the woods, avoid tick infestation in these ways:

★ Wear light-colored clothing so you can spot ticks before they bite.

★ Tuck your pant legs into your socks so ticks can't crawl inside your pant legs.

★ Apply permethrin repellent to boots and clothing. It will last for days.

★ Apply products containing DEET to skin; this treatment will last a few hours.

★ Conduct frequent body checks during tick season. Enlist a partner or use a hand-held or full-length mirror to view all parts of your body. Remove any tick you find on your body.

★ Check all clothing, pets, and horses carefully. Although RMSF does not affect pets and horses, they can carry the ticks to you, putting you at risk.

Tick Removal

If you find one, grasp the tick as close to the horse's skin as possible, using a tick remover or fine tweezers and then pulling straight up with a slow, steady force. If you pinch the tick with a thumb and forefinger and squish it as you pull it out, you could squirt the diseased material from the tick into the horse or onto you.

Once you've removed the ticks, seal them in a Zip-close bag and dispose of it. Apply an antiseptic (alcohol or antibiotic ointment) to the bite site and wash your hands.

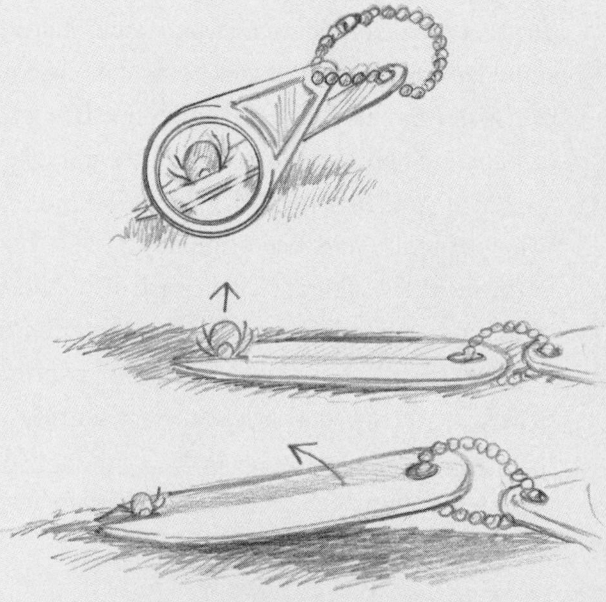

Grasp the tick as close to the horse's skin as possible, using a tick remover or fine tweezers, and then pull straight up with a slow, steady force.

invade the towns below us in droves on their way west up to the foothills. They spend one to two months at these higher elevations drinking nectar, then head east to lay eggs for the next cycle. There is no real control of these pests. We just try to keep buildings tightly closed and wait until the annoying migration is complete.

TENT CATERPILLARS

Several species of caterpillars feed on the chokecherry and mountain mahogany bushes, making a silken shelter (the tent) for themselves. They crawl out of their tents at night and eat, then go back in for the day. They enlarge the tent as they grow. Usually they are more unsightly than damaging, so it is often best to let the natural predators (birds, bugs, and wasps) control them. But some years, damage to trees and bushes is widespread and sustained, resulting in a high level of defoliation. In such cases, we walk around our property, each armed with a large paper feed bag, gloves, and clippers. We remove the tents from bush to bag, by hand or by pruning, and then burn the sacks.

> *Think, when we talk of horses,*
> that you see them
> Printing their proud hooves
> in the receiving earth;
> For 'tis your thoughts
> that now must deck our kings.
>
> — William Shakespeare, *Henry V*

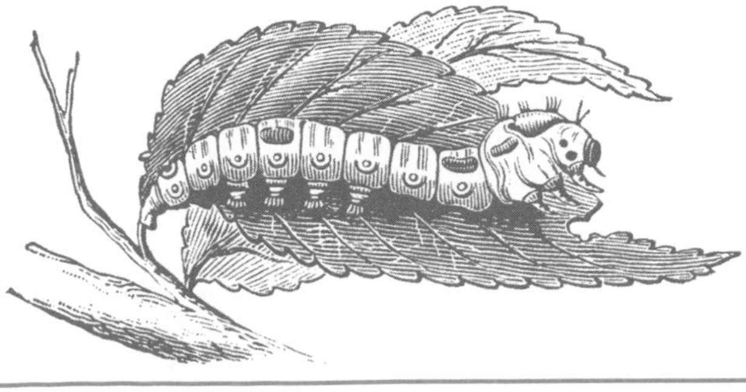

FYI

Miller Moths

Miller moths' name was inspired by the dusty scales on their wings, which brush off like powder or flour. A miller's clothing is often covered with a similar dust from flour grinding.

PASTURE PERFECT

MANAGEMENT GOALS

As mentioned, my goal is to have well-managed pastures. This time of year, I either have already harrowed or will do so before the grass begins to grow. I like to even out all of the pastures so they look smooth and ready to regenerate. Spraying with an herbicide before they emerge can reduce some of the early weeds.

IDEAL PASTURE

A good pasture has a stand of plants suitable for horses. The best kind of horse pasture is a well-drained grass mix with few weeds and no poisonous weeds, trees, or shrubs. If there is a good grass stand established, you have decent rainfall or access to irrigation, and you mow, harrow, and reseed as necessary, you should be able to keep one horse

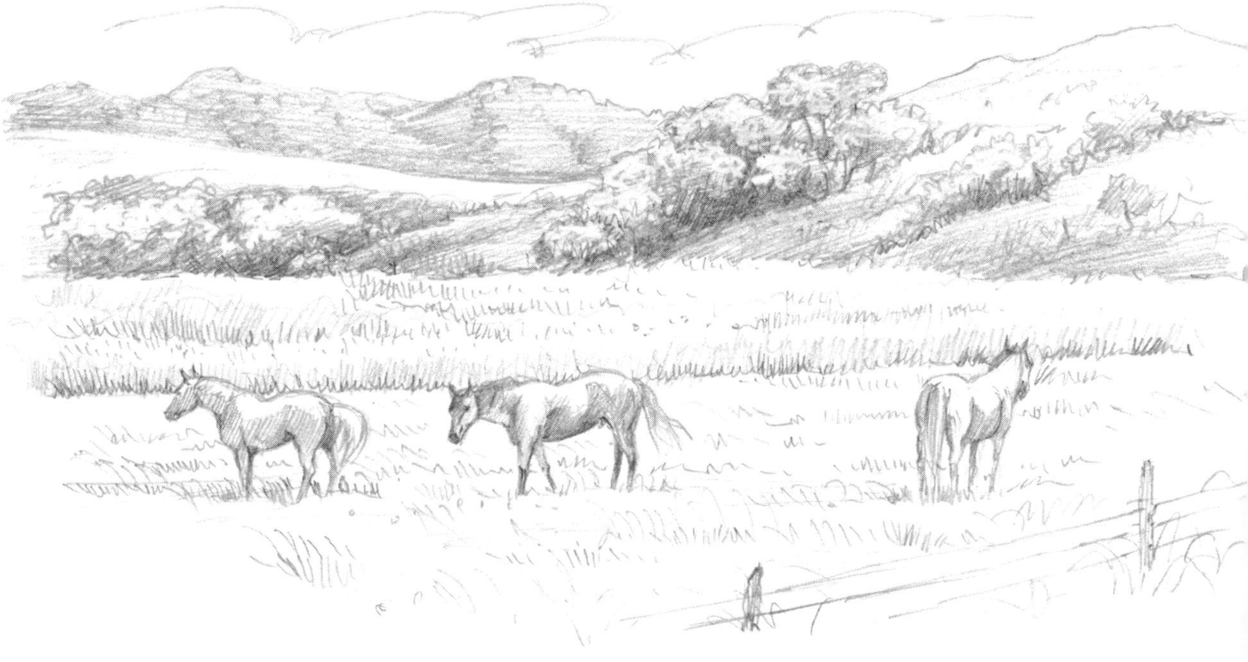

on an acre or two of pasture during the growing season. On the other hand, arid ranchland with minimal browse plants can require 20 acres or more to support a single horse. To get a better idea of the specific stocking rate for your property, contact your county extension agent.

SAFETY AND SECURITY. A pasture needs to be enclosed with safe fencing and gates; these should be at least 5 feet tall and well maintained to maximize the horses' safety and minimize the likelihood (and liability) of their escaping onto public or private property. Using electric fencing in conjunction with conventional fencing decreases the wear and tear on fences and adds to security, as long as the electric fence is checked daily to be sure it is working.

There should be no old dumps or farm equipment in a pasture; horses can easily get hurt on items that are hidden by tall grass.

Pastures should be well drained with no bogs, stagnant water, or sandy soil.

WATER. There should be easy and safe access to free-choice, good-quality water. Natural sources should be running, not stagnant. Know the source of the water your horse drinks. If it contains agricultural runoff, it could be high in nitrates. A trough or automatic waterer should be kept clean and situated to minimize mud and to prevent a horse from being crowded into a corner or against a fence.

SHELTER. The pasture should provide shelter — either natural (trees, rocks, or terrain) or man-made (a shed or windbreak) to ward off sun, wind, cold precipitation, and insects.

MINERALS. There should be free-choice salt and mineral blocks at all times.

Pasture Priorities

A good pasture:

★ has a stand of plants suitable for horses;

★ is enclosed with safe fencing and gates;

★ offers easy and safe access to free-choice, good-quality water;

★ contains no old dumps or farm equipment;

★ provides shelter against the elements;

★ is well drained;

★ offers free-choice salt and mineral blocks at all times.

If there is a good grass stand established, you have decent rainfall or access to irrigation, and you mow, harrow, and reseed as necessary, you should be able to keep one horse on an acre or two of pasture during the growing season.

SPRING: APRIL

Herbicide Pointers

Points to remember when using herbicides:

★ Get an applicator's license if required.

★ Mix according to directions.

★ Keep animals (including dogs and cats) away from the sprayed area as long as directions indicate.

★ Watch for wind drift or you could damage your fruit trees or your neighbor's garden.

★ Keep all pesticides away from streams and other water sources unless they are approved herbicides for riparian areas.

★ Wear a respirator, rubber boots (not leather shoes or boots), and rubber gloves.

SPRING PASTURE TUNE-UP

HARROWING. The principle behind harrowing a pasture after a grazing period is that it evens out rough spots and distributes manure clumps. If you are in a dry, sunny climate, this is a good practice because it dries the manure and helps to kill the parasite eggs. In humid climates, however, harrowing the manure in pastures just spreads the parasite eggs over a larger area while still allowing them to be viable, and so in effect increases a horse's chances of reinfestation. In such a situation, collecting manure and composting it would be best.

MOWING. Mowing can impair weed growth by removing the larger-leaved, more vigorous weeds that shade the developing desirable plants. If the plants are cut before the seedpods are mature, it can also prevent the start of a new cycle of weeds. Most fields tend to clean themselves of weeds with strategically timed pasture mowing or after the first cutting of hay during the second year.

BURNING. Burning eliminates mature vegetation and seeds and kills some parasites, but it can be a safety hazard and an air polluter. It is usually done in the spring. Check to see if your local ordinances require a burning permit.

USING HERBICIDES. It is difficult to control weeds chemically in a legume/grass hay field or pasture, as many of the herbicides would kill the desirable plants as well as the weeds. Herbicides can be used very effectively, however, in grass pastures. You will need to choose a selective herbicide specifically for your situation. Try to control your weeds by other means, but if you must use herbicides, carefully monitor every step or you can end up with a much greater problem than a few weeds.

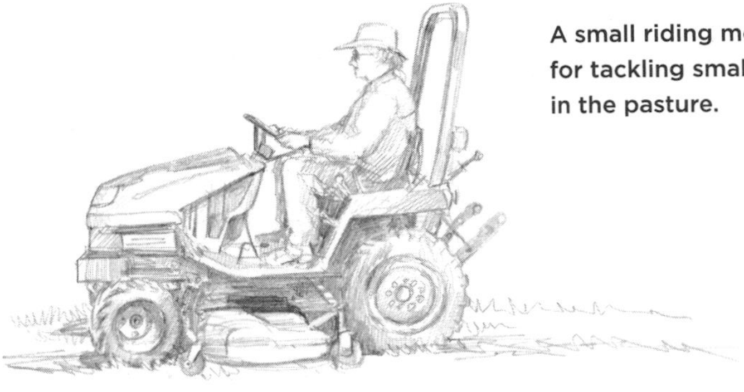

A small riding mower is handy for tackling small weed spots in the pasture.

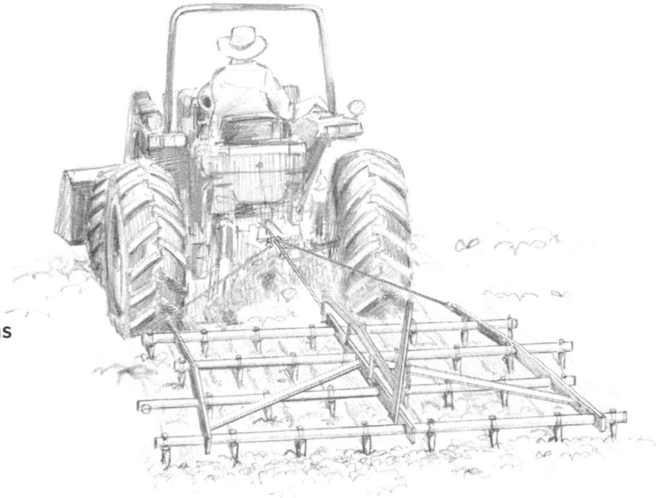

Spring harrowing smooths out rough spots and breaks up manure piles before the pasture grass begins to grow.

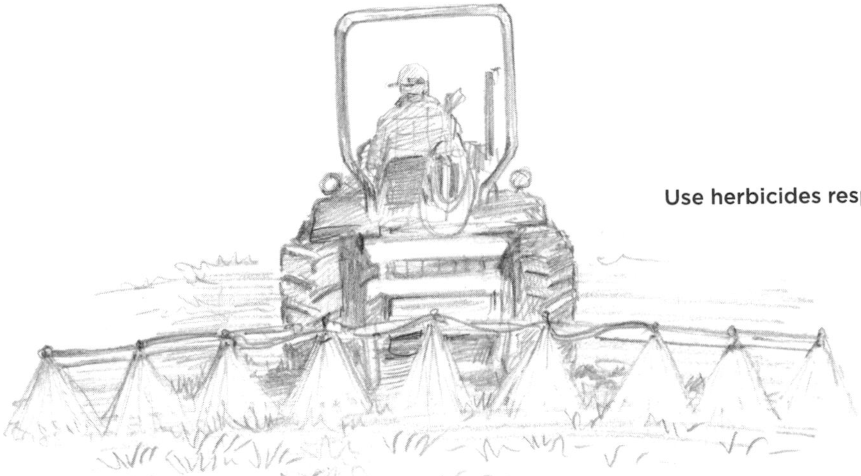

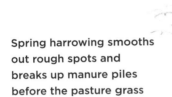

Use herbicides responsibly.

CLEAN-UP CREW

Four Ways to Deal with Manure

- ★ Leave it
- ★ Haul it
- ★ Spread it
- ★ Compost it (best)

HANDLING MANURE

There are four basic ways to manage manure, and you might use several methods on your farm or ranch: leave it, haul it, spread it, and compost it. Leaving the manure where it lies works best on very large pastures. The other three manure management options are more suitable to smaller horse farms and ranchettes and begin with daily or twice-daily collection. Once you've collected the manure, you can haul it away, spread it immediately on a hay field or cropland, or compost it for later distribution as humus.

LEAVE IT. If you have very large pastures, manure can stay where it is deposited. Four horses on 100 acres tend to create areas where they defecate, areas where they lie down and rest, and areas where they prefer to graze. Generally, given enough room, horses do not contaminate their eating areas.

On medium-sized horse operations, larger groups of horses tend to be turned out on smaller pastures. When nine head are turned out on 2 acres, even for a few hours each day, the manure accumulates quickly, yet it is impractical to manually pick up manure on a daily basis from that size pasture. The best option might be to let it lie where it fell.

If you can afford to leave a pasture vacant for a year, you can harrow the manure to spread it more evenly over the pasture. You wouldn't want to do this and then immediately use the pasture for grazing, however, because you would have just have helped parasites continue their life cycles by distributing their eggs and larvae over the entire pasture.

Agronomy 101

Agronomy is the science of land management. Agronomic rates of fertilizer application vary according to local conditions; your county extension agent will be able to help you determine the optimum for the land, the environment, and your operation.

HAUL IT AWAY. Some refuse collection services handle manure in a specially designated dumpster, which is emptied weekly or biweekly. Note that manure that is hauled off to a landfill soon becomes buried, so without access to oxygen, it won't decompose. Instead it generates methane gas, which is not a good contribution to our environment.

SPREAD IT. Spreading fresh manure daily is not an environmentally responsible choice, either. Fresh horse manure can burn plant tissue of newly seeded hay fields, pastures, gardens, or newly planted trees. If manure must be spread daily, it should be distributed on land that will not be grazed by horses for at least a year, and it should be spread thinly or harrowed to encourage rapid drying to eliminate favorable conditions for fly larvae and to decrease odor.

Many small horse operations produce more manure than their cropland or pastures require for fertilization. If you have four horses and a one-acre pasture, your pasture does not need and should not receive all of the manure the four horses produce.

COMPOST IT. The most ideal and environmentally friendly method of dealing with horse manure on a small acreage is daily collection and composting. (See May Cleanup Crew for more on composting.)

It is ideal to have at least three compost piles going at all times: one to which fresh manure is being added daily, one that is in the process of decomposing, and one that is fully composted and ready to spread. Each month will have a monthly manure task associated with each of the piles.

APRIL
Manure Pile Maintenance

PILE A
Turn twice, water as needed.

PILE B
Sell, store, or spread.

PILE C
Turn once, water as needed.

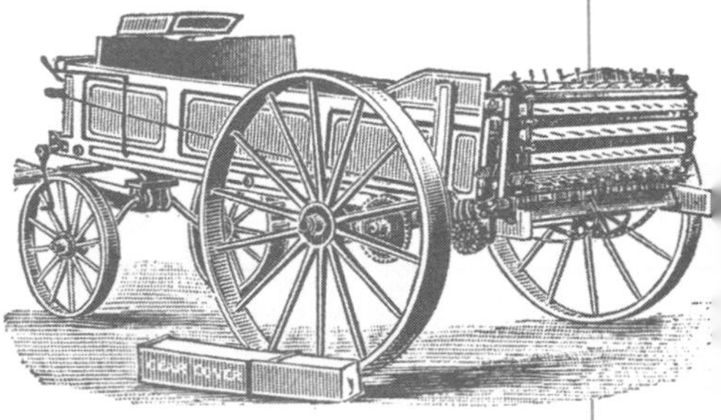

A horse loves freedom, and the weariest old work horse will roll on the ground or break into a lumbering gallop when he is turned loose into the open.

— Gerald Raferty

VACUUM

During three phases of the year, my grooming vacuum really comes in handy: spring shedding, our dusty summer, and fall shedding. You can use a canister vacuum, a heavy-duty livestock vacuum, or a shop vacuum, all of which vent near where you are working, or you can install a central vacuum, which vents outside the barn. If you are going to use a portable vacuum, choose one on wheels with an extra-long hose.

Horse, Meet Vacuum

1. Before you turn on the power, let your horse become accustomed to the sight and smell of the vacuum.
2. Then groom him with the hand tool to let him get used to the feel of it and the sight of the hose wiggling around and passing over his back.
3. Finally, turn the vacuum on. When you first start grooming him, begin at his shoulder and work your way around his body. (See annual barn cleaning in January Fine Facilities for more on vacuums.)

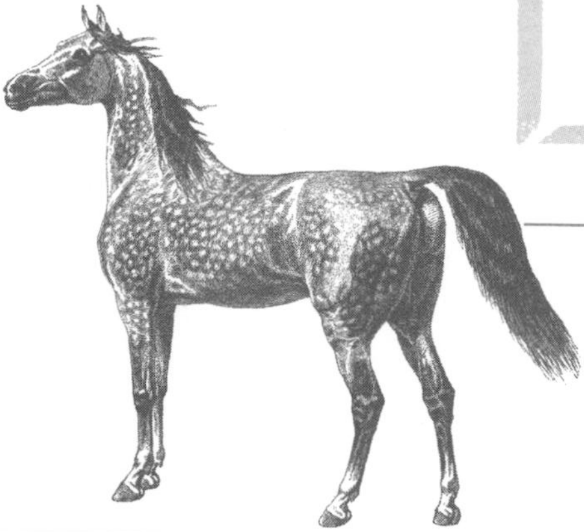

HELMETS

It is a good idea to wear a safety helmet whenever you ride or work around horses. A helmet will protect your head if you fall or if a horse bumps into you or hits you with a hoof. Don't think that a safety helmet is necessary only for jumping. You should wear one for all types of riding and sometimes when you are handling horses from the ground, too. If you are going to a show, check the rules of the association governing the show to see what type of helmet is required and allowed.

Although you can buy many types of helmets, not all are constructed to absorb the concussion from a fall. Helmets approved by the U.S. Pony Club, the United States Equestrian Federation, and the United States Eventing Association are labeled "ASTM/SEI" to show they have passed strict tests that prove they will protect your head.

Be careful when buying a used helmet, because you cannot tell whether the helmet has been damaged in an accident. A used helmet could look perfectly fine even though the inside protective layer may have been damaged and won't protect your head in case of a fall.

BACK IN THE SADDLE

If winter weather has kept you from riding, design and implement a program to wake up those ligaments and muscles. You might combine walking with some weight work, or tai chi or yoga with aerobics. Target specific areas of your body with exercises designed specifically for riders.

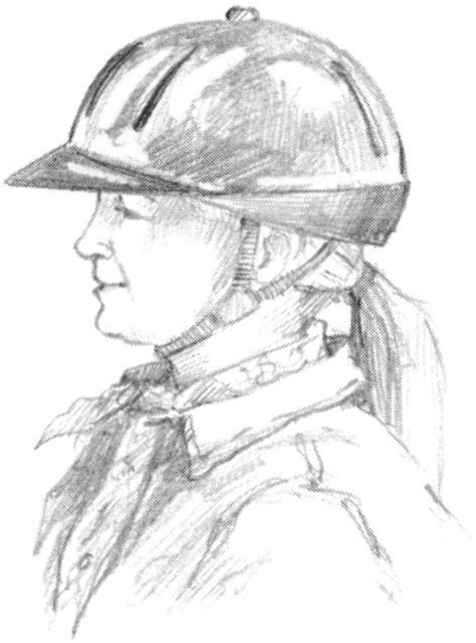

A safety helmet around horses just makes sense.

FYI

ASTM & SEI

The letters ASTM on your safety helmet stand for American Society for Testing and Materials, which sets the standard for safety equipment. SEI stands for Safety Equipment Institute, an independent laboratory that tests helmets to be sure they meet the ASTM standard.

CLOTHES HORSE

RAIN SHEETS

Since April brings showers, it's a good time to talk about rain sheets. Raincoats for horses come in two basic styles: cooler style and turnout style.

The cooler style is a large, loose cover that can be used, for example, on a tacked horse that is tied to a trailer. Like a cooler, the sheet covers the horse from poll to tail. Some have features that allow them to be used while riding.

The turnout style is for use in a pasture or pen, so it is basically a waterproof, breathable turnout sheet. It needs to be made of tough fabric because horses plus mud equals abrasion. It is also important that the sheet is waterproof and breathable. A waterproof and breathable fabric has a semipermeable membrane, which means that it keeps water out but allows moisture from normal respiration and sweat to escape through special pores. Skin is a perfect example of a waterproof-breathable material, and we can keep our horses' skin healthy by using skin-friendly sheet and blanket materials.

> **FYI**
>
> **Is It Waterproof?**
>
> A waterproof sheet is not only made of waterproof material, but in addition all seams are taped and sealed. A water-repellent sheet might be made of either waterproof or water-repellent material, but if the seams are rolled and sewn but not taped and sealed, water can seep through the stitching holes.

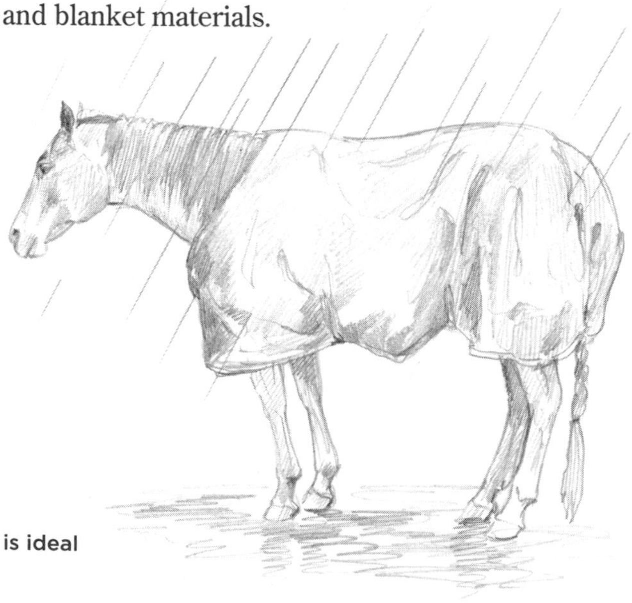

A waterproof, breathable rainsheet is ideal for those cool April showers.

When you remove a waterproof, nonbreathable blanket, a distinct sour odor means that the horse has been sweating. Waterproof and breathable sheets and blankets are much healthier and more comfortable for the horses and easier for us to take care of.

CHECK TEMPERATURE. Even if made of the world's best waterproof-breathable material, a sheet that is too warm for the ambient temperature will cause a horse to sweat. Once a horse sweats fairly heavily, it will take quite a bit of time for the sweat to evaporate even through a breathable material, so rain sheets should be used only in cool weather.

BE FLEXIBLE. Because turnout rain sheets are used in wet weather when a horse just loves to roll in the mud, a sheet should have areas of give. Elastic inserts in the chest and surcingle area are great. Most important are adjustable, heavy-duty elastic leg straps with swivel snaps on both ends so you can remove them easily for washing.

"A gyuen horse may not be loked in the tethe."

— Vulgaria Standbrigi, 1510

MODERN TRANSLATION: Don't look a gift horse in the mouth. If a horse was given to you as a gift, it would be ill mannered to examine his teeth to determine his age.

— Cherry Hill

Look Before You Leak

A well-fitted sheet should act like a gasket against the environment in the neck area, not an open invitation to rain seepage. A regular or high-cut neck is better than a cut-back withers style at keeping water from leaking into the shoulder area.

Sheets that are cut out of one piece of material do not have a center back seam, which makes them potentially more waterproof; however, sheets of this type are often not very form-fitting and tend to have a baggy, saggy look. Sheets that are made of fitted pieces with a center seam, shoulder panels, and hindquarter darts have a great-looking fit and stay put, but if every single seam is not taped and sealed, there will be leakage.

To prevent leakage around straps, choose low-set surcingles or belly bands and hind-leg straps that connect with D rings on the hem line rather than through slots in the side of the rain sheet.

FARM OFFICE

BUYING A HORSE

It just makes sense that the time of year when many people want to buy a horse is the beginning of riding season. In many parts of the United States, that is spring. (Conversely, I've noticed that when people decide to sell a horse, it is often in the fall, just before winter, which requires feeding hay — a significant cost. See September Farm Office for information on selling horses.) The following factors affect price and should be ranked in order of importance to you.

Temperament is the general consistency with which a horse behaves. Although a good disposition helps any rider, the single most important requirement of a novice's horse is a willing and cooperative temperament. Such a horse needs to be calm and sensible, yet responsive. A keen horse is alert and ready to work but under control at all times.

Soundness is mandatory for a performance horse. A sound horse has no defect, visible or unseen, that affects its serviceability. Although a horse may be declared unsound from a breeding standpoint, it may be perfectly useable as a working horse, and vice-versa. Unsoundness will be indicated in a pre-purchase exam.

Conformation is the overall structure of a horse as compared to a standard of perfection. (See Conformation in this month's More In Depth.)

A **breed** is a group of individuals with a common ancestry, exhibiting the characteristics outlined by the breed's governing association. **Type** refers to a particular style of horse of any breed, which has certain characteristics that contribute to its value and suitability for a particular use. Some competitions are open to only one particular breed, while others accept horses of all breeds and mixtures of breeds. Whether you are choosing within a breed or within

Odd Words

soundness. An absence of lameness or any other permanent condition that prevents a horse from working.

unsoundness. A defect that may or may not be visible, but that does affect a horse's serviceability. Most unsoundness is permanent.

blemish. A visible defect that does not affect serviceability. Some perfectly sound horses have blemishes or scars that might look bad but don't affect how the horse moves or works.

"*When you are buying a horse,* take care not to fall in love with him, for when this passion hath once seized you, you are no longer in a condition to judge his imperfections."

— Sieur de Sollesell, 17th century

a type, be sure to select a horse that is best suited for your intended use.

Manners make up a code of conduct, both inherited and learned. How a horse behaves in the privacy of his stall and as he is handled from the ground may not directly affect his performance, but it sure can make the owner's life pleasant or miserable. Vices may lower a horse's price but they might be more hassle than the discount is worth. Horses that are grouchy to bathe or cinch, but perform beautifully under saddle, may be an acceptable bargain. Realize, however, that the prospective horse's bad habit may be at its lowest intensity because of a professional's guidance, and the habit may worsen with handling by a novice or a new owner. (See Vices and Bad Habits in June.)

Gender affects price. Geldings usually make the most suitable horse for a novice because castrated males are reputably more steady and controllable than stallions. Mares often make brilliant performers but can be periodically silly, irritable, or fussy due to hormonal vacillations of the estrous cycle.

Health means the freedom from any temporary or chronic disease or debilitating condition. Although an ill horse may be purchased at a discount, what is saved in purchase price may be spent many-fold in time, labor, and supplies. There is also a chance that veterinary bills will be excessive or that the horse may experience complications or develop a chronic condition. Some health problems are permanent and require a lifetime of care. Be sure that you have a pre-purchase exam done on any horse you are seriously considering buying.

Age moves price. Horses in their prime, from five to eight years of age, usually command the highest prices. They have matured, mentally and physically, and if trained properly, have many years of service left. Younger horses often cost less because of their lack of training and experience and because of the risk of unsoundness. The future

Three Common Buying Errors

1. Do not be in a hurry.

2. Do not put a square peg in a round hole, but choose a horse to fit the use you have in mind. It would be more difficult to make a Saddlebred into a cutting horse than it would be to start with a Quarter Horse that is bred to work with cattle.

3. Do not pair a green horse with a green rider so they can learn together. A novice needs a well-seasoned, dependable mount. If you have a good deal of experience, however, you might want to take advantage of the usually lower prices on untrained young horses.

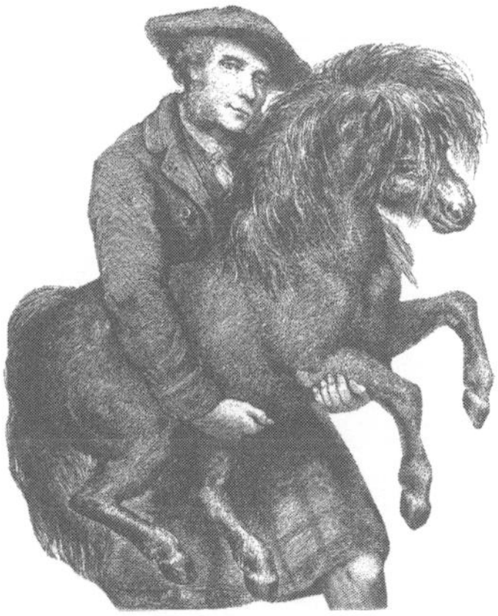

What Do You Want in a Horse?

Here are the criteria to keep in mind when shopping for a horse. Rank them in the order that matters most to you.

- ★ Temperament
- ★ Soundness
- ★ Conformation
- ★ Breed
- ★ Manners
- ★ Gender
- ★ Health
- ★ Age
- ★ Level of training and accomplishments
- ★ Size
- ★ Quality
- ★ Blemishes
- ★ Pedigree
- ★ Color and markings

soundness of a two-year-old cannot be predicted accurately. It is a good sign if a horse has been used regularly to age five or older and is still sound.

A horse's **level of performance training** and his accomplishments can greatly increase his price. Training is time, and time is money. A horse capable of performing consistently at the novice or nonprofessional levels, and especially one who has a record to prove it, has great worth. Although awards and points earned in competitions are impressive, there are many excellent horses that have never seen a show ring.

Size may affect price in either direction. In most situations, tall horses generally command a higher price than small horses because they can accommodate a wider variety of rider sizes. Exceptions might be the cutting horse or the youth horse. When considering a small horse, be sure to note whether your legs are positioned properly for effective use of the aids. Ask your instructor to help you determine what size horse is suitable for you.

A **quality horse** will cost more than a coarse horse. Refinement, class, and presence all increase a horse's price. Finely chiseled features, smooth hair coat, clean bone, and charisma all contribute to the horse saying "Look at me!" Since more people do look at a pretty horse, the price goes up. Because pride of ownership is a large part of the reason behind buying a horse in the first place, choose a horse that is attractive to you.

Blemishes (scars and irregularities that do not affect the serviceability of an animal) may or may not affect a horse's price. Although a blemish is not considered an unsoundness, it can lower the price of a horse. Old cuts, burns, and scars, small muscle atrophies, and white spots from old injuries may detract from the horse's appearance but may save the buyer money.

Some **pedigrees** are costly. The bloodlines of a horse's ancestors dictate, in large part, his quality and suitability for a particular event. Using the family name as the sole selection criterion is a poor system, but combining it with other observations can be helpful. Be sure you have a good horse in front of you first, and then look at the pedigree.

Certain **colors and markings** can increase a horse's price. Although often the first thing one notices about a horse is his body color and markings, it is really one of the least important considerations for selection unless you are purchasing the horse for use in halter classes in one of the color breeds.

Finely chiseled features, smooth hair coat, clean bone, and charisma all contribute to the horse saying "Look at me!"

BUYER BEWARE

It is always a good idea to have the seller give a demonstration of the horse's training. Then, if appropriate, the buyer can take a test ride. If the buyer is interested, then next step is to make an offer. If accepted, the seller might require a pre-purchase agreement with down payment so that while contingencies are being met and the horse is off the market, the seller is assured you are a serious buyer.

Horses are sold "as is." If a horse has a bad characteristic (such as a bad habit or physical defect), the seller should disclose that to potential buyers. Then when a buyer purchases the horse, the seller should have the buyer sign that

NO WAY!

Historical Horsekeeping

"It is a saying as trite as it is old that any color is good in a good horse. Yet a horse, however good otherwise, should be invariably rejected if his color is bad. For instance, it would essentially mark both an ignorant and vulgar person who would select a piebald, spotted, or otherwise extraordinary color for a carriage horse. It would savor of the circus or show ring."

— Gleason's Horse Book *by Prof. Oscar R. Gleason, 1892*

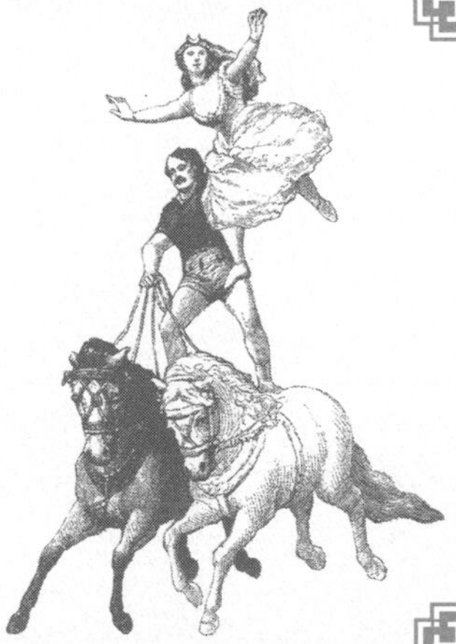

he purchased the horse knowing of this characteristic. See Recommended Reading for more information.

AUCTIONS

A good place to see a lot of horses in one place at one time, auctions are the combined effort of a sale manager and an auction company (often the same person or company) that presents a group of horses to buyers. Many very fine horses are sold at auction each year — and it is even possible to get a bargain if you are lucky. You'd probably be most likely to get a bargain at an absolute sale, one in which all horses sell, no matter what price is raised. Sales at which the seller has placed a reserve price on the horse will rarely yield a great bargain, because if the price is very low, the seller just says "no sale," pays the consignment fee, and takes the horse home.

> **Horse Buyer's Tip**
>
> It is almost always a good idea to have a pre-purchase veterinary exam performed. Veterinarians usually won't pass or fail a horse, so the exam won't have a specific outcome, but it will reveal things you can discuss with the veterinarian in order to help you make your decision.

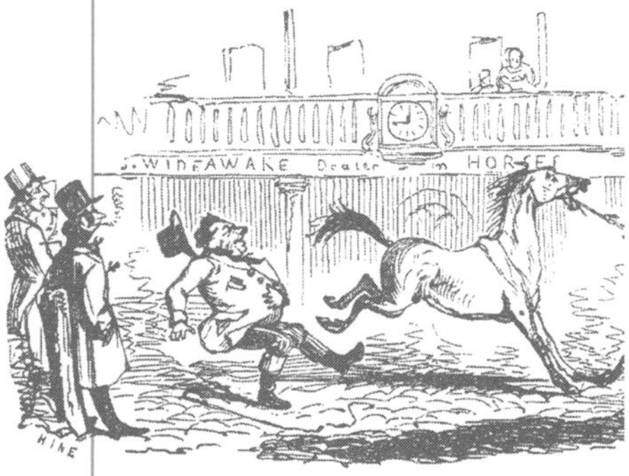

TYPES OF AUCTIONS. There are various types of horse auctions, and here are some brief descriptions.

The weekly miscellaneous horse and tack sale at the local sale barn usually has a low consignment fee (what the seller pays the auction company to sell the horse). If the horse sells, the auction company also gets a commission on the sale, something like 5 to 15 percent of the sale price. So if you pay $800 for a horse and the commission is 10 percent, the auctioneer receives $80 of your money and the seller $720. These types of sales generally attract low-priced horses or those heading to slaughterhouses.

A registered sale is usually confined to one breed and, depending on the quality of horses, the consignment fee will run somewhere between $100 and $300 plus the commission (often 10 percent).

A select sale is a group of horses that have been previewed by the sale manager to meet certain standards before being accepted into the sale. Usually the selection process is completed one to two months before the sale to allow time to print and distribute the sale flyer or catalog. Often such sales have a performance preview the day before the sale. Consignments and commissions are similar to those of the registered sales.

A dispersal sale is a complete sale of a ranch or farm, usually due to financial problems or the ranch going out of business. Often these sales are held on the ranch rather than at a sale barn.

PAPERWORK. It is important to deal with a registered and bonded auction company, because you will be assured that you will receive registration papers in good order. Find out ahead of time what type of payment is acceptable. Cash, cashier's check, or money order are usually acceptable anywhere. You will need to find out the individual sale's policy on personal bank checks and credit cards.

Occasionally, such as at some dispersal or production sales, contracts are offered by the seller to entice people to buy. You might have to put 30 percent down and have one to two years to pay the balance at a rate lower than the current bank rate. Of course, if that is your plan, you will need to have your credit approved before the sale.

ATTENDING AN AUCTION. When you arrive at a sale, register and get a buyer's number. You must provide your name, address, driver's license, and possibly bank information. Read carefully anything you sign when registering.

Some auctions accept sealed bids or telephone bids. Sometimes you will be required to send a certified check beforehand to back up the bids. Sealed bids are handled differently by each auction house, so you will need to check into their procedures. Phone bids allow someone who cannot attend the sale to participate in the bidding along with those present.

"Going, Going . . ."

Sellers choose to use auctions primarily for the convenience. Some feel it is simply too time-consuming to answer the phone and show horses to buyers. Some are too remote to expect to attract many buyers. Other sellers might be trying to get rid of a lame or dangerous horse, or they are desperate for money so need to sell quickly.

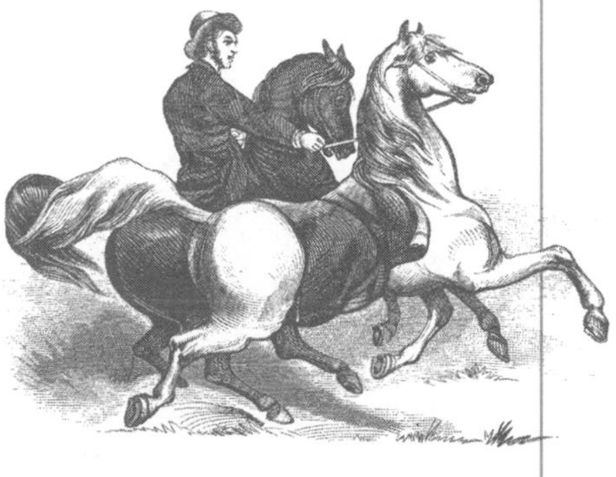

SPRING: *APRIL*

Auction Prices

Auction sales usually have a wide range of prices and a variety of sale averages. Some actual examples:

★ **Weekly.** 42 head from $200 to $1,000 with $400 sale average

★ **Breed.** 258 head with a high-selling horse of $8,100 and sale average of $2,169

★ **Select.** 301 head with a high-selling horse of $35,000 and sale average of $5,061

★ **Dispersal.** 185 head with a high-selling horse of $7,300 and sale average of $2,141.

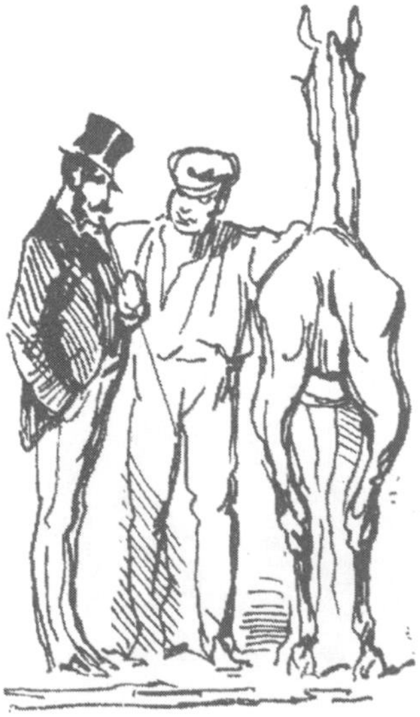

TERMS AND CONDITIONS. Be sure to read the terms and conditions in the sale catalog thoroughly. They will be different according to the state the sale is held in and the rules of the specific auction company. For example, the catalog will state what happens if there is a bidding dispute: two people think they bought a particular horse, or the auctioneer calls the horse sold just as your bid is accepted by a bid spotter. Will the bidding be started all over again, will it be reopened for a more advanced bid, or does the auctioneer have the right to settle a dispute as he sees fit?

Most auctions state that the horse is the buyer's risk and responsibility at the time the auctioneer's hammer falls; others state that it is when the buyer actually signs the acknowledgment of purchase. In some auctions, the document is passed up to you in the bleachers, and in other cases you sign it in the office. When you do, read it carefully, as that is when the title passes from the seller to you.

Horses are sold according to the laws in that state. Horses at auctions have not been vet-checked, and there are no guarantees of any kind. All information that is in the catalog or is announced prior to the sale is claimed to be reliable according to what was told to the auctioneer, but you as the buyer have no recourse against the auction company if the information is not true. So if a mare is said to be pregnant (according to the information given to the auctioneer) and is found not to be pregnant after you buy her, you have no recourse unless you want to go after the consignor.

Therefore, never rely on the catalog or what the auctioneer says about a horse. Be sure to look at the horse and have a vet examine the horse if appropriate. Test-ride a saddle horse before you consider bidding on it.

BUYING AND REGISTERING A HORSE. After signing the sales ticket, make settlement for the horse in the office. Check to be sure your name and address are correct on all paperwork. If you are a member of a breed association, use your name exactly as it appears on the membership. If you are not an association member, you will probably have to pay a membership fee to be able to transfer registration of the horse to your name. Be sure all is in order before you pay.

In most situations, after you pay for the horse, you are given the registration papers and the current transfer form, and you pay the transfer fee and send it in to the breed registry. If you pay by a personal check, the auction company may hold the paperwork until your check clears (usually three to 30 days).

In some cases, some horses sold at auction have been sold several times without the registration papers being transferred. In such cases, it will take time and money to straighten this out because all people involved in the previous transactions must be located, must be current members or pay membership fees to update, and must sign a transfer form in accordance with the particular breed association. In addition, there can be late fees assessed for transfers that are delinquent. If there is more than one transfer of ownership, the auction company should straighten it out and deduct the cost from the consignor's price.

No Guarantee

It is hard to have a thorough veterinary exam performed at an auction, and it is impossible to have a blood test run to check for drugs because it takes too long to get the results. The auction company is the middleman in the sale and the consignor (owner) is not directly involved in the sale to the buyer. Horses are often sold "as is" with no return. If a buyer is dissatisfied with a purchase, he or she generally has no recourse against the auctioneer or the seller.

Auction Etiquette

★ Set a price limit for yourself.

★ Never bid on impulse.

★ Never bid on a horse that you didn't examine before the sale but looks just fantastic from the bleachers.

★ Sometimes the last portion of the sale yields the best prices for a buyer.

★ If, at any time during the sale, you aren't sure what the bid is or who has it, don't be shy — ask the bid spotter nearest you.

★ If you buy a horse, don't immediately jump up to follow him out of the ring, because the sales ticket might be on its way up to you to sign.

★ In your excitement, be sure to read all information carefully.

HEADING ON OUT. From the moment you sign the sales ticket, you own the horse and are responsible for providing feed and water at the auction facility. You must remove the horse by a stipulated deadline. Some sales make transportation available for buyers who do not bring trailers to the sale. Commercial hauling rates will vary according to region and current fuel prices.

He was so learned that he could name a horse in nine languages; so ignorant that he bought a cow to ride on.
— Benjamin Franklin

Video Sales

Video sales are becoming more popular for private treaty sales. Sometimes the sale is made without the buyer actually seeing the horse in person. In other cases, the video provides a preliminary way for a buyer to narrow the field, especially with very specialized or high-priced horses. As a buyer, you should realize that a video can showcase a horse's strong points and downplay his faults, which the company is under no obligation to reveal.

STILL TRUE TODAY

Historical Horsekeeping

"There are several ways in which horses may be purchased, as, for instance, from a horse-dealer, from a farmer who breeds or who buys colts and breaks them, at an auction, at a fair, from persons who advertise in the newspapers, from a friend, who happens to have to sell the sort of animal you want. Respectable horse dealers never buy an unsound horse if they know it; and when they take a horse that makes a little noise, or has some other defect, within the list of what makes a "useful screw," they generally send it to be sold as a screw, at a screw price."

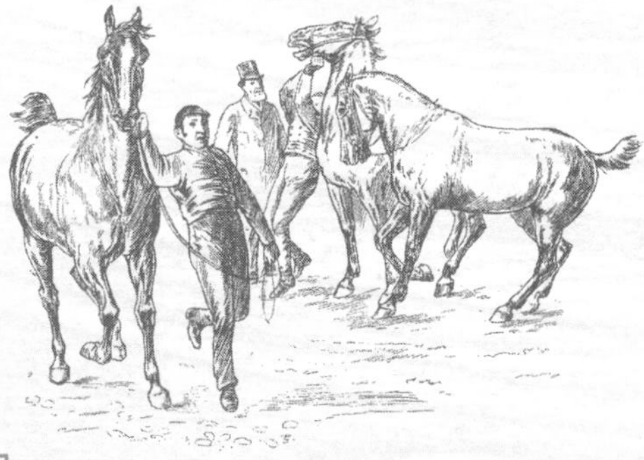

— The Book of the Horse *by Samuel Sidney, 1880*

GROUND TRAINING REVIEW

No matter how old your horse or how simple the exercises might be, it is a good idea to conduct a thorough in-hand review every spring to make sure your horse remembers all of his lessons.

TURNING LOOSE. I turn a horse loose in a specific way. To maintain control and keep a horse from developing the bad habit of bolting, I use safe techniques when turning loose.

1. I put a loop of lead rope around the horse's neck.
2. I unbuckle the halter, drop the noseband, and hold him momentarily. To prevent anticipation, I vary the length of time I hold the horse.
3. I remove the rope loop and again hold him momentarily, with my fingers on the off side of his neck.
4. When I release my horse, I want to be the first one to move away.

Odd Words

near side. Horse's left side.

off side. Horse's right side.

forehand. Shoulders and front legs.

hindquarters. Hips and rear legs.

LEADING. The safest and most effective place for you to be when leading a horse is between the middle of his neck and his shoulder. When leading from the near (left) side, hold the lead rope in your right hand 18 to 30 inches from the snap. Hold the rest of the lead rope in your left hand, not in a dangerous, hand-trapping coil, but either hanging straight down or in a figure-eight.

OFF SIDE. I practice all in-hand work on both sides of the horse. This keeps my horses and me from becoming "one-sided." The more ambidextrous you and your horse are, the easier and safer it will be for you to tack up and ride your horse and lead him from the off side, and for your veterinarian or your farrier to work on either side of him.

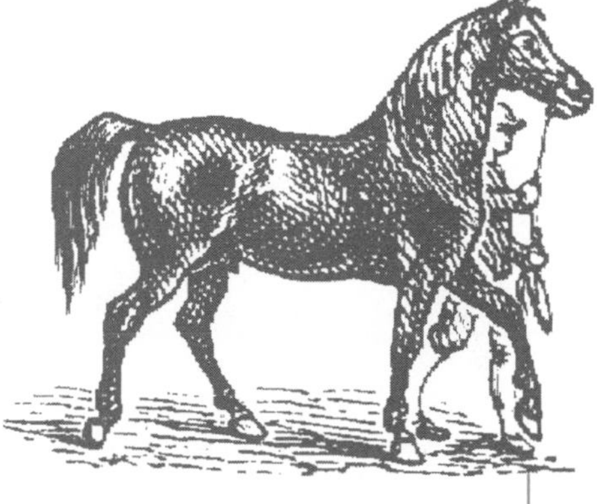

In-Hand Whip

I prefer to carry an in-hand whip to use as a visual aid when working a horse on the ground. I use it as a visual signal, a cueing device for forward movement, and a positioning guide to keep a horse tracking straight and to initiate sideways movement. A good length for an in-hand whip is 48 to 54 inches.

Of my two in-hand whips, one is a 48-inch dressage whip with a mushroom end-cap, which keeps the whip from slipping out of my hand. I do not leave this one outside because it has a leather cover and cotton stitching, which would be damaged by moisture and sun. My other whip is 54 inches long and had previously been a longeing whip that has seen better days. I was ready to discard it, so I cut it to length for an in-hand whip. I do not mind leaving it out in the arena or round pen because it is made entirely of synthetic materials. You can purchase in-hand whips from 42 to 60 inches long for horses of all sizes.

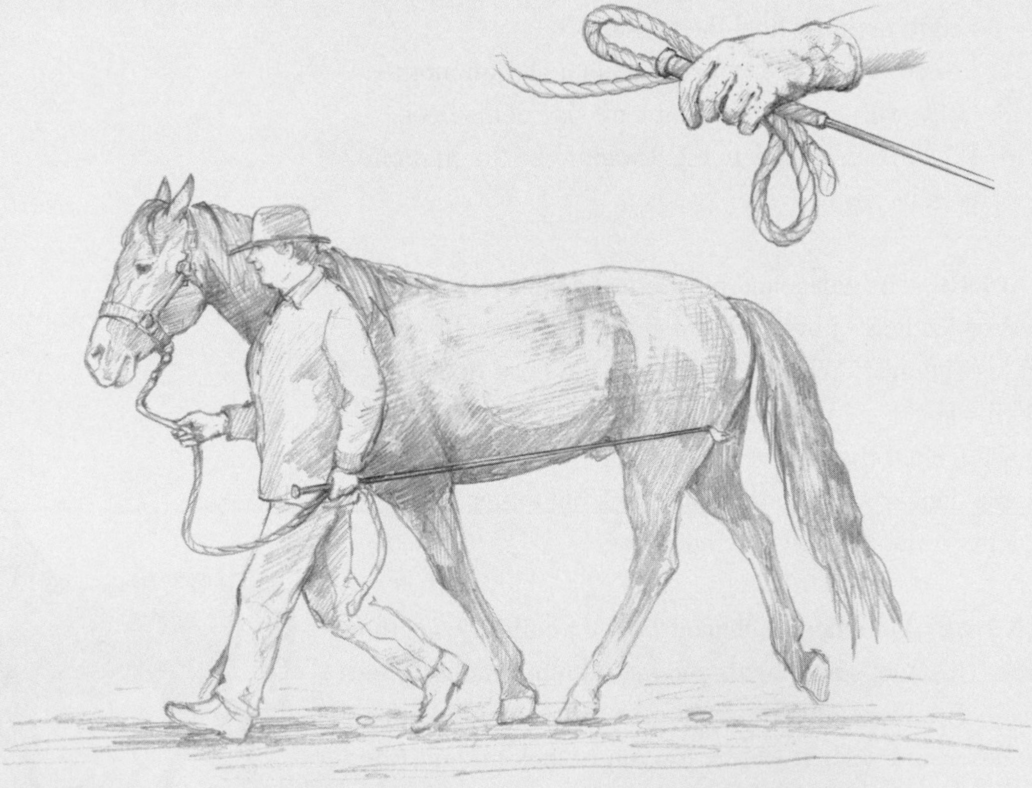

A 48″ whip allows you to guide your horse's hindquarters while still staying in proper position at his shoulder.

TURN ON THE FOREHAND. The turn on the forehand has recently been called yielding the hindquarters by a number of clinicians. It is an essential safety and control skill that I use many times every day, such as moving a horse over while tied, going through a gate, or positioning a horse for turnout. In a turn on the forehand, the horse's forehand (shoulders and front legs) remains relatively stationary while the hindquarters (hips and rear legs) rotate around it. Basically, you want the forehand to stop and the hindquarters to go. Here's how.

1. Stabilize the horse's forehand with body language, halter pressure, or a voice command, such as "whoa" to stop the horse or "stand" to remind him to stand.
2. Then move the hindquarters by the use of a finger, rope, whip butt, body language, or a voice command such as "over."
3. The forehand shouldn't move and the hind leg nearest you should cross over and in front of the hind leg farthest from you.

WHOA. I want my horses to stop when I say "whoa." That is why I teach whoa on a long line, requiring my horse to stop and stand still and square (with cannons vertical and hooves at the corners of a rectangle) on a 15- to 20-foot lead. Your eventual goal might be for him to stand absolutely square for three minutes, but at first, ask him to stand somewhat square and only for a few seconds. Gradually require him to stand more square and for longer periods of time. In between, move off and work on something else.

When you are perfecting "whoa" on the long line, stay close to your horse's forehand so you can quickly correct him with a tug on the halter and a verbal noise (such as "uh-uh" or "stand") as you return him to his original position. Soon he will learn what you want. Gradually go farther away, and then go out of his direct line of vision entirely.

Horse Sense and Safety

Respecting a Horse

★ Let the horse know that you are confident and firm, but will treat him fairly. Control your temper.

★ Don't surprise a horse. Let him know what you intend to do by talking to him and touching him firmly. (Soft, feathery touches make a horse's skin twitch, and he will often move away.)

Odd Word

standing square. Standing with cannons vertical and hooves at the corners of a rectangle.

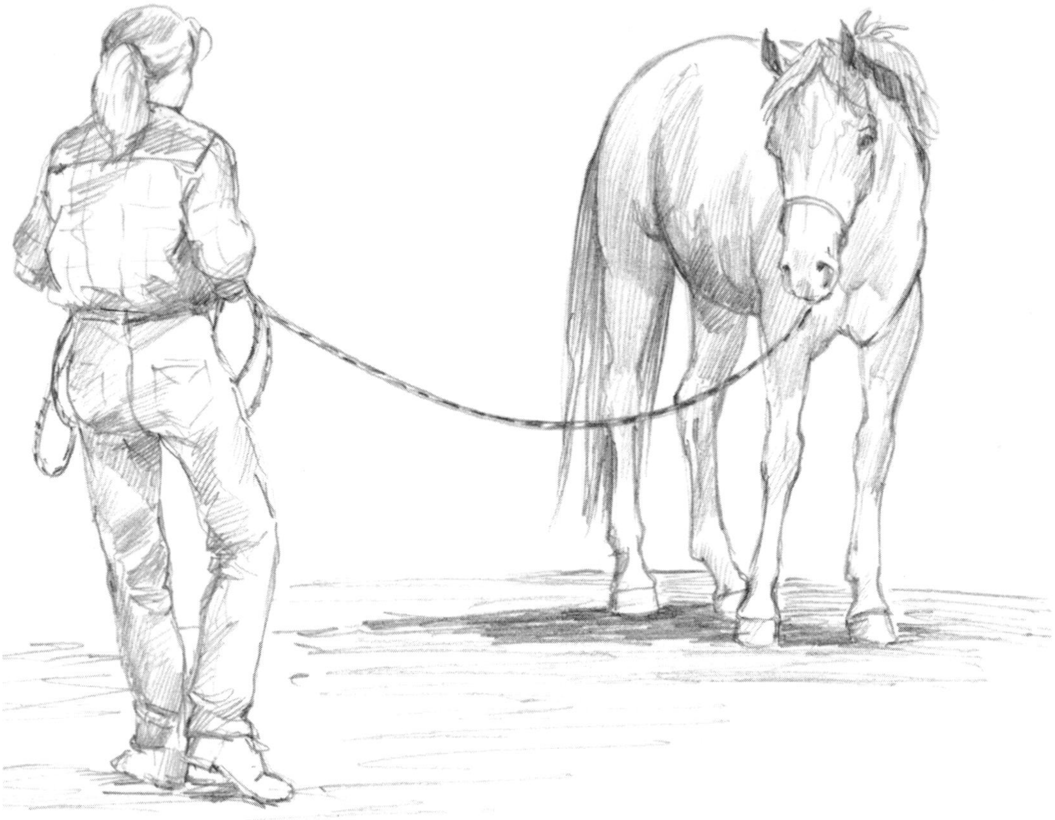

The best way to teach "Whoa" is by using a long line and requiring the horse to stand for gradually increasing time periods.

STILL TRUE TODAY

Historical Horsekeeping

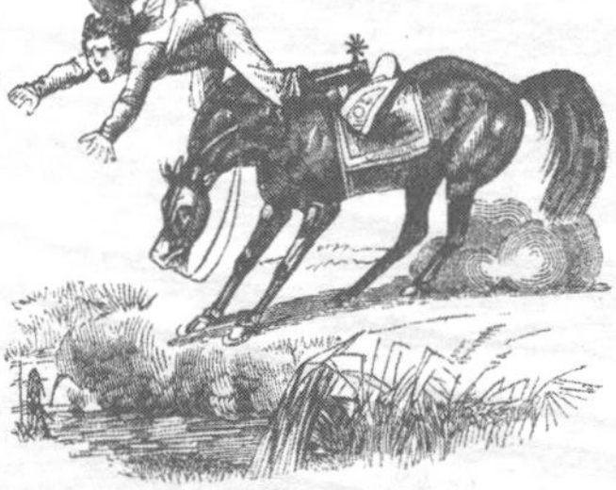

"Whoa,' as I understand the use of the word, is to bring the horse to a standstill, yet how many people when they walk up to a horse in the stall say 'Whoa' when they walk away. Another 'Whoa' when they put the bit in his mouth, and when they lift his tail up to crupper it, still another 'Whoa.' The word 'Steady' should be used and not 'Whoa,' the horse already being 'Whoa-ed.' "

— The Horse *by Sydney Galvayne, 1888*

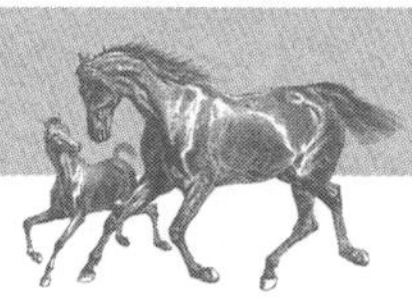

PREDICTING FOALING

You might know the date your mare was bred, and you know that the gestation period of a mare can range from 305 to 400 days, the average being 335 days. But when is your mare going to foal?

Predicting foaling is both an art and a science. The best approach is to get to know your mare. By about the third foal, you should have a pretty good idea. But I have been fooled, big time! Although I had predicted and witnessed almost all of Sassy's midnight foals, when she had her very last foal, I was tricked into turning her out for exercise one May afternoon. She didn't show me any of her normal signs of impending parturition, so I led her out of her luxurious, deeply bedded double stall and put her in a nice pasture for a stretch break.

Gestation length and time of foaling vary among mares.

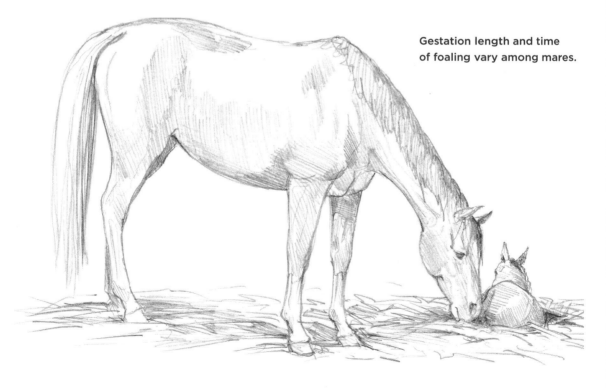

Minutes later, a hailstorm blew over the hill and rattled down on the building I was in. I immediately ran to bring Sassy in, but by then she was in the process of foaling. I called to Richard and we assisted her, all the while being pelted severely with Rocky Mountain hailstones.

The foaling was quick and the foal vigorous, so as soon as Sassy stood, I tied up the placenta so it wouldn't drag and led her back to the barn while Richard carried the foal. We were all soaking wet, so we stood under the radiant heat lamp that covers the wash rack and warmed up as I toweled off the mare and foal.

At less than an hour old, the foal walked all over the barn and explored every stall and nook, all the time carrying an oversized bath towel across his back like a cooler. This was certainly one of the most memorable foaling experiences we have had — a little nerve-wracking and yet amusing at the same time.

Signs a Mare Is Due to Foal

During the last trimester:

★ The abdomen enlarges.

During the last few weeks:

★ The abdomen drops and widens.

★ The udder shows marked fullness and development.

48 hours before foaling:

★ The muscles relax significantly over the tail head, the pelvic ligaments, and the vulva.

★ The udder will be full with milk.

★ The teats will wax (exude sticky colostrum at the end of the teats).

A few hours before foaling:

★ The milk will increase in calcium, which can be tested using a kit.

Just before foaling:

★ Milk will start streaming.

STILL TRUE TODAY

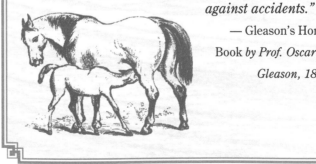

Historical Horsekeeping

Two days (and in some mares only one) before foaling, a sort of sticky substance will be found protruding from each teat, somewhat resembling drops of milk. She should be removed from other animals, and a careful person should see to her often enough to guard against accidents."

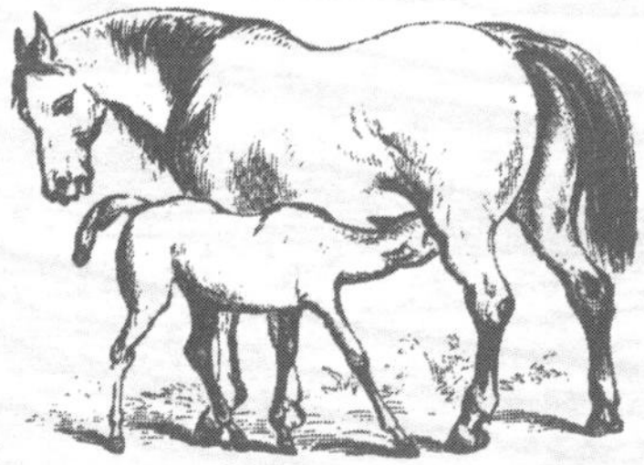

— Gleason's Horse Book *by Prof. Oscar R. Gleason, 1892*

FINE FACILITIES

HAZARDOUS WASTES

Because horses like to investigate unknown things by nibbling and tasting, it is essential to guard against chemical poisoning. All toxic substances must be stored in tight, well-labeled containers. Be sure to read all product labels thoroughly and follow directions carefully. Any unlabeled substance should be discarded in a safe manner. Chemical poisoning can often occur unknowingly.

Don't feed treated grain or seeds that were meant for planting, because you may give your horse a dose of mercury. Although treated grains often have a pink or reddish hue, sometimes they look just like feed grain. Be sure that grain treated for weevil infestation is safe to feed. Don't give a horse feed that was meant for cattle, sheep, or goats. Often these ruminant feeds contain urea, a source of non-protein nitrogen designed for ruminants, which should not be fed to horses. And some cattle feeds may contain growth stimulants that can be permanently damaging to the nervous system of the horse.

Don't let horses near junk or vehicles. Using lips and teeth to inspect things, they may ingest toxic paints, antifreeze, or battery fluids. Protect horses from all fumes from vehicles, paints, and solvents. Don't apply insecticides or herbicides near feed or water areas, and be aware of wind drift when you are spraying.

FYI

Toxic Substances

These include rodent poison, insecticides, herbicides, antifreeze, and lead-based paints. Although lead-based paints are no longer sold, you might find them on older horse buildings or fences, and horses should be prevented from contacting them.

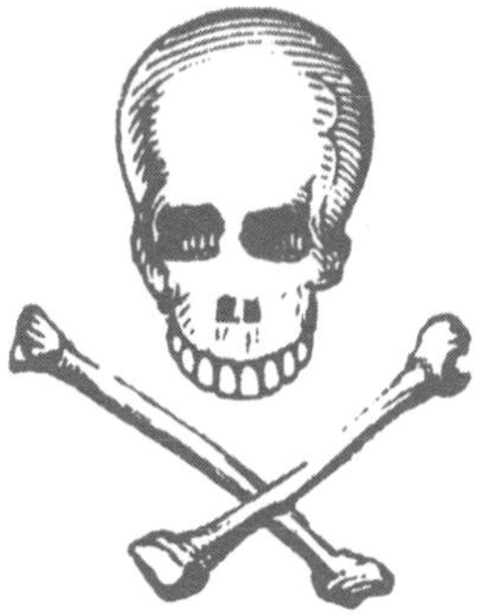

GATES AND LATCHES. There are different styles and widths of gates. Most gate styles are available in 2-foot increments.

Latches should be horseproof, safe when open or closed, and easy to use one-handed while leading a horse. When the gate is open, the latch should not have a portion

en español

tornado. Comes from *tornar*, meaning 'to turn', and *la tronada*, meaning 'thunderstorm'.

Horse sense is the thing a horse has which keeps it from betting on people.
— W.C. Fields

(such as a protruding pin) that could snag a coat or horse blanket. Latches with a feature to secure the latch, such as a hole for a snap or padlock, are useful for mouthy horses. When in doubt, secure gate latches with a short piece of chain and a double-ended snap or another means appropriate for the specific latch.

SPRING CLEANUP

April is when we usually do a cleanup of the creek area. Depending on the snowfall and spring rush, sometimes debris is deposited quite high above the creek banks. And invariably, some trees have fallen over during the winter. We head down with tractor, mower, chain saw and other tools. I usually mow while Richard tackles the deadfall.

We also check all of our pastures for any debris that might have blown in from neighboring ranches. One year we found an old dump site on our land, and the more we dug, the more old cans and bottles we found. Although some items were very old and interesting, most of the trash was broken glass, rusted cans, and even several sets of old bed springs, all horrible traps for horses.

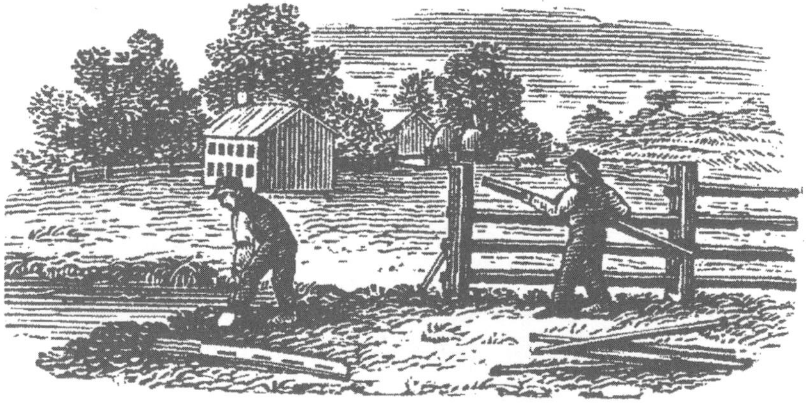

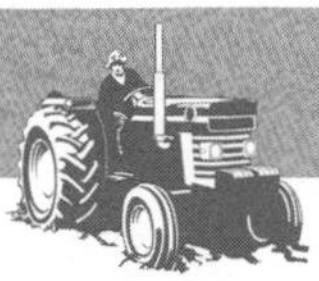

SPRING VEHICLE MAINTENANCE

You do certain things every time you hook up your rig to haul. Other things you keep an eye on and repair or replace as necessary. But it is a good idea to check some items annually, ahead of your busy towing season so you have time to make repairs or perform annual maintenance and service. We give the following a good going-over every spring: general structure, hitch, wheel bearings, and brakes.

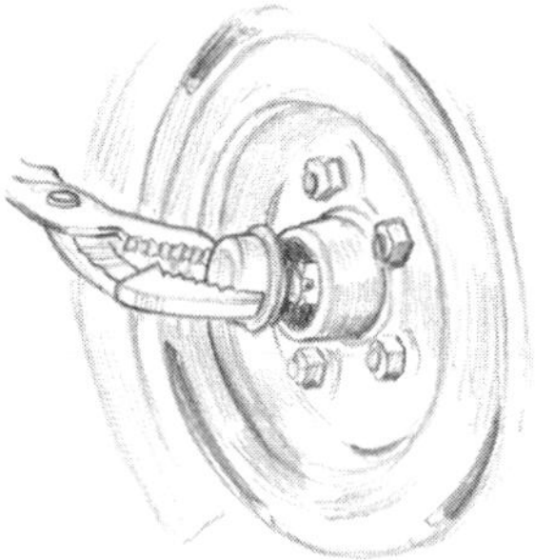

Check wheel bearings annually.

GENERAL STRUCTURE. Be sure that the hitch, safety chains, chest bars, tail bars, dividers, doors, and windows all work properly. You should be checking all of these things each time you use your trailer, and fix and repair as necessary. Check safety chains for worn links or cracked welds. Especially if you live in a humid climate, you'll need to clean and oil the teeth of the hitch jack so it moves up and down easily. Grease or soap the ball frequently to keep it moving freely in the coupler. Lubricate the moving parts of the coupler as necessary.

Use spray lubricant on any hinges, latches, or other moving parts that do not function freely.

Check rubber gaskets and molding around windows and doors to be sure it makes a complete seal against rain and weather. Replace when necessary.

TRAILER HITCH. Be sure that the hitch is not cracked or rusted and does not have loose parts, that the trailer coupler can be securely seated over the ball, and that the locking mechanism will engage. Inspect the truck's hitch, receiver, ball mount, and ball. Make sure the chains are in good shape and that the brakes work.

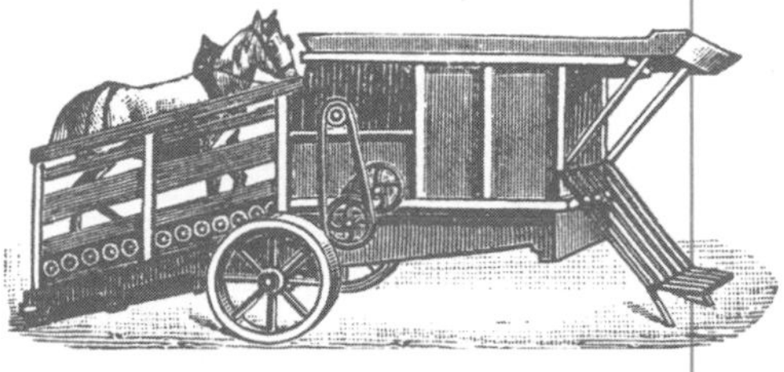

WHEEL BEARINGS. Have the wheel bearings cleaned and repacked with grease annually, or every 3,000 miles. Replace the seals at the same time.

BRAKES. Inspect the brakes on a new trailer after 200 miles of travel, and then plan to service or adjust them every 3,000 miles or according to the instructions in your trailer manual.

Check the pads for wear and replace if necessary.

If you have hydraulic brakes, be sure all fluid lines are in good condition and are not leaking.

Test Your Brakes

Several times each year, perform a brake test and adjustment. The test should be performed with an empty trailer and with a loaded trailer. A dry, hard, level roadway is ideal for this test.

Brake Test

Accelerate to 10 miles per hour and then brake. Have a knowledgeable observer on the ground tell you if a particular wheel is either locking up or rolling free in relation to the others.

If necessary, the noncompliant brake will need to be adjusted. This may involve crawling under the trailer and using a screwdriver-type tool to adjust a tensioning screw within the brake drum. If you are not experienced with this, have your trailer dealer make the adjustment for you.

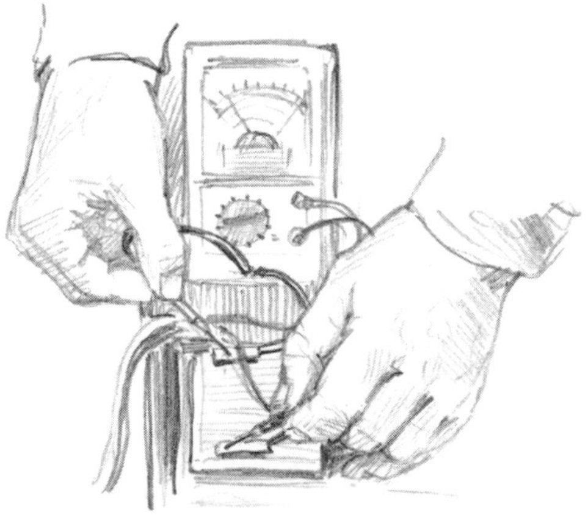

To guarantee that the emergency trailer brake battery is fully charged and operational, use a voltmeter to test it. It should read 12 volts.

PILL PASTE

If you need to give your horse a bitter pill, such as phenylbutazone, here's a way to cover the taste of the pill so he will not resent or avoid future dosing. Ahead of time, wash an old dewormer tube thoroughly, and remove the label or mark it clearly so that no one will think it is still dewormer. Put the cap back on the syringe.

1. Grind or crush the pills.
2. Put about one tablespoon of cake-frosting mix into the syringe, add the medicine powder, and top with one more tablespoon of frosting. Mix with a chopstick.
3. Now remove the cap, insert the plunger, and invert the syringe. The frosting will settle and air will escape.
4. When you dose the horse, the frosting will stick to his mouth and the sweet taste will cover up any bitter taste the medication might have.

What flavor frosting should you use? Well, you might find your horse prefers pistachio or cherry, but it is a safe bet to start with vanilla.

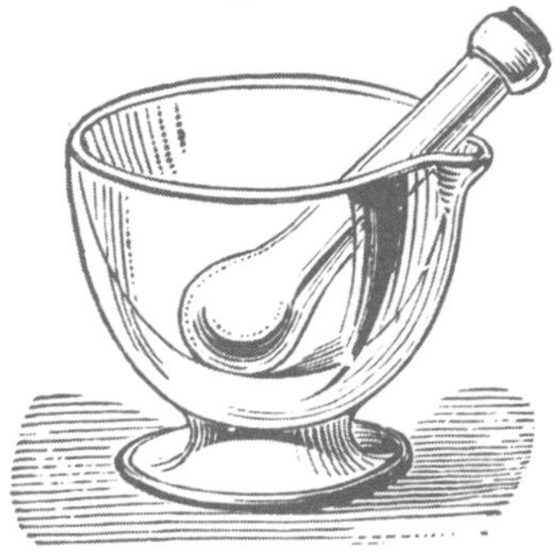

Horses' Favorite Flavors

Recent research showed that test horses ranked favorite flavors in this order: fenugreek, banana, cherry, rosemary, cumin, carrot, peppermint, oregano. Apple, ginger, and garlic were acceptable. But they just said no to echinacea, coriander, and nutmeg.

MORE IN DEPTH

Movie of the Month

***JEREMIAH JOHNSON* (1972)**

Almost a silent film, considering the small number of lines delivered by Robert Redford, yet full of vivid scenes shot in breathtaking Utah. One of my favorites shows a cold and hungry Jeremiah Johnson fishing barehanded in a frozen stream, suddenly looking up to see a handsome Sioux and his well-fed Paint horse, laden with furs and a string of a dozen fresh trout.

HORSE COLORS

- **Bay.** Body color ranges from tan to reddish brown coat with black mane, tail and, usually, lower legs.
- **Black.** True black over the entire body, including the flank and muzzle, except there may be white leg and face markings. The mane and tail are black.
- **Blue roan.** A uniform mixture of black and white hairs all over the horse's body. The horse is born this way and stays this color all its life, not getting lighter as he ages the way a gray horse does. The head and legs are usually darker than the body. There can be a few red hairs in the mixture.
- **Brown.** Mixed black and brown hair with black mane, tail, and legs. Often the horse appears black but has light areas around the eyes, muzzle, flank, and inside upper legs.
- **Buckskin.** Tan, yellow, or gold with black mane and tail and black lower legs. Buckskins do not have dorsal stripes the way duns do.

STILL TRUE TODAY

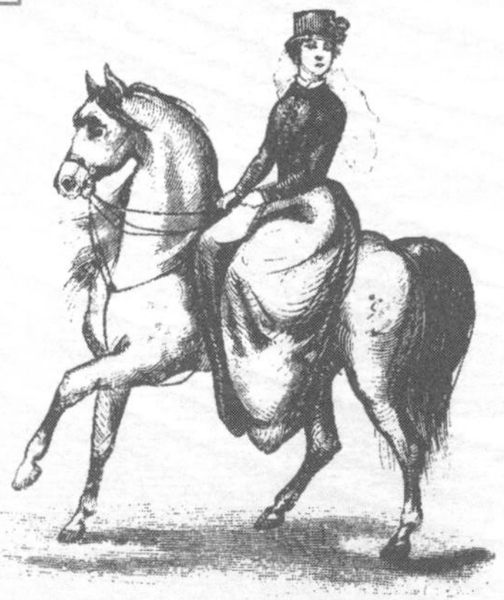

Historical Horsekeeping

"Saddle Horses of all Gaits. Lately, thoroughly trained saddle horses are much sought after in our cities, and certainly there is no place where they may be so perfectly trained as in the West. Twelve months training will put them in form. For good wear-and-tear, compact, able as a good leaper, of fine form, and undoubted bottom for any distance . . . will give an idea of what a saddle horse should be."

— Gleason's Horse Book *by Prof. Oscar R. Gleason, 1892*

- **Chestnut.** Body, mane, and tail are various shades of golden brown from sunny gold to reddish brown; some have manes and tails that are the same color as the body. When the mane and tail are lighter than the body they are referred to as flaxen.
- **Dun.** Yellow or gold body and leg color, often with black or brown mane and tail; usually has dorsal stripe (a dark stripe down the back), zebra stripes on the legs, and stripes over the withers.
- **Flaxen.** Describes the coloring of a golden mane or tail on a darker-bodied horse.
- **Gray.** Black skin with a mixture of black and white hairs. The horse is usually born dark (black or charcoal gray) and turns a lighter gray each year until it is almost white.
- **Grullo.** Smoky or mouse-colored body (each hair is this color; it is not a mixture of dark and light hairs); usually has dorsal stripe, and mane, tail, and lower legs are usually black.
- **Liver chestnut.** A very dark red chestnut color; mane, tail, and legs either same color as body or flaxen.
- **Palomino.** Golden coat with white mane and tail.
- **Red dun.** Yellowish, light red, or tan-colored body; mane and tail are reddish, flaxen, white, or mixed; has a red dorsal stripe and usually red stripes on legs and withers.
- **Sorrel.** A Western term used to describe a reddish or copper-red body with mane and tail either the same color as body or flaxen.
- **Strawberry roan or red roan.** A mixture of red and white hairs all over the horse's body but usually darker on the head and legs; can have red, black, or flaxen mane or tail.

See more about choosing a color on page 185.

Odd Word

ergot. This word has two farm meanings. The ergots on the backs of a horse's fetlocks are callous-like growths that may be vestigial remnants of toes or small hooves from the horse's ancestors. And the ergot fungus that can grow in mature grass and cereal-grain seed heads during moist conditions, if eaten, can lead to alkaloid toxicity, neurological problems, and abortion.

FYI

Coat Patterns

Besides colors and markings, some horses have distinctive coat patterns, which might qualify a horse to be registered in a breed or color registry. Paints and Pintos have large blocks of color over their entire body: white with black or brown. Appaloosas have spotted coat patterns, most commonly leopard (spots all over), blanketed (spotted on the rump), and frosted all over.

FYI

Balance

Balance refers to the relationship between the forehand and hindquarters, between the limbs and the trunk of the body, and between the right and the left sides of the horse.

CONFORMATION

Conformation refers to the physical appearance of a horse as dictated primarily by his bone and muscle structures and his outline. It is impractical to set a single standard of perfection or to specifically define ideal or normal conformation because the guidelines depend on the classification, type, breed, and intended use of a horse. A conformation evaluation should always relate to specific function.

BALANCE. A well-balanced horse can move more efficiently with less stress. The center of gravity is a theoretical point in the horse's body around which the mass of the horse is equally distributed. At a standstill, this is the point of intersection of a vertical line dropped from the highest point of the withers, and a line from the point of the shoulder to the point of the buttock.

Although the center of gravity remains relatively constant when a well-balanced horse moves, most horses must learn to rebalance their weight (and that of the rider and tack) when ridden. In order to simply pick up a front foot to step forward, the horse must shift his weight rearward.

How much the weight must shift to the hindquarters depends on the horse's conformation, the position of the

A horse's right and left sides should be symmetrical when viewed from front and back.

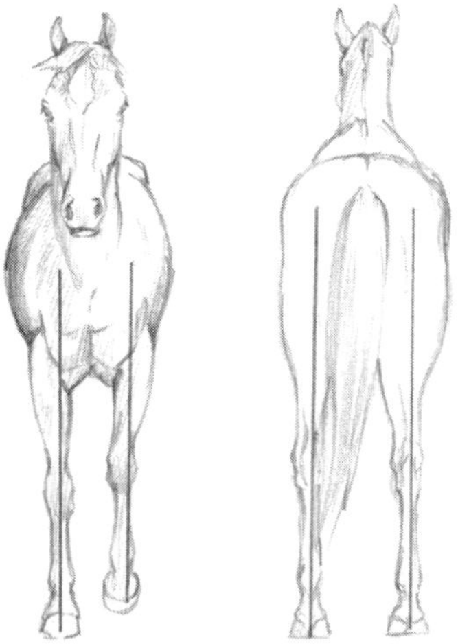

The center of gravity is usually a spot behind the elbow and about two thirds of the distance down from the topline of the back.

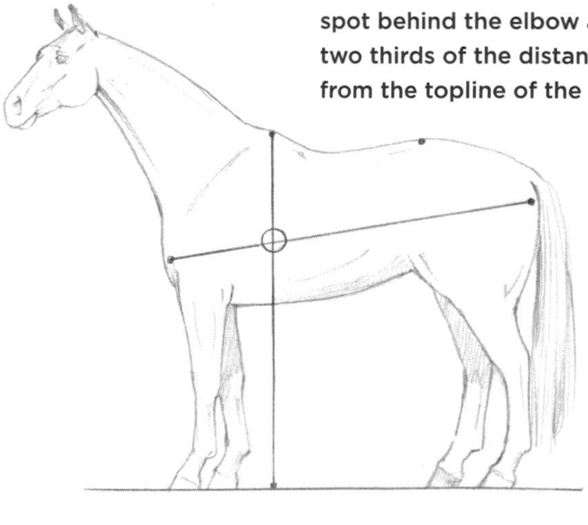

Looking at Horses: Assessing Balance

Here are some points to observe when evaluating a horse.

★ The lower limb length of the front legs (measured from the chest floor to the ground) should be equal to the distance from the chest floor to the top of the withers. Proportionately shorter lower limbs are associated with a choppy stride.

★ The horse's height or overall limb length (from the point of the withers to the ground) should approximate the length of the horse's body (from the point of the shoulder to the point of the buttock). A horse with a body a great deal longer than its height often experiences difficulty in synchronization and coordination of movement. A horse with limbs proportionately longer than the body may be predisposed to forging, over-reaching, and other gait defects.

★ When viewing a horse overall, the right side of the horse should be symmetric to the left side.

rider, the gait, the degree of collection, and the style of the performance. The more a horse collects, the more he steps under his center of gravity with his hind limbs.

If the forehand is proportionately larger than the hindquarters, especially if it is associated with a downhill topline, the horse's center of gravity tends to be forward. This causes the horse to travel heavily on his front feet, setting the stage for increased concussion, stress, and lameness. When the forehand and hindquarters are balanced and the withers are level with or higher than the level of the croup, the horse's center of gravity is located more rearward. Such a horse can carry more weight with his hindquarters, thus move in balance and exhibit a lighter, freer motion with his forehand than the horse with withers lower than the croup.

Cowboy Code

Never touch another's horse, tack, or hat.

Tornado Disaster Kit

If you live in tornado country, store a disaster kit in your horse trailer. If you must evacuate your horses, you will have everything you need. Include:

★ an extra halter and lead rope

★ feed

★ paperwork such as ownership papers, ID, or brand certificate

★ buckets and a hose

★ flashlight or lanterns

★ first-aid kit

MIDWEST TORNADO SEASON

Although tornados are more likely to occur in certain areas of North America than others, they can happen anytime, just about anywhere. Most often, the weather patterns favorable for tornado formation occur in the central United States in an area commonly known as Tornado Alley (see Map). The tornado season in the United States can begin as early as February in the Midwest, but most twisters are spawned during April, May, and June.

Tornados are rated according to the Fujita Damage Scale. Those with an F2 rating or higher are considered significant, and those of F4 or F5 are classified as violent and cause millions of dollars of damage.

Find out ahead of time how to get updates if your power goes out. A crank-operated weather radio is often your best bet. Make arrangements for someone to care for your animals should your facility be destroyed. See page 255 for more on tornados.

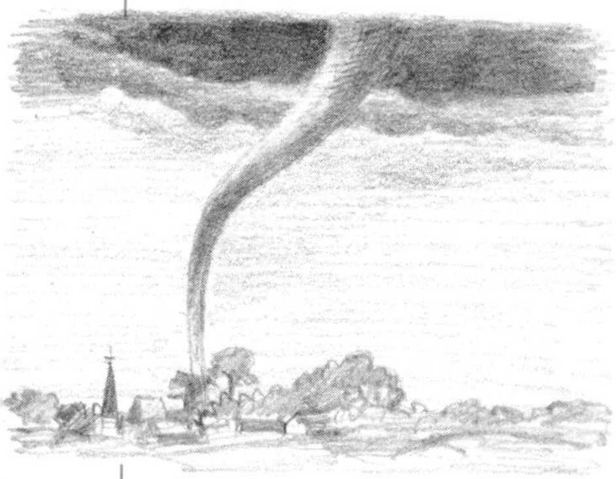

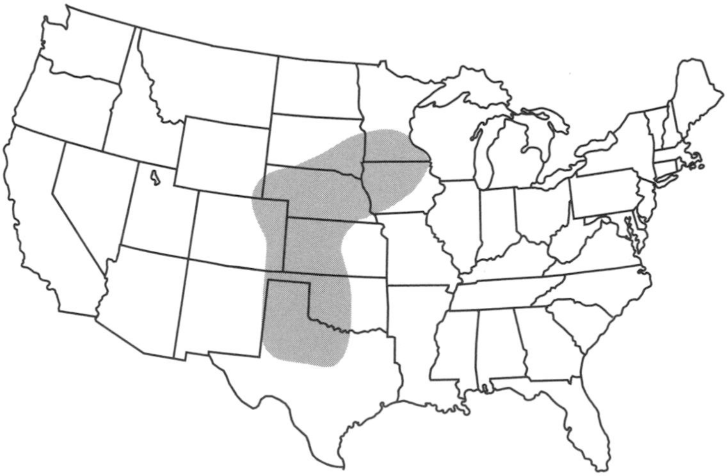

Tornado Alley includes Texas, Oklahoma, Kansas, Nebraska, Iowa, and parts of Colorado, South Dakota, and Minnesota.

MAY

Depending on the year, May marks the time when I first turn the horses out on pasture. I like to wait until the grass is at least 6 inches tall, which not only protects the pasture but also prevents a horse from eating too much of the early spring green growth. When a horse unaccustomed to green grass is suddenly turned out on pasture, or when any horse is allowed too much green grass, he can experience digestive and circulatory problems leading to colic and/or laminitis. (See more on pastures in Pasture Perfect.)

Day Length in Hours

Latitude	Date: May 1	Date: May 16	Date: June 1
60°N	51.57	16.81	17.88
55°N	14.91	15.87	16.67
50°N	14.41	15.19	15.81
45°N	14.01	14.65	15.16
40°N	13.68	14.21	14.63
35°N	13.4	13.84	14.18
30°N	13.15	13.51	13.79

See page 22 to find your latitude.

To Do

- ❑ Deworm
- ❑ Take a hay inventory
- ❑ Hoof trim and shoe
- ❑ Work arena
- ❑ Clip legs
- ❑ Make chore map
- ❑ Update feed board
- ❑ Scrub feed tubs and buckets
- ❑ Move hay to barns
- ❑ Wash saddle pads
- ❑ Review trailer loading

To Buy

- ❑ Beet pulp pellets
- ❑ Senior feed
- ❑ West Nile Virus vaccine
- ❑ Salt and mineral blocks
- ❑ Corn oil
- ❑ Shampoo

BEWARE OF HAIL

Here in the foothills of the Rockies, we have a fairly focused hail season that usually spans May to July but can start earlier or end later. Hail is super-cooled rain that forms into balls in the updraft of cumulonimbus thunderstorm clouds. Falling in swaths from a few feet to 100 miles long, it can range from a granule to the size of a grapefruit and has been reported to pile up 6 feet deep. Although radar can predict hail 15 minutes before it falls, it would be unlikely we would hear the warning in time to do anything.

Of most significance to horsekeepers are damage to property, such as vehicles or crops, and possible injury when riding. Hail does one billion dollars of damage to property and crops each year in the United States. The costliest hailstorm in U.S. history occurred in Denver in July 1990, causing damages of $625 million. If you have a storage building, park all vehicles, tractors, and trailers inside it.

Hail can also contribute to accidents while you are driving or riding. Often when driving across Wyoming I've seen a hail swath being laid across the road just ahead or behind me, but whether it is best to stop or keep going is a gamble. Although hail might startle a horse and the repeated pummeling is not a pleasant physical sensation, horses aren't usually injured from hailstorms. A rider can be injured, however, if her horse panics and bolts. Know your horse and head for cover if possible.

Vet Clinic

Coggins

A negative Coggins test is often required for a horse that will be traveling, shown, or bred, or will be anywhere horses are congregated, such as at a group trail ride. A positive Coggins test indicates the presence of antibodies for Equine Infectious Anemia (EIA) or "swamp fever," which means that the horse has been exposed to the disease and has formed antibodies to it.

The disease is spread by blood-sucking insects like deerflies and horseflies. Many horses that are positive show no clinical signs but are infected for life, so they are a potential threat to other horses. Therefore, positive horses are either quarantined or euthanized. State regulations vary but many require a negative Coggins test within 12 months.

Health Certificate

Horses that are traveling interstate or off the farm for showing or breeding within the state will also require a Veterinarian's Certificate of Health. The certificate of veterinary inspection will vary according to state and situation but usually must be dated within 30 days. It certifies that the horse has been examined by an accredited veterinarian and must include an accurate and complete description of the animal including age, sex, color, and markings.

Registered horses may be identified by registration name and number. When required, the EIA test date and the name of the laboratory must be recorded on the certificate of veterinary inspection.

FOOT NOTES

TO SHOE OR NOT TO SHOE

This is the time of year to decide which horses will be worked during the spring, summer, and fall and need shoes, and which will remain barefoot. Just because a horse is in work doesn't mean he absolutely requires shoes, and just because another horse is retired doesn't mean she will be most comfortable barefoot.

Ranch Notes

May 1. Made a hay inventory.

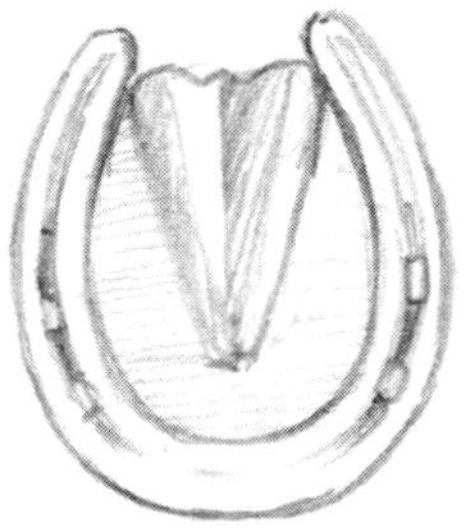

A shod foot from the bottom.

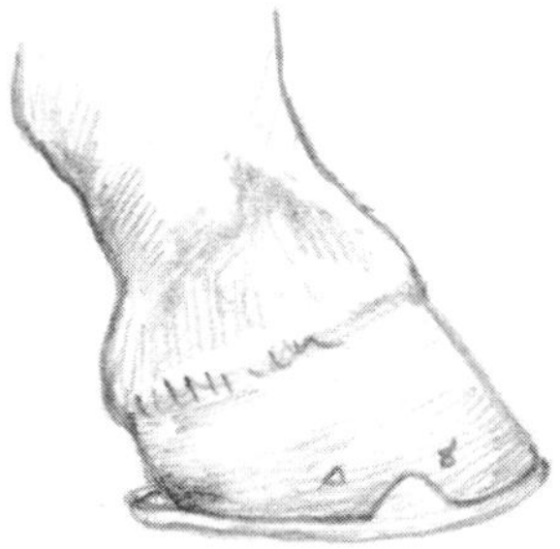

A shod foot from the side.

Whether or not you have your horse shod and with what type of shoes depend on what the horse is used for. A competitive trail horse will most likely require shoes that provide good traction and resist wear, while a broodmare will more likely be barefoot. A horse with a hoof or limb defect or hoof health problem, on the other hand, may require shoes no matter what the use. (See November Foot Notes to read about the barefoot horse and to help determine if your horse needs shoes.)

All domestic horses need regular trimming, and many are helped by good shoeing. Here are the three ways farriers approach their work.

- **Preventive** trimming and shoeing emphasize balance, support, and protection. The goals of preventive shoeing are long-term soundness and performance longevity.
- **Corrective** trimming and shoeing consist of altering the hoof to improve or correct stance or stride. Properly employed corrective shoeing generally does not force a limb into an abnormal position; instead it allows the hoof and limb to attain a desirable configuration and achieve sound movement.
- **Therapeutic** shoeing is often a part of lameness treatment designed to protect and/or support a damaged hoof or limb or to prevent or encourage a particular movement until healing can take place.

Corrective and therapeutic shoeing may be helpful in the treatment of some lameness but may have no beneficial effect in others. Preventive trimming and shoeing, however, should be part of every horse's routine hoof-care program.

Shod vs. Bare Feet

The barefoot hoof should be properly trimmed approximately every six weeks. It can be difficult to maintain the balance of a bare hoof, however, because it is not protected from hoof-wall wear and often wears unevenly, throwing the hoof out of balance. The wall can wear so excessively that the horse is walking on his soles, which often results in sole bruises and sole abscesses.

It is difficult to meet a horse's specialized corrective, therapeutic, or performance needs when he is barefoot. In the case of cracks, for example, a shoe can stabilize the hoof as it heals and grows an entire new, balanced hoof of solid horn. Other problems, such as laminitis, navicular disease syndrome, under-run heels, and fractured coffin bones, can be hard to treat without appropriate shoes.

The equine hoof evolved to carry the horse's own weight in a semiarid environment. The wild horse's free movement over dry terrain encouraged the hooves to become very tough and resistant to abrasion. Natural selection eliminated horses with unsound feet, but once human selection took over, horses with poor feet (but a pretty head or color) were protected and kept in the gene pool. Furthermore, domestic horses are usually restricted to a small, moist environment that softens the hooves and allows them to grow very long and deformed, and ultimately break off in chunks.

Movie of the Month

***THE HORSE WHISPERER* (1998)** Beginning with the slow motion accident sequence, the cinematography in this movie is excellent. Although I am not completely aligned with the horse training aspects of the book/movie, and many things are far-fetched and Hollywoodized, the movie works for me more in a symbolic rather than literal sense. The entire cast is excellent and the story very well told.

Purposes of Shoeing

As man's dependence on the horse for transport and war decreased, it seems that emphasis on hoof quality also decreased. Today the domestic horse often inherits poor feet, is fed too generously, and is then required to perform, carrying its overweight body plus an extra two hundred pounds of tack and rider. Appropriate shoes, knowledgeably applied, can help provide the support and protection to help an over-taxed horse to be functional without going lame.

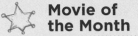

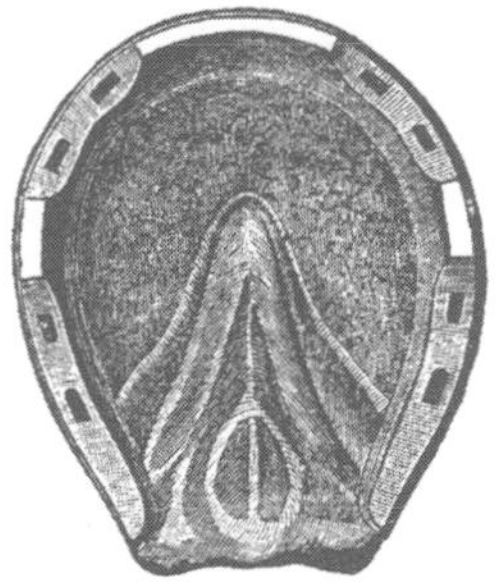

SHOEING PROTECTS. In a domestic environment, the growth rate of a horse's hooves is rarely equivalent to the

en español

corral. Comes from *el corral,* meaning 'an enclosure for confining livestock'.

wear. The hooves either wear away faster than they grow, making the horse tender-footed, or they grow faster than they wear, become very long, then crack or break off in chunks, possibly causing lameness and long-term hoof problems. Shoes can protect hooves and allow the horse to function comfortably and remain sound.

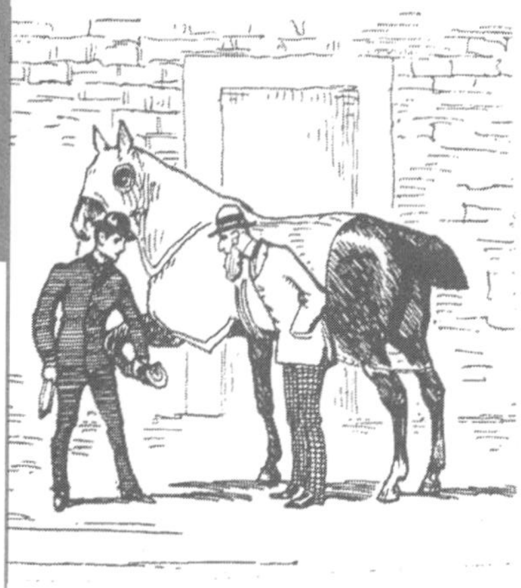

SHOEING HELPS MAINTAIN BALANCE. A domestic environment drastically changes the horse's natural patterns and rhythms of movement. Consequently, the hooves often wear in an unbalanced fashion. This puts uneven stress on the joints and support structures of the limb and can lead to lameness. Shoes can help to maintain hoof balance and minimize unsoundness.

SHOEING PROVIDES SUPPORT. Domestic breeding and unnatural environment have resulted in a greater number of horses that have feet either too small or too weak to hold up under the demands placed upon them. When the foundation of the horse breaks down, lameness is inevitable. Properly applied shoes can optimize the support of the limb and help stabilize the hoof.

See November for more on traction and bare feet.

SHOEING PROVIDES TRACTION. To perform safely, confidently, and without unnecessary exertion, a horse needs appropriate traction for his activity. Bare feet offer good traction but if a horse needs extra traction, it can be provided with shoes. A horse's traction requirements will depend on his use and the footing. Traction is affected by the type of shoes and nails used and by the addition of caulks or carbide chips to the shoes. Optimal traction can increase a horse's feeling of security so that he will stride normally, help him keep his balance in unstable footing such as mud, ice, snow, or rock, and minimize fatigue, all of which will add to horse and rider safety.

FINE FACILITIES

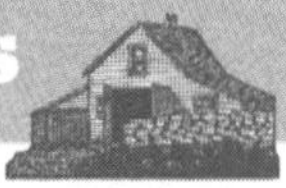

SUMMER CARETAKER

During May we try to set things up so that it is easy for a caretaker to do chores for us. (That is, if we get to take a summer vacation. For some reason, that doesn't often happen to us horsekeepers, but I think that is because our entire life is a vacation!) I try to make things as easy and simple as possible for the caretaker.

The map below is an example of what I might provide for a summer caretaker, with location of horses and water troughs marked.

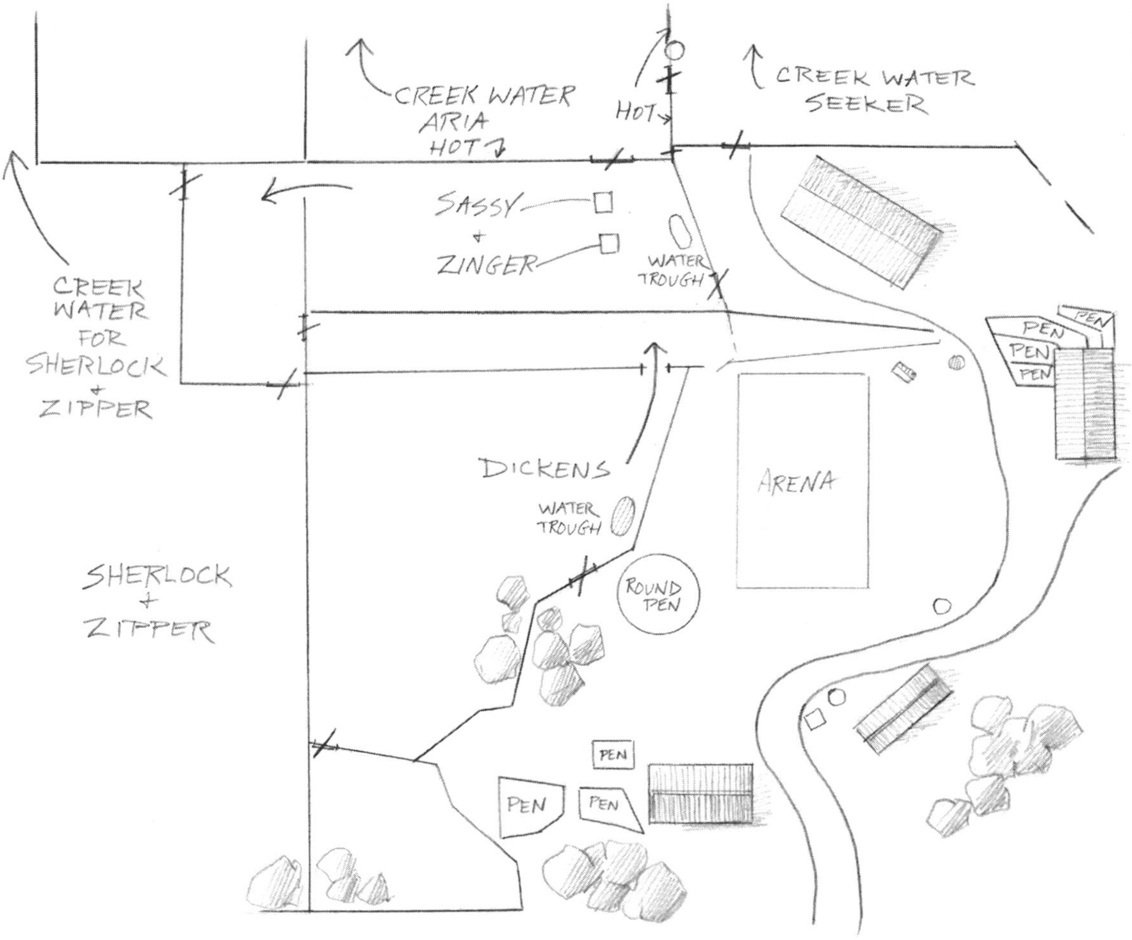

SPRING: MAY

Here's what I do to make it possible to take a (relatively) carefree vacation.

- Try to plan our vacation for a month when the horses can be out on pasture.
- Take all sheets off horses to minimize risk and to eliminate the possibility of shifting sheets, unbuckled leg straps, and so on.
- Simplify the ration or measure up special supplements ahead of time. Our middle-aged horses require only good pasture, salt, and water. Young or senior horses will usually continue receiving their grain mixture twice a day, so I mix everything ahead of time (except for the water). I leave a tower of labeled buckets.
- Make the feeding directions clear on the feed board.
- Make a map of the property (see the Caretaker Map on page 213), noting which horse is where and where halters are hanging for each horse. For the caretaker's convenience, I attach a separate sheet with feeding instructions for each horse. This makes a handy pocket reference.
- Provide an information sheet with our 24-hour contact information, our veterinarian's name and phone numbers, and our farrier's name and phone number.

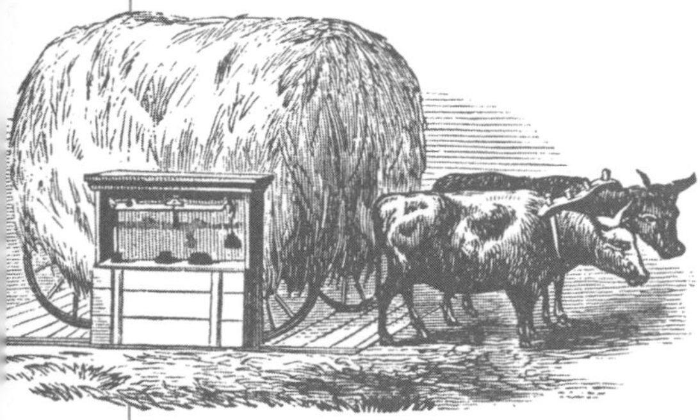

LOOKING AT HORSES

Muzzle Conformation

The horse's muzzle can be trim, but if it is too small, the nostrils may be pinched and there may be inadequate space for the incisors, resulting in dental misalignments. The incisors should meet evenly with no overhang of the upper incisors (parrot mouth) or jutting out of lower incisors. The width of the cheekbones indicates the space for molars; adequate room is required for the sideways grinding of food.

FEED BAG

GIVING HORSES TREATS

Normally, I do not use treats with my horses, but the exception is when I am training a horse to have good turnout manners and to come in from pasture when I call. Horses should be rewarded when they are good.

Many commercial products try to convince you that feeding your horse treats from your hand is the way to reward. If you want your horse to be a treat-seeking missile, just hand-feed him treats often. It takes only a few treats to turn a horse into a pocket pest or a dangerous finger nibbler. Horses can get greedy, pushy, and in a hurry and not be discriminating in what they grab with their teeth. If you don't want your horse to be a pest but you do want him to come when you call, use other forms of reward such as a scratch, a stroke, or a soothing voice such as "Gooooood Girl."

Treats do come in handy is when turning a horse out. If he bolts or pulls away, you could get trampled or kicked. (Bolting is when a horse wheels or races away suddenly, often kicking or bucking as he goes. Bolting also refers to a horse gulping his feed. Both indicate he is in a hurry!) You can use treats to encourage a horse to put his head down and relax rather than taking off when turned loose.

Here's how I add treats to the turning-loose routine. After I unhalter the horse, but before I release him, I drop a few treats on the ground, slightly ahead of him where he can see them. I use a few of the horse's normal complete feed wafers because they are cheaper than official horse treats. The first few times, I let him smell them before I drop them. Then I follow my normal turning-loose procedure. The horse develops the habit of putting his head down to find the treats and is preoccupied with eating them. I am the first to leave.

How do you catch a loose horse? Make a noise like a carrot.

— British Cavalry joke

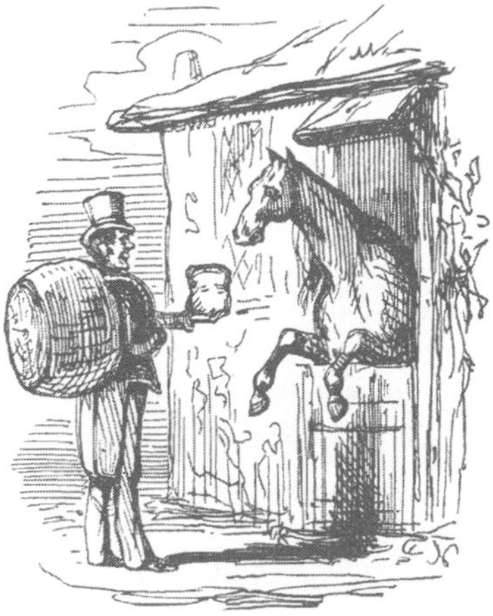

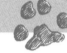

WILD LIFE

GOOD SNAKES

There are so many beautiful, beneficial snakes. One of my fondest pasture walk experiences was coming across a 5-foot-long bull snake (also known as a gopher snake) who very elegantly and calmly was working his way through the grass in front of me. Neither hurrying nor stopping, he glistened and glided, the sun highlighting the yellow in his body.

Because there are quite a few mimics or "lookalikes" in the snake world, good snakes can unfortunately be mistaken for poisonous snakes (see Pest Patrol). Garter snakes (the most widespread snake in the United States), king snakes, water snakes, rat snakes, and bull (AKA gopher) snakes are beneficial. As some of their names indicate, they eat rodents and insects. They are classified as non-game wildlife and are protected by law, which means it is illegal to kill them.

Bull, Gopher, and Pine Snakes

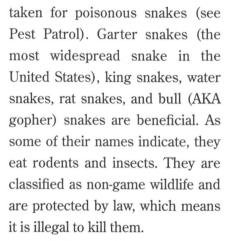

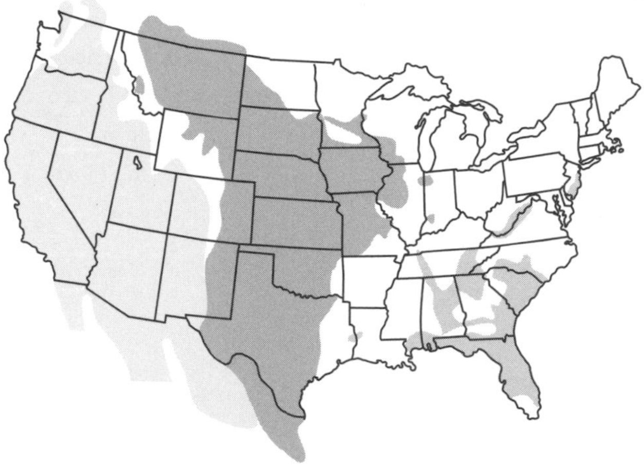

Poisonous Snakes by Region				
	Snake			
Region	Copperhead	Cottonmouth	Rattlesnake	Coral
Southwest	x	x	x	x
Northwest	x		x	x
Midwest	x	x	x	
Plains	x		x	x
Southwest Desert	x		x	x
Rocky Mountain			x	
Great Basin			x	
West Coast			x	

PEST PATROL

POISONOUS SNAKES

Two types of venomous snakes live in the United States: pit vipers and coral snakes. Pit vipers, which include rattlesnakes, cottonmouths, and copperheads, have elliptical pupils and heat-sensing pits on the side of the face between eyes and nostril. Coral snakes, with round pupils and no pits, are red, yellow and black.

To decrease snake habitat near your house and buildings, avoid the following:

- Landscape rocks (snake welcome mats).
- Crawl spaces under buildings.
- Dense vegetation near buildings (a fire hazard, too).
- If you have a hay barn full of mice, a snake might soon move in, so keep rodents under control. There are plenty for snakes to dine on out in the pastures!
- If you encounter a poisonous snake, back off slowly and smoothly. Snakes detect presence by heat and movement. Normally there is no need to kill a poisonous snake but if you are in danger, it is legal to do so in most states.

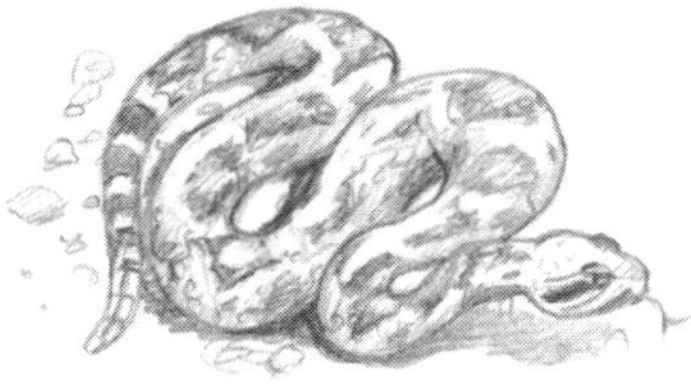

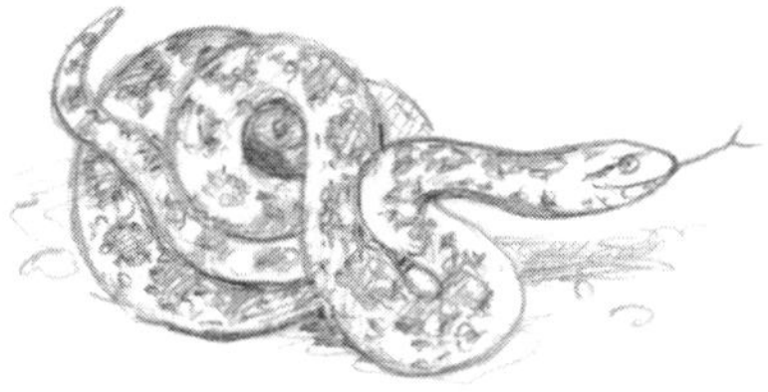

Don't confuse a rattlesnake (above) with a bullsnake (below).

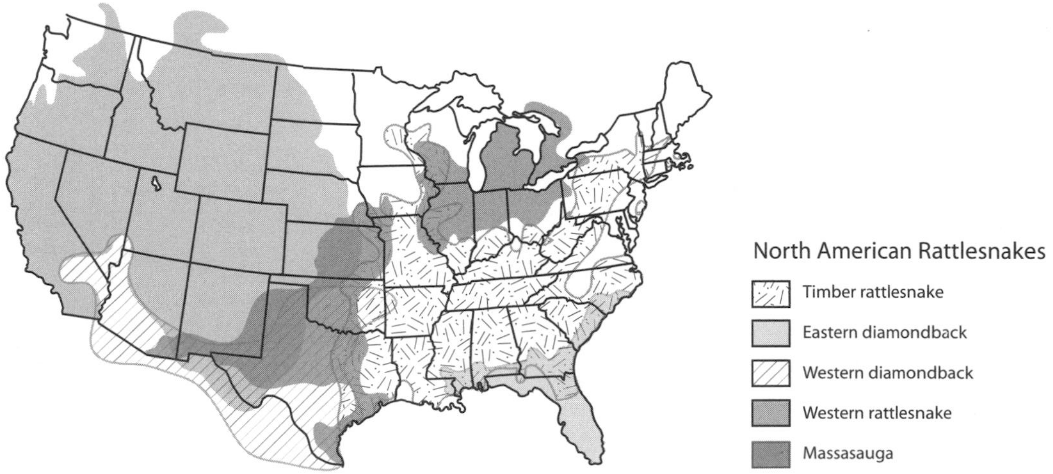

PASTURE PERFECT

SPRING PASTURE

Things are greening up and it is tempting to let the horses graze, but I err on the side of caution when it comes to early grazing in order to protect both my horses and the land. Horses go for the young plant growth and succulent roots, letting weeds go to seed and mature plants go to waste. They defecate in certain areas and then will never consider eating the plants growing there unless forced to by starvation. In addition, during wet periods (natural and irrigated) especially, their hooves ruin root structure and can turn a field into a sea of mud and then a plain of dirt when it dries. Horses left on a pasture too long paw to reach tender roots, thereby destroying a plant's ability to rejuvenate.

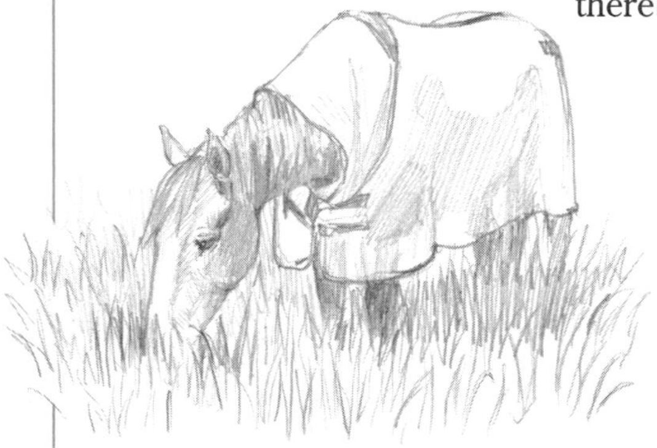

Horses should be put on pasture when it is 6–8″ high.

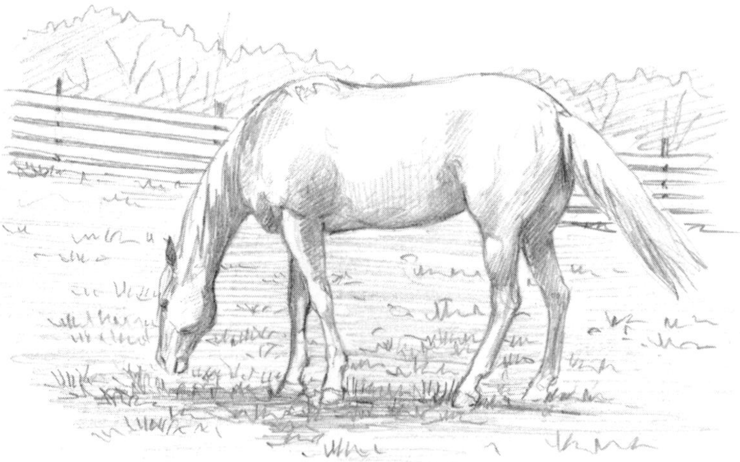

Remove horses when 50 percent of forage has been ingested or damaged.

Horses should therefore be put on pasture or hay fields when the growth is optimal — about 6 to 8 inches high depending on the grass species. After that the plant growth should be closely monitored. Remove the horses when 50 percent of the forage has been ingested or damaged.

MAINTAINING PASTURE QUALITY. Rapid pasture growth occurs early and then slows. By about 12 weeks into the season, most plants have matured and gone to seed. Mow weeds before they go to seed to help encourage re-growth and more desirable plants to take over. Reseed bare spots and protect them from traffic and grazing by removing horses or installing temporary electric fencing.

MONITORING GRAZING. Overgrazing causes pasture damage that costs much more in the long run to repair than the feed costs it saved. If the horses' grazing rate is greater than the field's ability to regrow, they should be put on another pasture so the grazed field can rest until it returns to the 6–8-inch height. After the first cut of hay is taken off a grass field, if the season isn't such that a second cut can be expected, grazing the field for several months in the late summer and early fall is often cost-effective and won't harm the field if it is not overstocked.

Ranch Notes

May 12. We saw a golden eagle take Yoda.

When you are on a great horse, you have the best seat you will ever have.

— Winston Churchill

STILL TRUE TODAY

Historical Horsekeeping

"The horse, having a very small stomach, should be fed frequently, but in small feeds. I have watched horses grazing, and, mind you, in this particular instance the pasture was thickly grassed, but I am sure they did not cease to feed for more than four hours out of the twenty-four."

— *From* The Horse *by Sydney Galvayne, 1888*

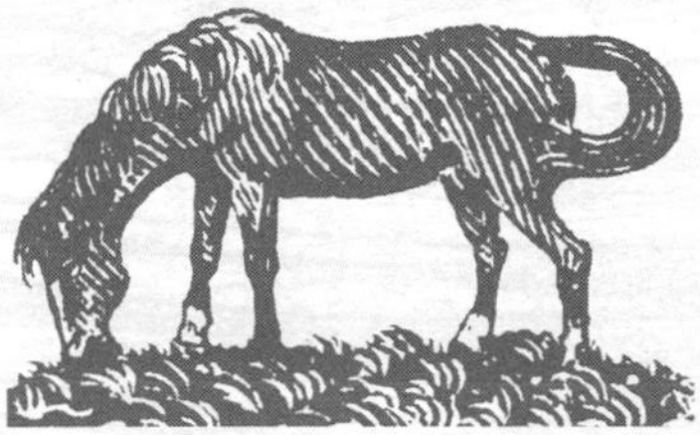

SPRING: MAY

ELIMINATING WEED TROUBLE SPOTS. At this time of year, we use our riding lawnmower and gas-powered weed-eater to spot-mow weed trouble spots. If a small area of broad-leaved weeds is cropping up, we lop off the tops to give the grass a better chance to use the soil nutrients and moisture to proliferate.

MOWING FOR A PURPOSE. We mow yards, lanes, pasture paths, and fire strips weekly for aesthetics as well as health and safety. Insects and rodents like tall grass, so although we try to leave much of our land as natural habitat, we try to minimize tall grass near our buildings. In addition, we keep a fire strip mowed around all buildings. And since we walk out to our pastures twice a day to check on horses, we mow "snake lanes": that is, 6-foot-wide paths that will let us easily spot a snake before stepping on it.

Adding a New Horse

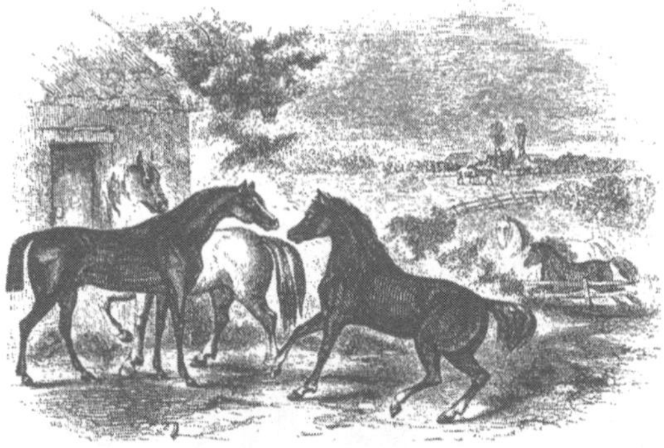

Pecking order is most evident at feeding time. Whenever a new horse is introduced into a herd, a band, or a barn, things will mix up a bit as the pecking order is established. That's why, in order to prevent injury, it is important to introduce new horses gradually. Put the new horse near but not across a fence from the old group for several days so they can see and smell each other. After a few days, turn the new horse out with some of the group members that are most agreeable, and then gradually add others back to the group.

CLEAN-UP CREW

COMPOSTING

A properly composted manure pile is efficient, convenient, and environmentally responsible. As mentioned, we recommend three compost piles: one to which fresh manure is being added daily; one that is in the process of decomposing; and one that is ready to spread.

LOCATING YOUR PILE. Before starting a pile, check your local zoning ordinances. Be sure the pile is out of sight and smell of residences and downwind from your stable and house. It should be located at least 150 feet away from waterways including streams, irrigation ditches, and wells.

Situate the pile so that it is convenient for daily dumping, periodic hauling, and regular watering with a hose. The ideal location for a manure pile is on a sloped concrete floor with 4-foot walls.

COVERING. The fresh pile is usually left uncovered for convenient daily addition, but an open pile is subject to drying by the sun and leaching of nutrients by rain and melting snow. A dry pile dehydrates the beneficial microorganisms; a soggy heap smothers them.

Whether you cover your composting and composted piles will depend on your local precipitations. Since compost should have moisture content of 50 percent (which you'll learn to estimate), the pile can be left uncovered in arid or semiarid climates so it can benefit from any precipitation, and you can add water as needed. In very wet regions, the compost pile could become too soggy, so might do better under a cover.

Plastic covers retard oxygen exchange and smother the bacteria. Earth covers are too heavy and so weight down

Eight Reasons to Compost

A properly composted manure pile:

1. Does not have to be hauled away every day.
2. Reduces bulk by up to 50 percent while concentrating nutrients.
3. Releases nitrogen and other nutrients slowly, so little nitrogen and phosphorus leach into the soil, minimizing environmental pollution.
4. Does not have an unpleasant odor.
5. Is pleasant to handle.
6. Will kill parasite eggs and many weed seeds.
7. Prevents flies from breeding.
8. Results in a good-quality soil enhancer and fertilizer.

Ideal Size Pile

An open compost pile should be about 4 feet high and 4 to 6 feet wide, or sized so that you can reach it with a fork to turn the compost. Once the pile has been formed, especially if you have room for windrows, you can add to its length, but should not add another layer on top. That way, when the compost process is completed at one end, it is ready for use.

the compost reducing necessary pore space. Open piles or those with geotextile fabric covers seem to fare the best.

SECRETS TO GREAT COMPOST. Decomposition of manure begins with the formation of ammonia as urinary nitrogen decomposes. The effectiveness of composting depends on the size and shape of the pile, the degree of compaction, the moisture content, and the aeration of the manure pile.

- A large pile with a flat or concave top is ideal because it retains its own heat and the top captures moisture from precipitation.
- A small pile with a dome would not hold its own heat as well, and its rounded top would shed water.
- A fluffy pile, turned every couple of weeks for aeration, makes the best environment for the aerobic composting microorganisms. Aeration can be accomplished by hand with a fork or by using the loader on a tractor.

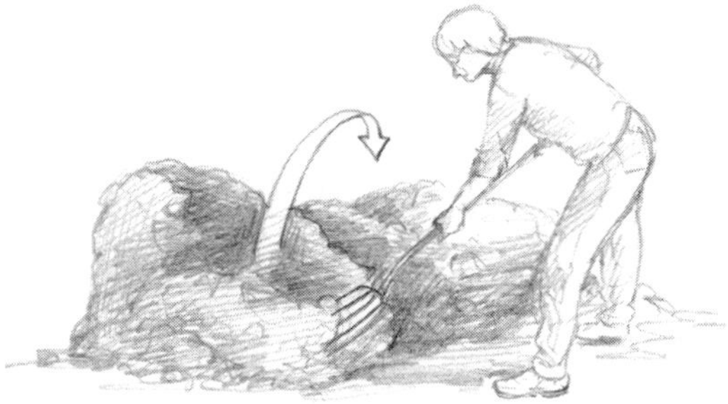

Depending on the size of your manure pile, you can aerate by hand or by tractor.

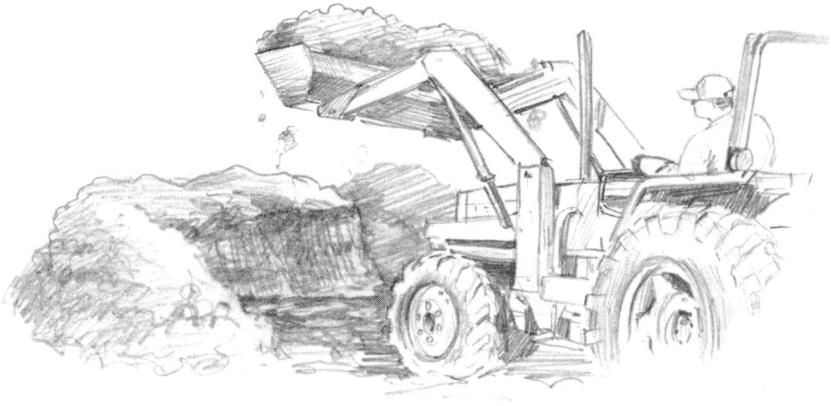

A carbon-to-nitrogen (C:N) ratio between 25:1 and 30:1 is optimal for composting. The lower the ratio, the hotter the compost. Horse manure has a C:N ratio of 30:1 to 50:1. If you add sawdust (400:1) or straw (80:1) as bedding, the C:N ratio will be higher (cooler). To keep the ratio in the ideal range, select an amendment with a lower carbon content or higher nitrogen content. Grass clippings, at 17:1, make a good addition to lower the C:N.

Hydrated lime used to dry stall floors will not affect a manure pile significantly one way or another.

TAKING TEMPERATURE. To kill most parasite eggs, the heat of the manure pile should be kept at 145 degrees Fahrenheit for at least two weeks, or lower for longer periods of time. The only way to know if a manure pile is properly composting is to take its temperature using a compost thermometer. If the pile is too cool, it may be too dry. If it is too hot, you can moderate its heat so the composting cycle lasts longer by adding leaves or bedding.

CURING. The final phase of composting is a curing stage of about a month, when the microorganisms finish degrading the more complex organic compounds and useful soil-nitrifying bacteria repopulate the compost. As the bacteria die and decompose, they release their stored nitrogen. As the fiber breaks down, carbon dioxide and water are released, decreasing the bulk of the manure by up to one-half.

HUMUS. The end product of composting is humus, the dark, uniform, finely textured, odorless product of the decomposition of organic matter that is so valuable as a soil conditioner and additive.

The process of decomposition of a manure pile can take anywhere from three to six months and the quality of the resulting humus varies.

FYI

Black Gold

Composting horse manure could become a lucrative cash by-product of your horse operation because landscapers, mushroom growers, and worm farmers seek good-quality humus. You could also use it to enhance the soil on your property — humus improves plant growth, makes the soil softer and more aerated, and increases the soil's ability to hold water.

MAY
Manure Pile Maintenance

PILE A
Turn twice, water as needed

PILE B
Sell, store, or spread

PILE C
Turn once, water as needed

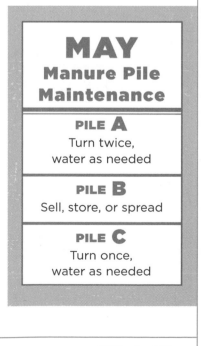

SPRING OVERHAUL

When the first of May hits, it's time for me to spend a week in the wash rack and clipping salon. Each horse receives a spring bath. I take tails out of winter storage and shampoo, condition, and trim them. Legs and bridle paths are clipped. The beauty shop is booked solid!

At Long Tail Ranch we bathe our horses three times a year: in mid- to late spring, midsummer, and late fall.

HOW OFTEN TO BATHE. My horses get three baths per year: one toward the end of spring shedding, one in midsummer, and one in late fall, just before they start to grow their long winter coats. Too many baths are not good for a horse: they can actually dry out his skin and hair, leading to further problems, and the repeated wet/dry cycles can cause hooves to deteriorate.

Sebum protects the skin (see FYI), but it also attracts dirt. I try to strike a balance in bathing frequency so that the sebum can do its job but does not become too heavy in the coat.

In addition, repeatedly wetting the legs and hooves can cause the hoof wall to become soft and punky, poorly shaped, and unable to hold nails and shoes. Saturated hooves are also an open invitation for thrush and white line disease, which can destroy hoof quality.

An alternative to bathing is a vigorous currying and vacuuming.

> FYI
>
> **Sebum Is Precious**
>
> The sebaceous glands of the skin produce sebum, an oily substance that repels water, lubricates the skin, inhibits undesirable bacterial and fungal growth, and creates the shine on a horse's coat.

BATHING IN COLD WEATHER. Generally, you can safely bathe a horse when the temperature is above 50°F and he is bathed and dried out of the wind. You can bathe in weather as low as 30°F, if you do it quickly in a shelter, preferably with an overhead heater, dry the horse vigorously and thoroughly with large towels, and cover him with one or two closely fitted wool coolers. Tie the horse for one to two hours while he dries, in case the cooler should shift and get stepped on.

When the moisture has wicked to the outside of the cooler (often appearing as frost), replace it with a dry, warm cooler. Once the horse is entirely dry, cover him with a warm, clean winter blanket.

PREPARATION. An indoor, well-drained wash rack is the ideal place to bathe a horse. The floor of the wash area should be texturized to prevent slipping. If you prefer to wash outdoors, choose a place that won't get muddy. A well-drained concrete pad or rubber-matted area in close proximity to a water hydrant is best.

Try to locate your bathing area near a source of hot water. If you do not have hot tap water in your barn, draw three or four 5-gallon buckets of water and set them out in the sun to warm. If the sun is not strong enough to warm the water within a few hours, it probably is not warm enough to give a bath. Warm water is not just nicer for your horse, but it also does a better job of cleaning his coat by dissolving oils and dirt more easily than cold water does.

Assemble your tools (see Bathing Equipment).

SHAMPOOS, CONDITIONERS, AND RINSES. For most situations, choose a mild, nondetergent shampoo. Detergents are too harsh and will dry the hair coat and may irritate the skin. At least once a year, use a medicated shampoo, such as one specially formulated with iodine, to cut down on rubbing caused by the irritation of fungal and bacterial skin conditions.

Horse shampoos and conditioners can contain a wide variety of ingredients. Proteins such as collagen, oils such as coconut oil or lanolin, and other substances such as aloe

Bathing Equipment

- ★ Clean halter
- ★ Wool cooler
- ★ Hose
- ★ Hose brush
- ★ Sponge
- ★ Rubber mitt
- ★ Sweat scraper
- ★ Large towels
- ★ Shampoo
- ★ Conditioner
- ★ Liniment

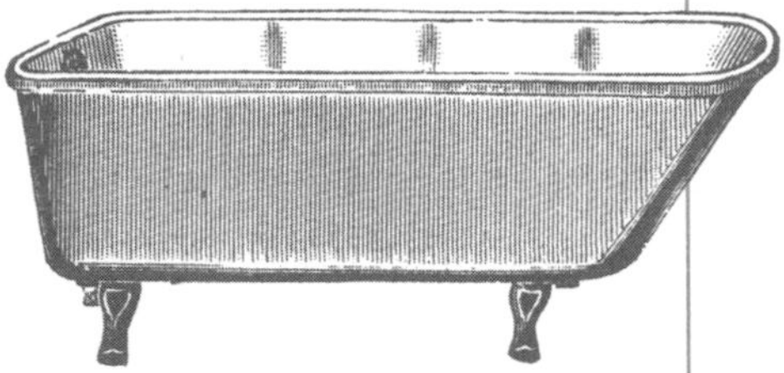

> **TIPS & TECHNIQUES**
>
> **Shine**
>
> If you are preparing a horse for a show, photo session, or presentation for sale, bathe him the day before the occasion and keep him blanketed. A freshly shampooed coat "stares" — that is, the individual hairs stand out from the horse's body. Given 24 hours, the sebum has a chance to coat each hair, causing it to lie flat, reflect light, and make the coat shine.

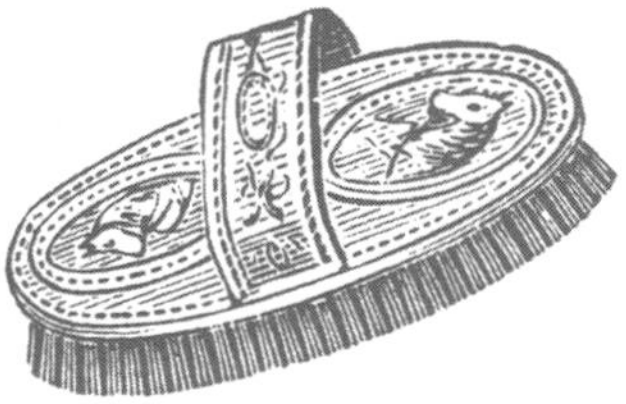

vera are added to condition and coat the rough surface (cuticle) of each hair shaft so that it lies smoothly against the next conditioned hair. Shampoos designed for white or gray horses usually contain a bluing agent, which transforms yellow stains, caused by urine and leather, to a whiter hue.

Final rinses are designed to carry away the shampoo film to leave the coat squeaky clean. Sodium hexametaphosphate, a water softener sold under the trade name of Calgon (not Calgonite), removes the graying dullness caused by previously deposited soap or shampoo residues. It has a superior ability to combine with and sequester oily and greasy substances and prevent them from reacting with the horse's skin.

Finishers, if desired, are applied last, often sprayed on. Those containing silicone are designed to give each hair a dazzling shine that lasts up to one week, repelling stains and moisture. Other finishers contain relatively long-lasting sunscreens to prevent the hair coat from becoming bleached.

How to Bathe a Horse

1. **PREPARING THE HORSE.** First, groom your horse very thoroughly to loosen the dirt and move it toward the surface of the hair where the shampoo will have a better chance of carrying it away. Before bathing, use scissors to cut the heavy fetlock hair or bridle path and winter throat hairs. (If you use clippers on dirty hair, the blades will become dull very quickly. Save clipping for after the bath.) If the horse is shedding, remove as much hair as possible by grooming before bathing. If you have put the horse's tail up for the winter, take it down and finger through it to separate it for washing.

2. **WET THE LEGS.** To accustom your horse to the sensation and temperature of the water, wet his legs

first, although they will be the last portion of his body that you will actually wash.

3. **MANE AND TAIL FIRST.** Start the bath by shampooing the mane and tail so you can spend ample time scrubbing them. If you wash the body first, your horse may chill while you spend the time necessary to do a good job on the mane and tail. Also, shampooing the mane and tail after the body has been washed and rinsed would cause soapy water to once again be washed over the previously rinsed body.

Wet the mane and tail with clear water using a hose or a sponge, taking care not to spray the horse's face when wetting the mane. Thoroughly wet the tail by dunking the end into a bucket of water and lifting the bucket upward. Accustom your horse ahead of time to this activity with an empty bucket or you may find that you are the one who gets the bath!

Squirt shampoo solution (see page 422) into the base of the mane and all along the dock of the tail, deep into the hairs. Scrub every inch of the crest and dock (including the underside); add a little water to reactivate the suds; scrub some more. Strip the clouds of suds with your hands and then rinse using sponge, bucket, or hose until you can no longer entice even one bubble to appear. Thorough

Steps in Bathing

1. Groom the horse
2. Wet his legs to accustom him to the water
3. Shampoo the mane and tail first
4. Wash the body
5. Wash the head, legs, and hooves
6. Rinse well
7. Apply a conditioning rinse; remove with a sweat scraper
8. Dry the legs and hooves thoroughly
9. Allow the horse to dry, wearing a wool cooler or standing in a warm place out of the sun
10. Put a clean sheet on him and place him in his stall

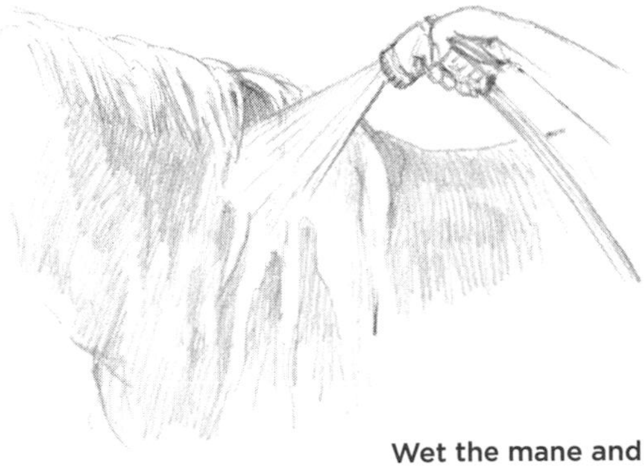

Wet the mane and tail.

rinsing is imperative or your horse may develop dermatitis, a generalized flaky skin condition, which commonly leads to rubbing.

4. **THE BODY WASH.** Next use the hose or sponge to wet one part of the horse's body. Add shampoo solution, scrub, rewet, rescrub, and rinse, rinse, rinse. Use this procedure all around the horse's body, following a system that works best for you. Try starting with the neck on the near side, then the chest and shoulder, then the back and barrel, finally the hindquarters. Move to the opposite side and repeat the pattern. Don't forget to clean the throat, the area between and immediately behind the front legs, the area between the hind legs, the belly, the anus, and the sheath or udder (see August Beauty Shop).

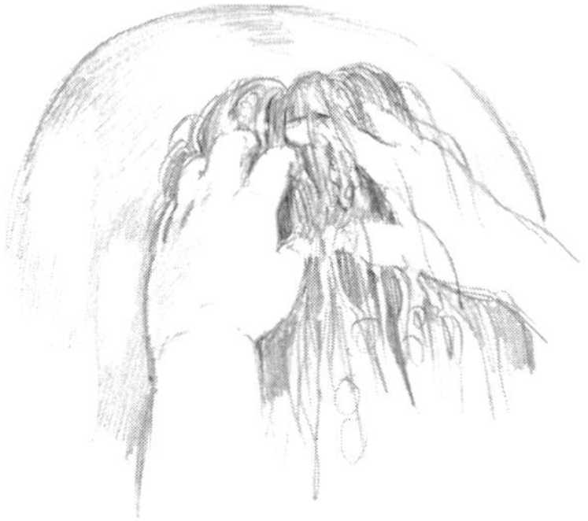

Scrub the base of the mane and tail thoroughly.

5. **HEAD, LEGS, AND HOOVES.** With a wet sponge, using more elbow grease than shampoo, clean the head, taking care not to get soap or water in the horse's eyes, ears, or nostrils. Rinse the head with a clear, wet sponge repeatedly until all dirt and shampoo have been removed. Be careful about spraying a horse's head with a hose. Some horses regard it as threatening and dangerous. The horse could get water in his eyes, ears, or nostrils. Once the head is rinsed, buff it with a towel. Finally, scrub the legs and hooves.

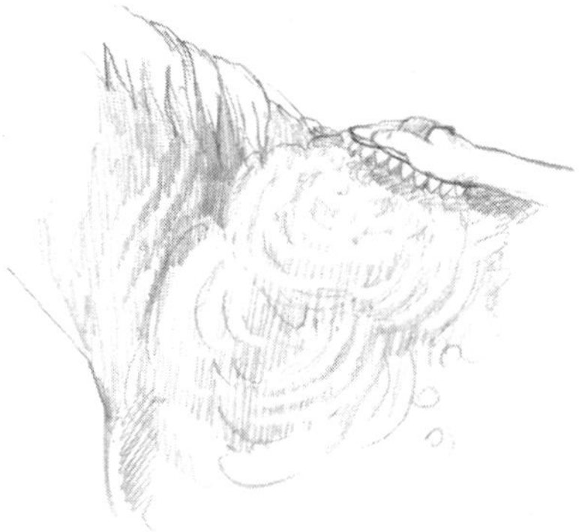

Scrub the body with shampoo solution.

6. **RINSE WELL.** Pour a commercial or customized rinse solution (such as diluted apple cider vinegar, liniment, or Calgon) over the horse's body (except for the head) including the mane and tail, until it runs off clear. Use a sweat scraper or your hands to remove as much water from the body as possible.

7. **CONDITIONING.** Then apply the conditioning rinse in a similar fashion. Thoroughly remove the conditioning rinse water from the coat with a sweat scraper. If the mane and tail require additional moisturizing, apply a very light coat of baby oil or a specialized product.

8. **DRYING AND FINISHING.** Dry the legs and hooves thoroughly with towels to discourage scratches, hoof deterioration, and chapped heels.

Spray on a coat finisher such as silicone, if desired, and lightly brush or finger through the mane, tail, and coat to distribute it. Avoid spraying silicone on the saddle area, as it would make it extremely slippery.

9. **DRYING THE COAT.** Then, depending on the weather, either cover your horse with a wool cooler or let him stand in a warm, draft-free place out of the direct rays of the sun while his coat dries. You can also hand walk him, but this will likely dirty his legs. As he is drying, periodically brush through his coat, mane, and tail.

10. **FINISHING.** Once dry, put a clean sheet on your horse and place him in his stall. If you turn out a freshly bathed horse, nine times out of 10 he will immediately roll. If you must turn your horse out after his bath, do so in a grassy pasture where he will be less likely to dirty himself while rolling.

Wet the head with a sponge.

Rinse, rinse, rinse, and then rinse some more.

Clipping

When and how much to clip the legs, bridle path, jaw, and ears depends on the weather and the intended use of the horse. The hairs in the ears and under the jaw provide valuable fly protection.

The thick hair surrounding the fetlock affords some protection from bumps and abrasions. In addition, the long

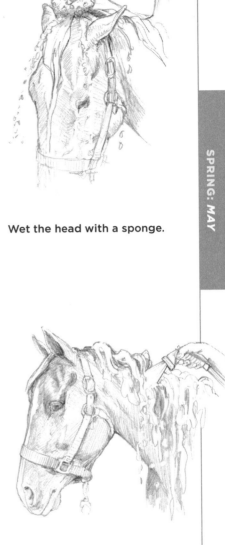

FYI

No-Clip Zone

Certain places on a horse's body have extra hair for a reason. During the summer, your horse will shed the hair on the outside of the ears, but the fine hair on the inside remains to protect him from flies and gnats. Unless you really need to clip your horse for the show ring, leave the hair inside the ears for protection.

hairs on the fetlocks keep spring moisture away from the sensitive heels and pasterns. If you want your horse to have the added protection of fetlock hair, then leave the fetlocks long. During wet weather, however, sometimes the fetlock hair never really dries out and can lead to problems. So, for sanitation reasons, it is often best to thin, shorten, or completely remove the fetlock hairs. A stabled horse often fares best if fetlock hairs are removed year-round.

The fetlock and pastern areas of some horses, especially those with white markings and long fetlock hairs (like some Warmbloods and cold-blooded draft breeds) and those living in wet, dirty conditions or hot, humid climates, can suffer a condition called scratches (see April Vet Clinic).

BRIDLE PATH. One thing that can really improve a horse's appearance is a tidy bridle path. This is a space of hair removed between the forelock and the mane to make a neater place for the crownpiece of a halter or a bridle to rest.

The length of the bridle path depends on the breed of your horse and your personal preference. Start short; you

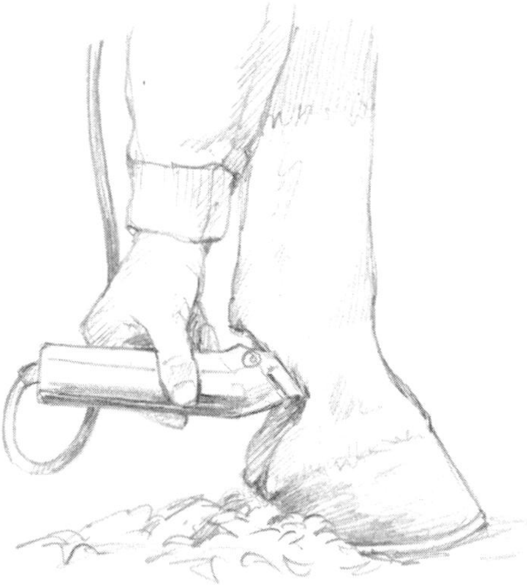

Remove winter fetlock hair by clipping with the hair, not against it.

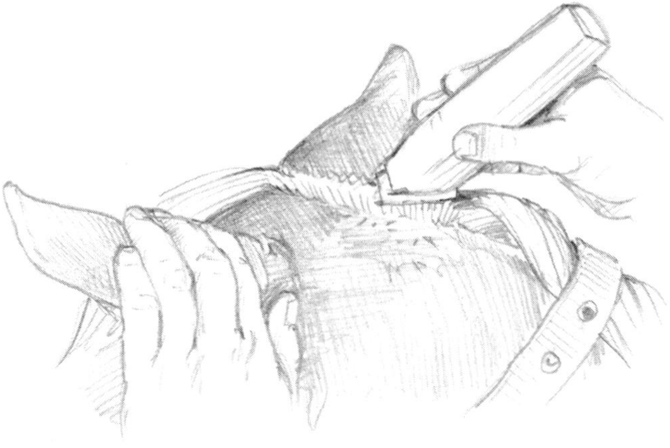

Start with a 2–3" bridle path. You can always make it longer.

can always make it longer. A good rule of thumb is 3 to 4 inches, or not longer than the length of the horse's ear.

CLIPPER BLADES. Clipper blades stay sharper and last longer if you clip only clean hair and keep the blades clean and well oiled. I store some small brushes, blade wash, clipper oil, and a cloth near my clipping area. When I am clipping, I stop periodically to brush hairs out of the blades. If the blades are accumulating a sticky buildup, dip the tips of the blades in blade wash (available through vet suppliers and tack catalogs) with the clippers running. Then turn them off and wipe them with a cloth. Turn them back on and add a drop of three-in-one oil or clipper oil, turn them off, and wipe again. Then resume clipping. When finished clipping, clean the blades once more before hanging them up.

Brushing a Tail

Here at Long Tail Ranch, I brush out a tail only when it is clean and dry. If you brush a dirty or wet tail, a lot of hair will be lost to snags and tangles. Always condition manes and tails after a bath, and mist the clean, dry tail with a detangler before brushing: both practices further protect the tail from breakage. When brushing, start at the bottom, brush out a few inches of the tail at a time, and work your way up to the top of the tail.

You can buy sturdy hairbrushes with wide-set bristles at a drug store or discount department store. Never use a comb, which tends to grab hair and pull it out.

Banging a Tail

To keep a tail thick, trim it regularly. The straight, blunt cut called a banged tail is my favorite because it is tidy and it makes the tail look healthy and strong.

Clipping the Bridle Path

1. Slip the halter back to hold the mane out of the way
2. Decide how long you want the bridle path
3. Remove most of the hair by clipping forward
4. Then turn the clippers around and clip backwards
5. Tidy up by clipping down one side of the bridle path and then the other

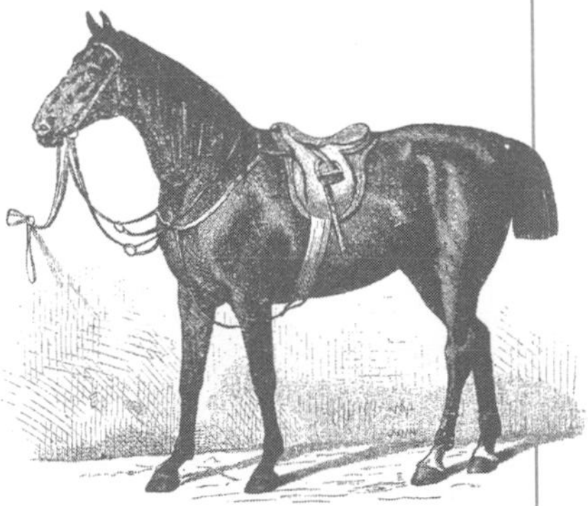

Horse Sense and Safety

Handling a Horse

★ Stand near the shoulder rather than in front of the horse when clipping and braiding. Stand next to the hindquarters rather than directly behind a horse when working on his tail.

Although the longer the tail, the better it performs as a fly swatter, a very long tail often ends up very thin. A tail at fetlock level or above has less of a chance of being stepped on when the horse backs up, straightens up after resting a hind, or gets up after lying down. I've found that if I cut a tail to the level of the fetlock when it is relaxed, it will be just above the fetlock when the horse is working or exercising.

Before you bang a tail, shampoo it well with a conditioning shampoo, rinse it very thoroughly, and brush it out completely. Start at the bottom and work your way up. Be sure to stand the horse square on a level surface, and then follow these steps.

1. Slide your hand down the tail until you reach fetlock level so you can gauge how much will have to be removed.
2. Raise the tail up to a more comfortable cutting level.
3. Cut off the amount that needs to be removed.
4. Let the tail back down and brush it out again.
5. Check to see that your cut was level and that there are no long stragglers.

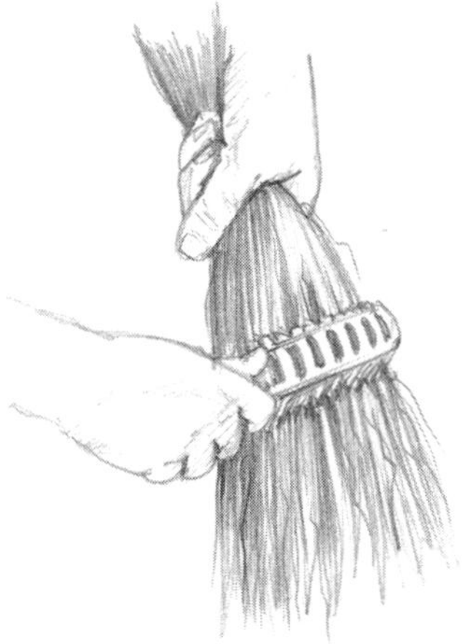

When brushing, start at the bottom, brush out a few inches of the tail at a time, and work your way up to the top of the tail.

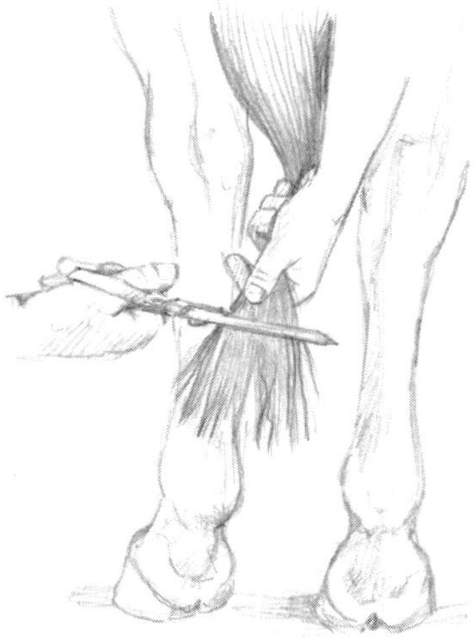

A banged tail is a safe but attractive tail style for both English and Western horses.

SADDLE PAD CARE

A saddle pad is essential for a safe and comfortable ride. Keep it clean. This means having both a clean pad and a clean horse. Check the pad or blanket for hard spots, dried sweat, dirt, sand, matted hair, burrs, twigs, and other foreign objects. Thoroughly groom the horse's back and cinch area, because dirt and sand embedded in the horse's coat can work loose during a ride to irritate and rub him raw. Matted hair that collects on a pad can make it slip, so remove it by brushing or vacuuming before each use.

After use, rather than spreading the blanket wet-side-up over a saddle to dry, hang it wet-side-out on a blanket rod so that air can reach all sides of the pad. Thick pads can get stiff because they absorb horse sweat, which contains salt and other minerals and also conducts dirt from the horse's coat into the pad. The sweat evaporates and the dirt and minerals accumulate, making the pad stiff and crusty.

One way to avoid this is to use a washable liner (underpad) next to the horse. A thin blanket or felt pad works well. Having several liners on hand ensures that a horse's main pad or blanket stays cleaner, especially during shedding season.

TIPS & TECHNIQUES

Keeping Burrs at Bay

When you ride through brush or woods, it's easy for sticks, leaves, pine needles, and burrs to find their way under the pad. Make an occasional stop to check for debris, especially if your horse's behavior suddenly changes.

Before washing a saddle pad, remove hair using one of your old bristled hairbrushes.

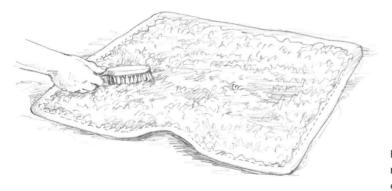

LOOKING AT HORSES

The Eyes Have It

A horse's eye should be prominent without bulging. The expression of the eye should indicate a quiet, tractable temperament. The shape of the nasal bone and forehead is largely a matter of breed and personal preference.

CLEANING PADS. When I do have to clean a pad, I brush and vacuum it, which increases its life and maximizes the time between washings. A sarvis-style brush (a plastic curry made to be attached to a hose) or a hairbrush for humans with little balls on the bristle ends works well on felt, woven fabrics, and short fleece. A brush with hard steel bristles is often too sharp and can cut or fray felt and blanket material. However, a steel dog-grooming brush works well for brushing out long fleece pads.

WASHING PADS. Thick, woven Western pads and long-panel dressage pads are often too large and too stiff to fit into a conventional washing machine. What's more, they often have wear leathers and fancy additions that wouldn't stand up to the agitation. You can take pads to a dry cleaner or Laundromat but not all welcome horse hair and sweat, and if they do, the cost can be substantial. (You might even see a sign in a window that says "No horse equipment allowed.")

WASHING WOOL. To wash a wool blanket or pad, soak it for an hour in water (most manufacturers recommend cold or lukewarm). Squeeze the blanket to remove as much water as you can and hang the blanket over a rail. Lightly brush it on both sides. Let the blanket air-dry completely and then slap it against a solid surface, such as a clean, smooth wall, until it feels soft as new.

If you choose to add a cleaner to the water, be careful. Alkaline solutions can damage wool, so it's best to use a pH-balanced shampoo (between 5.5 and 8) or a non-sudsing blanket wash specially designed for washing wool blankets and pads. Use very little detergent, and make sure to rinse every trace from the blanket or pad. Otherwise, soap can work out of the pad when a horse sweats, and can irritate and sore the horse's back.

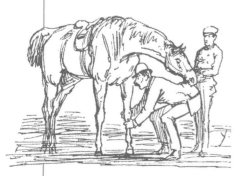

Time to Clean Your Pad

Pressure Washing at Home

I like to wash pads at home with a pressure washer and no soap. You especially do not want soap residue on a saddle pad, as it could be very irritating to your horse's back. Before washing a pad, remove all hair and dirt with a vacuum or brush.

1. Lay the pad, dirty side down, on a clean, flat surface.

2. Spray to wet it from the top side, so dirt and sweat aren't forced into the pad.

3. Let the pad soak, and then hang it up on a rail.

4. Spray the top side again, then flip the pad. When you spray the dirty side, direct the stream of water sideways to send the dirt off the pad rather than into it.

5. Let the pad drip-dry.

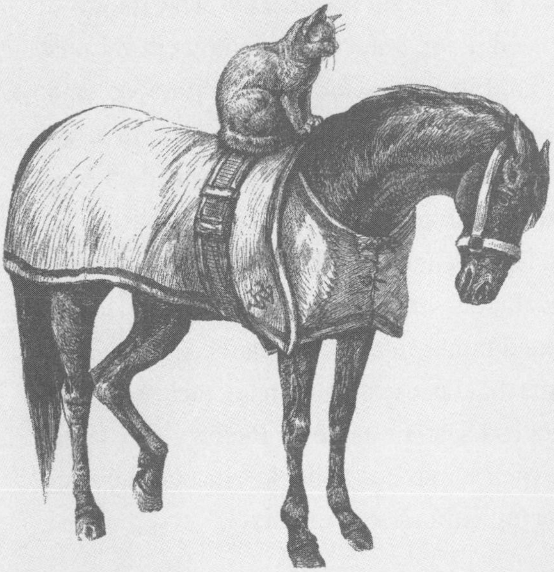

Car-Wash Technique

If you do not have a power washer, you can wash pads at a self-serve car wash.

1. Use the floor mat clips to hang your pad.

2. Select the rinse cycle, so you do not drive automotive detergent into your pad. Let the water flow for a minute or so to be sure there is no soap left in the wand from the previous customer.

3. When the pad is clean, put it in a plastic bag, bring it home, and hang it to dry.

Maintenance

★ After a blanket has dried from a ride, if it is very dirty, first slap it against a post or panel to knock the dried dirt, sweat, and hair loose.

★ Place the pad or blanket bottom side up on a firm, flat surface.

★ Brush in a circular motion to raise the nap of the material, loosen crusty areas, and remove the majority of the hair.

★ After brushing, vacuum to remove scurf and dirt embedded in the material.

SPRING: MAY

TIPS & TECHNIQUES

Rinse Cycle

Whether washing by hand or by machine, add a cup of white vinegar or a half cup of Calgon to the rinse water to help flush out the soap.

When machine-washing blankets and pads, run them through an additional heavy wash cycle using only water, no soap, to be sure they are rinsed thoroughly.

CLEANING FOAM PADS. Open-cell foam, the absorbent, sponge-like padding used in some pads, can be soaked in warm water, squeezed or pressed to remove the water and dirt, and then air-dried in the shade to protect it from damage by the sun's ultraviolet rays. Soap can be extremely difficult to rinse completely from open-cell foam, so use very little or none. Closed-cell foam, such as neoprene, is nonabsorbent so washing with soap is not a problem, but usually isn't necessary since this material usually wipes or rinses clean with plain water.

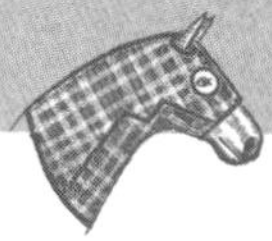

CLOTHES HORSE

BLANKET STORAGE

Before I put horse blankets away for the season, I make sure they are clean and in good repair. That way, they will be ready when I need them. I store the blankets in various locations. Those that I won't use for a while either go on a high shelf in my dust-free, rodent-free tack room; in large trunks; in plastic bags on a high shelf in my rodent-free feed room; or in metal cabinets in the aisle of the barn. For added protection, I keep a few mothballs in these cabinets. Even though the cabinets seal very well and our barn is virtually mouse free, I'd rather not take a chance.

I store the items that I use regularly in my tack room, on a swinging blanket rod system made by Richard (see page 475). In addition, each horse has a blanket bar on the stall door where I hang an extra sheet or blanket.

Ranch Notes

May 22. Get 3 geldings used to pasture gradually.

LESSONS

If you are thinking of giving lessons at your farm or ranch, consider liability and income-tax implications. Become a certified instructor and join an organization that will help you develop your business. See the appendix for helpful Web sites.

LEASING

You might someday be on one side or the other of leasing a horse, so it is a good idea to know how it works. If you don't want to sell a horse but you need help paying for his expenses, you might want to offer your horse on a full lease or a half-lease (share-a-horse). Or if you don't have the money to buy a horse or are not sure if he is the horse for you, you might want to lease him to test him out before buying.

Usually someone who agrees to a full lease expects to take the horse to her own facility and care for and use him exclusively. However, if you have the facilities and room but you just need help with costs, consider a full lease that allows the lessee to keep the horse at your place. A horse on a shared lease would most likely reside at the owner's facility and the half-lessee would share the costs and use of the horse.

Most lessors (owners) require the horse to be fully insured by the lessee during a lease. The lease agreement should specifically spell out what occurs if the horse becomes seriously ill or injured. Would the lease be automatically canceled? Or would the lessee be responsible for caring for the horse during lay-up?

Some owners (generally of less expensive horses) are very flexible about lease arrangements and may lease the horse for a much lower cost, might absorb some maintenance costs, and might even provide some tack to use. Some leases have an option-to-buy clause.

FYI

Leasing Costs

Most leases are made for a period of a year at a time. The lessee pays the horse's owner an annual lease fee, usually a third of the value of the horse, due at the time of agreement. For a $9,000 horse, expect to pay $3,000 to lease the horse for the year.

A full lease allows the lessee to use the horse for purposes agreed with the owner. However, the lessee is usually responsible for all maintenance costs: feed, board, farrier, and veterinary maintenance.

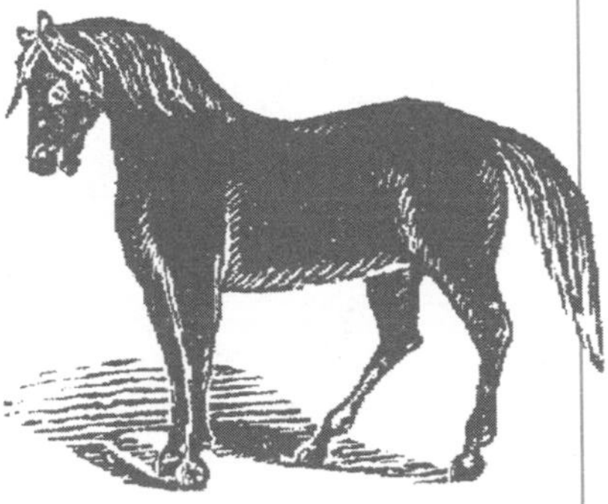

Common Lease Problems

★ No written contract

★ Length of time not specified

★ No restrictions listed on horse use, where or how the horse is kept, or who can handle him

★ Liability responsibility is not specified if someone gets hurt

★ Liability is not assigned if horse is injured, ill, or dies

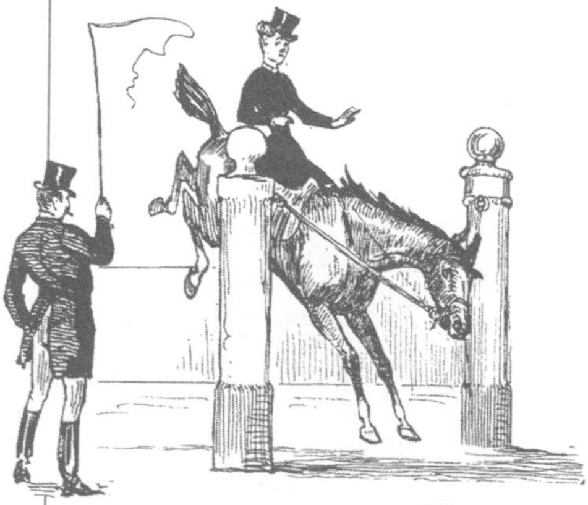

INSPECTION. When leasing a horse, be sure to inspect it just as thoroughly as you would if purchasing the horse. If you are leasing a broodmare, be sure to have a thorough reproductive exam performed.

TERMS OF AGREEMENT. A lease agreement should contain the following:

- Names and addresses of lessor (owner) and lessee (person leasing the horse)
- Full and complete description of the horse
- Purpose of the lease; proposed use of the horse; limitations on use
- Length of the lease
- Whether the lessee has the right to sub-lease
- The cost of the lease and when payment is due
- Insurance arrangements including mortality, major medical, surgical, and liability
- An outline of care of the horse
- Who pays when bills exceed a certain amount
- Whether the lease is still in effect if horse is seriously ill or injured
- Circumstances under which the lessor may cancel the lease
- Circumstances under which the lessee may cancel the lease
- Warranty by lessor as to ownership, horse's health, suitability, and so on
- Any other specific arrangements such as option to buy, delivery arrangements, right of lessor to sell horse during lease and if lessee has the right of first refusal, if there is a sole rider, driver, or handler stipulated, if there is a trade of formal training of the horse in exchange for the lease fee, if the horse can be used as a school horse, and automatic renewal option
- Signatures of both parties with dates and witness

TAKE A HAY INVENTORY

Since hay is the single largest purchase I make each year, I keep a close eye on my hay supply. I take an inventory of hay on May 1, and then monthly thereafter. (For your budget, you might want to do this in March; see March Farm Office.) I use my inventory to determine how much hay I need to buy for the next year. I always like to have extra on hand, which I call my "buffer" in case we have a drought, hay prices go sky high, or I add a horse to our band.

In my first inventory, I calculate how long the hay I have on hand will last me, feeding every horse at full feed. However, the pasture months are just beginning, so hay usage will start to go down, which means my supply on hand will last longer.

Starting in May, the horses eat part hay and part pasture. During June, July, and August, most horses are on pasture full time, so hay usage drops dramatically. In September, most horses are back on partial hay rations and then all horses are usually on full hay rations starting in October. Of course, depending on the weather, we might have lush or sparse pasture, so that will make a difference in the hay usage. That's why I take inventory at the beginning of each month from May until October.

Estimating Consumption

A safe estimate is that each horse can consume 20 pounds of hay per day on full feed.

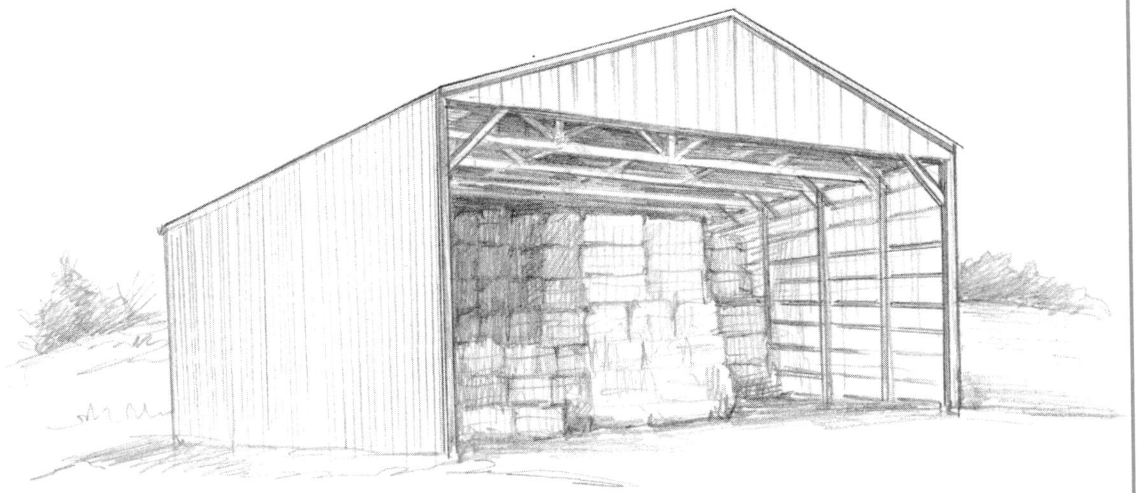

A separate hay storage area away from the main horse barn is the ideal way to store hay.

Extra Hay

Figuring 20 pounds per day, per hourse, is a generous estimate. Most horses will receive 15 pounds per day. The extra hay might be used during very cold winter weather, and some hay might need to be discarded due to weeds or spoilage.

Opposite is a sample worksheet for three horses to help you design your own worksheet.

Figure 20 pounds of hay per horse per day on full feed. For three horses, that totals 60 pounds of hay per day. The total of 17,352 pounds of hay would be enough for 289 days, or approximately 9½ months, lasting until mid-February.

BUDGET FOR HAY PURCHASE. Knowing the consumption rate, to have enough hay to last until midsummer next year, I'd need to buy four months' worth, or 120 days × 60 pounds per day, a total of 7,200 pounds, or 3.6 tons. Purchase this amount of hay to get you through to hay time next year. If you don't need to feed it all because you have pasture, sell a horse, or so on, the leftover will be your "buffer" hay for the next year.

TAKE INVENTORY EACH MONTH TO TRACK USAGE. The example below will show you how your hay supply stretches if you have pasture.

During May, the horses are on part hay and part pasture. According to the June 1 inventory figures, the horses have consumed 16 bales. Looking ahead, for three horses on full feed, at a total of 60 pounds of hay per day, there is enough for 273 days, or approximately nine months, lasting until March 1.

During June, the horses are on pasture. That's why the July 1 inventory shows the same amount of hay as last month. Feeding three horses at 60 pounds of hay per day would still be enough for 273 days, or approximately nine months, now lasting until April 1.

During July, the horses are on pasture full time so the August 1 inventory is the same. Hay for three horses at 60 pounds per day would now last until May 1.

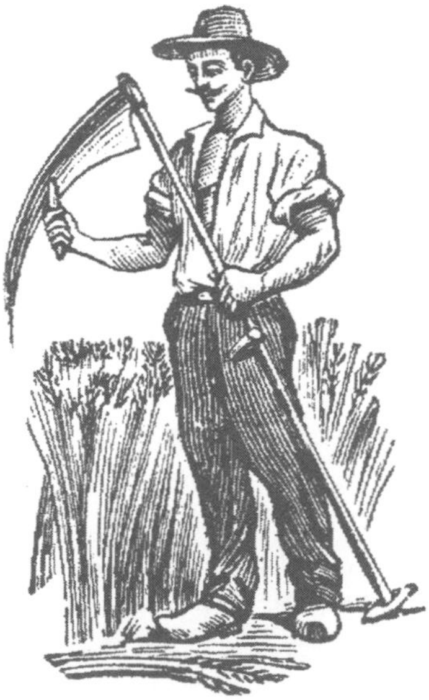

During August, the horses are still on pasture. Purchasing 7200 pounds (125 bales) of hay increases the September 1 inventory so that (for three horses at 60 pounds per day) there is enough for 394 days (about 13 months), lasting until next year's October 1.

During September, the horses are on pasture but supplemented with half-rations of hay. At the October 1 inventory, 16 bales have been used and there is now enough for 379 days, or approximately 12½ months, lasting until mid-October of next year.

Conclusion: Purchase the hay you need in the summer and keep a "buffer" to carry you through the next hay season.

Sample Hay Inventory

	Type of Hay	Weight per Bale	Number of Bales	Total Weight
May 1	Alfalfa, first cut	60	63	3,780
	Grass, first cut	58	234	13,572
	Total hay on hand	enough until mid-Feb.		17,352
June 1	Alfalfa, first cut	60	63	3,780
	Grass, first cut	58	218	12,644
	Total hay on hand	enough until March 1		16,424
July 1	Alfalfa, first cut	60	63	3,780
	Grass, first cut	58	218	12,644
	Total hay on hand	enough until April 1		16,424
Aug 1	Alfalfa, first cut	60	63	3,780
	Grass, first cut	58	218	12,644
	Total hay on hand	enough until May 1		16,424
Sept 1	Alfalfa, first cut	60	63	3,780
	Grass, first cut	58	218 + 125 = 343	12,644 + 7,200 = 19,844
	Total hay on hand	enough until Oct. 1 of next year		23,624
Oct 1	Alfalfa, first cut	60	63	3,780
	Grass, first cut	58	327	18,966
	Total hay on hand	enough until mid-Oct. of next year		22,746

In-Hand Checklist

- ❑ Catch in stall, pen, paddock, and pasture
- ❑ Halter without fussing
- ❑ Unhalter without pulling away
- ❑ Turn loose without galloping away
- ❑ Walk forward promptly and in proper position
- ❑ Turn left from light cues
- ❑ Turn right from light cues
- ❑ Stop without requiring strong cues
- ❑ Back without requiring strong cues
- ❑ Stand on a long line without moving while trainer moves around
- ❑ Move sideways from light cues
- ❑ Turn on the forehand from each side
- ❑ Turn on the hindquarters from each side

TRAILER LOADING

Before you review trailer loading, review in-hand work from the near and off sides. Then, trailer loading will go more easily.

PREPARING TO LOAD. When you review trailer loading, attach the trailer to a towing vehicle or a heavy tractor to prevent it shifting when the horse steps in. Then follow these steps.

1. Open the manger doors or drop-down head doors and fasten them into position. This will allow more light and air into the trailer so it won't appear as confining to the horse.
2. Open the rear doors as far as they will open and fasten them securely in the open position.
3. In a slant load, fasten all dividers securely against the wall. In a straight load, you can move or remove the center divider to give the horse more room.
4. Place a railroad tie under the rear of the trailer to

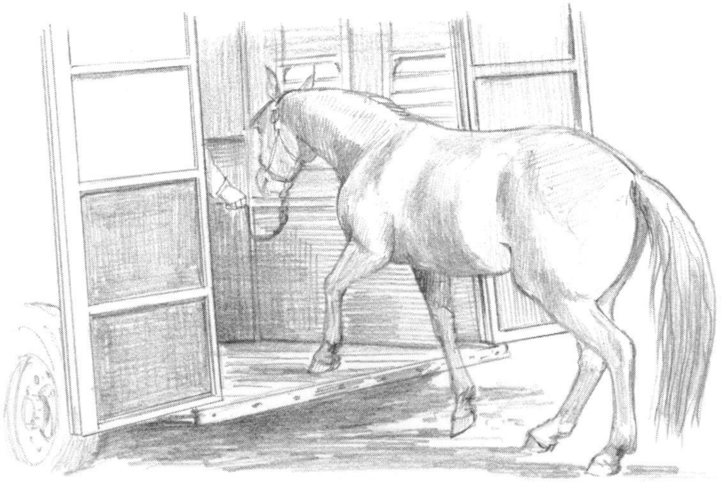

Before show or trail-ride season, review trailer loading.

prevent a horse's hind leg from slipping under when unloading.

5. Place a treat in the manger or feed bag of the trailer so the horse will instantly be rewarded for loading. (Don't use treats or feed to bribe a horse into the trailer, but let the horse discover the treat when he has stepped fully into the trailer.)

For more on trailer training, see Recommended Reading in the appendix.

REPRODUCTION ROUNDUP

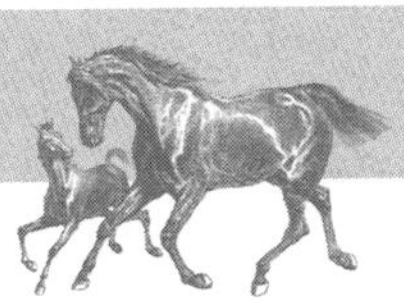

FOALING

You have your foaling kit (see page 55), and you've been watching your mare for signs indicating that foaling is near (see page 196). To understand what to do at foaling time, refer to Recommended Reading in the appendix for books devoted solely to this subject.

EARLY HANDLING. One of the questions I am most frequently asked is whether I imprint my foals. Academically, the answer is no. That's because my definition of imprinting is really species bonding, something that happens between the mare and foal. The first type of learning that a foal experiences is imprinting. This is the process of dam and species bonding that takes place during the first few hours after birth. The odors of the placental fluids and the sounds exchanged between foal and dam confirm innate behaviors in the foal.

Human interference can cause long-lasting disorientation in the foal. Some youngsters inadvertently imprinted with human smells and sounds have trouble locating their dam, or worse yet, experience difficulty relating to their species in general.

The old mare
watched the
tractor work,
A thing of rubber and
steel,
Ready to follow
the slightest wish
Of the man who held
the wheel.
She said to herself
as it passed by,
You gave me an
awful jolt,
But there's still one
thing you can't do,
You cannot raise
a colt.

— George Rupp

Odd Word

scurf. The flaky buildup on an ungroomed horse's skin that is the result of natural skin-cell shedding, oil production, and dirt accumulation. It can cause a horse to itch and can make him look dull and dirty. Rolling, bathing, and regular grooming remove scurf.

So, when a foal is born at my place, besides making sure all is going well with the birthing, the only time I handle the foal the first night is to quickly slip into the stall to dip its navel in iodine and give it an enema. (I also will tie up the mare's afterbirth if necessary.) For the mare's sake and the foal's, give them plenty of privacy and time to remain lying down, establish their bond, and begin their routines.

I choose to postpone handling until the foal's first day, and then provide regular handling. I think that "regular" is the key here. Poor handling at any age can make the foal pushy and disrespectful toward people. Good handling at any age encourages respect, curiosity, and friendliness.

WHAT IS A FOAL LIKE AT BIRTH? A foal is born with needs like a human infant's: hunger, thirst, sleep, and comfort. Within hours, however, it has the physical ability and mechanical skills of a two-year-old human.

Twenty-four hours after birth the foal is able to run, using legs that are 90 percent as long as an adult horse's. Coupled with keen instincts, this physical advantage has helped the young horse survive over the millennia. Sometimes this physical strength and vigor are expressed too exuberantly

STILL TRUE TODAY

Historical Horsekeeping

"The udder continues to increase until wax appears; this is a yellow substance which remains on the fronts of the teats about a day, and when it drops off, milk beings to show, and continues dropping away; and as a rule, the mare will foal within ten hours of the change from wax to milk."

— *From* The Horse *by Sydney Galvayne, 1888*

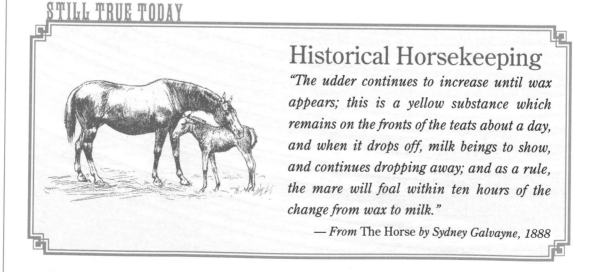

Reproduction Roundup

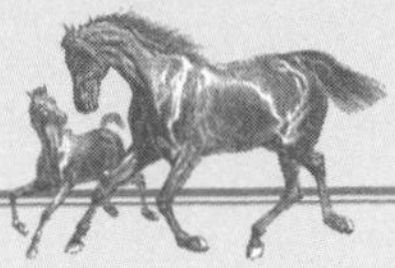

A Foal's First Week

My foal-handling program is systematic early handling. I move on when the foal is ready to progress and I don't dwell on a particular stage if the foal is ready to learn something new. It usually goes something like this:

Day 1 Apply iodine to navel. Give enema.

Day 2 Catch and release. Catch and hold with one arm around chest and one around rump, with no pressure unless foal is trying to leave. When foal stands still, there should be no pressure from your arms. Release the foal. The foal learns to accept restraint without fighting and to stand still on his own. Begin desensitization (see Day 3). Foal will have a strong suckle reflex at this time, so discourage nibbling. Frequent, short lessons are best.

Day 3 Desensitization: head, leg, and body handling. I like to override some of the foal's reflexes such as head flipping when the poll or the bridge of the nose is touched, head shaking when the ears or mouth are handled, kicking when the rump is pressed, and overall fidgeting when topline is stroked from poll to tail. I handle all legs from the barrel all the way to the hoof. I handle the belly, girth area, and flank, and lift the tail and touch the anus. If the foal is doing well, I may begin to teach haltering (see Day 4). Frequent, short (five-minute) lessons throughout the day.

Day 4 Haltering: halter and unhalter to get foal used to the object coming up in his line of vision from front and sides. Just put the halter on and take it off. Do not attach a lead rope at this time.

Day 5 Attach a lead and use it as a combination lead rope, chest rope, and butt rope to teach the foal to lead. Two sessions per day. Include lifting each leg so you can look at the bottom of the hoof.

Day 6 Remove the foal's butt rope and with a helper leading the dam, lead the foal behind the dam using only the halter and lead rope in a normal fashion. (You might need to go back to the butt rope a few times for review.)

Day 7 Lead the foal with only the halter with the dam confined nearby.

This concludes what I call "early handling." Now the foal's training progresses into an overall ground-training program, which over the next months includes in-hand maneuvers, obstacles, tying, and trailer loading.

and foals overstress themselves, especially when they are turned out following extended confinement.

In spite of their apparent vigor, foals are fragile, both mentally and physically, and need close contact and security from their dam. The suckling foal is characteristically inquisitive yet timid; fractious yet vulnerable; feisty yet fearful. Although it is advantageous to handle the youngster before he gets unwieldy, it is best to make the sessions short, firm, fair, and to the point.

FINE FACILITIES

THE IDEAL ROUND PEN SIZE

I've found that a diameter of 66 feet (20 meters) is an ideal size for most of my round pen training. It is small enough to allow me to teach a horse about human/horse body language, such as turning to face me. Yet it is large enough for active longeing lessons without stressing the horse's legs. Working a horse in small circles can damage his joints and tendons. A 66-foot pen is ideal for early long-lining or ground-driving lessons too. I can even drive the horse in a figure-eight change of rein at a trot in my round pen. And a 66-foot round pen is big enough to lope a horse in.

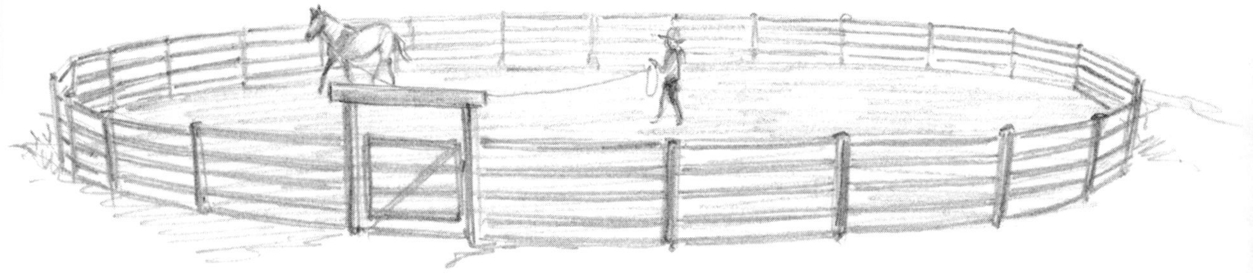

FIRE STRIPS

Depending where you live, the grass might be tall about now and if you are like us, you are already in full mow. We try to keep at least a 30-foot fire strip mowed around all buildings so if a grass fire starts, it can't burn up to the buildings. There are no trees or bushes in the fire strip either. The defensible zone will depend on where you live, the slope of your land and the fire danger. (See more on Fire in August.)

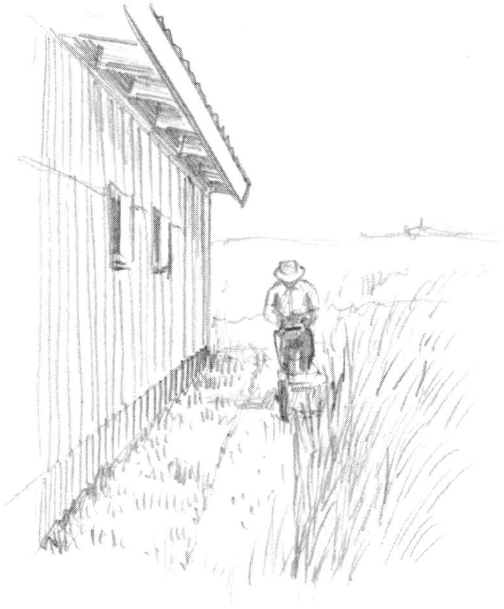

RPMS & PTOS

SERVICING EQUIPMENT

Now that the weather is a little warmer, it is a good time for those tinkering jobs, such as finding the pesky leak on the tractor or servicing the rotary harrow to make sure it is ready for another season of arena grooming. For tractor service, refer to January RPMs & PTOs.

ROTARY HARROW

Capable of both aerating and smoothing the soil, a rotary harrow is ideal for working up the footing in an arena. The three-point hitch can be adjusted so that the harrow works flat, tipped to one side, or tipped to the front or back. When adjusted flat, the harrow doesn't rotate, while tipping it slightly to one side causes it to turn as it is pulled forward. Set at its most aggressive tilt, a rotary harrow can dig 4 to 5 inches into soil, if the soil is not too compacted.

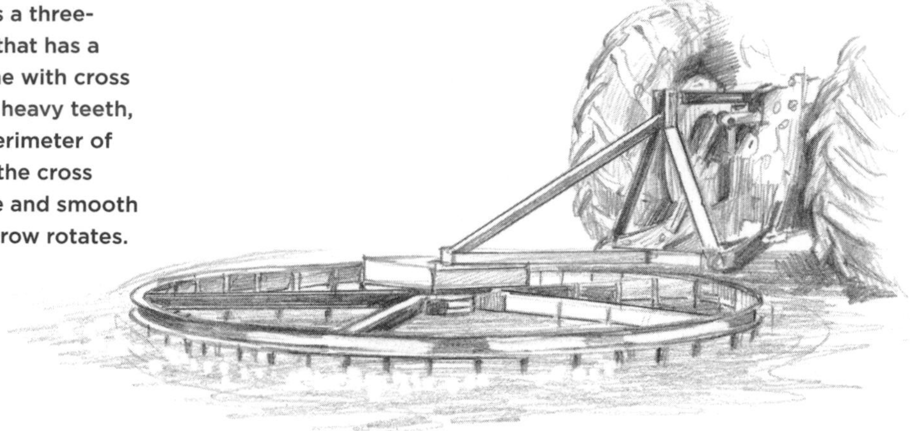

A rotary harrow is a three-point implement that has a rigid circular frame with cross braces. There are heavy teeth, or tines, on the perimeter of the circle and on the cross braces that aerate and smooth the soil as the harrow rotates.

The teeth are welded or bolted on. When tines wear down, bolted tines can be easily replaced, while welded tines must have new tines welded next to the old ones.

MORE IN DEPTH

CORRECT WEIGHT

Here is how to determine if your horse is at the proper weight. A horse's weight is considered about right when he scores in the middle of a body condition scale, as follows:

- Using a scale from 1 to 9, 1 represents emaciated and 9 represents extremely obese.
- A horse that is determined to be between 5 and 7 is usually at an optimal weight.
- Horses that have a body condition score of less than 4 have less energy, lower resistance to disease, and may have trouble breeding.
- Horses with scores of 8 to 9 are just a step away from colic or laminitis. Obese horses also have low energy and reproductive problems.

See January for information on weighing horses.

Before we get to the scoring itself, I should note that some horses and some breeds of horses have bonier withers

Ranch Recipes

Flavored Water

If you travel with your horse, he will have to drink unfamiliar water. Every horse's tastes and tolerances are different in this regard. Some horses drink water from almost any source; others are so finicky that you will have to devise a means of disguising water from a non-home source.

It is almost impossible to carry enough water to satisfy a horse's requirements for more than a day or so. Water is simply too heavy and bulky to haul very much of it. Nevertheless, one of the leading causes of travel colic is dehydration, so keep a close eye on your horse's water intake before and during all trips.

You can prevent dehydration by preparing him in advance for possible changes in smell or taste of water. The trick is to flavor his water ahead of time, at home. Using trial and error, you can find what works for your horse. Start with apple juice, which has a pleasant but distinctive smell and taste.

1. Begin adding an ounce or two to your horse's water bucket at home for a week before traveling.
2. Work up to a full 8-ounce cup per bucket if you anticipate encountering very odd water on your trip.
3. If your horse is drinking well with the apple juice at home, you can use it to flavor the water on your trips to keep him drinking and hydrated.

Other substances that can be used to flavor water include vinegar, molasses, flavored powdered electrolytes, oil of peppermint or wintergreen, vanilla extract (just one or two drops per bucket), a sprinkling of Kool-Aid or Jell-O, or in an emergency, a splash of soda pop.

Often the sweetness will encourage a horse to drink. But be sure to find out what your horse likes *before* a trip.

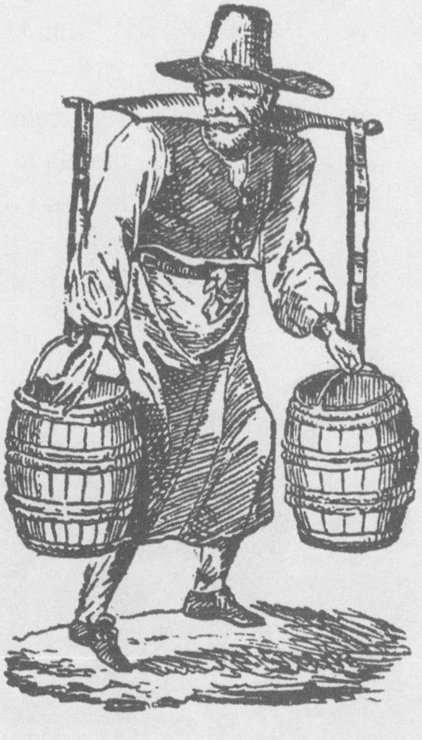

and show more rib naturally. Thoroughbreds, Saddlebreds, and some Tennessee Walkers might fall into this category. They might be of an ideal weight but show some of the signs of a horse that would be classified as underweight.

Conversely, some Quarter Horses can be in good weight but exhibit some of the characteristics of an overweight horse. To determine your horse's score, inspect him from each side, the front, and the rear from about 20 feet away. Is your overall impression that the horse is too fat, too thin, or just about right?

Then, get specific. If you can see a horse's ribs, he will score 4 or lower. If you can't see the ribs, he will score 5 or higher. If the horse's hair is too long or thick to see the ribs, feel the ribcage. At 5, you can feel the ribs but not see them. At 7, the spaces start to fill in with fat between the ribs.

Next, look for fat deposits on the back, ribs, neck, shoulders, withers, and tailhead. Compare what you find to the descriptions listed on the Horse Body Condition Criteria.

Aim to keep your horse at optimal weight year-round. The exception to the rule is that if you live in an area with very cold winters, allow your horse to gain a little fat in the fall to help insulate him in the winter. For example, if he is normally a 6, let him move up to a 7 in October and maintain that weight until spring, when increased work will bring him back to his normal working condition of 6.

"Their horses were of great stature, strong and clean-limbed; their grey coats glistened, their long tails flowed in the wind, their manes were braided on their proud necks."

— J. R. R. Tolkien, *The Lord of the Rings*, Book 3, Chapter 2

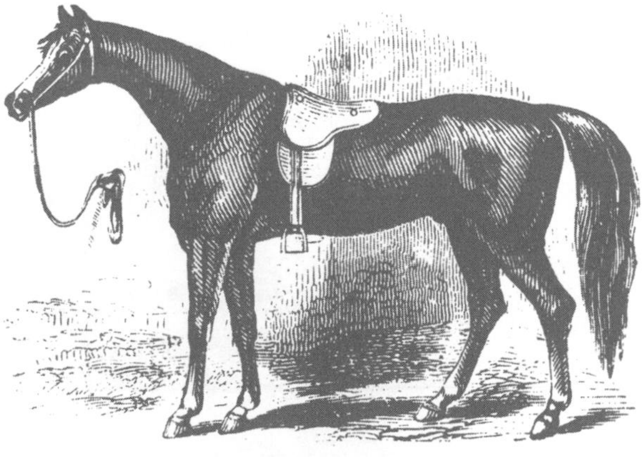

Horse Body Condition Criteria

SCORE	DESCRIPTION
1 POOR	Horse is extremely emaciated. The spine, ribs, hip bones, tailhead, and pelvic bones project prominently. Bone structure of the withers, shoulders, and neck easily noticeable. No fatty tissues can be felt.
2 VERY THIN	Horse is emaciated. Slight fat covering over vertebrae. Backbone, ribs, tailhead, and hip bones are prominent. Withers, shoulders, and neck structures are discernible.
3 THIN	Fat built up about halfway on vertebrae. Slight fat layer can be felt over ribs, but ribs easily discernible. The tailhead is evident, but individual vertebrae cannot be seen. The hip bones cannot be seen, but withers, shoulder, and neck are emphasized.
4 MODERATELY THIN	Slight ridge along back. Faint outline of ribs can be seen. Fat can be felt along tailhead. Hip bones cannot be seen. Withers, neck and shoulders not obviously thin.
5 MODERATE	Back is level with no crease or ridge. Ribs can be felt but not easily seen. Fat around tailhead beginning to feel spongy. Withers are rounded, and shoulders and neck blend smoothly into the body.
6 MODERATELY FLESHY	May have a slight crease down the back. Fat on the tailhead feels soft. Fat over the ribs feels spongy. Fat beginning to be deposited along the sides of the withers, behind the shoulders and along the sides of the neck.
7 FLESHY	A crease is often seen down the back. Individual ribs can be felt, but noticeable filling between ribs with fat. Fat around tailhead is soft. Noticeable fat deposited along the withers, behind the shoulders, and along the neck.
8 FAT	Crease down back is prominent. Ribs difficult to feel due to fat in between. Fat around tailhead very soft. Area along withers filled with fat. Area behind shoulders filled in flush with the barrel of the body. Noticeable thickening of neck. Fat deposited along the inner thighs.
9 EXTREMELY FAT	Obvious crease down back. Fat is in patches over rib area, with bulging fat over tailhead, withers, neck, and behind shoulders. Fat along inner thighs may rub together. Flank is filled in flush with the barrel of the body.

FYI

Mold = Misery

Mold contributes to allergies, asthma, and other respiratory problems for both humans and horses. It destroys property, such as feed, tack, and buildings.

MOLD AND MILDEW IN THE SOUTHEAST

Mold is a fuzzy surface growth of fungus that forms on stale, damp, or decaying matter. As horsekeepers, we need to be concerned about mold for specific reasons, including moldy feed, tack, and environment. Areas of high humidity, such as the southeastern United States, are particularly prone to develop mold and mildew.

MOLDY HAY. When hay is baled too damp, or when it gets wet from precipitation or ground moisture, it can mold. Mold spores can be irritating to a horse's respiratory system and lead to coughing, heaves, or colic. You can recognize moldy hay by its gray, dusty appearance and its rank smell. Don't feed moldy hay to your horses.

A neighbor with cows might be able to use the hay because most ruminants, such as mature cattle, are not bothered by mold the way horses are. Ruminants are cud chewers with four stomachs. Cud is undigested food that has been regurgitated to be re-chewed. As cows masticate, regurgitate, ruminate, and eructate, their special microorganisms detoxify and transform molds and mycotoxins into less harmful substances. Horses are not ruminants, and have only one stomach. They should never be fed moldy hay.

Clover, alfalfa hay, and some grains can be affected with molds and fungus while growing. Alflatoxins in infected corn are poisonous carcinogens that can cause blind staggers. An ergot fungus in grains and tall fescue can cause abortion. If you feed fescue, you can have it tested for ergot. Buy grain from a reputable dealer.

They can turn on a dime and give you back nine cents change.

— Common saying about the Quarter Horse

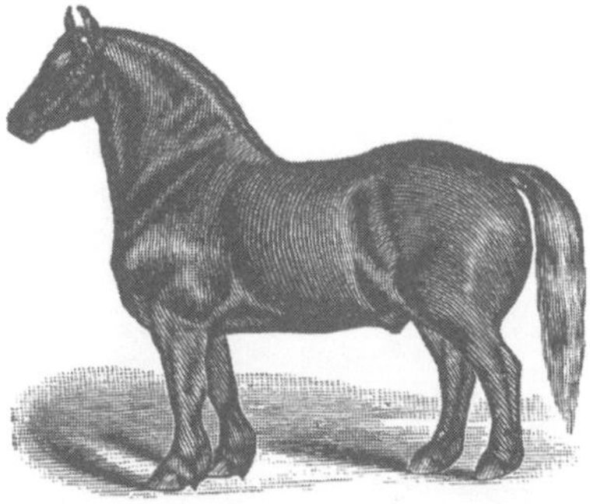

Feed Freshness

Paying attention to freshness of feed is especially important if it contains molasses or if you live in a hot or humid climate. Even in semiarid Colorado, we store our various horse feeds in large, plastic garbage cans with tight-fitting lids. I feed from the barrels until they are almost empty. Then I dump out the old feed, Richard fills the barrel with a new batch, and I put the leftovers back on top. That way, my horse's grain stays fresh and it is protected from rodents and insects.

LEATHER TACK RESTORATION. If leather tack has been saturated, such as by flooding, you'll have the best luck with restoration if you can begin before the leather dries out. Remove all dirt and then apply leather conditioner while still very damp. To prevent the spread of mold and mildew on leather and other items in your barn, clean moldy tack outdoors with plenty of ventilation. When you handle a moldy item, spores are released into the air and settle inside your nose and on other items. When cleaning, use cloths or rags that you will throw away. Flush the moldy items repeatedly with clear water and wipe.

Once the mold is visibly gone, it is time to start cleaning! Using clean water and a water-based pH-neutral cleaner and a toothbrush, clean all surfaces, crevices, tooling, and so on. Let the item dry in the sun. Before completely dry, apply a pH-neutral conditioner.

Other tack items that are moldy can be washed in hot, soapy water with bleach, depending on the item.

TIPS & TECHNIQUES

Controlling Mold

To control mold, you need to control moisture. Here are some strategies:

★ Reduce humidity in buildings to 30 to 60 percent.

★ Add vents and a vent dryer to the outside of the building.

★ Use a dehumidifier in tack and feed rooms.

★ Use floor, overhead, and exhaust fans.

★ Prevent condensation by insulating barns and buildings with a vapor barrier.

★ Avoid carpet in mold-prone areas.

★ Consider installing more windows and skylights to let in more sunlight.

A CONTINENT OF PASTURES

Horses will eat, trample, or otherwise damage approximately 1,000 pounds of air-dry forage per month. What this means is that while an improved 2-acre pasture might support a horse during the growing season, if the horse were to live year-round on pasture, he might require five acres of improved pasture; 30 to 65 acres of dry rangeland; or 200 acres or more of desert.

In the southwest United States, Bermuda grass is popular and it can be grown with or without irrigation, but it requires fertilization to thrive. In the West, pastures are mostly rangeland, with very little improved, irrigated pasture. Due to limited precipitation, drought-resistant plants such as brome and wheatgrass tend to do best. In the East and Midwest, pastures flourish due to natural precipitation, so improved pastures are common and include bluegrass, brome, and timothy.

In the South, beware of tall fescue pasture or hay that is infected with an endophyte (an organism living in another plant) fungus, which can be toxic to broodmares and young horses. This fungus produces an alkaloid substance that is toxic to grazing animals, yet it makes plants hardier and parasite resistant, so soon it becomes dominant in a pasture. Although endophyte-free seed is available, it is hard to establish and maintain an endophyte-free pasture, especially in the South. In close cooperation with your vet, plan to remove mares from tall fescue pastures no later than 300 days into pregnancy.

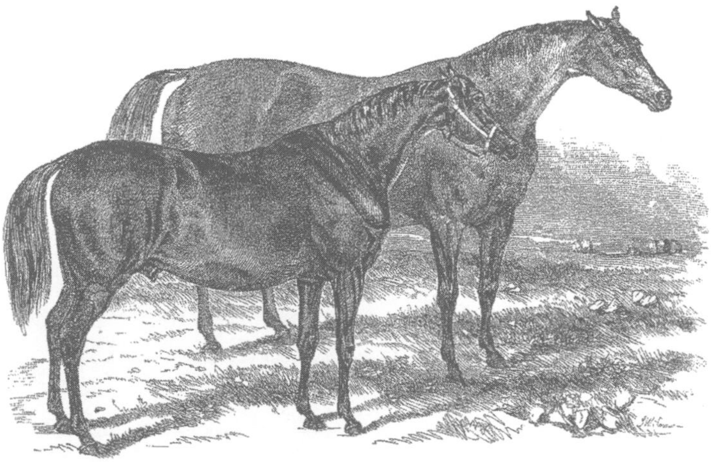

Ask Cherry

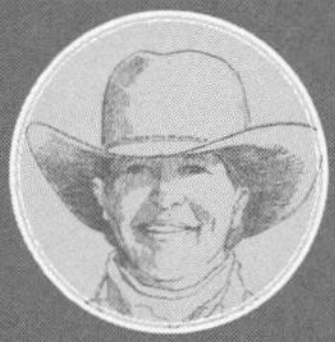

Complete Feed Wafers

Q You have referred to complete feed wafers. What are they and where do I find them?

A Complete feed wafers are processed and compressed hay, grain, and supplements. Pellets are the small versions; wafers are a larger version and can be round or flat — ½–1-inch thick and 1–2 inches long. They are the shape and size of a horse treat. I add a handful of these to the grain ration of eager eaters to slow them down because they have to chew rather than gulp. Most feed companies manufacture a product like this. I also use them for turnout treats.

Age to Begin Training

Q My horse turned two years old this past March. Is she too young to begin training and riding? Thanks so much for any and all advice.

A If a horse turns two early in the spring the way yours did, I often do longeing and long-lining training during the summer and do some light riding training in the fall. I then turn the horse out for the winter and resume in the spring when the horse is three. It depends a lot on the breed and size of the horse and the maturity of the limbs — you might want to have your veterinarian look at your filly's knees to determine if the growth plates are "closed," that is, mature enough to begin training.

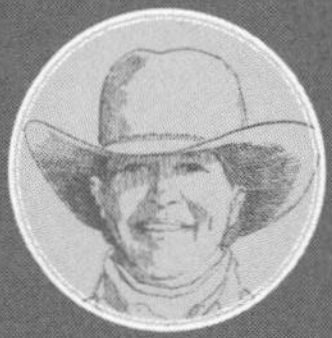

Ask Cherry

Wash Rack /Work Area

Q

My indoor wash rack will also be my only indoor tack, groom, vet, and farrier area. I was wondering about the advantages and disadvantages of permanently installing enclosed stocks in this area. Are stocks a safe place for young horses and for first-time bathers? What is the ideal size for enclosed stocks to accommodate small ponies (10 hands) to Warmbloods? I will have a variety of other tie areas outside and in the stalls, but no aisles in the barn for tying. Will an infrared heater installed above the stocks 11 feet from the ground provide sufficient heat? If not, how can I safely move it closer to the horse without risking having the horse hit it if he rears?

A

I'd suggest leaving the wash rack as an open work area with crossties at both ends. It will make bathing, shoeing, grooming, and tacking up much more convenient and safer. To keep horses away from the shelves, counter, and so on, install a heavy pipe guardrail around the perimeter of the stall. If you need stocks for vet work or breeding, you can have a set installed outdoors on a concrete pad. The stocks can also be used as a training area for first-time baths. It would be great to set the outdoor stocks under a roof overhang or under a tree for shade and shelter.

No stocks will perfectly accommodate small ponies to Warmbloods. You can choose stocks that fit the largest horse and then make provisions to adjust to smaller horses (not as easy as it sounds) or you could purchase an adjustable stock.

An infrared heater over your wash rack would probably provide adequate warmth at 11 feet, and it would be risky to mount it lower. Hanging a heater from the ceiling or rafters by a chain is a safer option, because even if a horse did contact it, it would swing out of the way.

SUMMER

JUNE TO AUGUST

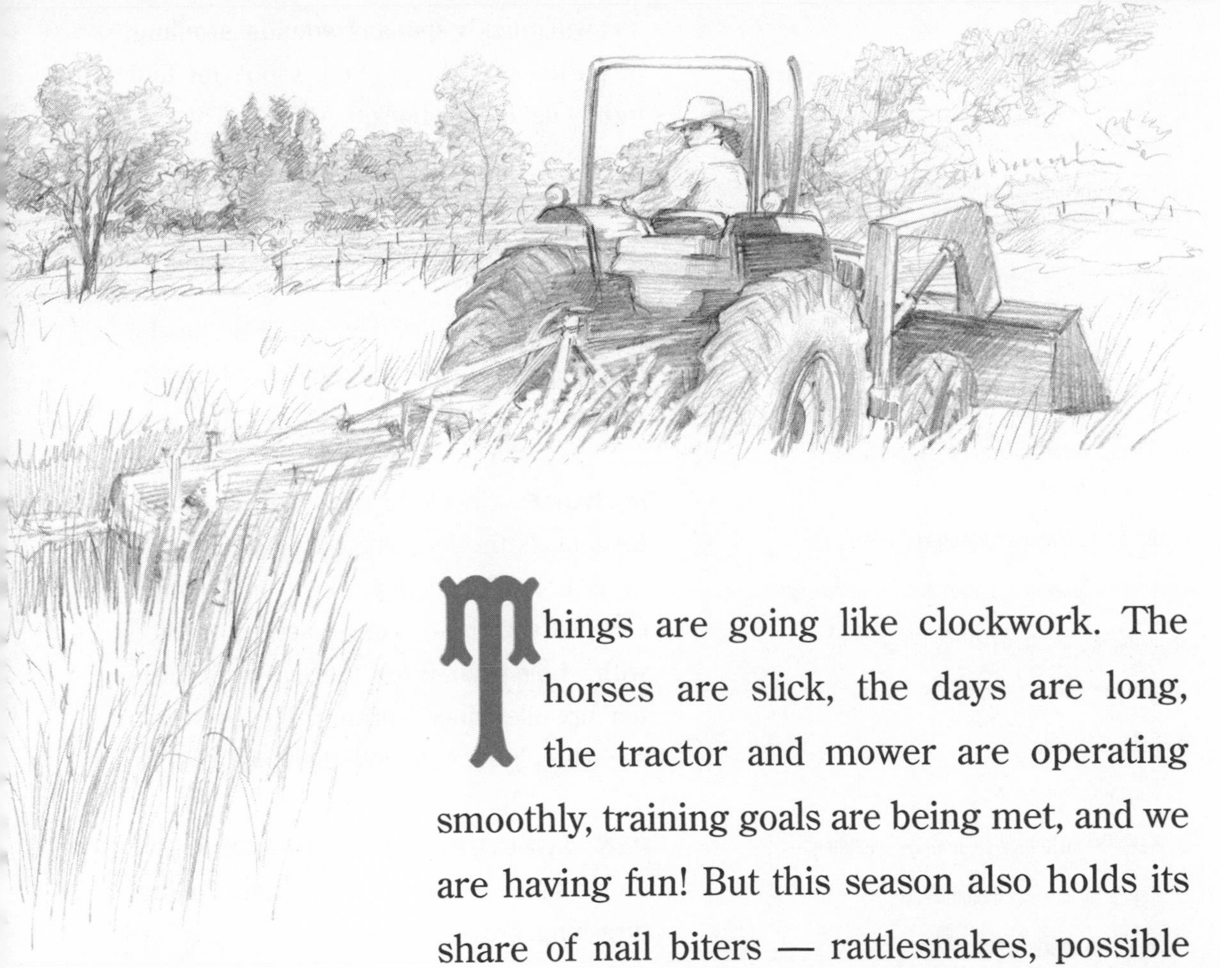

Things are going like clockwork. The horses are slick, the days are long, the tractor and mower are operating smoothly, training goals are being met, and we are having fun! But this season also holds its share of nail biters — rattlesnakes, possible drought and fire, and the annual worry about securing a year's supply of hay.

Weekly Tasks

- ❑ Restock hay supply in horse barns
- ❑ Check grain supply
- ❑ Check bedding supply
- ❑ Take hay inventory
- ❑ Dump and scrub all waterers, troughs, tanks, tubs, and buckets
- ❑ Mow walking paths
- ❑ Scrub feed dishes
- ❑ Check veterinary and grooming supply needs
- ❑ Check upcoming farrier and veterinarian appointments and prepare for them

Seasonal Tasks

- ❑ Monitor pasture until grass is 4 to 6 inches tall
- ❑ Set out salt and mineral blocks on pasture
- ❑ Set out water troughs on pasture or check creek or pond
- ❑ Introduce horses to pasture gradually
- ❑ Monitor grazing so horses don't get overweight
- ❑ Monitor grazing so pasture isn't overgrazed
- ❑ Assign fly sheets and masks
- ❑ Set out fly traps
- ❑ Mow weeds in pasture
- ❑ Keep fire strip mowed around all buildings
- ❑ Repair facilities and paint fences
- ❑ Purchase year's supply of hay
- ❑ Ride!
- ❑ Protect horses from the sun and insects
- ❑ Make sure winter blankets are ready to go — it won't be long!

Summer Visual Exam

OVERALL STANCE AND ATTITUDE. As I approach a horse in the pasture, does he have his head up, are his eyes bright, and is he eager for feed — or is he lethargic, inattentive, or anxious?

LEGS. I look at the horse from both sides so I will quickly spot any wounds, swelling, or puffiness. If he is shod, I look for four tightly nailed-on shoes.

APPETITE. Does the horse begin eating when I put him in his pen?

WATER. Is there evidence that he has he taken in a sufficient amount of water from the pasture trough?

MANURE. Check in the evening before turnout. Is the fecal material well formed, or is it hard and dry, loose and sloppy, covered with mucus or parasites, or filled with whole grains? Are there at least three manure piles since morning? This is easy to see when horses live in individual pens.

PEN, SHELTER, STALL, OR BODY. Are there signs of pawing, rubbing, rolling, thrashing, or wood chewing?

✳	My Day	A Horse's Day
5:00 AM		Stand near pasture gate.
5:30 AM	Rise.	
6:00 AM	Bring horses in from pasture, give visual exam, feed hay to barn horses. Give visual exam to pasture horses. Feed grain to barn horses.	Be led into pen and eat a small amount of hay.
6:30 AM		Eat grain.
7:00 AM	Eat breakfast.	
8:00 AM	Work in office.	Walk over to the water tub for a drink.
8:15 AM		Return to the feed area to vacuum up the dregs.
9:00 AM	Head to the barn, round pen, and arena for training and riding.	
10:00 AM		Exercise and training (if not in afternoon) or doze or lie down.
12:00 PM	Chores, then lunch.	Eat.
1:00 PM	Work in office or barn, do domestic duties, or sometimes take a nap in my recliner.	
2:00 PM		Drink.
2:15 PM		Doze, lie down.
5:00 PM	Back to the barn, round pen, and arena for training and riding.	
5:30 PM		Exercise or training if not in morning.
7:00 PM	Light feed to those that need it; light supper for horsekeepers.	Eat small meal or nothing depending on individual.
8:00 PM	Turn out horses.	Turnout on pasture.
8:15 PM		Mosey, grazing until dawn, keeping alert for unusual sights or sounds.
8:30 PM	Nightly movie.	
10:30 PM	Go to bed.	

JUNE

In a good year, the horses are now enjoying belly-deep smooth brome in some of our pastures, while I keep the broad-leaved weeds under control in others. Mowing is a satisfying Zen-like task for me. When I'm outfitted with sun-protective clothing and a Thermos of cold yerba mate, the job goes quickly. The horses sport their fly sheets and masks for protection from insects and UV rays. We partner up in the early morning or late afternoon for a ride.

Day Length in Hours

Latitude	Date: June 1	June 16	July 1
60°N	17.88	18.43	18.38
55°N	16.67	17.06	17.03
50°N	15.81	16.12	16.09
45°N	15.16	15.4	15.38
40°N	14.63	14.82	14.81
35°N	14.18	14.34	14.33
30°N	13.79	13.92	13.91

See page 22 to find your latitude.

WACKY WONDERFUL WEATHER

IT'S HURRICANE SEASON

The storm surges associated with hurricanes can be devastating to horse farms, so disaster preparedness is essential. See more about hurricanes in this month's Horsekeeping Across America.

LONGEST DAY, SHORTEST NIGHT

The summer solstice is an astronomical term that refers to the position of the sun in relation to the celestial equator. The summer solstice is the day of the year with the longest daylight period and hence the shortest night. This day usually occurs on June 21 or 22 in the Northern Hemisphere and on December 21 or 22 in the Southern Hemisphere.

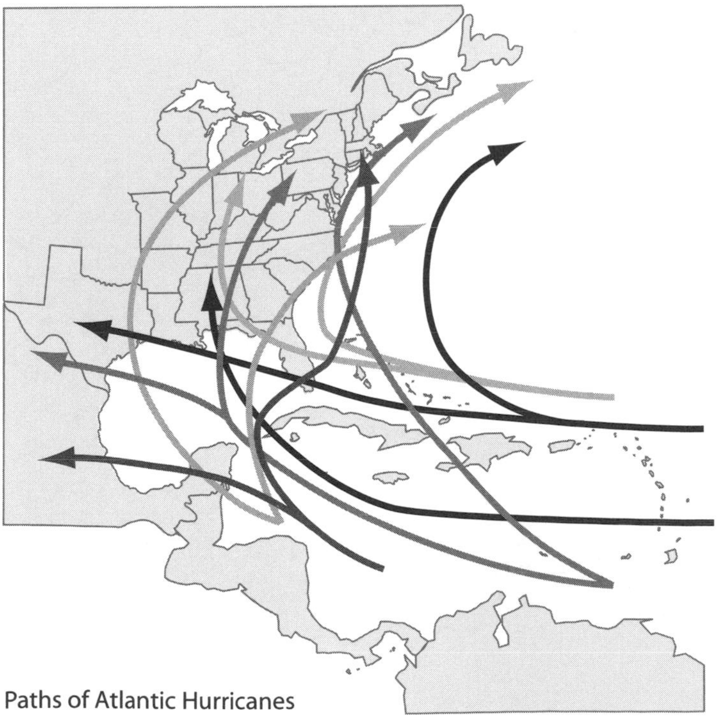

Paths of Atlantic Hurricanes

To Do

- ❑ Take stock of all hoses — check ends, fix leaks, repair, or replace
- ❑ Vaccinate for West Nile virus
- ❑ Work arena
- ❑ Scrub feed tubs and buckets
- ❑ Move hay to barns
- ❑ Restock pasture kit
- ❑ Mosquito control
- ❑ Fence work
- ❑ Conditioning

To Buy

- ❑ Complete feed wafers
- ❑ Grain
- ❑ Hoof supplement
- ❑ Dewormer
- ❑ Psyllium

"*Old minds are* like old horses; you must exercise them if you wish to keep them in working order."

— John Adams

WEST NILE VIRUS

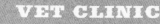

West Nile virus (WNV) is a mosquito-borne virus that was first detected in the United States in 1999 and is now permanently established in the Western Hemisphere. Humans and horses may be infected by the virus, which causes encephalitis (inflammation of the brain). Clinical signs of WNV in horses include ataxia (stumbling or incoordination), weakness of limbs, partial paralysis, and death.

Most often, WNV is spread when a mosquito feeds on an infected bird and then bites a human or other animal. It is not spread through casual contact such as touching or kissing a person with the virus, and infected horses can't

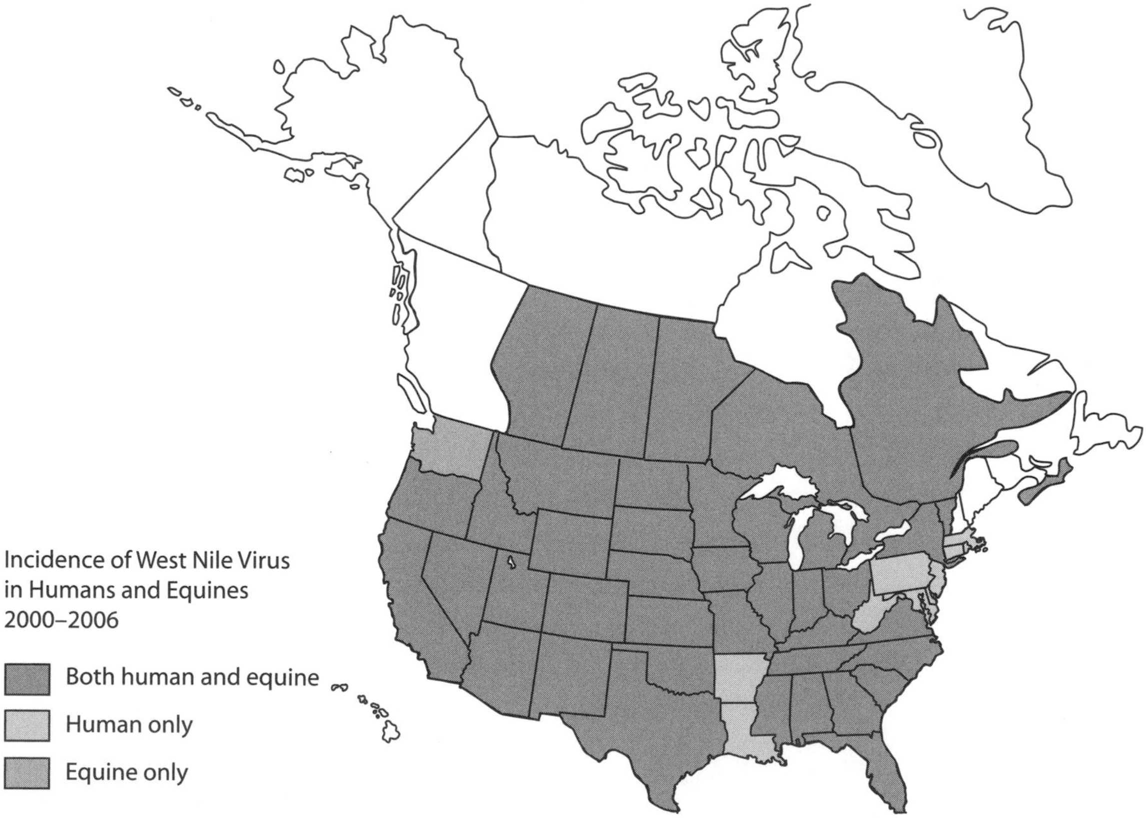
Incidence of West Nile Virus in Humans and Equines 2000–2006
Both human and equine
Human only
Equine only

spread the virus to uninfected horses or to other animals or people. Certain migrating birds (such as the corvids, which include crows, ravens, magpies, and jays) appear to play a role in spreading the disease. In the temperate zone of the world (i.e., between latitudes 23.5° and 66.5° north and south), WNV cases occur primarily in the late summer or early fall. In the southern climates where temperatures are milder, West Nile virus can be transmitted year-round.

When WNV became a threat to our horses, I became very concerned and took all precautions, but didn't give as much thought to the possibility of Richard and I being at risk — that is, until some elderly people died of the disease in the nearest town. So when you are outdoors, use insect repellent containing an EPA-registered active ingredient. Since many mosquitoes are most active at dusk and dawn, use insect repellent and wear long sleeves and pants, or consider staying indoors, during these hours. Make sure you have good screens on your windows and doors to keep mosquitoes out.

Since many mosquitoes are most active at dusk and dawn, use insect repellent and wear long sleeves and pants, or consider staying indoors, during these hours.

Preventing West Nile

WNV prevention on farms and ranches focuses on reducing mosquito breeding sites (see this month's Pest Patrol). Reducing the mosquito population can help prevent or eliminate the virus. Here are some additional strategies.

- ★ Try to decrease horses' exposure to adult mosquitoes. In some high-risk situations, screened stables might be the answer, as long as no mosquitoes are inside the building.
- ★ Where risk is lower, fans can help by keeping air moving in the barn.
- ★ Turn horses out for exercise when mosquitoes don't feed. This may mean keeping horses in the barn from dusk to dawn.
- ★ Insect repellents, fly sheets, and masks can help but are not absolute protection.
- ★ A WNV vaccine for horses became available in 2002. Ask your vet when the most strategic month for you to vaccinate is. Here, it is no earlier than June.

Recognizing Laminitis

Signs of laminitis, which most frequently affects the front feet, include:

- ★ Sore soles and a reluctance to walk
- ★ Sensitivity to hoof testers in the toe area
- ★ Increased digital pulse rate
- ★ Hot feet
- ★ Shifting weight or standing with front legs extended

Severe laminitis results in misalignment of the bones within the hoof and is called founder.

LAMINITIS

Laminitis is an acute inflammation of the sensitive laminae in the hoof, that can be caused by a wide variety of factors, including overeating of grain or rich pasture, trauma, and foaling complications. Severe laminitis results in misalignment of the bones within the hoof and is called founder.

Foundered horses are unlikely to ever return to their previous level of performance. That's why it is important to prevent it with good management. Since laminitis is the second leading cause (next to colic) of equine death, prevention is essential. Monitor your horse's weight closely, be certain he cannot get into the feed room, and carefully select and monitor the horses you turn out on pasture.

Drought-stressed, slower-growing pastures tend to concentrate their nutrients, so they often provide more sugars than fast-growing pastures. Irrigated pastures tend to be fast growing and can be more "diluted," containing lower amounts of nutrients. Either type of pasture can cause laminitis due to carbohydrate overload — as can a binge in the grain bin. Certain plants seem to contribute more than others to laminitis, and research is underway to determine which. Some horses, due to age, breed, diet, level of exercise, and other factors are more susceptible to laminitis (see the Safergrass Web site in the appendix).

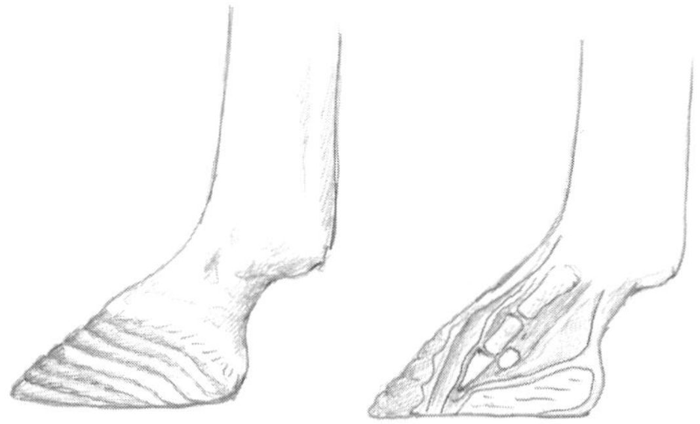

A foundered hoof has rings on the wall, and in severe cases the coffin bone has rotated downward.

SAND COLIC

Sand colic occurs when a horse ingests sand (or decomposed granite, dirt, or small gravel) with his feed and the sand blocks his intestines. Although most common in California, Florida, and the southwestern United States, it can occur anywhere that horses graze on sandy pastures or are fed on sandy ground.

Horses naturally rid their intestines of a certain amount of sand with the feces. However, when the amount of sand ingested is greater than the natural elimination process can handle, mechanical obstruction or inflammation of the junction of the large and small colon can occur. To help prevent sand colic, I have covered the ground of all feeding areas with rubber mats and I keep them swept clean. I let the horses in only at eating time and lock them out at other times. This makes it easier to keep their eating areas clean.

DOES YOUR HORSE EAT SAND? One way to find out if he does is to collect one fecal pile that has not contacted the soil. This is best accomplished from a stall with rubber mats (it's okay if bedding is stuck to the feces, but not

Ranch Notes

June 6. While taking Mom around the "spread" in a borrowed golf car, the batteries caught on fire! Something we will always remember! Luckily, Richard and a fire extinguisher were not far away.

Sand colic occurs when a horse ingests sand with his feed and the sand blocks his intestines.

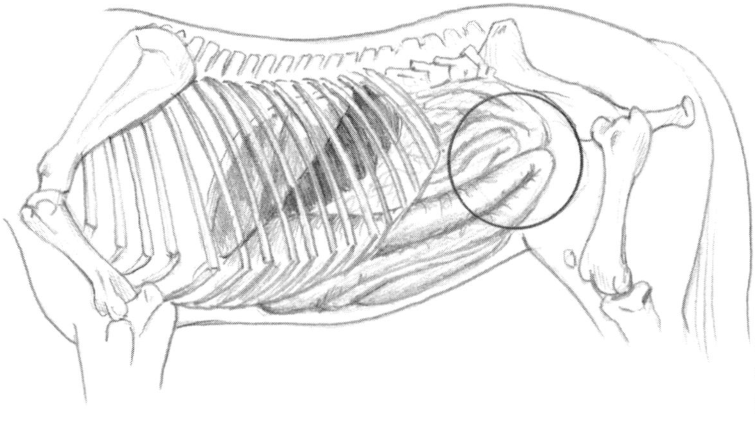

Another place sand blockage can occur is in the pelvic flexure.

Odd Words

colic. A general term for any intestinal upset.

Recognizing Sand Colic

- ★ Symptoms of chronic sand colic are usually mild: depression and slightly elevated heart and respiratory rates.
- ★ There may be diarrhea, restlessness, pawing, laying down, rolling, kicking, biting flanks or abdomen, or sweating and yawning.
- ★ The horse might assume the urination posture without urinating or might not eat, drink, or have normal bowel movements.
- ★ Acute sand colic symptoms are an intensification of the above symptoms. A veterinarian should be called in all cases of acute colic. Diagnostics include radiographs, auscultation (listening to gut sounds), and ultrasound.

dirt) or when the horse is in cross-ties on mats. Place the feces in a 5-gallon pail and fill it with water. Stir with a sweat scraper until the feces has broken apart and is uniformly distributed through the water. Tip the bucket, letting the green slurry spill out. Stop when you reach the solid material toward the bottom of the bucket. Repeat the washing and dumping process until all that you have is sand at the bottom of the pail.

If you come up with an eighth of a cup of sand or more from one bowel movement, it shows your horse *is* ingesting sand and able to rid his intestines of some of it. Identify areas in your feeding management that could use improvement and consider feeding psyllium.

PSYLLIUM

Many veterinarians in the sandy areas of the Pacific Coast, Florida, and the Southwest prescribe periodic doses of psyllium-husk products as a preventive measure. Because psyllium hydrophilic mucilloid contains 80 percent water-soluble fiber, it has the potential to capture and move sand through a horse's digestive system. Although there is no research to date that proves or disproves the effectiveness of psyllium in collecting and removing sand from the intestines, many veterinarians (including mine) say that besides proper management, psyllium is the only tool we have to manage sand colic.

On contact with fluids, psyllium swells and becomes a bulky, mucous mass. That's why grain should never be wetted in an attempt to get the psyllium to "stick" to it. The result would be an ineffective gluey mass, which 99 percent of all horses would refuse anyway. The hydrophilic characteristic of psyllium is also the reason feeders require more cleaning when psyllium products are fed. The horse's saliva starts the gel-making process and the feeders invariably get a tapioca-like coating.

PROVIDING PSYLLIUM. To prevent choke when feeding any psyllium product, be sure your horse has access to water. Horses that bolt their grain should be slowed down with large stones or wafers in the feed. Store psyllium products at a temperature below 86°F, and seal the jar or bucket tightly to prevent moisture absorption from humidity. The psyllium regimen I use is 4 ounces per day, five days in a row, once a month.

Psyllium comes in pellets, crumbles, flakes, or powder. Pellets are convenient, but some horses sort them out or refuse the entire grain ration. Powder can sift to the bottom and is often left in the feed dish. You can bind psyllium flakes or powder to the grain ration with 2 ounces of molasses or corn oil, but never use water or you'll get a gluey mess.

The best approach is to measure the grain or a fluffy, moist mash into a pail, add oil and other supplements, stir so they are distributed uniformly, and then add the psyllium flakes or power. Stir and feed immediately.

I suggest you buy a small amount of a psyllium product at your feed store, tack store, or through a mail order veterinary supply catalog. Try it out on your horse to be sure he will eat it before you purchase a large quantity.

I've been asked if you can use the human product Metamucil. You can, but it is more expensive and might not be palatable for your horse. There are a number of equine psyllium products on the market that are more cost effective. Once you find a product that works for you, you can buy it in 20- to 50-pound containers.

After a five-day regimen of feeding psyllium, be sure to scrub all grain pails and feeders.

GRAZING

As you've no doubt noticed, I tend to be cautious about allowing my horses to graze too much too early in the season. I

Handy Oil Pump

To apply corn oil to grain so the psyllium flakes stick, set up a 40- or 50-ounce ketchup bottle with a large pump. Keep your eye on the large ketchup bottles in your grocery store. Sometimes they come with a pump taped to the side of the bottle. Other times there will be an offer for you to send a dollar for a pump to fit the bottle. It is a handy way to serve up a measure of oil without mess.

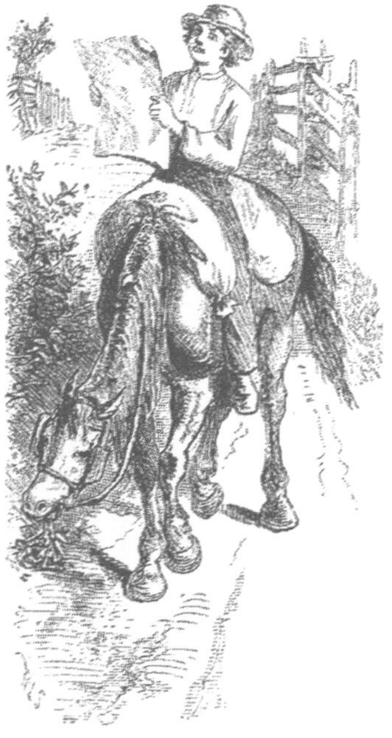

Grazing Guidelines

- ★ Make the best use of pasture by grazing it when it is 4–6 inches tall.
- ★ Before turning a horse out to pasture for the first time, give him a full feed of hay.
- ★ Limit grazing to one half hour per day for the first two days; then one half hour twice a day for two days; then one hour twice a day, and so on.
- ★ As soon as it is grazed down, move the horse to another pasture.

am mainly concerned about my horses' health; I don't want them to colic or founder. But by being a good pasture manager, I keep the pastures healthier as well.

Pasture horses can quickly become overweight or founder from too much lush pasture. During certain times of year, such as spring and early summer or other times of lush growth, the high sugar content of pasture grasses is more likely to cause founder.

I have a moveable pen set up on our "front lawn" (if such a thing exists in the Colorado mountains), which is composed of eight 12-foot panels and a gate. In order to get my horses accustomed to green feed in the spring, I put them in the grazing pen for an increasingly longer time every day. I usually start them out with 10 minutes in the grazing pen, although I know that some of my horses can go longer with no problem. I increase the time by five minutes a day until by the end of two weeks, the horses can be out for an hour or more. I keep a close eye on each horse for subtle signs of intestinal discomfort or hoof tenderness, both of which can be signs of impending laminitis.

Here in the semiarid Colorado foothills, we don't ever have really lush grass — not like we did back in Iowa, for

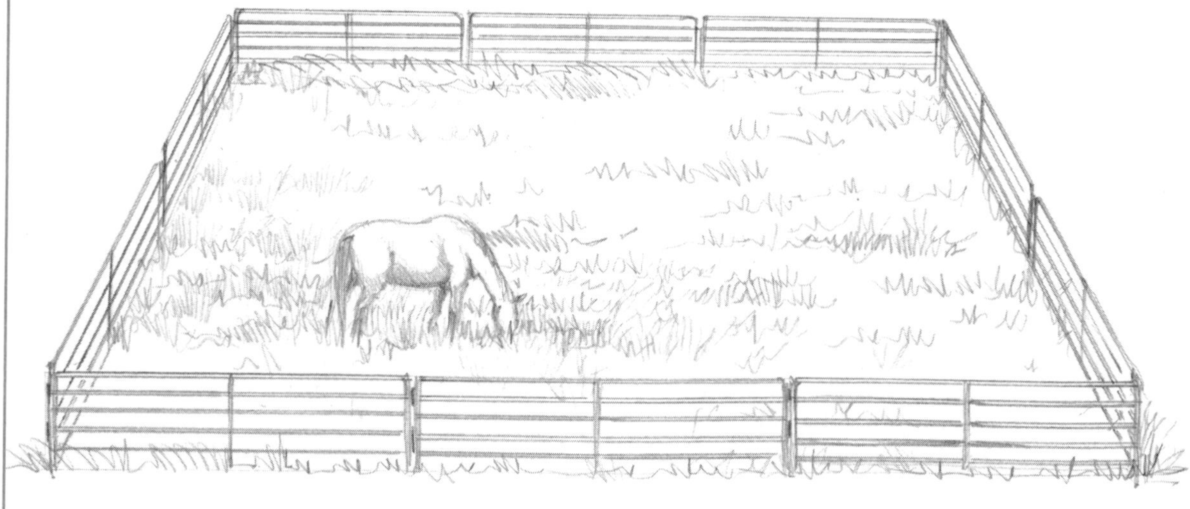

A small grazing pen, made of panels or electric fencing, can be easily moved.

example. So the risk for laminitis is relatively low, but I still don't take any chances. Having seen some sad cases over the 17 years that Richard was a farrier, I urge you to be very careful with how long you let your horse be on pasture. Watch your horse's weight carefully; an overweight horse is much more likely to founder.

WILD LIFE

GOPHERS, PRAIRIE DOGS, MOLES, AND MORE

These burrowing, tunneling creatures can be darling to observe but very destructive when they overrun a pasture or yard. Not only do they disturb and eat the vegetation, but they also create dangerous holes, which can make an area unsafe to ride, exercise, or turn out horses.

Prairie dogs (ground squirrels) are rodents that live socially, mainly in western North America. They are 14 to 17 inches long and have a network of tunnels with a large mound opening. They live in large groups and are active during the day. Omnivorous, they eat both plants and insects. Many other animals, such as birds and snakes, use prairie dog burrows as homes.

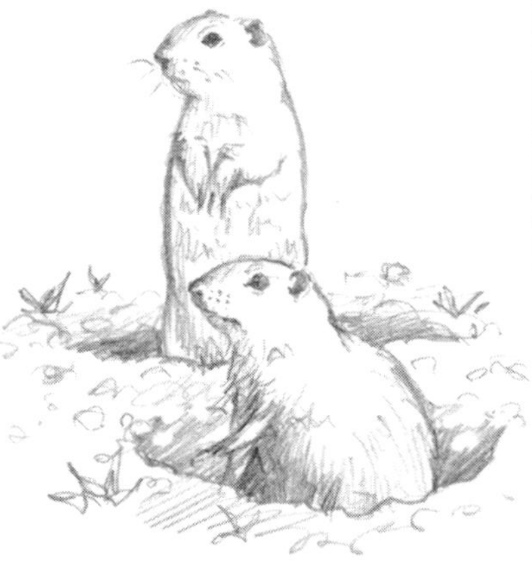

Prairie dog holes can ruin a pasture and create a safety hazard for you and your horses.

Gophers are rodents that live solitarily and eat pasture vegetation, including some weeds. They are 6 to 10 inches long and dig their tunnels 1 to 2 feet below the surface. You usually see evidence of their location as mounded ridges of soil. This tunneling provides some aeration benefits to the soil. The surface mounds are usually spokes from the main tunnel. If you want to find the main tunnel, you'll need to probe. Control methods include natural predators, cats and some dogs, poison, and flooding.

Moles are small, burrowing mammals with pointed

Artificial Nectar for Hummingbird Feeders

- ★ 4 cups water
- ★ 1 cup white table sugar (sucrose)

Heat water to boiling. Let cool somewhat. Add sugar and stir to dissolve. Let cool completely to room temperature. Fill hummingbird feeder. Store the rest in the refrigerator.

Every time you fill the feeder, flush it with hot water, no soap. Never add red food coloring to artificial nectar. It is not necessary and could do the hummers harm.

snouts, rudimentary eyes, and broad feet with long, powerful claws on the front feet. Their diet consists primarily of insect larvae, worms, and beetles, so they thrive in moist, fertile soil. They are 6 to 8 inches long. Having a few moles around is not a problem at all, but if you happen to have ideal conditions, they could become a nuisance. Traps seem to work best for decreasing the mole population.

FAWNS

Those darling little spotted Bambis start appearing in June, although most were born in May. See October Wild Life for more on deer.

HUMMINGBIRDS

Broadtail hummers have been buzzing our house begging for nectar water. By the end of the month, the bossy, noisy, but spectacularly showy rufous hummingbirds arrive.

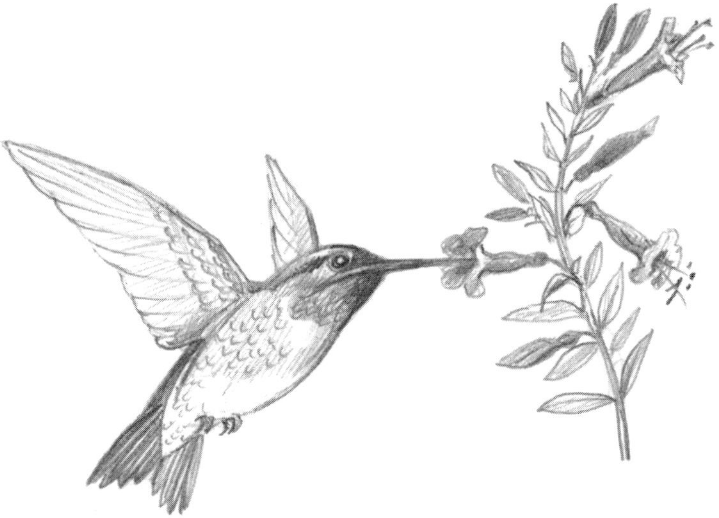

When hummingbirds arrive, treat them like the royalty they are.

PEST PATROL

GNATS AND MIDGES

Will the real culprit please fly away! Horse owners often incorrectly refer to biting midges as gnats. Biting midges (Ceratopogonidae) are tiny, about 2 to 3 millimeters long. They are also sometimes referred to as no-see-ums, punkies, or sand flies (a misnomer). True gnats generally don't bite humans, but just swarm in bothersome clouds.

Certain species of biting midges are very troublesome for horses and can be for people, too. These small, blood-feeding flies feed around the face, particularly the eyes. Although they have sponging mouthparts, these are spiny sponges that abrade membranes, sometimes leading to disease transmission and infection.

Biting midges cause the skin condition sweet itch, in which affected horses have an allergic reaction to the bites. Horses housed or pastured side by side may have varying reactions: Some will show little, if any reaction. Others will be possessed, constantly rubbing and biting to relieve the itch, and end up with bald patches or open, weeping sores. Biting midges generally thrive near marshy or swampy areas, but springs, creeks, and ponds can be a source as well. It is nearly impossible to eliminate midges, so it is best to try to protect horses from bites using repellents. An allergy treatment is available from your veterinarian.

Controlling Rodents

Rodents are a part of the ecosystem, but when their natural predators (bobcats, coyotes, owls, hawks, eagles, snakes, dogs, and cats) are few and far between, rodents procreate exuberantly and take over.

Encourage natural predators by providing habitat for them, and keep farm cats to help control the rodent population. Cats are often a better option than trapping or shooting. (Contact the Department of Wildlife for the legalities of rodent control.)

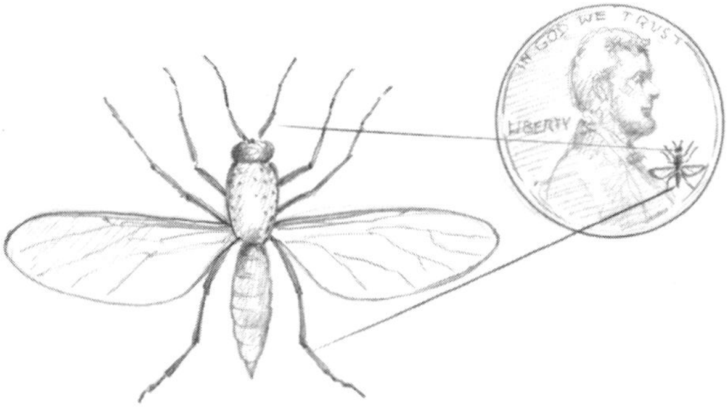

Midges may be tiny, but a swarm of them can bring big misery to your horse.

Controlling Mosquitoes

To eliminate or reduce mosquito breeding areas, you can:

★ Throw out old tires that tend to collect rainwater and make ideal mosquito breeding conditions.

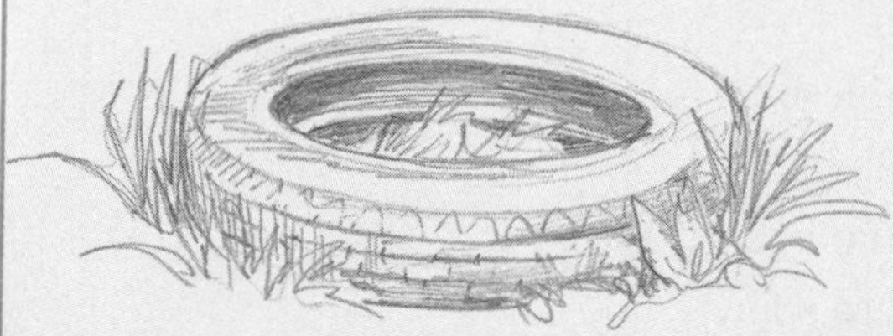

Old tires collect rainwater. Discard them.

★ Discard or empty tin cans, buckets, drums, bottles, old tires, wheelbarrows, or any vessel that can hold water.

★ Fill in or drain any low spots that turn into puddles.

★ Regularly check drains, ditches, and culverts to ensure they are clean of weeds and trash, so water will drain properly.

★ Repair leaky pipes and outdoor faucets.

★ Manage swimming pools or wading pools responsibly; turn plastic wading pools over when they are not in use.

★ Aerate ornamental pools or stock them with fish. Clean and apply chlorine to swimming pools that are not in use. (Mosquitoes can breed in water collecting on pool covers.)

★ Keep grass mowed and shrubbery trimmed around the barn and house, so adult mosquitoes will not find refuge there.

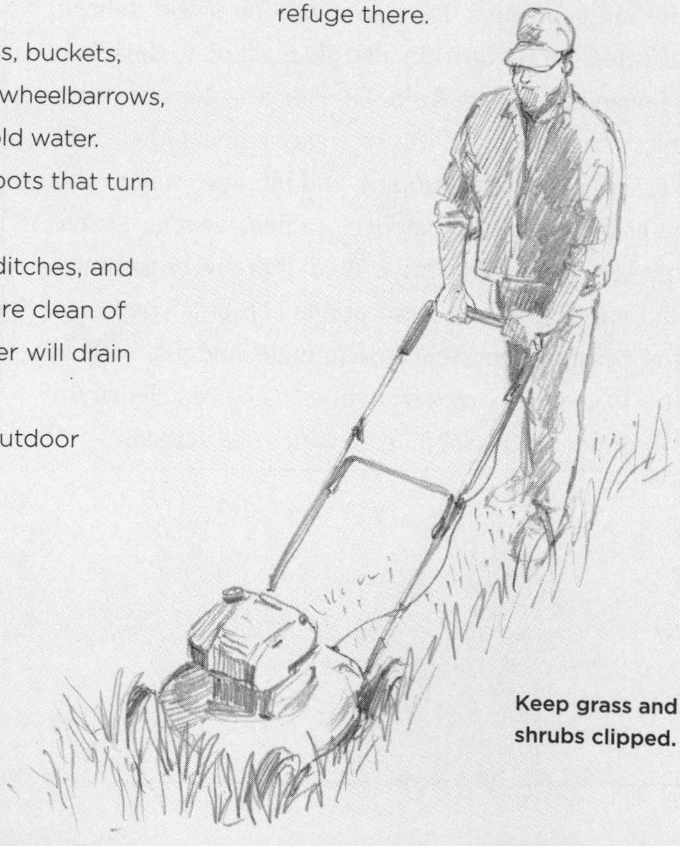

Keep grass and shrubs clipped.

★ Change water in birdbaths regularly so it doesn't become stagnant, and empty plant-pot drip trays at least once a week.
★ Keep gutters clean and free of debris and leaves so they drain completely.
★ Flush fresh water through any barn drains at least weekly.
★ Clean out and refill watering troughs at least once a week.
★ Contact your local extension agent for other suggestions suitable to your particular location.

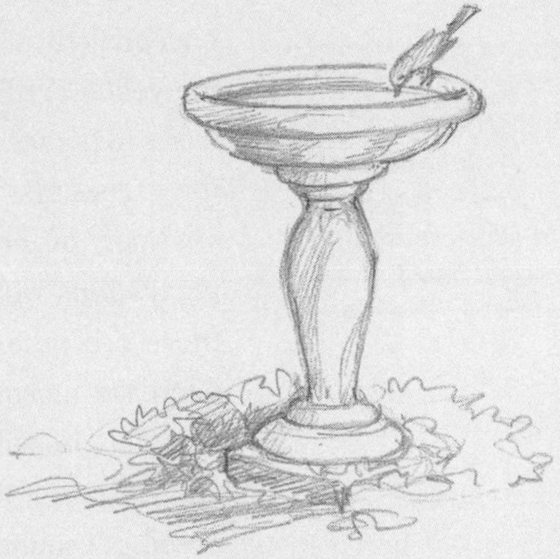

Keep birdbath water fresh.

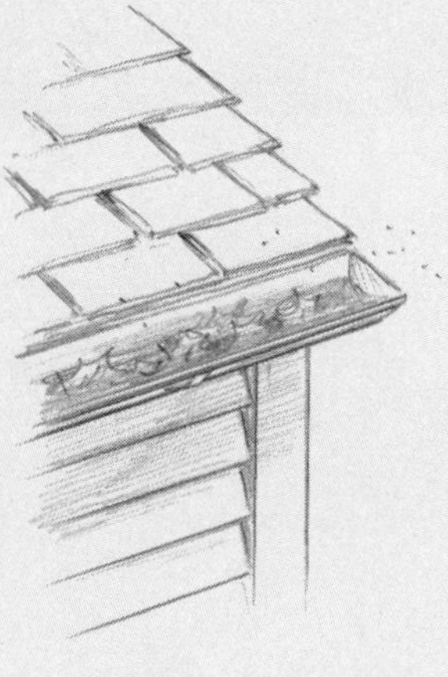

Clean gutters so they drain properly.

Don't let the water trough overflow and create a muddy mess.

MOSQUITOES

Birds and rodents are reservoirs for West Nile virus (WNV), western equine encephalomyelitis (WEE), eastern equine encephalomyelitis (EEE), and Venezuelan equine encephalomyelitis (VEE), and mosquitoes can transmit these diseases to horses. Fortunately, there are vaccinations against these diseases; however, sanitation is key to prevention.

The most important step property owners can take is to remove all potential sources of stagnant water in which mosquitoes might breed.

Many of the good sanitation practices that reduce fly populations will also discourage mosquito breeding. But there are other specific practices that can significantly decrease mosquito breeding grounds. The most important step property owners can take is to remove all potential sources of stagnant water in which mosquitoes might breed. Mosquitoes can breed in any puddle that lasts more than four days.

PASTURE PERFECT

POISONOUS PLANTS AND WEEDS

I've spent a number of hours on my tractor this month mowing the first crop of weeds that appeared in our pastures. With a wet spring, everything grows well, including weeds that have been dormant, not only from the last year, but sometimes for years. Weeds are opportunistic. They can lay low and become a real problem when conditions are ripe.

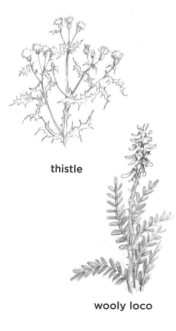

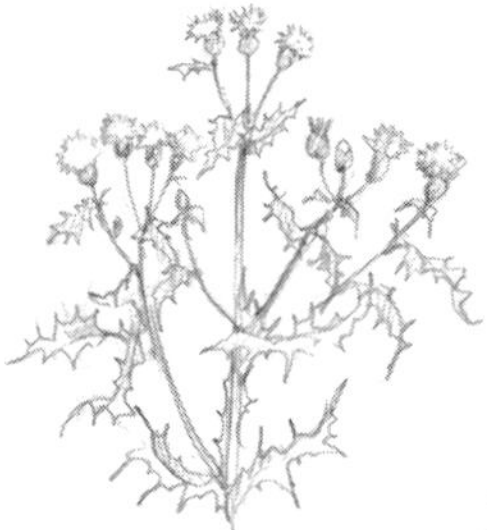

thistle

wooly loco

Our usual toxic culprits — wooly loco, larkspur, and lupine — are well under control. When we purchased this property 20 years ago, it was basically a weed and cactus patch with an occasional blade of grass here and there. With judicious spraying and mowing, along with reseeding and some luck, we have improved the pastures. This time of year, I am ever-vigilant for new patches of weeds.

Virtues of Fencing

Good fencing is necessary for many practical, safety, legal, and aesthetic reasons:

★ Fences keep horses separated and in a particular place, away from the residence, lawns, crops, vehicles, buildings, and roads.

★ Fences maintain boundaries and property lines, and thus promote good relationships between neighbors.

★ Fences decrease liability because they lessen the chance of a horse doing damage to others' property, decrease the chance of a horse getting on the road and causing an accident, and keep people (especially children) and animals (especially dogs and other horses) off the property.

★ And, finally, attractive fencing can visually set off acreage and add to the value of the property.

In addition to the poisonous plants, I try to stay informed of any plants that might cause my horses to be photosensitive or get a skin irritation. This task is greatly helped by local experts and reference books. (See Recommended Reading.)

MOWING

This is a good time to mow because the taller, broad-leafed weeds are taller than the grass. I can set my mower high and lop the tops off the weeds, leaving the precious grass to flourish. That is enough to stop certain weeds in our climate for the summer. Those that regrow will be mowed again later in the summer.

High Mowing

Just as with overgrazing, it weakens pasture grasses to mow them too short, because it results in shallow roots. Weeds are likely to take over more easily. Leave all grasses at least 3 to 4 inches tall. Your goal is to lop off the tops of broad-leaved weeds. When in doubt, mow higher rather than lower.

FENCING

Good fencing is designed to keep horses from getting hurt, whether the horses are turned out or being trained. Besides being safe, good horse fencing is sturdy, low maintenance, highly visible, attractive, and affordable.

FYI

Barbed Wire

Barbed wire is not a suitable horse fence because the sharp points, coupled with a horse's natural propensity to fight when tangled and flee when frightened, can lead to horrible injuries. Do not use barbed wire for horse fences.

When choosing fencing, make sure it fits your situation and budget. Probably, no one type of fencing will be suitable for all of your needs. You might choose different fencing for your pens, paddocks, runs, pastures, round pen, and arena, ending up with five or more types of fencing on your farm or ranch.

PLANNING. To make a fence plan for your acreage, draw a scale map of your land on graph paper. Design a complete perimeter fence with entrance gates that can easily be closed and locked, so that loose horses are kept off your property and your horses are kept on your property. Draw on the map all permanent structures and objects, including such things as trees, water, large rocks, and buildings. Draw current and proposed traffic patterns. Locate places where gateways would be convenient, and decide if they should be man gates, horse gates, or equipment gates. Then draw in fence lines on your map, including cross fencing that you may plan for the future.

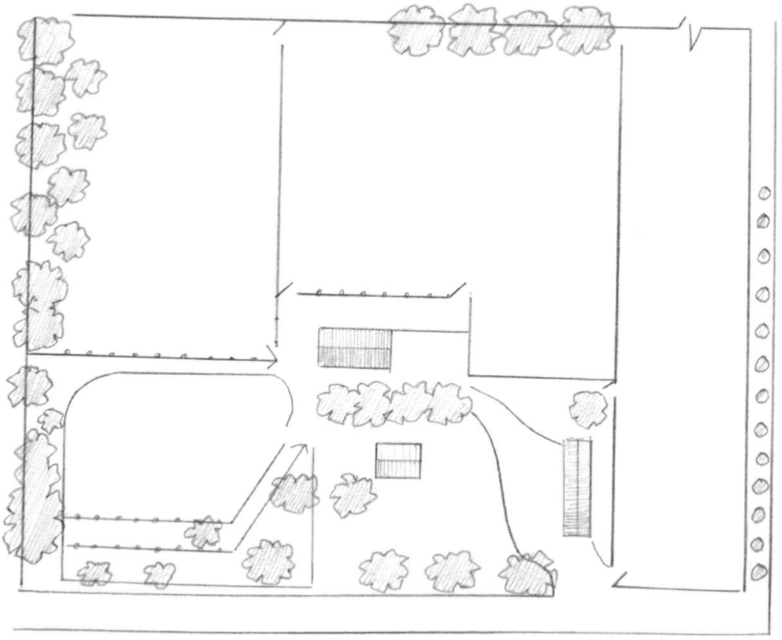

When laying out fence lines, avoid acute angles where a horse can become cornered by other members of the herd, even if only in play.

TRY IT OUT. Once you have your fence map drawn, use rocks, boards, or stakes and flags as markers to translate the proposed plan from paper to the land itself. Make adjustments. When you have found a layout that will work, mark your postholes (marking paint works well for this). Finally, calculate the number of feet and amount of materials necessary: corner posts, brace materials, line posts, gates, fencing material (such as planks, rails, or rolls of wire), and miscellaneous supplies such as bracing wire, insulators, and electric wire.

FENCE HEIGHT. When horses are running, whether from fright or exuberance, they can go through or over fences. Four and a half feet is the absolute minimum fence height that you should consider to discourage horses from jumping. Aim for a finished fence height of 5 to 6 feet, especially for stallions, larger breeds, or those specifically bred and trained for jumping. For smaller horses and ponies, a fence that is just a bit higher than the withers is usually safe. Fence height refers to the height of the top strand or board and includes the height of all horizontal elements of the fence including gates.

TIPS & TECHNIQUES

Fence Footage

How much fence will you need to enclose a particular parcel of land?

★ 20 acres require 1½ miles of fence, or 3,960 feet

★ 10 acres require 2,640 feet

★ 5 acres require 1,980 feet

★ 2½ acres require 1,320 feet

★ 1½ acres require 990 feet

★ Fencing is typically sold in 20- or 80-rod rolls (10 rods = 165 feet) and 100-foot rolls.

NO WAY!

Historical Horsekeeping

"For a severe case [of founder] draw about one gallon of blood from the neck, then drench with linseed oil, one quart; rub the forelegs with water as hot as can be borne without scalding, continue the washing till the horse is perfectly limber."

— A New System of Horse Training or Horse Education, *as taught by Prof. H. D. Brush, Fingal, Ontario, 1902*

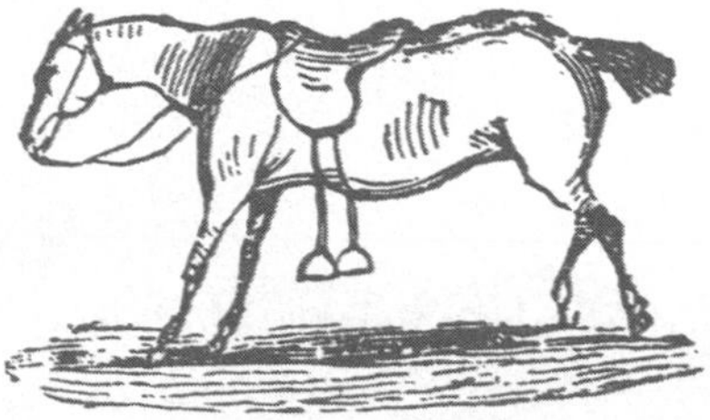

CLEAN-UP CREW

MULTIPLE MANURE PILES

As you've noticed through the months, we've devised a manure-handling system that we highly recommend: multiple piles. There are several reasons this system works. If you try to do all of your composting in one manure pile, it might be difficult. The pile might get too large and not fully decompose. You might find that the inside is still raw manure or dry fecal balls if you live in an arid or semiarid climate. It is best to have multiple piles and care for them. That way, you can tend to each pile's needs specifically, adding moisture, turning, letting rest, or spreading.

We like to use "manure forts," which are dugouts in the hill below our barn. The earthen cave is lined with railroad ties to keep the soil walls from collapsing inward. It is easy to dump a cart over the edge of the manure fort.

"I must not forget to thank the difficult horses who made my life miserable, but who were better teachers than the well-behaved school horses who raised no problems."

— Alois Podhajsky, director of the Spanish Riding School, 1939

JUNE
Manure Pile Maintenance

JUNE Manure Pile Maintenance
PILE A Turn once, water as needed
PILE B Sell, store, or spread
PILE C Turn once, water as needed

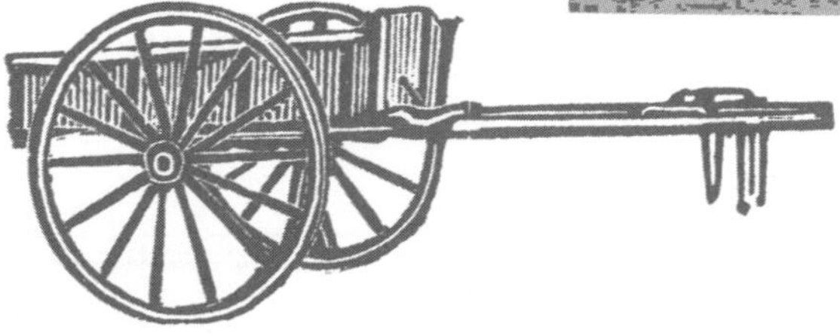

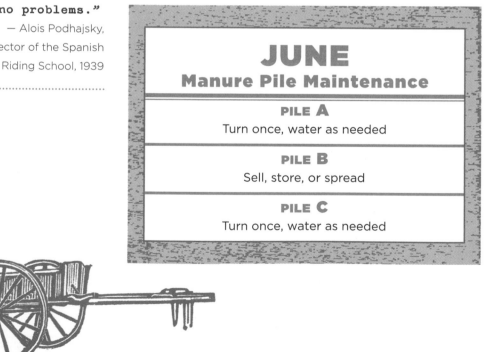

BEAUTY SHOP

GROOMING ON THE GO

During the summer, for horses on pasture, I groom on the go. Even with a gentle and well-trained horse, a halter and lead come in handy if I need to stabilize her while removing a branch that has become entangled in her tail. I've taught my horses to come to a certain spot when I whistle or call. Just as they arrive, I drop a few feed wafers on the ground in several spots. As the horses nibble, I give them a thorough visual exam (see Summer Seasonal Opener).

Daily Visual Checklist

Besides the visual exam I give all horses, I do the following with pasture horses:

- I look for discharge from the eyes; head shaking or ears held at an odd angle; and all signs of fly problems.
- I remove any burrs or sticks in the mane or tail and look for any damage from mutual grooming to the mane or sheet.
- I make sure all blanket and leg straps are fastened. I take care of most things right out on pasture.
- For anything that requires closer attention, I halter the horse and lead him back to the barn.

Weekly Check

Every day if a horse is wearing a sheet and at least once a week if he is not, I halter each pasture horse and give him a thorough hands-on check. Here's what I do weekly:

- I remove the blanket and mask and look for any obvious problems such as wounds, scabs from fly bites, blanket or mask rub marks, sores, or lumps, which could indicate an abscess.

TIPS & TECHNIQUES

Pasture Kit

Put together a pasture kit for daily checks so you can tend to little things before they become big problems. Here is what is in my kit:

- ★ Halter and lead rope
- ★ Fly spray, cream, and wipes
- ★ Gloves
- ★ Mane detangler
- ★ Treats or carrots
- ★ Wound ointment
- ★ Zinc oxide
- ★ Extra fly mask
- ★ Extra leg strap for sheet or blanket

- I run my hands from throatlatch to shoulder down both sides of the horse's neck, paying special attention to the crest of the mane, where there might be signs of rubbing, and under the mane, where there might be skin problems or ticks.
- I do the same for the horse's entire body, paying special attention to the junction of the neck and chest and in front of the sheath or udder, two places where flies love to feast.
- I keep an eye out for rough bumps under the coat, which could indicate rain rot.
- I examine the inside of the hind legs to see if there have been any abrasions from leg straps.

Blanket Donuts

Many blankets have surcingle-style buckles on belly bands and leg straps. These buckles fit together with a lot of play in them, so when a horse lies down or rolls, they often come unfastened. The dangling straps can be stepped on, causing the blanket to shift terribly or be torn. To keep buckles buckled, I use blanket donuts. I borrow blanket donuts from another farm use — they are actually tail docking or castrating bands. These green rubber "donuts" come in packages of 100 for about two bucks. They are made of natural latex rubber, so if they are stored on a sunny windowsill, they will dry and crack quickly. Instead, store your stash in a tight container in a dark, cool place to preserve their elasticity. At about 3⁄16-inch thick, they are the perfect size to slip over the tongue of the surcingle buckle to take up the slack and keep them fastened, yet the buckles are still easy to operate. They are super cheap insurance to prevent ruined blankets.

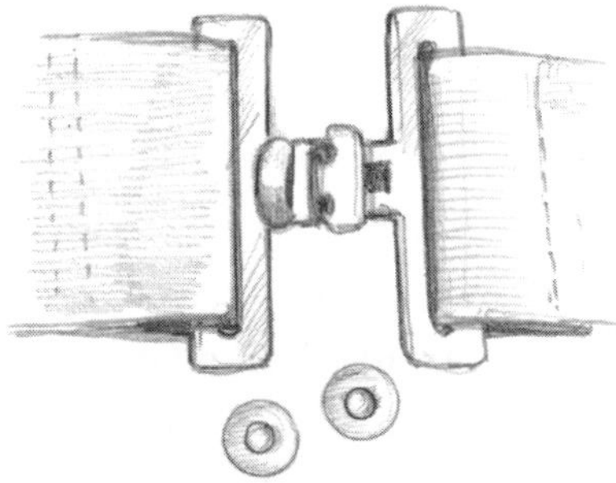

- I examine by palpation and visual exam every inch of the legs and hooves, making note of any nicks or bumps, roughness under the hair of the legs that could indicate rain rot, scabs at the back of the pastern that could be scratches, loose shoes, hoof chips or cracks, or sticks or stones stuck in the frog.
- I give the tail a once-over, removing any embedded burrs or branches.
- I check the tailhead, another favorite site for ticks.
- I apply a detangler, sunscreen spray, or leave-in conditioner to the tail as needed.

TACK ROOM

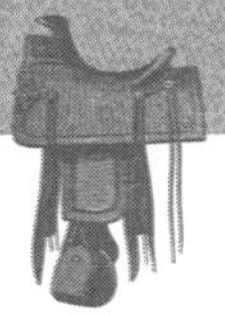

KNOTS

Part of being a horseman is knowing how to tie knots. In this knot roundup, I've included four knots you should master: the quick release knot, the bowline, the half hitch, and the sheet bend.

QUICK-RELEASE KNOT. As the name implies, this knot can be released quickly with a pull on the tail of the rope. It is used to tie a horse to a hitch rail or post, or to a horse trailer. You can also use it to tie individual reins to a surcingle or to rigging rings on a Western saddle. Also called a manger knot, it was the knot used to tie horses at their mangers when horses were kept in tie stalls. With practice, you can tie the quick release knot without hesitation and keep your fingers out of the loops while tying.

Weekly Head Check

- ❑ When I examine each horse I finish off with the head, running my fingers inside the ears and noting if he is sensitive or if there are scabs or red spots inside from gnats.
- ❑ I look carefully around the eyes for small dings or rub marks from the fly mask.
- ❑ I make sure the eyes and nostrils are clear.
- ❑ I run my hand between the lower jawbones and over the fleshy portion of the throatlatch, two more favorite places for fly feasting.
- ❑ Finally, I open the horse's mouth, looking for any evidence of barbed plant awns or sticks lodged in the horse's gums or lips.
- ❑ If a horse seems out of sorts, I check his vital signs and take appropriate action.

Quick-Release Knot

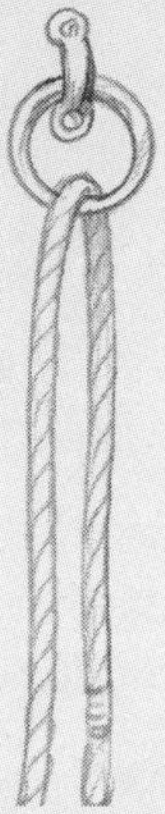

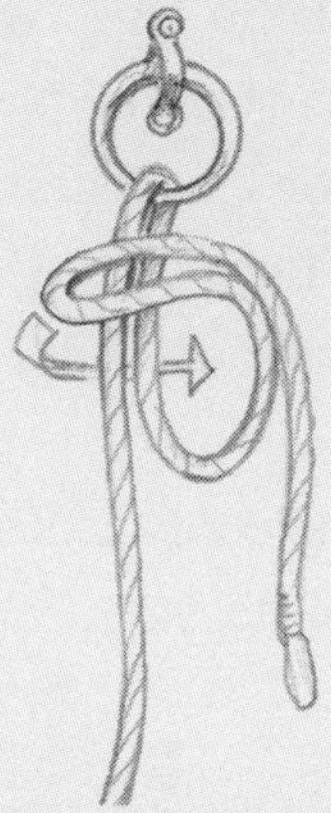

1 Run the tail of the rope (called the free end) over the rail or through the tie ring. Hold the standing end (the portion attached to the horse) and the free end together in your left hand.

2 With your right hand, pick up a portion of the free end of the rope and make a fold (bight) in it. Cross the fold over the two ropes you are holding in your left hand and through the loop that has formed. (Take care not to let your fingers get inside any of the loops, because if your horse were to pull at this point, your fingers could get trapped in the loops.)

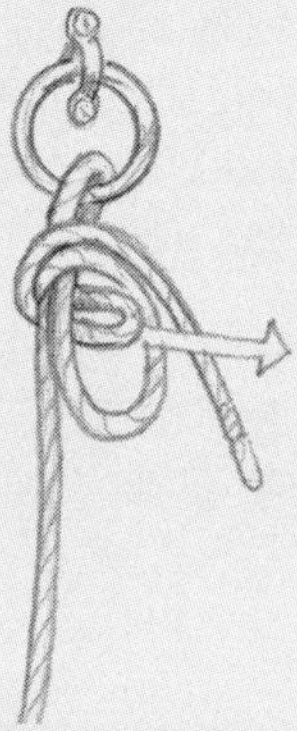

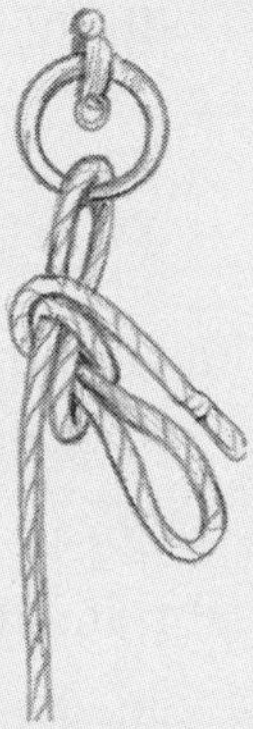

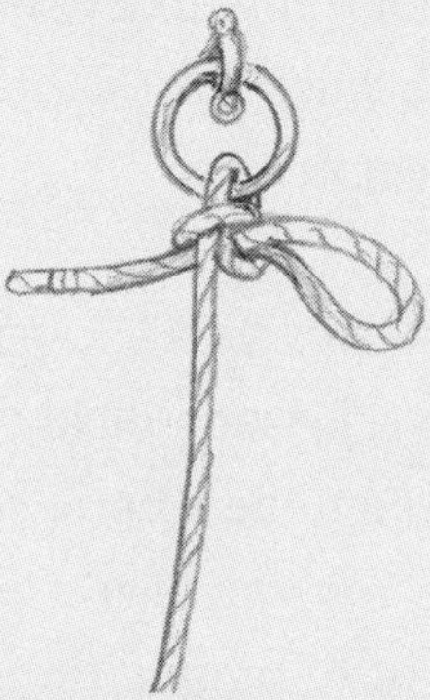

3 Grab the bight and pull it through the loop. Pull until the U-shaped bight is about 6 inches long and the knot is snug.

4 Grasp the standing portion of the lead rope with your left hand and the knot with your right hand. As you pull with your left hand, slide the knot up to the ring or the rail with your right hand.

5 To release, just pull the free end. If your horse has learned how to nibble the quick-release knot and free himself, you will have to "horseproof" the knot by dropping the tail of the rope through the loop. In order to release a horseproof knot, you must first remove the tail from the loop.

Bowline Knot

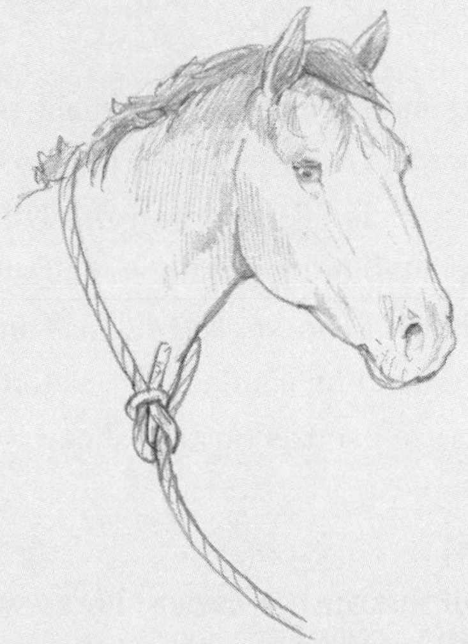

This is a non-tightening knot that is safe to use as a neck rope or in restraint.

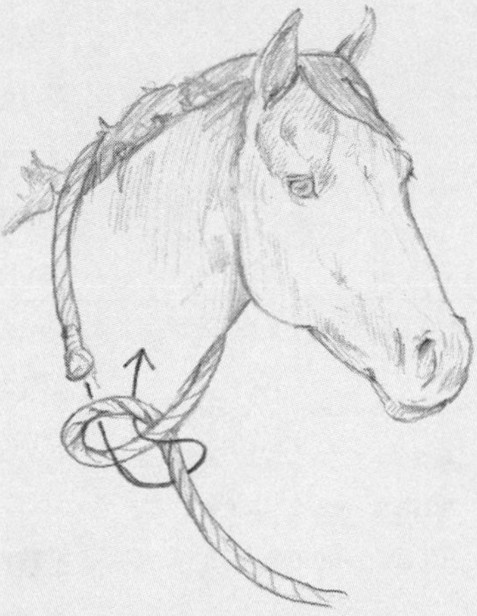

The rabbit runs out of the hole, around the tree, and back into the hole.

Half Hitch

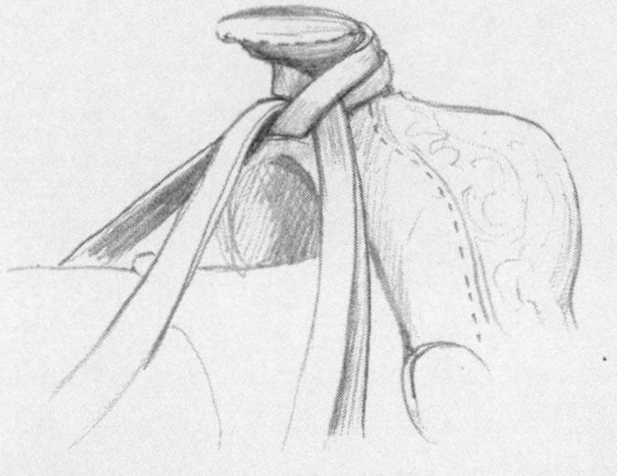

Not actually a knot, the half hitch is made by looping a rope or strap around an object and then back around itself. Useful to fasten a pair of reins over a Western saddle horn; to fasten the leading end of a mecate to a Western saddle horn; and to secure a quick-release knot.

Sheet Bend

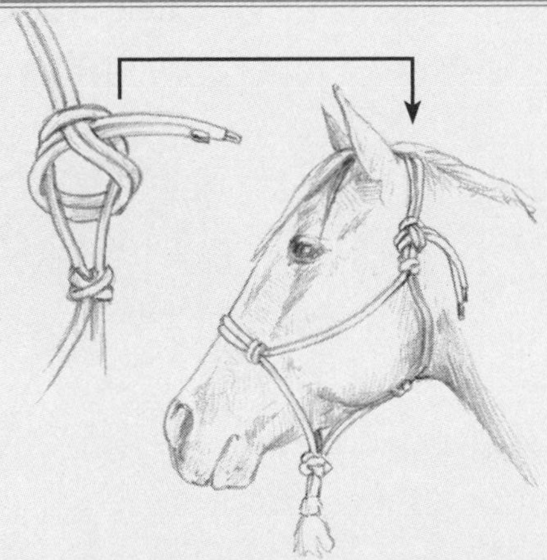

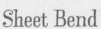

The sheet bend is used to fasten a rope halter or a fiador (rope throatlatch on a bosal) onto a horse.

CLOTHES HORSE

FLY SHEETS

When the weather is hot and the flies are unusually pesky during the summer months, use a fly sheet to give your horses relief. A fly sheet repels flies and provides UV protection. It must be comfortable for the horse and sturdy enough to withstand normal horse activities. Thin fly sheets, called scrims, are used on stabled horses; tougher PVC-coated mesh sheets are used as turnout sheets.

Show me your horse and I will tell you what you are.
— Old English saying

Fly Sheet Priorities

A fly sheet must be cool, because a sweaty horse would only attract more flies. It must be made of fabric that is tough enough to withstand the occasional bite at the side or chest made by a horse's reflex action to chase a pesky fly. It must have safe, functional leg straps, because a horse stomps and rolls in fly season. The sheet must be held in place, but the legs straps should be elastic so they have give.

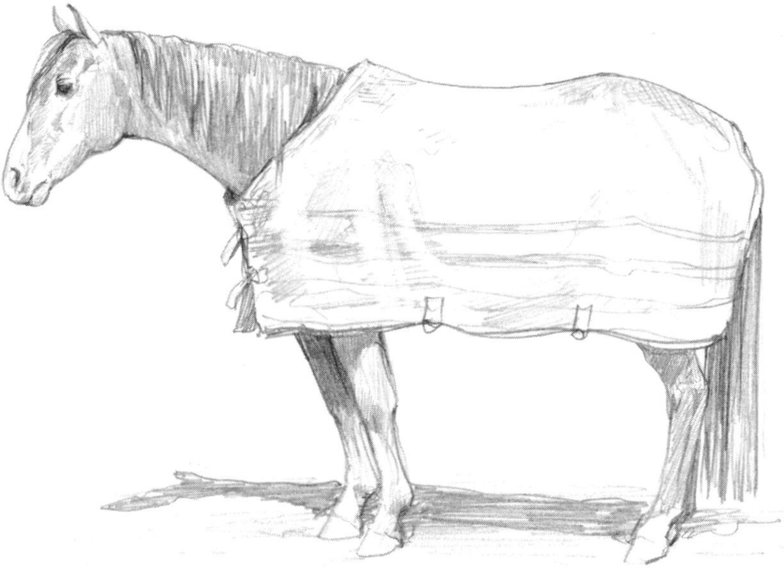

A fly sheet can eliminate stomping and swishing and bring your horse peace.

FARM OFFICE

VEHICLE INSURANCE

Your farm truck's vehicle insurance is important. Do not let it lapse. Talk to your agent to determine how much coverage you need for your horse trailer. Your tractor should be covered by your homeowner's or farm or ranch business policy from loss by fire or theft. Be sure you have factored your vehicles into the building contents totals if necessary.

PROPERTY BOUNDARIES

Summer is a good time to have any necessary surveys done. Property lines are important, as they determine where fences, buildings, and other facilities can be placed. Your building and zoning commission dictates where you can locate buildings in relation to boundaries, street rights-of-way, and your home.

FENCING. Boundary fencing is also important. Usually a state statute covers fence laws. Often, state laws say that a person has the duty to fence animals in and his neighbors do not have the responsibility to fence them out. In contrast, some open-range states, like Colorado, require landowners to fence out free-roaming livestock.

If you share a division fence with a neighbor and the fence is put on the property boundary, state law will usually dictate whether you share the cost of installation. Adjoining owners usually cannot legally force one another to erect a fence of a particular height or materials. Once a boundary fence is built, depending on your laws, you might be required to maintain the half of the fence to your right as you stand on your property at the midpoint of the fence facing the division line, and your neighbor would be required to maintain the half of the fence to his right. If you can't

RPMs & PTOs

Truck Inspection

Every time you use your rig, you should follow an inspection routine. June happens to be the month my truck and trailer license tags are renewed, so here's my list.

- ❑ Tire pressure
- ❑ Wheel lugs
- ❑ Hitch
- ❑ Running lights, turn signals, and brake lights
- ❑ Trailer brakes
- ❑ Emergency trailer breakaway system
- ❑ Oil
- ❑ Power steering fluid
- ❑ Transmission fluid
- ❑ Brake fluid
- ❑ Coolant in both radiator and recovery reservoir
- ❑ Windshield washer fluid
- ❑ Wiper blades
- ❑ Air filter (especially if you drive in dusty conditions)
- ❑ Battery terminals clean of corrosion
- ❑ Fill tanks with gas either beforehand or at your earliest convenience

come to an agreement with a neighbor on the type of fence or cost sharing, set the fence 2 to 6 inches inside the property line, so it becomes your fence and your responsibility. Note, however, that once so placed, in many states, over time the fence becomes the boundary between the properties. Although we all hope that good fences make good neighbors, it is always a good idea to have any fence agreements with your neighbors in writing.

No matter who does the work on your land, buildings, or fences, it is ultimately your responsibility to comply with all legal codes and regulations. Check the local zoning regulations. These restrictions are designed to control the growth and development of communities by establishing particular areas for certain uses such as residential, commercial, industrial, and agricultural. These laws define the type of building you can construct and the type of activity that can take place on your land. Zoning laws may also dictate building height and size, property size, legal distance from road or neighbors, and appearance of facilities. You may need to get approval from the zoning committee for your plans.

RPMs & PTOs

Trailer Inspection

- ❑ Hitch
- ❑ Lights and wiring
- ❑ Floor
- ❑ Emergency breakaway brake
- ❑ Tires
- ❑ Doors
- ❑ Frame
- ❑ Body, waxing or acid wash
- ❑ Suspension
- ❑ Latches and fasteners
- ❑ Trim
- ❑ Tire pressure
- ❑ Wheel lugs
- ❑ Bearings (checked in April)
- ❑ Brakes (checked in April)

Your Boundary Fence

A property boundary line should be determined exactly by an official survey. Check your local and state fence laws to determine whether your perimeter fence should be set on the property line, and whether the installation and maintenance costs should be shared by you and your neighbors, OR whether your fence should be set inside the property line on your land and paid for and maintained entirely by you. This is an important distinction that should be decided before you dig your first posthole. Errors can be costly and disputes can get ugly.

I let my neighbor
know beyond the hill;
And on a day we meet
to walk the line
And set the wall
between us once again.
He only says, "Good
fences make good
neighbors."

— Robert Frost,
"Mending Wall"

SADDLING REVIEW

Be sure a horse is well groomed before saddling. Check the horse, the saddle, and the blanket for foreign objects, such as burrs, hay, or dirt. Place the blanket in front of the withers and slide it back into position. If you put it on and slide it forward into position, you will ruffle the horse's hair and make him uncomfortable.

Place the saddle on the blanket. Peak the blanket up in the gullet of the saddle so the blanket won't put pressure on the horse's withers. Buckle the girth.

With an English saddle, attach the breast collar and accessories to the girth before buckling the girth. Reverse the order when unsaddling.

With a Western saddle, fasten the front cinch first, then the back cinch, then the breast collar and accessories. Reverse the order when unsaddling. If a horse were to spook with just a rear cinch fastened, the saddle could slip under his belly and cause him to buck, resulting in possible injury to himself and damage to the saddle. Buckle the rear cinch so that it is snug but not tight. Tighten all cinches and girths gradually.

Check saddle tightness several times before mounting and again after riding a short while.

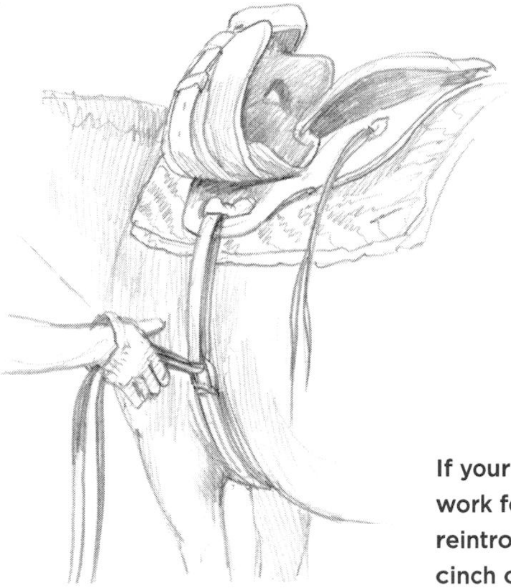

If your horse has been out of work for a while, gradually reintroduce the pressure of a cinch or girth.

Ranch Notes

June 25. While working in our office, we heard something bang against the wall outside. Peeking out, we saw two darling spotted fawns rough-housing just outside our door.

No matter who does the work on your land, buildings, or fences, it is ultimately your responsibility to comply with all legal codes and regulations. Check the local zoning regulations.

Ranch Recipes

Avoid the Alkaline

A horse's skin is slightly acidic (pH 4.5 to 6.0), so using an alkaline shampoo can strip his skin of natural oils, cause it to dry out and become itchy, and leave an open invitation for bacteria and parasites.

To prevent these problems, never use an alkaline soap or shampoo. Most human shampoos and all human soaps and detergents are alkaline. Use a very mild, specially designed horse shampoo in a very dilute solution. Then give your horse a vinegar rinse (see box opposite).

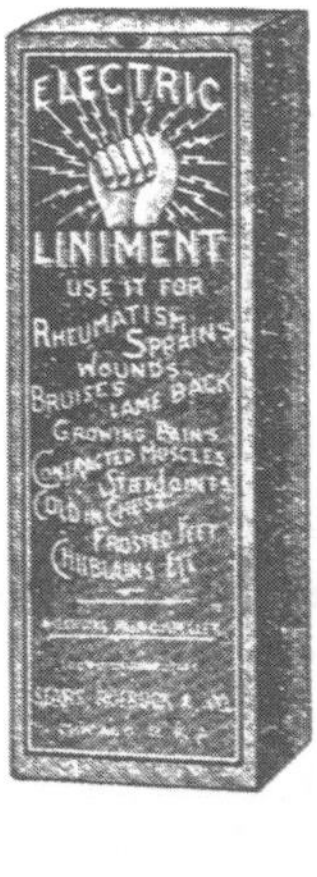

START CONDITIONING YOUR HORSE

A horse not only needs to be trained, but also conditioned. A physically fit horse feels better and performs better. Conditioned horses are more durable and useful and have less chance of injury and setback. Horses generally require less work, relatively speaking, than humans do to get fit, and once fit, they can maintain that particular fitness level with little work. But no matter what type of program is followed, a horse should have a minimum of three to a maximum of six scheduled work days per week, with free or light exercise on the other days. Knowledge of some conditioning concepts can help you keep your horse in shape.

WARM-UP AND COOL-DOWN. Each training session should begin with a warm-up period: a vigorous grooming, hand-walking, and longeing or riding on a loose rein. A warm-up dissipates the fluids in the legs and lungs, which have pooled during inactivity; it opens capillaries, lubricates joints, relaxes the horse, and sharpens the responses of the neuromuscular reflexes. After a work session, a cool-down period allows the muscles to expel lactic acid and heat. Light trotting on completion of strenuous exercise is a necessary part of a cool-down, and should be followed by walking and grooming.

BODY SYSTEMS. A horse should be relatively fit before you start him on a conditioning program — that is, not fat, underweight, parasite-ridden, or ill. Hooves and legs must be in a sound and healthy state so the horse is mechanically capable of complying with the conditioning program. Although a conditioning program affects the whole horse, certain body systems respond more quickly to exercise than others. And every horse has a system or a portion of a system that may be a little more delicate or slower to respond than the other systems. The time schedule of the entire conditioning program must be planned with a horse's weak link in mind. The metabolic system is comprised of the heart, blood vessels, muscles, digestive tract, respiratory tract, and the skin and sweating mechanism. A horse's performance is a series of contractions and relaxations of muscle cells. These cells must be properly nourished and detoxified. It is the combined efforts of the components of the horse's metabolic systems that accomplish this vital task.

The heart is the first to show great improvement after the first few months of exercise. The balance of the horse's metabolism may take up to a year or more to adapt to its new demands. During the early months of a properly designed conditioning program, the cardiac output increases, which in turn increases the number of circulating red blood cells. At the same time, since the horse's heart doesn't need to work as hard but accomplishes more, the resting pulse rate decreases.

After several months of exercise, the horse's muscle chemistry becomes more efficient. There is an increase in the number of capillaries in both the skeletal muscles and the heart, which allows more nutrients and oxygen to be distributed during work. Muscles become more tolerant of lactic acid buildup and more efficient at detoxification. Heat is dispersed more quickly.

SHOWING IMPROVEMENT. Based on average hoof growth rate of a quarter inch per month, it takes up to one year or more for the hooves to show their response to new exercise demands. The skeletal system, bones, joints, tendons, and ligaments require two to three years to fully adapt to the demands of a new sport.

Progressive conditioning can increase the ability of bones and joints to withstand loading and the torque associated with turning. Joints become more prominent with thicker articular cartilage and broader joint surfaces.

Ranch Recipes

Vinegar Rinse

I call this the "Pickle Bath" because my wash rack and my horses smell like a pickle for a few minutes. Using an empty 128-ounce ketchup bottle, put in 1/4 cup apple cider vinegar and fill it with water. Then gently invert the bottle and squirt the solution on your bathed and rinsed horse, especially on the itchy areas.

A horse should be relatively fit before you start him on a conditioning program — that is, not fat, underweight, parasite-ridden, or ill.

Bones can become denser. The bones of younger horses are more responsive to remodeling, but are also weaker and more easily damaged. As bones become stronger with age, they lose some of their flexibility as well as their remodeling capacities. With progressive exercise, tendons and ligaments become stronger and more resilient, able to accept a greater load and recover faster from the elastic deformity which accompanies hard work.

"It was a great treat to us to be turned out into the home paddock or the old orchard; the grass was so cool and soft to our feet, the air so sweet, and the freedom to do as we liked was so pleasant; to gallop, to lie down, and roll over on our backs, or to nibble the sweet grass.

— *Black Beauty*, by Anna Sewell

The last system to become finely honed to the demands of a sport is the nervous system. It can take as many as five or more years to develop the finesse and control needed to become a top-notch reining horse or dressage horse.

CONDITIONING PHASES. Conditioning programs are usually comprised of three phases: long, slow distance work, strenuous work, and maximal work.

Long, slow distance work is steady, aerobic training of a relatively long duration but below the horse's maximum speed. It results in lean, supple muscle mass and is designed to develop the long-distance trail horse and to provide a base for the future work of any horse.

Strenuous work is an anaerobic demand of high resistance in proportion to effort. It can be in the form of interval training, sprints, or repetitions. Interval training consists of controlled speed works of precise distances followed by partial recovery of the heart rate. Sprints are short, all-out bursts followed by full recovery. Repetitions are controlled speed works followed by full recovery. Strenuous work results in an increase in muscle bulk, strength, stamina, agility, range of motion, and brilliance. Such exercise is essential for the event horse and the all-around performance horse.

Maximal work is performed at the horse's highest level of exertion. It is anaerobic and is designed to develop speed and quickness. Maximal work results in an increase of fast-twitch fibers and is appropriate conditioning for events requiring explosive work, such as calf roping, reining, and sprinting.

CHANGING WORK LEVEL. During all three phases of conditioning, you can change certain parameters to increase or decrease the work:

- The intensity, or speed, of a workout: for example, the walk (4 miles per hour) versus the lope (12 miles per hour)
- The duration of each episode in the session: for example, walking interspersed with three 2-minute trots, versus three 10-minute trots
- The frequency of episodes during a session: for example, walking with one 10-minute lope versus ten 1-minute lopes
- The activity immediately preceding a strenuous episode: for example, breaking to a gallop from a standstill versus galloping from a trot after a long warm-up
- The changes in speed or direction: for example, galloping down a straight road versus galloping over a cross country course
- The weight the horse is carrying.

WEATHER AND TERRAIN. Various environmental factors also dictate the conditioning effect of a workout, namely weather and terrain. Heat and humidity can combine to make it tough for a horse's cooling system to operate effectively enough to allow him to continue working. A combined temperature and humidity value of more than 140 may make even a fit horse sweat a lot and have difficulty self-cooling.

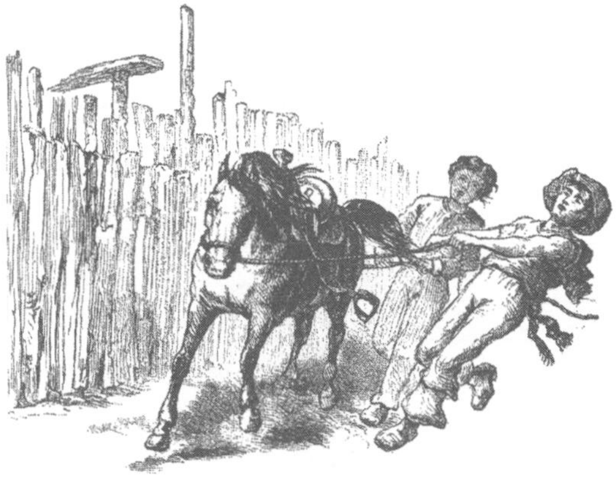

Horse Sense and Safety

Working Around a Horse

★ Learn simple means of control from a knowledgeable horseperson, and use them to control your horse when he becomes frightened or unruly.

★ Be calm and keep your balance.

★ Be very careful not to drop tools or tack underfoot. If you do drop something, nudge it into a safer area with your foot and then pick it up.

Is Your Terrain Too Challenging?

Some terrain can present dangerous situations, even for the fit horse. Any **increase in incline** represents more work, but steepness over 15 percent is considered strenuous. Traversing **deep footing**, such as sand, requires harder work than shallow footing such as sod. The **hardness of footing**, such as pasture versus blacktop, may not affect workload but can create excessive concussion for the legs and hooves. **Icy or muddy footing** can result in strains and sprains and may require much more muscular exertion to negotiate than dry ground. **Irregular footing,** such as that found on a cross-country course, make a horse work harder than does the even surface of an arena.

If the combined temperature and humidity value is higher than 150, especially if the humidity contributes half of the sum, sweating may not be effective and the horse may require cooling from external sources, such as cool water on the head, jugular furrows, and the large vessels of the legs and abdomen. Working a horse in a heat/humidity combination higher than 180 can be very dangerous.

MONITORING THE HORSE. Stress is a demand for adaptation. Failure can occur if a horse is asked to exert beyond his capacity. Therefore, it is important to closely monitor horses before, during, and after workouts. Before a conditioning program even begins, evaluate each horse thoroughly and record individual normal values for the following stress monitoring tests:

- **Vital signs (see January Vet Clinic).** Overall appearance and muscle tone.
- **Sweat.** As a horse becomes more fit, the sweat changes from a sticky, smelly paste to a thin, watery, odorless liquid.
- **Joint fillings and heat.** Palpate the joints for amount of fluid and accompanying heat. Compare with the horse's normal condition from before work and several hours after work.

EXERCISE OPTIONS. Not all types of exercise fulfill the requirements of a conditioning program. Vary a horse's exercise for the best results. Free exercise is natural and unconstrained and the least labor-intensive, but carries the risk of injury due to unregulated, overexuberant bursts. On the other hand, some horses spend most of their turnout time eating rather than exercising if the turnout area is a pasture.

Riding is an ideal way to exercise a horse and can include arena, cross-country, trail, and road riding.

Electric horse walkers are convenient and good for a short warm-up or cool-down, but lengthy sessions can create an attitude of disinterest and boredom. Thirty minutes of walking once or twice a week might be a good alternative if the horse would otherwise stand in the stall.

Hand-walking is labor-intensive but is a controlled warm-up, especially good for a young horse before turnout, longeing, or other work.

Longeing can provide exercise at all gaits, but can inflict damaging effects of torque if the horse is worked in a circle less than 60 feet in diameter.

A **treadmill** increases slow-twitch muscle mass and definition, but does not prepare a horse for strenuous or speed work. The horse must be gradually conditioned to a treadmill. The slope of the treadmill increases the work effort, and the workout is accomplished in about half the time as most other forms of exercise. A horse's hooves must be in balance for treadmill work — long toes would be devastating to the tendons.

Swimming loosens muscles, develops slow-twitch fibers, and minimizes the strain on legs and joints, but is counterproductive for tightening muscles and ineffective for developing speed.

Ponying (leading one horse while riding another) may require a bit more preparation, but is extremely valuable for the mental experience and physical development of a young horse. Ponying is a very good way to teach manners and provide exercise for a young horse. The pony horse must be calm and responsive to the rider and assertive toward the yearling without being aggressive. Although the horse being ponied may try to bite, rear, kick, or balk, the pony horse should just keep moving forward and not attempt to discipline. The best gait for pony work is the long trot.

Odd Word

flehmen. A behavioral response in reaction to a smell or taste; the horse raises the head and curls back the upper lip.

Movie of the Month

***THE MASK OF ZORRO* (1998)**

With Antonio Banderas . . . were there horses in this movie?! Oh. Yes, the black Andalusian Tornado and others. I particularly enjoyed the great tack and turnout and the fantastic stunt riding, including a great bit of Roman riding. There are more adventures in the 2005 sequel *Legend of Zorro.*

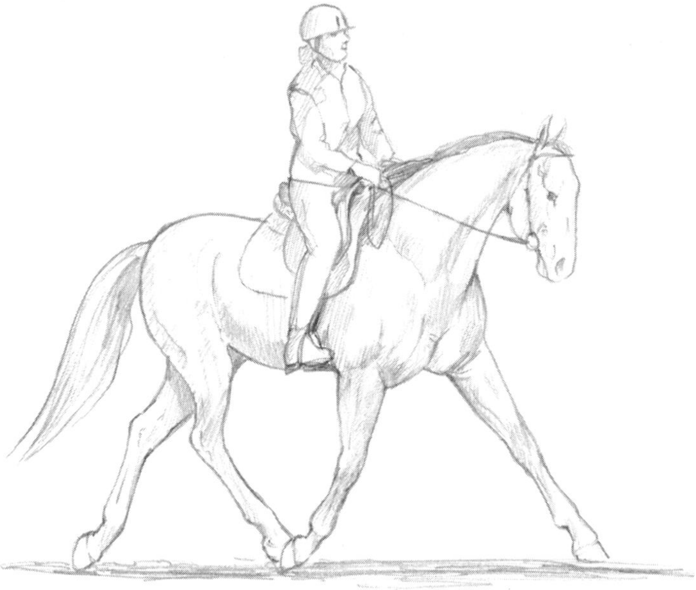

An energetic trot is one of the best forms of exercise for your horse.

PROVIDE VARIETY. An arena represents a controlled, regulated environment and can be very effective for skill development in the strenuous work phase, but can also breed boredom in horse and rider and result in a horse becoming a lazy mover. A road or track offers a level, straight stretch for endurance or speed work. Cross-country riding provides a variety of terrain that challenges the horse's systems and refreshes his interest in his work.

REPRODUCTION ROUNDUP

ESTROUS CYCLE, BREEDING, AND PMS

Mares are seasonally polyestrous, meaning they have estrous cycles many times per year during breeding season. Depending on where you live, this usually means during late spring, summer, and early fall. During those seasons, the mare will have a heat (estrous) cycle about once every 21 to 23 days and during that cycle, she will have from three to eight days of standing heat (estrus; note the difference in

Odd Words

estrous. The cycle during breeding season, lasting 21–23 days.

estrus. The period of standing heat, lasting 3–8 days

spelling between the cycle and the standing heat), during which she would be receptive to a stallion for breeding.

MARES AND THEIR CYCLES. Just like women, each mare is different about how she expresses her heat. Some have PMS — pouty mare syndrome! Not an official term or syndrome, but you get the idea. Some mares are grouchy just before estrus, some during, and some after. One of my mares behaves almost like a gelding. Another is a real "hormone queen" and can get quite anxious and irritable during her heat cycle. The others are more normal in their expression, without a big behavioral change.

Now that you are in the thick of breeding season, jot notes on a calendar. You might notice a pattern: your mare may be sweet, cooperative, and easy to work with on certain days and other days she is impatient, noisy, and preoccupied with something other than what you are doing with her, or even downright grouchy and mean. If you have a mare that is extreme, you might want to plan your training sessions around her worst days. Extra-grouchy mares might kick, bite, or swish their tails when you groom or handle them — so be alert for this. However, it is likely that your mare will show little change at all when she is in heat.

MARES WITH EXTREME PMS. If your mare is dangerous when in heat, confer with your veterinarian, who might suggest hormone therapy. Progesterone administered before the mare comes into heat can cause her to skip her cycle. The drug is injected, implanted, or given orally. If your vet leaves the medication for you to administer, be sure to wear rubber gloves.

Note that mares on this type of therapy can have reproductive problems later. Discuss this thoroughly with your veterinarian before starting your horse on any program.

TIPS & TECHNIQUES

Handling a Mare in Heat

You don't need to do anything special for her when she is in heat. Just be sure, as always, that you provide her with her normal ration, free-choice mineral salt, water, and daily exercise. If you were to leave a mare that is in heat cooped up, when you do take her out, you might have your hands full.

Mares are seasonally polyestrous, meaning they have estrous cycles many times per year during breeding season.

Signs of Estrus

A mare may show none, some, or all of the following signs when she is in heat:

- ★ Frequent urination and winking of the vulva
- ★ Interest in stallions and geldings; backing up and squatting near a male
- ★ Squealing, striking, and kicking in response to other horses coming near
- ★ Swishing tail
- ★ Irritability
- ★ Less cooperative, more excitable, antsy
- ★ Sore or sensitive in the loin area (over the ovaries)

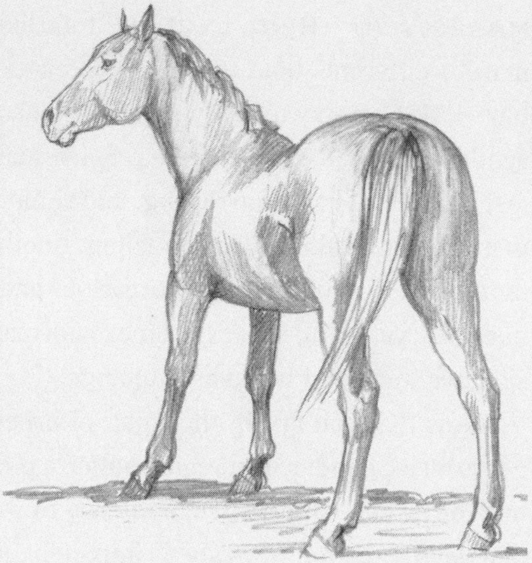

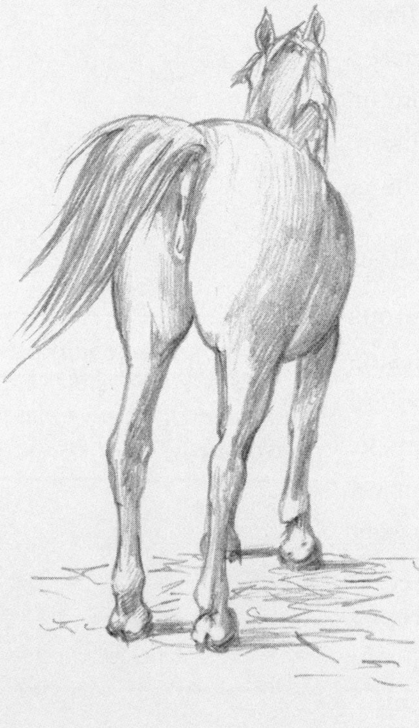

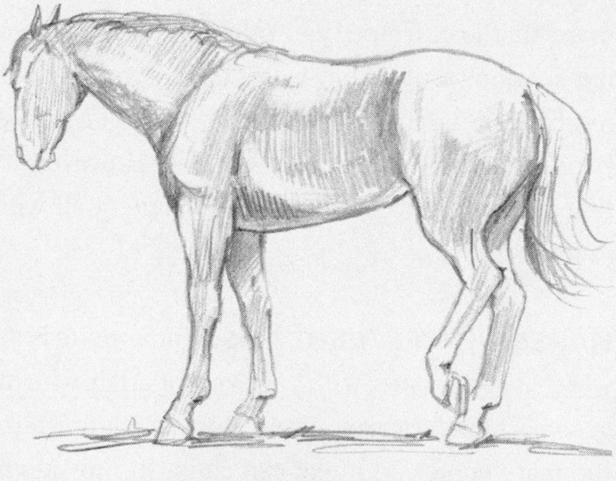

Body language of a mare in heat.

FINE FACILITIES

DESIGNING AN ARENA

The size and type of arena that is best for you depends on the type of riding you plan to do. Here are some guidelines for various activities:

- Dressage: Small size, 66 feet x 132 feet (20 meters x 40 meters); Large size, 66 feet x 198 feet (20 meters x 60 meters)
- Calf roping: 100 feet x 300 feet
- Team roping: 150 feet x 300 feet
- Pleasure riding: 100 feet x 200 feet
- Barrel racing: 150 feet x 260 feet
- Jumping: 150 feet x 300 feet

An arena fence at least six feet tall discourages horses from putting their heads over the rail as they are turning near the fence. The fencing should be very strong if you plan to ride young horses.

The shape of your arena depends on your training goals. Rectangles allow you to ride your horses deep into the corners and teach them to bend. Oval arenas or rectangles

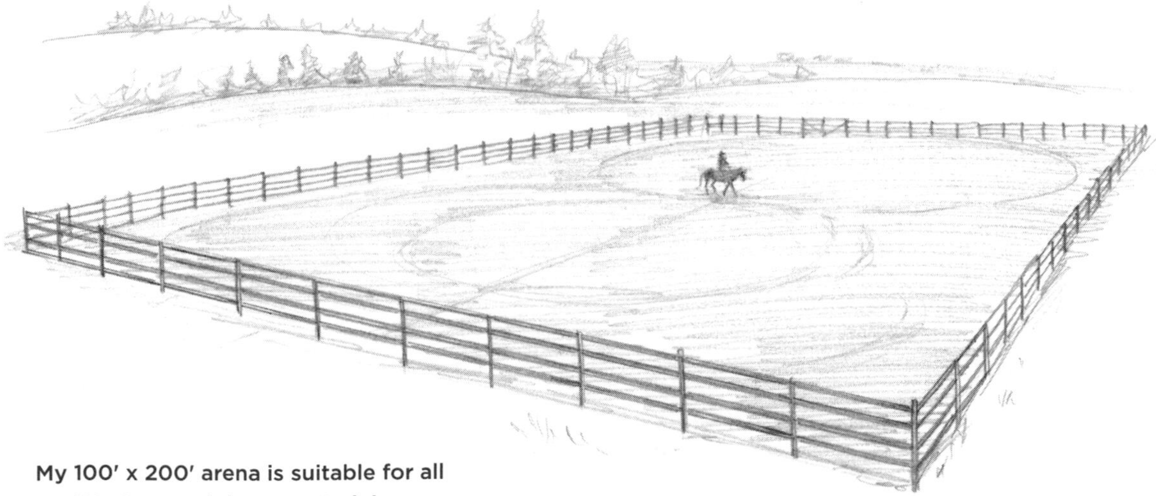

My 100′ x 200′ arena is suitable for all my Western and dressage training.

> ### Odd Word
> **"Rode hard and put up wet."** This phrase describes a horse that was worked until sweaty, then put away without cooling down or grooming. Today, busy people that are overworked, underpaid, and unappreciated use this phrase to describe themselves.

with rounded edges, however, are more appropriate for driving and jumping and are easier to disc and harrow. Gates should be flush on the inside of the arena and the latch should be operable from horseback.

SHAPING AND EXCAVATING. All arenas should either be crowned at the center or sloped gradually from one side to the other. Choose a site that requires minimal excavating. Bulldozing and grading are very expensive, and the less earth that has to be moved, the cheaper the final project will be. While the heavy equipment is there, you may need to install some ditches to divert surrounding drainage away from your arena. After excavation, the arena site will have to settle for six to 12 months, then be leveled periodically before you add any footing material on top of the base.

FOOTING. Footing must be well drained and of appropriate cushion. The type of footing you choose will depend on your climate, whether the arena is indoor or outdoor, and what type of activity you participate in. Jumpers require cushion without excessive depth. Speed events require a firm footing, such as a mixture including stone dust. Reining horses do best on a firm base with a slightly slick top of sandy loam. Dressage and pleasure

STILL TRUE TODAY

Historical Horsekeeping

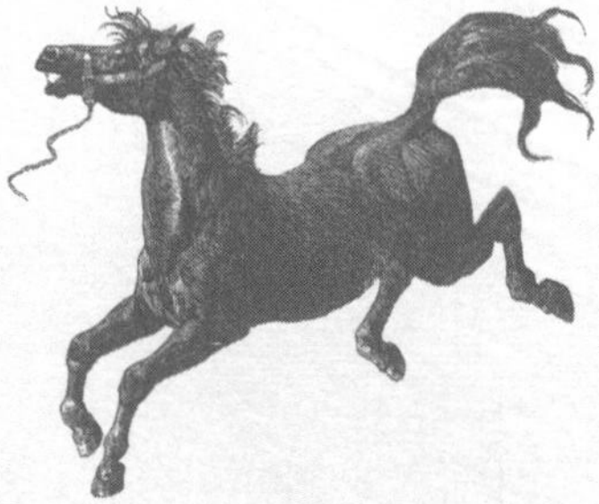

"The rogue is the horse of vices; he may take the bit in his mouth and run away, he will rear, back, kick, strike, bite and do twenty other unpleasant tricks, not always from pure vice, but often from exuberance of spirits, or from being crossed in some way. They generally perform well after they have found out that their rider is their master."

— Gleason's Horse Book *by Prof. Oscar R. Gleason, 1892*

horses work well on a resilient footing without excessive depth, such as some of the processed wood products. One of the most common ways of improving native soil is to disc sand or sawdust into the dirt. This lightens and loosens the soil and increases its drainage while adding to its cushion. It takes about 250 tons of sand to provide a 4-inch cover in a 100-foot x 200-foot arena. To firm up the footing, add stone dust, but only a little at a time until you reach the desired consistency. The total footing should probably consist of no more than 10 percent stone dust. Processed footings can be spread over a firm arena base, but they are better to use in an indoor arena. Tan bark, hardwood fiber, and wood chip products tend to freeze later and thaw sooner than the surrounding ground. They don't need to be disced, just lightly harrowed. However, besides the high expense of the footing itself, processed wood fiber footing requires a well-engineered drainage system in order for it to work at its optimum level.

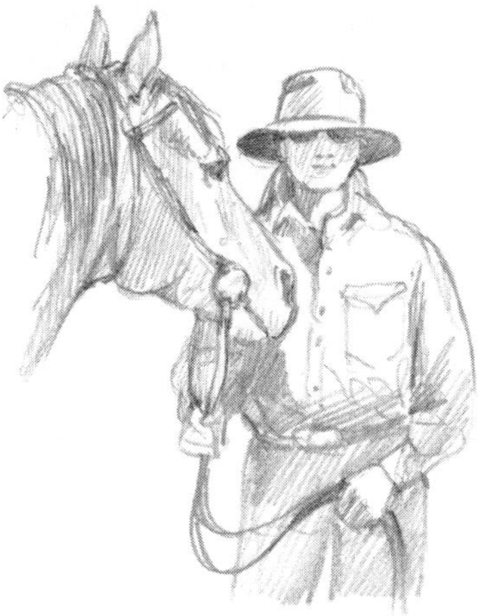

Sun damage is cumulative, so protect yourself every day.

SHELTER FROM UV RAYS

Although exposed skin allows for more evaporative cooling than covered skin, it also absorbs more ultraviolet (UV) rays. And even though a bit of sun can bring color to your cheeks, too much can be destructive to the skin. Get in the habit of wearing a broad-brimmed hat, a long-sleeved shirt with a collar that you can fold up to protect your neck, and gloves for sun protection. Use high-quality sunscreen regularly on your face, hands, and lips.

Take extra-good care of your eyes by making a pair of high-quality sunglasses an integral part of your riding outfit. Buy the ones that provide at least 98 percent protection from ultraviolet rays. Tinted lenses with less protection from UV rays may be worse than no sunglasses at all, because the dark lenses encourage the pupils to dilate, making them more susceptible to harmful rays.

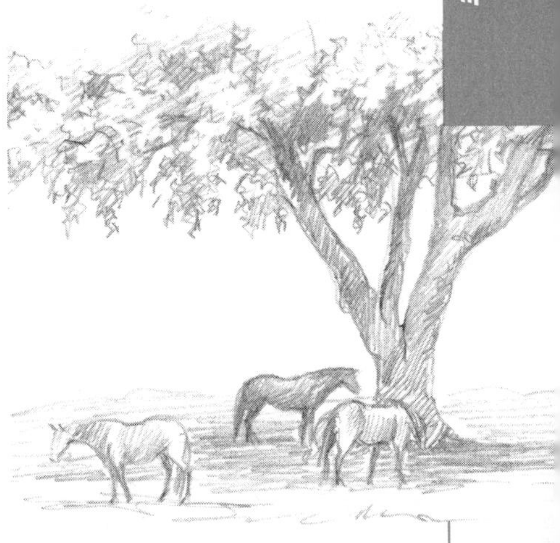

Outfit your horse with a fly sheet and mask when appropriate, and provide him shelter from the hot summer sun.

Get the Green Light

Make sure you have your building plans approved by your local building commission.

en español

hurricane. Comes from *el huracán*, meaning a 'severe tropical cyclone'.

SUMMER LOAFING SHEDS

A run-in shed or loafing shed can provide summer protection. They usually have three walls, with one of the long sides open. A shed can protect a horse's coat from bleaching; protect light-skinned horses that sunburn easily; and provide a place for horses to escape from flies.

I've never liked the word "shed," because it sounds flimsy, yet a run-in shed for horses must be anything but. It must be tough and safe, because horses are free to do whatever they want to it, often without anyone near enough to see. They will rub, kick, and chew; therefore, there should be no sharp edges, protruding fasteners, rough boards with splinters, extending metal roof edges, or anything else that might remotely be a source of injury.

One of the most common causes of severe foot and leg injuries on a shed is the bottom edge of metal siding. There should not be a gap between the siding and the ground

Shed Specs

Figure 12 feet by 12 feet for one horse; 12 feet by 24 feet for two; and so on. The ceiling at the back should be 8 feet high; with 11 feet of clearance at the open side. If a shed is permanent, the back wall should stop the prevailing winter wind, which means the opening would normally face east to southeast. If your shed is portable or on skids, you could move it so that it faces north for the summer, or if you have two sheds in one pasture, you could orient them in different directions for full shade during various times of the day. Locate the shed on high ground with good drainage. Plan for access to the shed for cleaning.

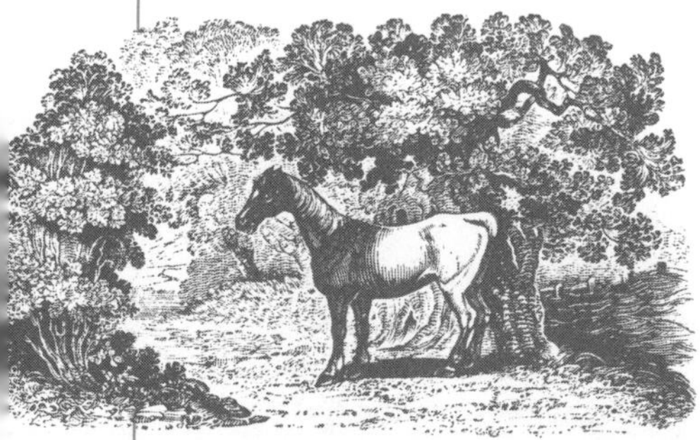

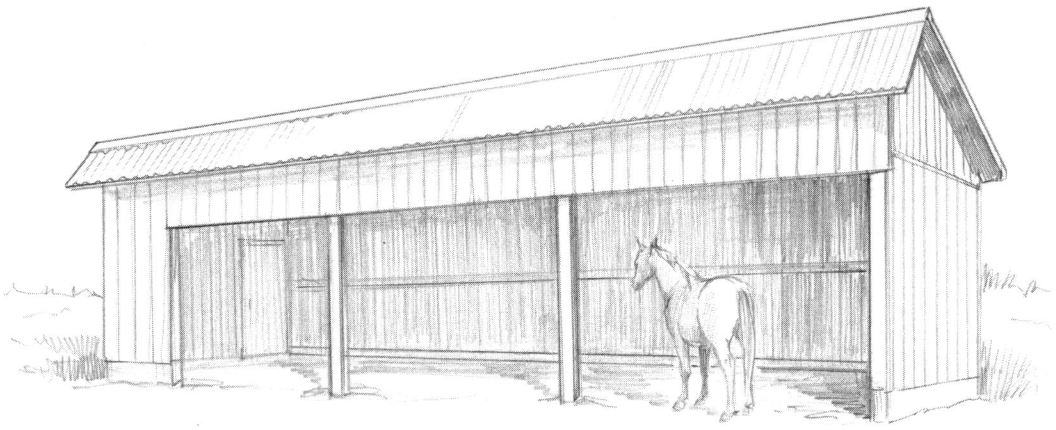

A loafing shed can provide shelter from UV rays and insects.

where a horse's hoof could slip under. The bottom edge of the siding needs to be securely attached to a wide skirt board. All exposed wooden edges of a shed (that a horse can reach with his teeth) should be covered with metal edging or treated regularly with a reliable anti-chew product. For siding, choose smooth surfaces that discourage rubbing and chewing, like steel or plywood panels.

Inside the shed, there should be a kick wall — a solid wall at least 4 feet high around the inside of the walls that prevents a horse from pushing or kicking the siding off from the inside and from rubbing and chewing on the shed framing. Use something like: two layers of ¾-inch plywood or oriented-strand board (OSB); one layer of 1⅛-inch plywood; a layer of ¾-inch plywood covered by rubber mats; 1½-inch tongue-and-groove boards; or 2-inch rough-sawn boards. If you use boards, space them close together. Leaving wide spaces between boards saves materials, but there are more edges for horses to chew on, and wide spaces could be leg traps.

Native soil can work for the floor a run-in shed, especially if it is a portable shed that you move frequently. A more permanent shed would benefit from 4 inches of sand or gravel, but adding footing just invites a horse to use this soft, no-splash area as a preferred place to defecate and urinate.

Steel Gauge

As with fence wire, the thickness of steel is described by gauge. The size most commonly used for horse panels is 15- or 16-gauge, because it is the best compromise between strength and weight. Thicker 14-gauge steel weighs more, so it would be more suitable for crowding cattle or housing rough stock. Thinner 18-gauge steel is lighter and can bend and dent fairly easily from normal horse activities.

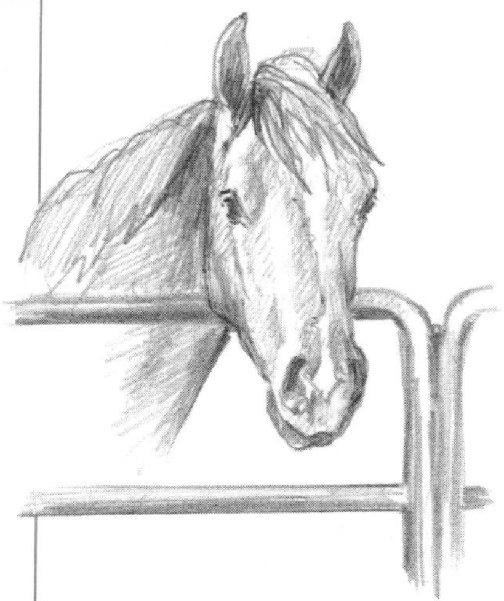

PANELS

We use metal panels in many ways around our ranch. They can be used to make "instant fence" enclosures of various shapes and sizes to house or train horses — round pens, turnout pens, runs, or outdoor covered "stalls." Their portability makes them ideal for a temporary situation as well as for long-term use. With panels, it is not necessary to dig postholes, as it is with permanent fencing.

When choosing panels, whether new or used, the first priority should always be safety. Reviewing their features carefully, because most manufacturers make several grades from utility to premium to heavy duty. Horse panels should be weather resistant and of strong construction. It's a plus if they are easily portable, attractive, and affordable, too.

Here are some features to consider.

- Connectors affect panels' safety, ease of set-up, and stability. Some require level ground underneath. The panel gap should be minimal so a hoof or leg cannot get caught. (See March Fine Facilities.) Three-way and four-way corners are optimal.
- Panel height. Taller panels cost more but are usually better for horses. I like 6-foot-tall panels.
- Panel length. The most popular horse panels are 12 feet long, because they can be moved by one person.
- Rails. Panels usually have five to seven rails (depending on the panel height) with 8 to 12 inches between the rails. An 8-inch space is ideal for housing adult horses. Panels with 12-inch spacing between rails are more suitable for riding pens and arenas.

The space between the last rail and the ground varies. A 16- to 20-inch space would allow a horse that rolled under a panel to get his legs free more easily, but it also allows a foal to roll completely out of his pen or a yearling to wedge his barrel under the bottom rail. Yet a smaller space isn't perfect either, as it would make it difficult for any horse to get untangled without hurting himself. Choose the larger spacing if you have only adult horses. For young horses, choose the smaller space and check them frequently.

MATERIALS. Most horse panels are made from either square, round, or oval steel tubing — usually 1⅝-inch or 2-inch stock. Oval steel tubing is round tubing that has been flattened. Oval tubing panels require less storage space when stacked, such as on the side of a trailer, so would be a good choice for a portable show or trail-riding pen. On the other hand, oval pipe panels can bend more easily than round pipe panels of an equivalent dimension and gauge.

WEIGHT. A horse panel should be substantial enough to stay in place and withstand normal horse activity, yet easy to move around. There is a great variety in the weight of 12-foot horse panels on the market today, from 53 to 107 pounds. If you need a truly portable pen, opt for lighter weight but realize that you are most likely sacrificing durability and perhaps safety. Especially if you are using panels to make fairly permanent pens or runs, choose heavy panels that will withstand rubbing and general horsing around.

FINISH. Horse panels are either galvanized or painted. Common colors are gray, brown, green, and galvanized silver. The finish must withstand horses rubbing, banging, and chewing, as well as the effects of sun and moisture.

PRICE. When it comes to price, it is important to compare similar heights, lengths, and quality of materials. Be sure you are not comparing the economy panel from one manufacturer with the premium panel of another. The final price you pay will also be affected by tax and delivery charges.

Sizing Gates

A 4-foot gate with a full 48-inch opening and at least a 7-foot head clearance provides a safe passage for blanketed horses and manure carts. A 6-foot wide gate with 9-foot head clearance is necessary for leading or riding a saddled horse through.

TIPS & TECHNIQUES

Corral Gates

If you are incorporating a pen or run attached to solid fence posts, or to a building that has posts, consider using corral gates (much less expensive than bow gates) that hang on the post from hinge pins. Corral gates are usually available in 2-foot increments from 4 feet to 16 feet.

MORE IN DEPTH

VICES AND BAD HABITS

A vice is an abnormal behavior that usually shows up in the barn or stable environment, resulting from confinement, improper management, or lack of exercise.

When horses do something we perceive as bad, it's usually due to poor management or training. To deal with vices and bad habits, we need to understand what causes them and then design our horse care and training programs to prevent them.

A vice is an abnormal behavior that usually shows up in the barn or stable environment, resulting from confinement, improper management, or lack of exercise. A vice can affect a horse's usefulness, dependability, and health. Examples are cribbing, weaving, and self-mutilation.

Pawing is destructive to facilities and hooves.

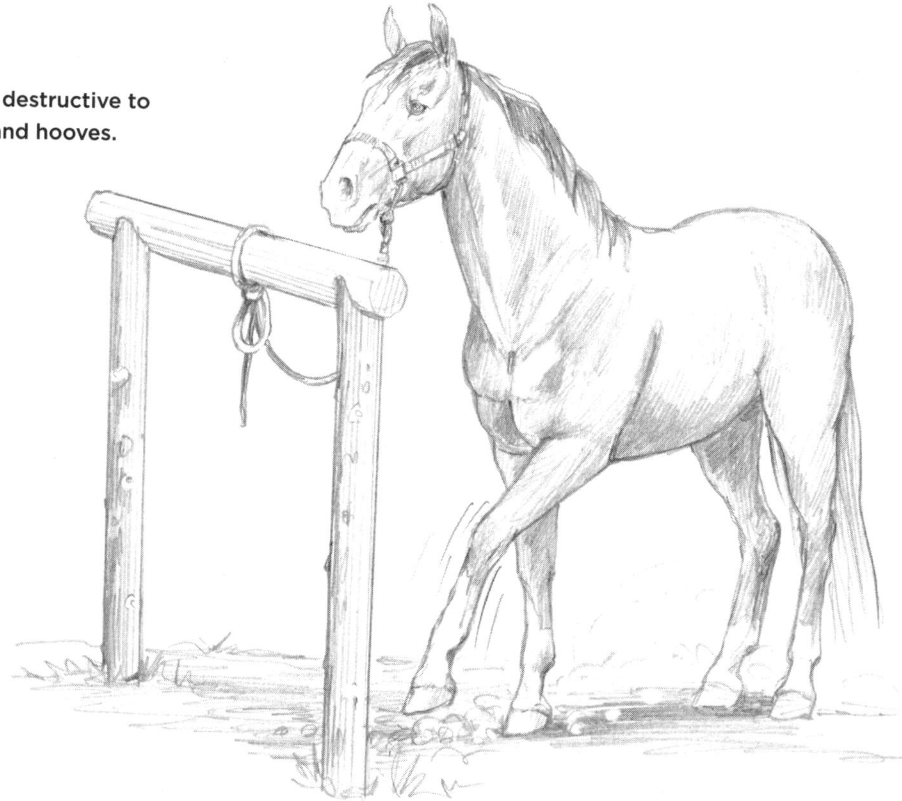

Handling Vices and Bad Habits

Vices and bad habits are best approached in a step-by-step manner:

1. Understand horse behavior and needs
2. Identify and describe the vice or bad habit
3. Determine the cause(s)
4. Make management changes (facilities, exercise, nutrition, conditioning, or grooming)
5. Implement appropriate training practices
6. Consider remedial training practices
7. Consider medical and surgical solutions.

A bad habit is an undesirable behavior that occurs during training or handling and is usually a result of poor techniques and a lack of understanding of horse behavior. Examples are rearing, halter pulling, striking, and kicking.

Certain horses have a predisposition to neurotic breakdown when faced with domestication pressures. This psychological frailty may be genetically inherited, formed from early experiences with the dam or training, or may develop later in life due to disease or trauma. Horses with neurotic tendencies often form vices. Most vices and bad habits are preventable, that is, with forethought and proper management and training, most of them can be avoided. Prevention is the desirable route because once certain habits are established, they can be much more difficult to change.

Some habits are manageable: that is, certain techniques and equipment can diminish negative effects, but the underlying habit is still there. If the equipment is not used, the habit resurfaces. A few habits are curable. With carefully planned, diligent efforts, some habits can be permanently changed. Some vices and bad habits are incurable.

A bad habit is an undesirable behavior that occurs during training or handling and is usually a result of poor techniques and a lack of understanding of horse behavior.

Whoever said a horse was dumb was dumb.

— Will Rogers

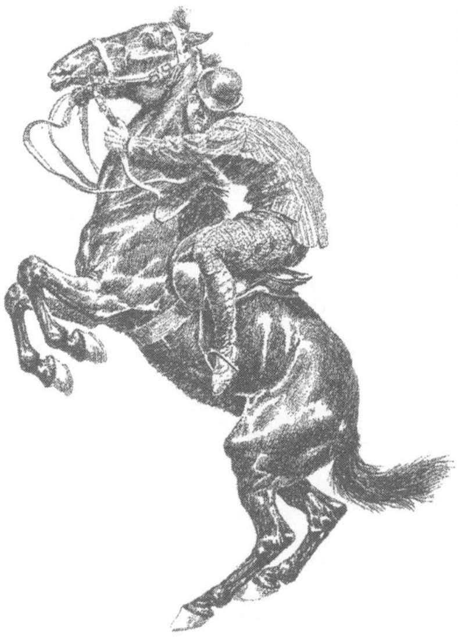

Bad Habits

Habit	Description	Causes	Treatment
BALKING	Refusal to go forward often followed by violent temper if rider insists.	Fear, heavy hands, stubbornness, extreme fatigue.	Curable. Review forward work with in-hand & longeing. Turn horse's head to untrack left or right. Strong driving aids with no conflicting restraining aids (no pull on bit). Do not try to force horse forward by pulling — you'll lose.
BARN SOUR HERD BOUND	Balking, rearing, swinging around, screaming and then rushing back to the barn or herd.	Separation from buddies or barn (food, comfort).	Curable, but stubborn cases require a professional. A confident, capable trainer that insists the horse leave the barn (herd) and then positively reinforces the horse's good behavior so horse develops confidence. The lessons GO and WHOA must both be reviewed.
BITING	Nibbling with lips or grabbing with teeth; especially young horses.	Greed (treats), playfulness (curiosity) or resentment (irritated or sore). Investigate things with mouth. Often from hand-feeding treats.	Curable. Handle lips, muzzle, and nostrils regularly in a business-like way; when horse nips, tug on nose chain, then resume as if nothing happened. Can also use thumb tack on sleeve; hold wire brush toward lips; use muzzle.
BOLTING	Wheels away suddenly before halter is fully removed.	Poor handling, anxious to exercise or join other horses.	Curable but dangerous, as horse often kicks as he wheels away. Use treats on ground before you remove halter; use rope around the neck.
BUCKING	Arching the back, lowering the head, kicking with hind legs or leaping.	High spirits, desire to get rid of rider or tack, sensitive or sore back, reaction to legs or spurs.	Monitor feed and exercise; proper progressive training; check tack fit.

Bad Habits continued

Habit	Description	Causes	Treatment
HARD TO CATCH	Avoids humans with halter and lead.	Fear, resentment, disrespect, bad habit.	Curable. Take time to properly train, use walk-down method in small area first, progress to larger. Remove other horses from pasture; treats on ground, never punish horse once caught.
WON'T ALLOW HANDLING OF FEET	Swaying, leaning, rearing, jerking foot away, kicking, striking.	Insufficient or improper training. Horse hasn't learned to cooperate, balance on three legs, take pressure and movement of farrier work.	Curable, but persistent cases require a professional. Thorough, systematic conditioning and restraint lessons: pick up foot, hold in both flexed & extended positions for several minutes while cleaning, grooming, rubbing leg, coronary band, or bulbs, etc.
HALTER PULLING	Rearing or setting back when tied, often until something breaks or horse falls and/or hangs by halter.	Rushed, poor halter training, using weak equipment or unsafe facilities so horse gets free by breaking something. Often horse was tied by bridle reins and broke free.	Can be curable but very dangerous and incurable in some chronic cases which require a professional. Might use stiff bristled broom on the rump or wither rope on advice of professional.
HEAD SHY	Moves head away during grooming, bridling, clipping, vet work.	Initially rough handling or insufficient conditioning, painful ears or mouth problems.	Curable. First eliminate medical reasons such as ear, tongue, lip or dental problems. Start from square one with handling; after horse allows touching, then teach him to put head down.
JIGGING WHEN RIDDEN	Short, stilted walk/jog with hollow back and high head.	Poor training attempt at collection, horse not trained to aids, too strong bridle aids, sore back.	Curable. Check tack fit, use aids properly including use of pressure/release (half halt) to bring horse to walk or use strong driving aids to push horse into active trot.

Bad Habits continued

Habit	Description	Causes	Treatment
KICKING	Lashing back at a person with one or both hind legs, also "cow kicking," which is lashing out to the side.	Initially a reflex to touching legs, then fear (defense) of rough handling, or to get rid of a threat or unwanted nuisance.	Might be curable but serious cases are very dangerous and require a professional to use remedial restraint methods. Unlikely to ever completely cure.
REARING	Standing on hind legs when led or ridden, sometimes falling over backwards.	Fear, rough handling, doesn't think he must go forward or is afraid to go forward into contact with bit; associated with balking; a response to collected work.	Can be curable but is a very dangerous habit that might be impossible to cure even by a professional. Check to be sure no mouth or back problems. Review going forward in-hand with a whip and review longeing.
RUNNING AWAY; BOLTING	Galloping out of control when ridden.	Fear, panic, (flight response), lack of training to the aids, overfeeding, under exercise, pain from poor fitting tack.	Might be curable but very dangerous; when horse panics, can run into traffic, over cliff, through fence, etc.; remedy is to pull (with pressure and release) the horse into a large circle, gradually decreasing the size.
SHYING	Spooking at real or imagined sights, sounds, smells, or occurrences.	Fear (of object or of trainer's reaction to horse's behavior), poor vision, head being forcibly held so horse can't see, playful habit.	Generally curable. Put horse on aids and guide and control his movement with driving and restraining aids.
STRIKING	Taking a swipe at a person with a front leg.	Reaction to clipping, first use of chain or twitch, restraint of head, dental work.	Curable but very dangerous especially if coupled with rearing as person's head could be struck. Review head handling (mouth, nostrils, ears); head down lesson; and thorough body handling and sacking out.
STUMBLING	Losing balance or catching the toe on the ground and missing a beat or falling.	Weakness, lack of coordination, lack of condition, young, lazy, long toe/low heel, delayed breakover of hooves, horse ridden on forehand, poor footing.	Curable. Have hoof balance assessed, check breakover, ride horse with more weight on the hindquarters (collect), conditioning horse properly.
TAIL WRINGING	Switching and/or rotating tail in an irritated or angry fashion.	Sore back from poor fitting tack, poorly balanced rider, injury, rushed training.	May not be curable once established. Proper saddle fit, rider lessons, massage and other medical therapy, proper warm-up and progressive, achievable training demands.

Vices

Vice	Description	Causes	Treatment
CRIBBING	Colic, poor keeper (prefers mind drugs over food). Anchoring of incisors on edge (post, stall ledge), arching neck, gulping air.	Theory: endorphins are released during the behavior; horse is addicted to endorphins, which stimulate pleasure center of brain.	Incurable. Cribbing strap prevents contraction of neck muscles; also available with clamps, spikes, electric shock; muzzle. Possible future drug or surgical treatment.
PAWING	Digs holes; tips over feeders and waterers; gets leg caught in fence; wears hooves away, loses shoes; most often young horses.	Confinement, boredom, excess feed.	Curable. Provide exercise, diversion, don't use ground feeders and waterers, use rubber mats, don't reinforce by feeding.Formal restraint lessons.
SELF MUTILATION	Bites flanks, front legs, chest, scrotal area with squealing, pawing, and kicking out.	Onset at two years, primarily stallions. Can be endorphin addiction similar to cribbing; can be triggered by confinement, lack of exercise, or sexual frustration.	Manageable/might be curable. Geld nonbreeding stallions; increase exercise, reduce confinement, stall companion or toy, neck cradle, muzzle, possible future pharmacological treatment
STALL KICKING	Smashing stall walls and doors with hind hooves resulting in facilities damage and hoof and leg injuries.	Confinement; doesn't like neighbor; gets attention.	Can be curable depending on how long-standing the habit. Increase exercise, change neighbors, pad stall walls or hooves, use kicking chains or kicking shoe, don't reinforce by feeding.
TAIL RUBBING	Rhythmically swaying the rear against a fence or stall wall.	Initially dirty udder, sheath, or tail; shedding HQ, pinworms, ticks and other external parasites or skin conditions. Later, just habit.	Manageable with grooming, cleaning sheath and udder, deworming, other medical treatments. For chronic habit, use electric fence.
WEAVING, PACING	Swaying back and forth often by stall door or pen gate. Repeatedly walking a path back and forth.	Confinement, boredom, excess feed, high strung or stressed horse.	Manageable. Turn out where he can see other horses. Use specially fitted stall door for weaver.
WOOD CHEWING	Gnawing of wood fences, feeders, stall walls, up to 3 pounds of wood per day.	Lack of course roughage in diet, boredom, teething.	Manageable. Increase roughage in diet. Decrease palatability of wood. Increase exercise and activity. More time out on pasture.

> "And God took a handful of southerly wind, blew his breath over it, and created the horse."
>
> — Bedouin legend

HURRICANE SEASON IN THE SOUTHEAST

Hurricanes are severe tropical storms that form in the Atlantic Ocean. The winds rotate counterclockwise around the eye and must be at least 74 miles per hour to qualify as a hurricane. Approximately six hurricanes per year affect the United States. Although the Eastern Pacific hurricane season generally runs from May 15 to November 30, the Atlantic, Caribbean, and Gulf of Mexico season begins June 1 and runs until the end of November. Hurricane threats include storm surge, wind, floods, and tornadoes.

The storm surge is the heavy waves that come ashore when the eye hits land. They can be 50 miles wide. The eyewall wind speeds can be 100 miles per hour at the coast, and have reached 175 miles per hour inland. Flooding occurs from the strong storm surge plus the heavy rain that often accompanies hurricanes. There is usually at least one tornado during the first three days after a hurricane has hit land. See more about tornadoes in April Horsekeeping Across America.

PLAN FOR THE WORST. If you live in a hurricane-prone area, have an evacuation plan that includes your horses. This might mean boarding your horses inland in a safe area for a few days ahead of each forecast storm, or for the entire season. Be sure they are up to date on all vaccinations and have current health papers and necessary identification. Have feed, water, and medical supplies packed and ready to roll. Keep paperwork in a waterproof container, including all pertinent phone numbers, photos and legal descriptions, brand papers, and anything else you need to identify your horse and prove ownership.

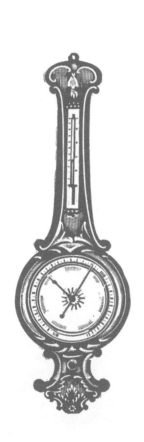

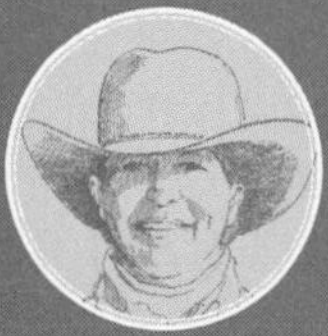

Ask Cherry

Outdoor Arena Fence

Q

I have leveled out a spot 170 feet by 70 feet for an outdoor arena. What size boards should I use? I am using railroad ties for the posts. I don't plan on turning horses loose in it. I want a riding arena that I can also use for trail horse obstacles. My posts will be 10 feet apart. Would 10-foot 2x6s work?

A

For a riding arena you need a visual barrier more than a strong physical barrier, so either 2-inch by 6-inch or 2-inch by 8-inch boards would work. You can put in from two to four boards. If you use two rails, they should be 36 inches and 54 inches high. The problem with spanning a 10-foot space with a 10-foot long 2x6, or even a 2x8, is that the board might warp and twist. It would be better to space the posts 8 feet apart and then span two spaces with 16-foot-long boards. That way, each board is attached to three posts and will stay straighter.

An option worth considering is high-tensile polymer (HTP) fence used with your railroad tie posts. It consists of high-tensile wire encased in polymer webbing, which makes up rails of various widths. HTP is comparable in price to wood rails and would likely be more cost effective in the long run, because you would never have to paint it or treat it. The posts could be spaced 10 feet apart or even wider with HTP. Another option is to use 10-foot-long vinyl-covered boards, which would not twist and warp, and would never need painting. However, they are quite expensive.

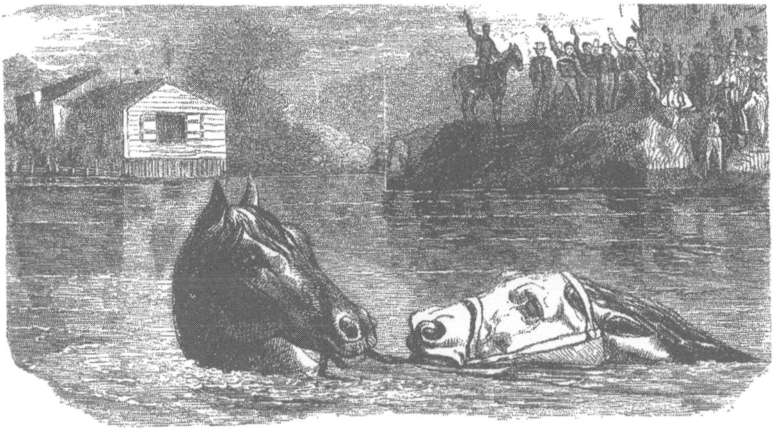

JULY

I always breathe a deep sigh of relief when we have our year's supply of grass hay put away in the hay barn, and this often happens in July. Usually it is hot and dusty work that quickly tells us which muscles we haven't used much since last year this time. But in spite of all the hay down my shirt and the seemingly endless supply of bales to be moved, each year I look forward to locating good hay and moving it in. It's security.

Day Length in Hours

		Date		
		July 1	July 16	Aug 1
Latitude	60°N	18.38	17.74	16.62
	55°N	17.03	16.57	15.73
	50°N	16.09	15.74	15.07
	45°N	15.38	15.1	14.56
	40°N	14.81	14.58	14.13
	35°N	14.33	14.14	13.77
	30°N	13.91	13.75	13.46

See page 22 to find your latitude.

MONSOON TIME

A monsoon is any wind that reverses its direction seasonally. The southwest United States is affected by the Mexican monsoon season, also known as the North American Monsoon System (NAMS), the Southwest U.S. monsoon, or the Arizona monsoon. U.S. states affected by the NAMS are Arizona, New Mexico, and Colorado.

Most of the year, winds aloft over the United States are from the west and northwest. During the summer, the winds shift to a south–southeast direction, carrying moisture into the southwest U.S. from the Pacific Ocean, the Gulf of California, and the Gulf of Mexico. As these moist winds move into the arid Southwest, thunderstorms form from the combination of the air being forced upward by the mountains, daytime heating by the sun, and weak upper-level disturbances across the region.

FYI

How Dew?

Dew point is the temperature to which air must be cooled for saturation (100 percent relative humidity) to occur.

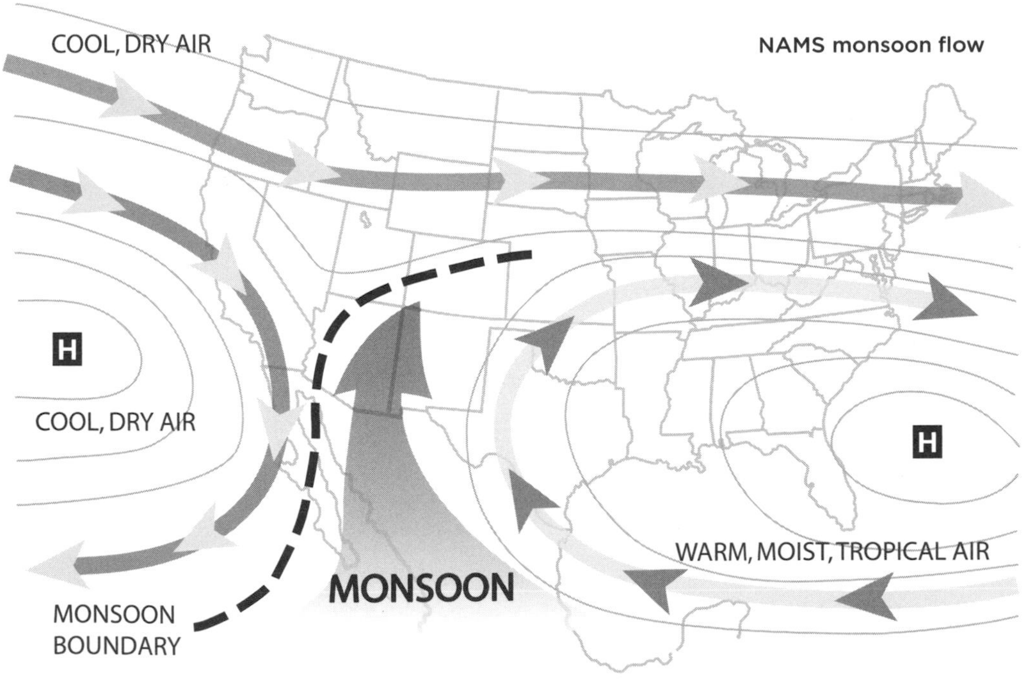

To Do

- ❑ Deworm
- ❑ Haul hay
- ❑ Cut tails
- ❑ Mark hay loads
- ❑ Trim and shoe horses
- ❑ Work arena
- ❑ Set up fly traps
- ❑ Scrub feed tubs and buckets
- ❑ Move hay to barns
- ❑ Thank farrier
- ❑ Rotate pastures
- ❑ Control dust

To Buy

- ❑ Hay
- ❑ Beet pulp pellets
- ❑ Senior feed
- ❑ Corn oil
- ❑ Hoof sealer
- ❑ Fly traps
- ❑ Fly spray

Arizona monsoons consist of early afternoon thunderstorms over the higher mountains. The rain cools and then moves to the desert, producing more thunderstorms, often over the Phoenix area during late afternoon and evening, usually ending by midnight. These storms can produce wind gusts of more than 50 miles per hour and have been recorded at as high as 115 miles per hour.

The NAMS produces 35 to 45 percent of Arizona's and New Mexico's annual precipitation and more than 60 percent of northern Mexico's. The monsoon season officially starts when there are three consecutive days when the dew point in southern Arizona or New Mexico reaches 55°F or higher.

The average start date of the monsoon season is July 7, and the end is September 13. Usually a very hot and dry period precedes the onset of the monsoon season. The rainfall from the monsoon is localized and often heavy, so some areas might receive flooding while others don't receive a drop. Lightning accompanying these fast-moving storms can be responsible for fires.

LOOKING AT HORSES

Forelegs

Both of a horse's forelegs should appear to be of equal length and size and to bear equal weight. A line dropped from the point of the shoulder to the ground should bisect the limb. The toes should point forward and the feet should be as far apart on the ground as the legs are at their origin in the chest.

Vet Clinic

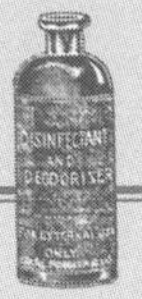

Lyme Disease

Lyme disease is caused by the bacterium *Borrelia burgdorfer* and is transmitted to horses, dogs, and humans by the bite of an infected black-legged (deer) tick. The ticks become infected when they drink blood from infected small mammals, often the white-footed mouse. Lyme disease occurs most often in the Northeast and Midwest United States.

HORSES. Since a tick must be attached for a number of hours before transmitting the disease, regular tick checks and removal go a long way toward preventing the disease. Although adult ticks are large enough to feel, see, and remove, the tick's nymph stage is quite small and easily missed. (See April Pest Patrol for tick removal techniques.) Symptoms in the horse include stiffness and lameness, swollen joints, fever, and lethargy. Diagnosis and treatment are difficult.

HUMANS. Typical symptoms in humans include fever, headache, fatigue, and a characteristic skin rash that resembles a red bulls-eye. Untreated, the infection can spread to joints, the heart, and the nervous system. Treatment with a few weeks of antibiotics is usually successful. Prevention includes use of insect repellent and protective clothing (such as long-sleeved shirts and long pants), removing ticks promptly, landscape modification, and pest management. The ticks that transmit Lyme disease can occasionally transmit other tick-borne diseases as well, including Rocky Mountain spotted fever (see April Pest Patrol).

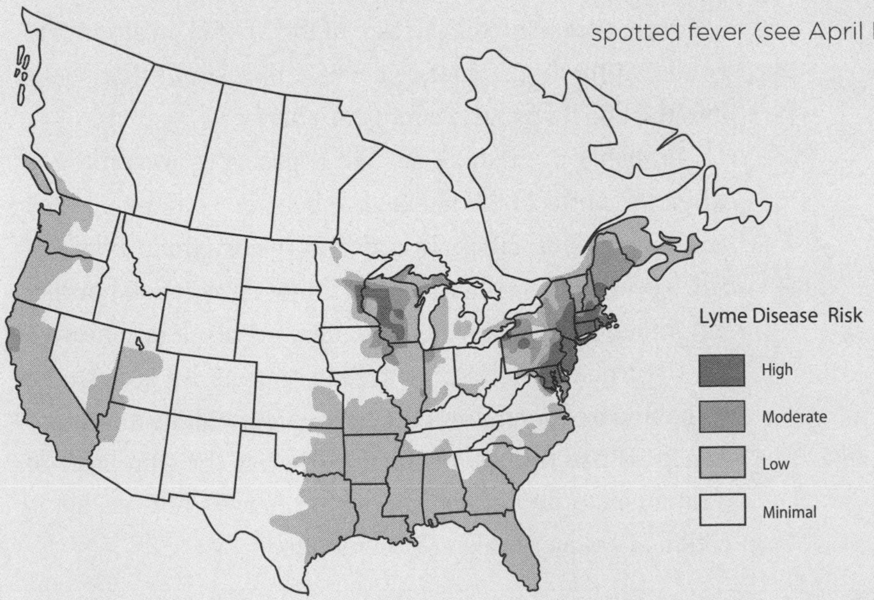

FOOT NOTES

Dry Hooves, Good Hooves

A horse's hoof is most healthy when it is in a consistently dry environment. The hoof has two natural protective coverings, the periople and the stratum tectorium, which retard moisture movement from either direction — from the outside environment into the hoof or from the inner layer of the hoof to the outside. In addition to keeping your horse's stall, pen, and pastures dry, use hoof dressing discriminately. Some greases and oils soften the hoof too much; others do nothing but lighten your wallet.

NATIONAL FARRIER WEEK

The second week of July is National Farrier Week, a perfect time to recognize the hard work and valuable skills provided by your horseshoer. Here are some ways to recognize his or her talents and dedication:

- Make all visits pleasant and safe by following the advice in January and February Foot Notes.
- Make an improvement to the shoeing area, such as an upgrade in the footing, lighting, or ease of access.
- Make a personalized card. A tip is optional.
- Bake a batch of his or her favorite cookies.
- Ask your farrier how you can improve the comfort and safety of his or her visit.

HOOF DRESSING AND SEALER

During the hot, dry weather of summer, many horse owners want to moisten their horses' hooves but often don't know how to do it. Understanding the difference between hoof dressing and sealer is a start. Hoof dressing is a grease or cream spread on the surface of the hoof in an attempt to condition the hoof. Hoof sealer is a thin liquid that soaks into the hoof to provide a moisture barrier.

Probably the only time hoof dressing is warranted is when the bulbs of the heels have become so dry that they are beginning to crack. In order to restore their pliability, rub a product containing animal fat (such as lanolin or fish oil) into the heels daily until the desired result is achieved.

Use a hoof sealer during the wet seasons, if a horse must be bathed frequently, or if the hooves show signs of surface cracks. When the farrier must rasp away the thin layer of stratum tectorium as he shapes your horse's hooves, application of a sealer is also recommended.

FOAL HOOF CARE

Unless you are very experienced in raising foals and are certain that your foal is normal, you should arrange for a veterinary examination the day after birth. This will allow your veterinarian to evaluate the foal's limbs and determine whether any deviations are normal or whether they will require close observation or treatment. For example, many foals are born with carpus valgus (knock-knees): that is, they stand with their knees closer together than their hooves. Because most newborn foals' chests are very narrow, the front limbs are very close together at the chest. The foal, in its attempt to stabilize itself when standing and grazing, widens its base of support by increasing the distance between its hooves and allowing the lower limb to rotate outward. This causes the limbs to bend inward, bringing the knees even closer together.

Most angular deformities greater than 15 degrees require immediate veterinary treatment; however, the majority of foals do not fall into this category. Many foals born with crooked limbs straighten without any formal treatment, and those that don't can often be corrected with care from a competent veterinarian and farrier and by proper management. Closure of the growth plates has an important bearing on the timing of corrective treatments.

A regular program of farrier care should begin when the foal is about one month of age. Avoid or minimize rasping, however. Radical rasping or trimming usually does more harm than good with the very young foal.

FEATHERY HOOVES. A foal is born with soft feathers of horn on the bottoms of its hooves. These normally wear off by the end of the first day. The neonate (baby) hoof is soft and waxy the first week but gradually hardens to more durable hoof horn. The last bit of neonate hoof will have grown down to ground level by about six months of age.

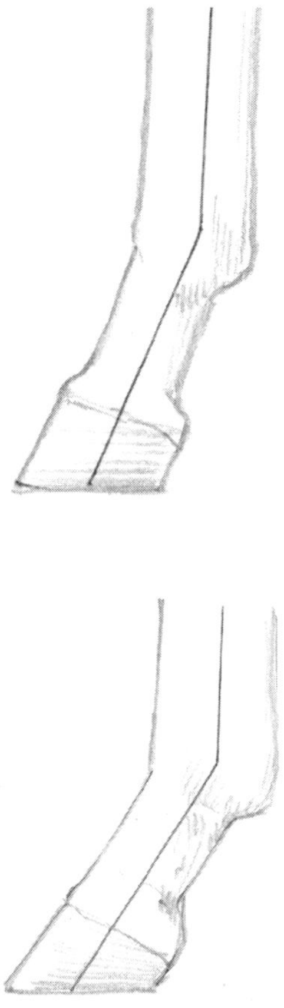

A foal's hooves and pasterns (top) are often more upright and with a higher heel than an adult horse's (bottom).

FEED BAG

Purchasing Hay

It is most economical to select and purchase a year's supply of hay all at once. See Choosing Good Hay in this month's More In Depth.

HAY DREGS

I rake or sweep hay dregs (leftovers) off the floor of my feeding areas after each feeding to keep dust and debris from spreading through the barn. I pick up the edible portion of the hay with a fork and put it in a small cart. In a few days, there is enough for one horse's ration.

The longer hay lies on the ground, the more likely it will be fouled by traffic, moisture, or dirt and the less likely a horse will be to eat it, so it is best to feed dregs regularly when they are fresh.

WILD LIFE

BIRDS

It is a rare treat when Mother Nature allows a brood of ducklings to be born on the North Fork of Rabbit Creek, and a great surprise when I manage to see them! Predators and spring floods make this an uncommon occurrence.

RAPTORS. The falcons and hawks in our area vary from season to season. The red-tailed hawk, prairie falcon, and American kestrel live here year-round. Other hawks winter here, then go elsewhere to breed, or winter elsewhere and come here to breed. I'm keeping my eye out for the Swainson's hawks coming in from Argentina, the Mississippi kites soaring in from Mexico, and the elusive peregrine falcons.

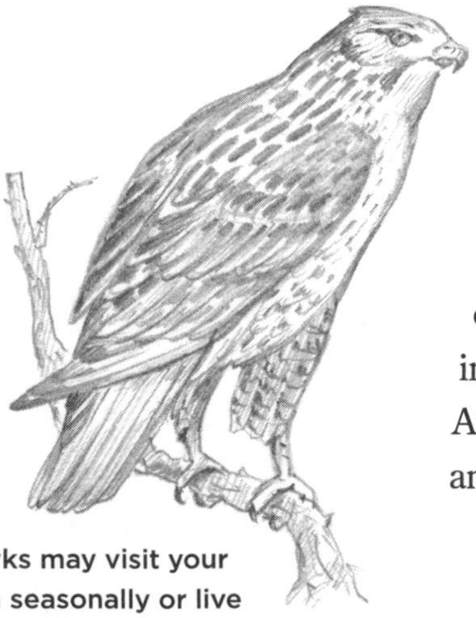

Hawks may visit your area seasonally or live there year round.

KESTRELS. Although the American kestrel is also called the sparrow hawk, we call them the mountain parrot because they are so vividly marked. Males are gunmetal blue, rusty red, and buff, with a red cap. Female kestrels are mainly reddish with lighter under-portions. Both have two distinctive streaks, or "sideburns," down each cheek.

The old name sparrow hawk is misleading because kestrels don't eat sparrows. They eat grasshoppers and insects during the spring and summer and mice, voles, and shrews in the winter.

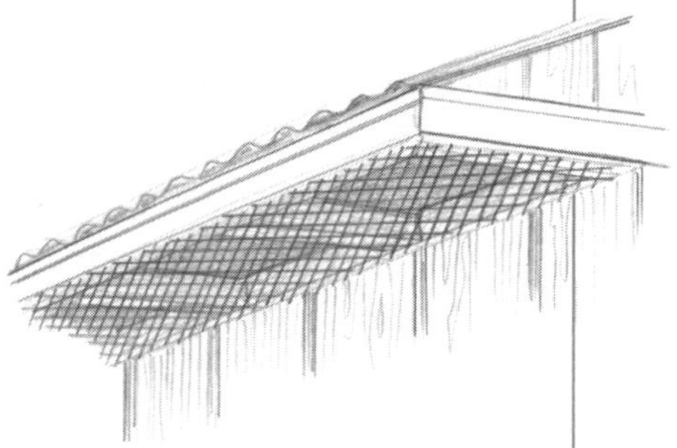

Wire mesh under barn eaves discourages nesting while still allowing ventilation.

BARN-DWELLING BIRDS. Birds are wonderful and I really do love them all, in moderation. When sparrows, starlings, or swallows become too numerous, however, they can be a real problem in a horse barn. Besides making a mess, with their droppings coating everything below their perches (which are often high in the barn rafters), birds carry disease, contaminate feed, and persist in nesting where we don't want them. Some horse barns are an engraved invitation for birds: doors and windows open during nesting season, and plenty of food, water, and nesting materials available — who wouldn't want to move in?

I've found that the most effective deterrent at our place is to keep the barn closed during nesting season. Since migratory birds are protected under federal law, you can't shoot or otherwise kill birds such as swallows, gulls, or pigeons. You'll need to devise ways to discourage them from taking up residence at your facilities. In case you feel as though you're in that Alfred Hitchcock movie, rest assured, you are not alone. There are many bird deterrent products on the market.

TIPS & TECHNIQUES

Keeping Birds Out of the Barn

Bird control methods include:

- ★ Construction that discourages roosting, such as wires above the roof peak
- ★ Sticky deterrents to discourage them from perching
- ★ Wires, mesh, or blocks under the eaves to discourage nesting
- ★ The use of sounds and objects to repel the birds

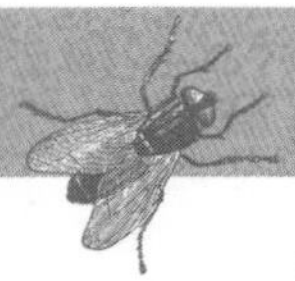

PEST PATROL

Who's Who?

The clouds of small flies on manure are often mistaken for immature stable flies, but in fact are a different type of fly that may play an important part in the decomposition of manure.

Five Steps in Fighting Flies

1. Prevent flies from breeding.

2. Prevent larvae from hatching.

3. Capture adult flies immediately.

4. Kill remaining flies.

5. Protect your horse.

WAGING WAR ON FLIES

1. PREVENT FLIES FROM BREEDING. Proper manure management and moisture control are the two biggest factors in keeping flies from breeding. Remove manure and wasted feed daily from stalls and pens and either spread it thinly to dry or compost it (see January and March Cleanup Crew). While a manure pile is fermenting, certain portions of it can make inviting fly-breeding grounds. One way to discourage flies from congregating is to sprinkle the wettest portions of the pile with hydrated lime. The lime speeds up the bacterial action of fermentation, and the "hotter" alkalizing action discourages flies from landing.

Managing a pile properly will kill the parasite eggs and larvae, prevent flies from breeding, and result in a good-quality fertilizer.

Moisture control strategies can include:

- Rake around feeders and waterers every day, removing the moist feed that has been dropped.
- Pick up grass clippings, keep grass and weeds mowed, and pick up trash regularly.
- Be sure there is proper drainage in all stalls, pens, paddocks, and pastures.
- Repair leaking faucets, hydrants, hoses, and waterers.
- Eliminate wet spots in stalls and pens by clearing the bedding away, sprinkling with an absorbent, and letting the ground dry out.

Barn designs that allow sunshine to dry the floors are best. Proper air circulation (via natural wind flow or fans) is essential. If possible, have an extra stall or pen so you can rotate each horse out of his regular stall for a day or two each month to let the floor dry.

Know Your Enemy

We have very few flies at our particular location, mainly due to the semiarid climate and our manure management program. If we do have a wet year, we might have flies in July, August, or September. In that case, we get out our fly traps early. There are many ways to control flies that don't include the use of chemicals.

Stable flies, horseflies, deerflies, horn flies, and face flies can be a health concern for your horse and can drive him crazy. Stable flies, by far the most common, are the same size as a house fly, but while the latter just feeds on garbage and spreads filth, stable flies (both males and females) suck your horse's blood. Common feeding sites include the lower legs, flanks, belly, under the jaw, and at the junction of the neck and the chest.

The bite of a blood-sucking fly is painful, and some horses have such a low fly tolerance that they can be driven into a snorting and striking frenzy or an injurious stampede. Even fairly tough horses, subjected to a large number of aggressive stable flies, might spend the entire day stomping alternate legs. This can cause damaging concussion to legs, joints, and hooves and result in loose shoes and loss of weight and condition.

When stable flies have finished feeding, they seek shelter to rest and digest. They lay their eggs in decaying organic matter: moist manure, wet hay, unclipped grassy areas, and other places where there is moist plant material are ideal sites. The life cycle is 21 to 25 days from egg to adult. A female often lays 20 batches of eggs during her 30-day life span, each batch containing between 40 and 80 eggs. When the eggs hatch, the adult flies emerge ready to breed. The number of flies produced by one pair of adults and their offspring in 30 days is a staggering figure in the millions. That's why fly prevention is the most important line of defense in your war against flies.

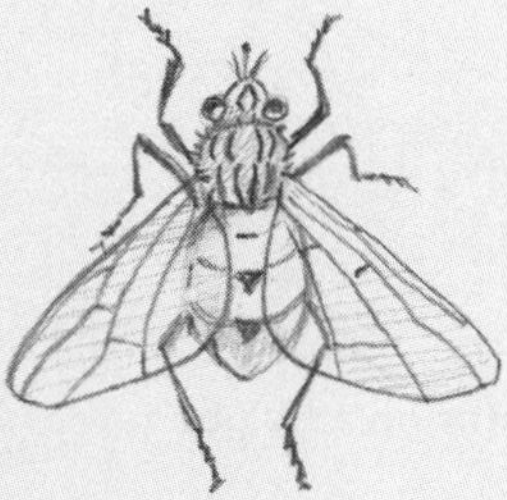

Stable fly

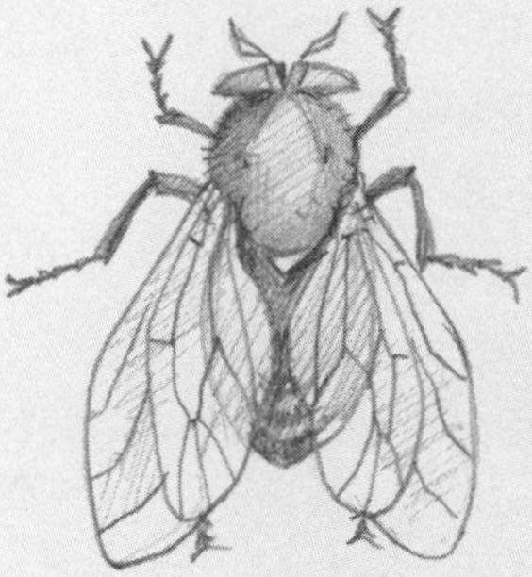

Horse fly

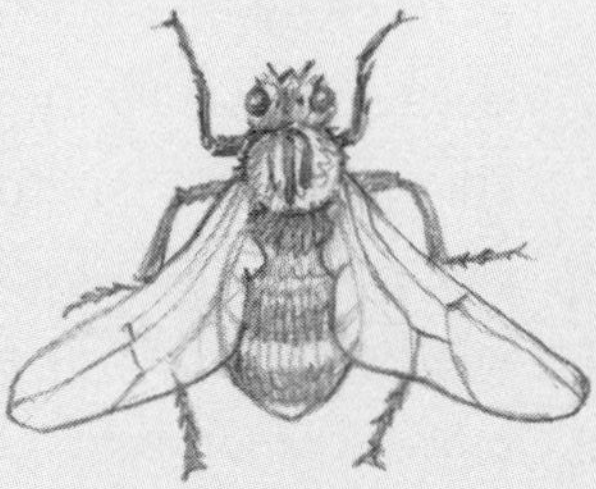

Horn fly

God in His wisdom made the fly
And then forgot to
tell us why.
— Ogden Nash

Prevention is the most important tactic in your war against flies.

2. **PREVENT LARVAE FROM HATCHING.** On large farms in warm, moist climates, it may be necessary to kill larvae. You can do this two ways. One is by using a feed-through oral larvicide daily during fly season. Feeding a fly-control product can prevent the development of flies in the manure, but the chemical that kills the larvae could also kill beneficial microorganisms such as the ones necessary for decomposing manure. In addition, some toxicity has been reported. As with all medical decisions, confer with your veterinarian before feeding a supplement that contains a chemical.

The other way to prevent flies from hatching is by using fly predators. Fly predators are naturally present wherever there are flies, but not in large enough numbers to control an aggressive stable-fly population. Commercially raised predators are available for purchase. They are most effective if released early in the fly season and every one to two weeks thereafter. The success of the approach depends on the severity of the fly problem, the number of predators released,

Fly Predators

Fly predators are tiny, nocturnal, stingless wasps that lay eggs in the pupa of the face fly, biting stable fly, horn fly, and house fly. The wasp eggs utilize the contents of the pupa as food, thereby killing the pupa before it can develop into a fly. The newly hatched wasps stay within 200 feet of their emergence site. Because fly predators are harmless to animals and people, they are a safe, nontoxic means of biological control.

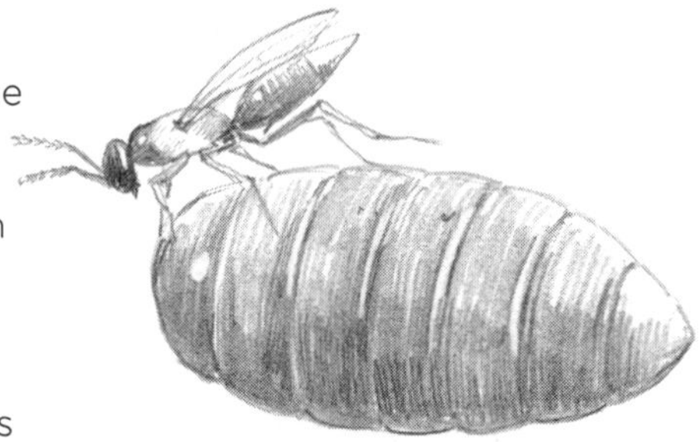

A fly predator on a fly pupa

and the management program. You must carefully monitor all methods of fly control involving insecticides or they will wipe out the predator population along with the flies.

3. **CAPTURE ADULT FLIES IMMEDIATELY AFTER HATCHING.** When flies do hatch, it is essential to capture the adults before they can breed. We set out jar and bag traps in July or August if necessary. Jar traps that utilize attractants can capture thousands of flies. Some systems utilize muscalure, a pheromone (sex attractant) to draw the flies. Others require the addition of fish or meat. These traps, commonly used with a 1 or 2½ gallon jar, can be smelly and must be emptied, then restocked. Disposable traps are available for a fifth the price of the jar traps. They are designed to be used with the supplied pheromone and water and claim to hold 10,000 flies.

Fly paper is generally an inexpensive, disposable way of mechanically catching flies. In our barn, we always have a sticky fly-tape system set up near the barn roof where flies like to rest. Fly paper is available in strips of several widths. Some types are designed to hang from the ceiling, while others are to be tacked across doorways or aisles or strung as narrow tape near the barn ceiling. Some contain pheromones, while others are merely sticky. A few brands contain insecticides, so it is important to read the label if you plan to use them around food or animals.

4. **KILL REMAINING FLIES.** For those flies that evade the traps, you can employ methods of killing the flies. Be sure, however, that your management practices are the very best they can be, and employ all strategies previously mentioned before investing in these methods.

A mechanical way of killing flies is to use an electric fly zapper. The flies are attracted to the light and are immediately killed upon contact.

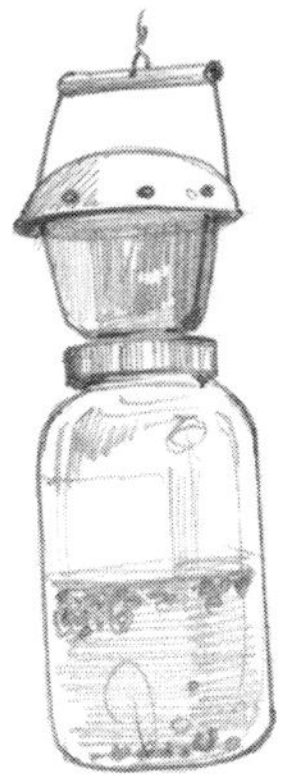

Reusable jar fly trap

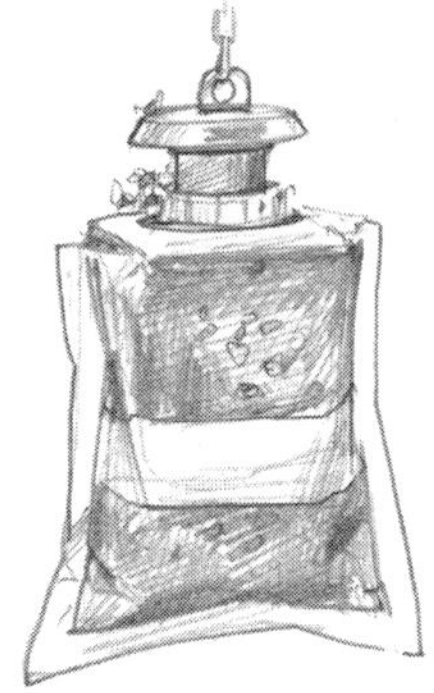

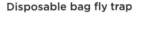

Disposable bag fly trap

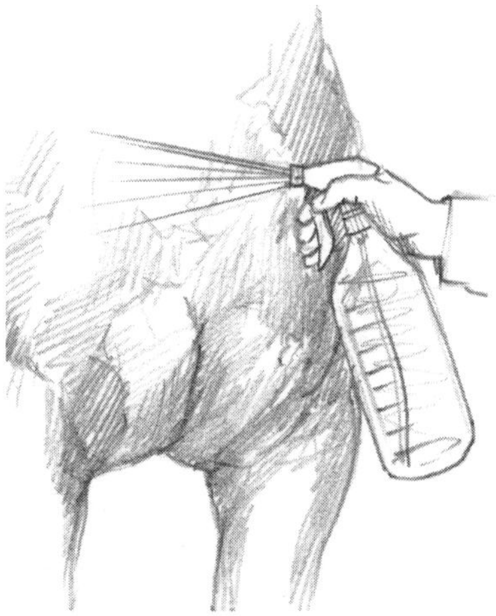

Insecticides and repellents should be used responsibly.

SUMMER: JULY

TIPS & TECHNIQUES

Use Insecticides with Caution

The use of insecticides (chemicals that kill insects) is often the first thing we think of, but really should be a last resort. While insecticides are an important part of many fly control programs, they are much less needed if manure and moisture are managed properly. Overuse of insecticide could result in resistant strains of flies and harm to horses, humans, and the environment.

What type and brand of insecticide will work best for you will depend on your weather, fly problem, style of management, and each horse's sensitivity. Finding the best one involves testing for effectiveness and allergic reactions (both human and horse).

Equine insecticides generally fall into four categories: pyrethrins ("natural" insecticides), permethrins (synthetic pyrethrins), carbamates, and organophosphates, listed in order from least toxic to most toxic and from least to most long-lasting. Insecticides are available in many forms for various applications.

Topical sprays can be purchased in ready-to-apply forms or concentrates that are usually diluted in a 1:7 ratio of insecticide to water for house flies or a stronger mix for other flies. Certain general livestock sprays are not safe for horses.

Anti-Fly Accessories

Fly strips and tags, impregnated with repellent, can be attached to breakaway halters. Also available is a collar/browband affair with a breakaway feature. These fly strips are particularly useful for controlling face flies and can last several months. Face flies have sponging mouth parts and feed on mucus around the eyes and nostrils, often causing inflammation and infection.

Some degree of relief can also be afforded a horse by using fly shakers (with or without repellent) attached to the crownpiece of a halter or browband of a bridle. These strips mechanically jiggle the flies off a horse's face when he shakes his head.

Fly masks are available in several styles. Some protect the eyes while others protect the eyes, ears, and jowls. Most are made of a mesh that allows the horse to see.

Cool, open-weave, mesh fly sheets keep flies from pestering the horse's body. Consider using a repellent on the legs, belly, and face in conjunction with a fly sheet.

Premises sprays are for use in and around buildings. Some are not safe to use on livestock, manure, or bedding. Long-term (up to six-week) residual insecticides are designed to be applied on fly resting sites such as on rafters or in bushes. Stable sprays are usually sold as concentrates, which are diluted and applied with sprayers that range in cost from $20 to $100. Foggers are disposable cans of insecticide designed for the interior of buildings. To use a fogger, close all doors, set the can to spray automatically until empty, keep the doors closed for 15 minutes, and then ventilate the building.

Automatic misters are available in several types. The disposable type uses an aerosol can set in a battery-operated automatic spray unit that delivers a spray every 15 minutes and lasts for about a month. One unit is required for every 6,000 square feet. Electric fogger/misters are available for about five times the price. Instead of using aerosol cans of insecticide, the electric misters have a reservoir that can be filled with a chosen solution. Barn-wide automatic mister systems are incorporated in some large barns. Since flies tend to congregate in certain places during certain times of the day, an effective use of misters is to aim them at the resting places and be sure they are functioning during fly siesta time.

Strips impregnated with insecticide are designed to keep approximately 1,000 square feet free of flies for about four months, so could be useful for enclosed areas such as tack rooms, feed rooms, and offices. However, since there is a variety on the market, it is essential to read the package carefully as some are not safe to be used in enclosed areas frequented by humans or in areas where food is present.

5. **PROTECT YOUR HORSE.** While an insecticide is a chemical that kills flies, a repellent is a substance that discourages flies from landing. You can buy

Fly Bait

The idea behind fly bait is to attract and entice flies to eat a specially prepared "food" that is laced with insecticides. To that end, some baits contain sex attractants plus a sugar-based feeding enticer. Fly bait can be used in hanging bait stations or as scatter bait on lawns and around buildings. It is important to note the potential danger of other animals (such as birds, puppies, or even children) eating the bait.

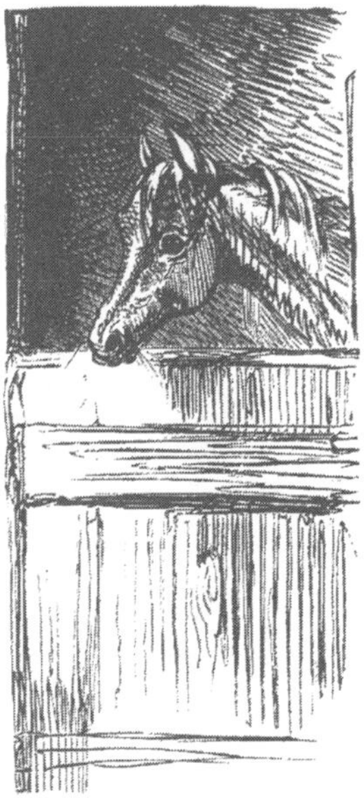

SUMMER: JULY

Sock Tip for Face Flies

To keep my horses comfortable I've found that socks make good applicators for fly products.

I wear the sock inside out, and over my hand like a mitten. I apply the product to the sock and rub it thoroughly under the horse's chin and jaw, around and on the ears, and on the poll. I make a light pass down the front of the horse's face, avoiding the muzzle. I store the socks in a plastic bag marked "Fly," and when one gets too dirty to use, I just pitch it.

I always wash my hands thoroughly after using any fly product. If your skin is sensitive or if you want added protection, wear a disposable Latex glove under the sock.

fly repellents as spray, lotion, wipe-on, gel, dusting powder, ointment, roll-on, shampoos, and towelettes. Repellents contain a substance irritating to flies, such as oil of citronella, and most contain some amount of insecticide (mostly pyrethrins and permethrins) as well.

Repellents can be water-, oil-, or alcohol-based. Oil-based repellents remain on the hair shaft longer, but the oil attracts dirt. Water-based repellents don't last as long, but attract less dirt. To increase the lasting effect, some water-based repellents are made with silicone, which coats the hair shaft and holds the repellent in place longer. Alcohol-based repellents dry quickly, so are good for a fast touch-up, but the alcohol can have a drying effect on the hair and skin.

In addition, repellents can contain sunscreen, coat conditioners (such as lanolin or aloe vera), and other products that increase lasting power. Claims of duration of protection range from one to 14 days. How long a repellent will last depends on the weather, the management, the exercise level of the horse (how much he sweats), grooming, blanketing, and whether the horse rolls.

OTHER PESTS

Some pests are not so obvious, but often summer is the time of year you will see their damage. There is a wide variety of miscellaneous pests, ranging from fungus to beetles to parasitic plants. These types of pests are often very localized, so consult your county extension office for more information.

In Colorado, the dwarf mistletoe grows in pine trees and ultimately causes the death of the affected tree. Since the plants disperse their seeds in August and September, now is the time to be informed and take action.

ROTATIONAL GRAZING

The practice of rotational grazing allows you to work with the natural cycle of pasture growth. Horses left on a pasture too long will paw to reach tender roots, thereby destroying a plant's ability to rejuvenate. Overgrazing causes pasture damage that costs much more in the long run to repair than the feed costs it saved. Horses should therefore be put on pasture or hay fields when the growth is optimal — about 4 to 8 inches high, depending on the grass species — and then the plant growth in the field should be closely monitored. Remove the horses when 50 percent of the forage has been ingested or damaged. If the horses' grazing rate is greater than the field's ability to regrow, they should be

Remove horses from a field when 50 percent of the forage has been ingested or damaged.

Mixing Livestock on Pasture

Horses can be mixed or rotated with other livestock to maximize the use of the pasture. If you run cattle and horses together, you do run the risk of aggressive horses chasing calves, or horned cattle going after meek horses, but more often there is no problem at all. If you rotate cattle with horses in a pasture, the bovines may clean up some of the mature grasses left behind by the equines.

Since horses and cattle have different parasites, the life cycles of horse parasites will be broken during the time the cattle are in the pasture. Sheep, on the other hand, which tend to eat the center of a plant and leave the tall, tough outer leaves, don't really contribute to the health of a horse pasture.

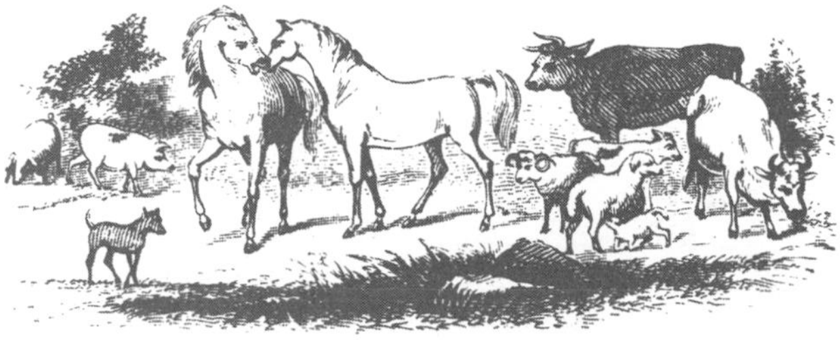

Movie of the Month

***MONTE WALSH* (2003)**
Riding both a great buckskin and red roan in this movie, Tom Selleck portrays the quickly disappearing cowboy lifestyle when he says, "I ain't doin' nothin' I can't do from the back of a horse." Tom Selleck has personal interest in the authenticity of dress and tack and it shows in this movie and his other Westerns: *Crossfire Trail, Quigly Down Under*, and *Last Stand at Sabre River*.

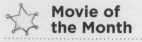

put on another pasture so the grazed field can rest until it returns to the 4- to 8-inch height.

Rapid pasture growth occurs early in the season, and then starts slowing until about 12 weeks into the season, when most plants have matured and gone to seed. In the meantime, weeds should be mowed before they go to seed to encourage desirable plants to take over. Bare spots should be reseeded and protected from traffic and grazing by removing horses or installing temporary electric fencing.

After the first cut of hay is taken off a grass field, if the season isn't such that a second cut can be expected, grazing the field for several months in the late summer and early fall is often cost effective and won't harm the field if it is not overstocked.

ROTATIONAL VS. CONTINUOUS GRAZING. Rotational grazing means that land must be divided up into more pieces, requiring more fences, waterers, and labor. It does, however, result in a higher stocking rate per acre of land. For example, 1 acre per horse could be sufficient if horses were rotated between three pastures or between two pastures and a set of holding pens.

Continuous grazing is typically practiced on farms or ranches with very large pastures. This minimizes the amount of fencing and waterers, but it can result in seasonal forage shortages and areas that are permanently contaminated with feces and permanently overgrazed. Moving the location of salt and water in such pastures will minimize spots of overgrazing. Continuous grazing yields a low stocking rate — one horse requires two to three times as many acres, or more, as it would for rotational grazing.

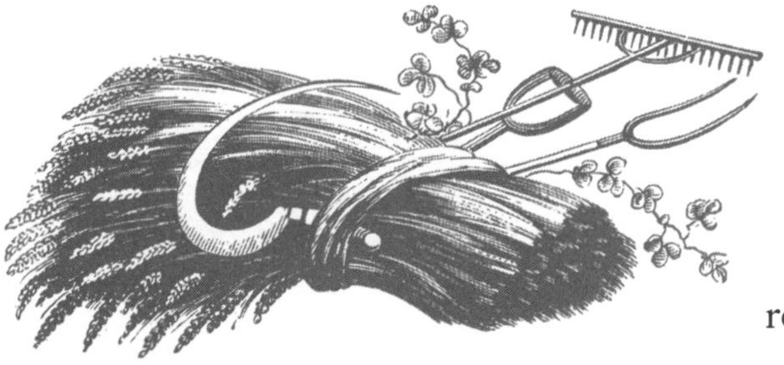

SPECIES AND VARIETIES OF GRASSES AND PASTURE PLANTS

Because our pastures are native, semiarid mountain pastures with no irrigation, native plant species are quite different than those in the irrigated pastures and hay fields east of us. Besides undesirable weeds mentioned elsewhere in this book, our pastures contain sage, sunflowers, wild geraniums and roses, yucca, prickly pear cactus, and numerous wildflowers, plus several varieties of wheatgrass, needlegrass, bluegrass, fescue, and grama grasses. Smooth brome also appears in places that have more moisture, such as sub-irrigated low-lying patches.

We've improved our pastures by seeding with several local mixes containing grasses that are drought resistant, trample resistant, high yield, late season, and early season. That seems to cover all of the bases. When one grass does poorly, another might thrive.

Grasses such as brome, bluegrass, timothy, rye, tall fescue, wheatgrass, and orchardgrass are hardy perennials

en español

chaps. Comes from *las chaparreras*, 'heavy leather trousers without a seat, worn over pants when riding'. Pronounced SHAPS.

Rocky Mountain Seed Mixes

Here are some examples of seed mixtures suited to the Colorado foothills. Your extension agent can help you find a seed dealer in your area that has a mix specially suited for your land.

Mountain Mix

- ★ 20 percent brome
- ★ 20 percent orchardgrass
- ★ 20 percent ryegrass
- ★ 20 percent winter rye
- ★ 10 percent bluegrass
- ★ 5 percent clover
- ★ 5 percent timothy

Dryland Pasture Mix

- ★ 28 percent tall wheatgrass
- ★ 19 percent smooth brome
- ★ 19 percent crested wheatgrass
- ★ 19 percent intermediate wheatgrass
- ★ 10 percent perennial ryegrass
- ★ 5 percent other

that usually decrease in digestible nutrients as they mature. Specifically:

- Tall fescue is widely adapted, has good tolerance to wet, dry, or alkaline soil conditions, and can withstand a lot of traffic.
- Orchardgrass produces excellent-quality forage but will not tolerate drought, wet, or alkaline soil.
- If irrigation water is not available for the entire season, smooth brome and wheatgrass can be used.
- Bermuda grass (in the south) and tall fescue (in the north and south) resist trampling, so are good varieties for "exercise" pastures; however, be aware of potential problems with fescue (see May Horsekeeping Across America).

Legumes such as alfalfa, clover, and bird's-foot trefoil are more nutritious and don't require nitrogen fertilizer, but they are less hardy and impractical when used alone for pasture. With pasture mixes, plants mature at different times and exhibit a range of abilities to withstand stresses such as drought, flood, heat, and cold. If a blend of grasses and alfalfa (or other legume) is preferred, the legumes should not exceed 25 percent of the mix.

Brome

Timothy

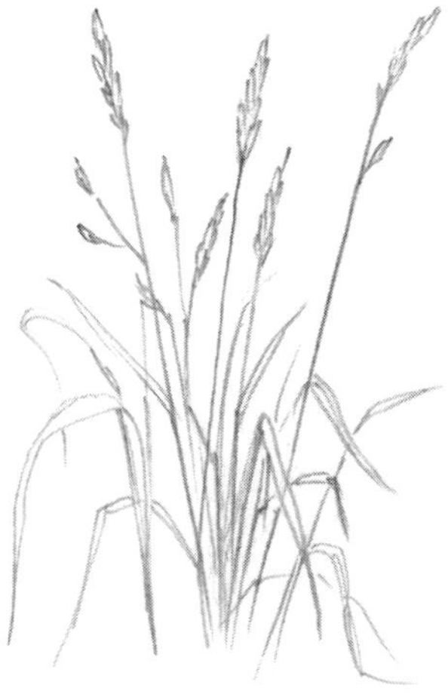

Orchardgrass

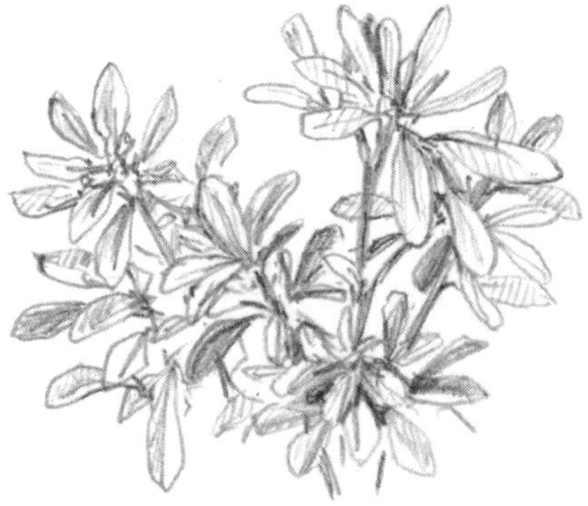

Alfalfa

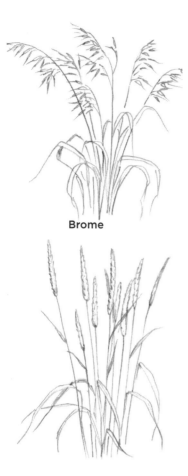

CLEAN-UP CREW

FUGITIVE DUST

Neighbor A has a heart of gold and lets 15 4-H kids and their horses come every Saturday to practice gymkhana for four hours in his outdoor arena. Neighbor B, downwind, gets all of the dust and although he hates to complain, who can blame him?

Fugitive dust is the term given to airborne particulate matter that rises from the ground. It is often a large part of the brown cloud that is seen in the air, which is caused not by smokestacks, vents, or chimneys, but by bare patches of earth including agricultural fields, school yards, vacant lots, overgrazed pastures, bare driveways, horse pens, round pens and arenas, and other bare-dirt areas. Areas with dry seasons tend to have more problems with fugitive dust than most, because the earth gets so dry that it just blows away. Fugitive dust is not only a nuisance, but it also is a great health concern to both humans and animals. Most states have regulations related to the emissions of fugitive dust.

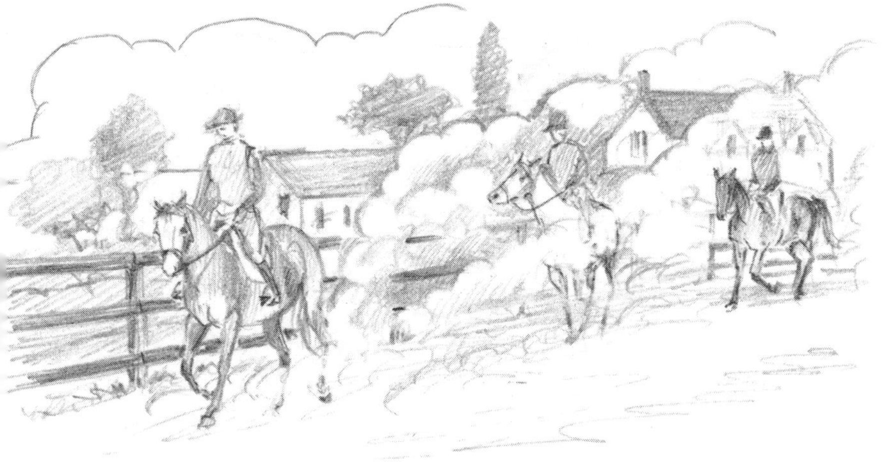

Use dust control measures in your arena.

TIPS & TECHNIQUES

Keeping Dust Down

★ Minimize the surface area disturbed. The less ground you disturb, the less dust you will raise as you work your horses or as they move around.

★ Try not to work on windy days.

★ Use dust-suppression measures when needed. Apply water and/or chemicals to control dust.

★ Pave or gravel driveways and paths.

★ Prevent overgrazing of paddocks and pastures. Plants hold the soil together.

★ When new construction is taking place on your farm or ranch, try to keep excavated areas as undisturbed as possible.

FYI

Overstocked

The more crowded and overgrazed a pasture, the worse the parasite recontamination problem. One horse on 5 acres won't have as large a parasite load as five horses on 1 acre.

PARASITES ON PASTURE

Horses shed parasite eggs in their feces, the larvae hatch on the pasture, and grazing horses ingest them. Parasite larvae are very tough and it takes extreme dryness, heat, or cold to kill them.

To reduce recontamination, manure can be removed, left where it falls, or harrowed, depending on pasture size.

SMALL PASTURES. Since a horse produces 50 pounds of manure per day, on small pastures and paddocks it is best if manure is picked up daily. It can be hauled away or it can be composted for one year and then spread on horse pastures.

LARGE PASTURES. Horses with plenty of room tend to allocate distinct areas for grazing, defecating, and lounging, thereby instinctively avoiding the parasites in their manure. In such pastures, it may be best to leave the manure piles where they are rather than harrow and spread the larvae throughout the pasture.

MIDSIZED PASTURES. In temperate climates, once you remove the horses in the fall or early winter, you can harrow the manure in the pastures to expose parasite eggs to freezing weather and to spread the manure more evenly so it decomposes over the winter. Otherwise, larvae that survive the winter immediately begin reinfecting horses in the spring, especially young stock.

In southern pastures, the timetable is flipped — the summer is the best time to keep horses off pasture and to harrow the pastures to expose the larvae to the hot, dry weather. When the horses are returned to the rested and harrowed pastures in November, the recontamination rate should be decreased.

JULY Manure Pile Maintenance
PILE A Quit adding, turn once
PILE B Start pile.
PILE C Sell, store, or spread.

TACK ROOM

SAFE CLOTHING

Proper clothing is an important part of safe handling and riding. Safe clothing includes boots or shoes, with hard toes and heels, and gloves.

FOOTWEAR. Always wear hard-toed boots or shoes when you are working around your horse. If you wear soft shoes or sandals and your horse accidentally steps on your foot, your toes could be seriously hurt. Also, your boots or shoes must have soles and heels that give you good grip on the ground. If you wear slippery shoes around your horse, you can lose your footing and slide underneath him, which puts you in a dangerous position, especially if he spooks because of your odd behavior. When riding, always wear a boot with a heel to prevent your foot from slipping through the stirrup.

GLOVES. Because you will need to hold onto a lead rope when handling your horse, you should get used to wearing gloves when you are working with your horse. If your horse suddenly darts to the side and the lead rope "zings" through your hand, it could leave a nasty rope burn behind. The heat from the friction of the rope moving so fast against your skin is as painful as a burn from a hot stove. Gloves will protect you in such a case.

Beauty Shop

MANE CARE

The best way to prevent tangled burrs in your horses' long manes is to keep your pastures clean of burdock and any other plants with sticky or spiny seeds or pods. Apply a slippery mane conditioner to the mane to make it less likely for a burr to stick and easier to take it out if it does. Finger through long manes and tails regularly.

MIDSUMMER TAIL

About this time of year, the horses' tails have grown so long that they could step on them when backing up or getting up after rolling, so I cut off 1–4 inches, depending on the horse. Some horses' tails seem barely to grow, while others grow ½–1 inch per month.

CLOTHES HORSE

TURNOUT SHEETS

A turnout sheet must be safe, nonslip, and tough. Whether a turnout sheet needs to be waterproof, water resistant, or just dirt resistant depends on its intended use. You might want to use turnout sheets for horses that are in work, kept in stalls, and given daily time out in a paddock and on horses that live full-time in pastures with partial shelter.

The primary purpose of a turnout sheet is to keep horses clean for sanitation reasons, as well as to minimize our grooming time and protect tack. A full-feature turnout sheet is also waterproof, but that is not always necessary or desirable. A waterproof sheet is usually warmer, sometimes less breathable, and more expensive, and requires more specialized care than a nonwaterproof sheet.

There is something about the outside of a horse that is good for the inside of a man.
— Sir Winston Churchill

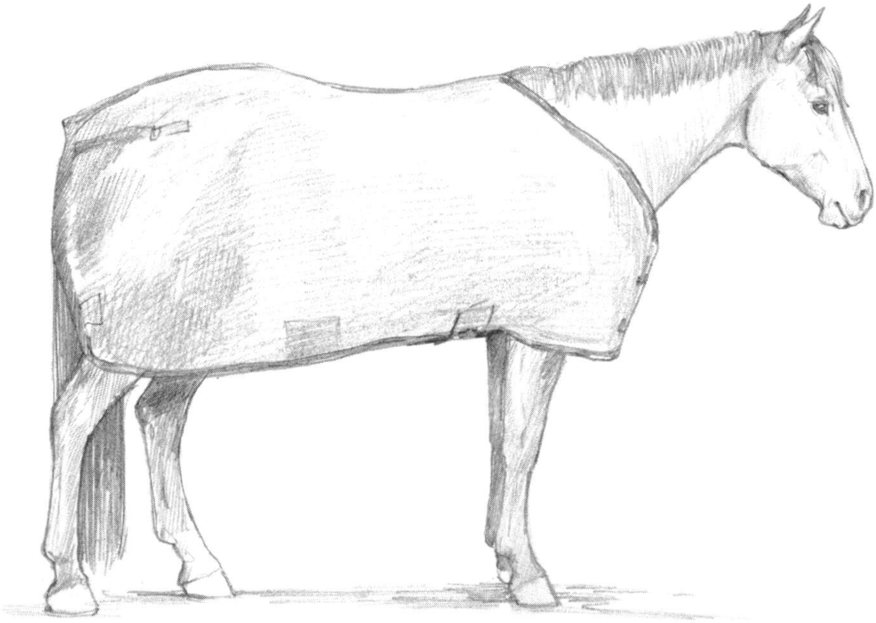

The purpose of a turnout sheet is to keep a horse clean.

SUMMER: JULY

Blanket Size

Here's how to measure your horse to figure out what size blanket he should wear. I use a 120-inch quilter's tape measure, which you can find at a sewing store.

★ Place one end of the tape at the midpoint of the horse's chest.

★ Run the tape over the point of the shoulder and horizontally along the horse's side. Continue horizontally to the hindquarters.

★ Take two measurements — one to the edge of the horse's tail and one to the midpoint of the tail.

Some blanket manufacturers suggest one measuring method and some the other. For example, some of my horses wear between a 78 and 80 blanket. Having both measurements on hand will help when you are blanket shopping.

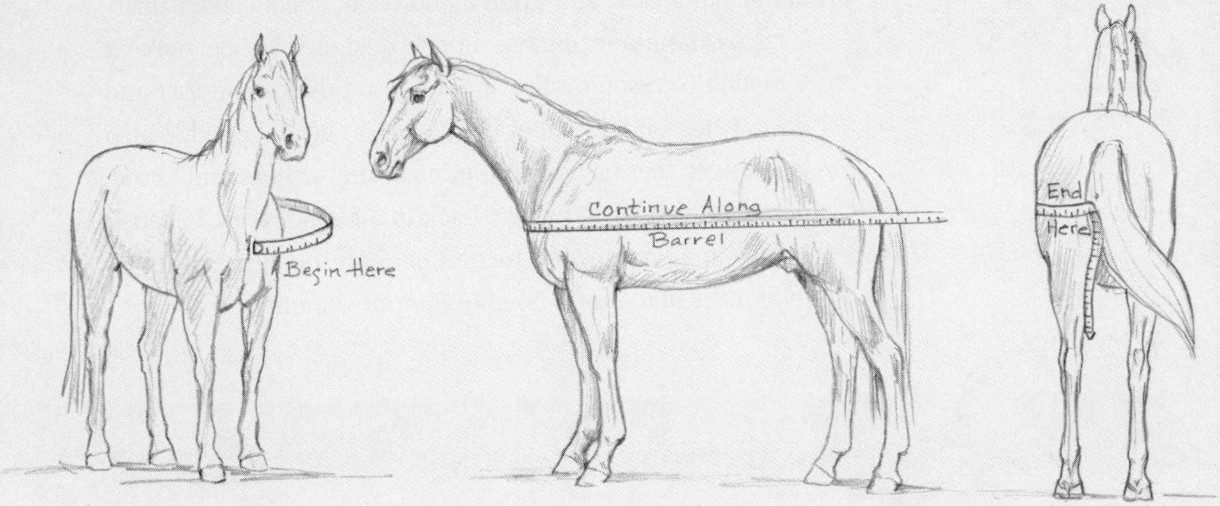

Any turnout sheet must be tough and well designed, because when horses are turned out, they are often very active, galloping, bucking, and rolling vigorously. I like to have a few waterproof turnout sheets at hand so I don't have to constantly change sheets during the fickle weather of spring and fall. However, I also use cotton turnout sheets for the warm, dry days of July so the horses are protected from dirt, sun, and insects.

SUMMER: JULY

TIPS & TECHNIQUES

Stall Sheets

Lightweight sheets made of cotton or polyester blends can be used to keep a stalled horse clean. They don't provide much warmth, because they are not insulated.

WHAT TO LOOK FOR. I prefer a turnout sheet that has wide, adjustable leg straps, elastic inserts, and an easy buckle front with overlapping front panels for good chest protection. It should be cut deep (long on the sides) to protect the horse's belly. In a waterproof turnout, a tail flap can add stability as well as extra protection. However, I've found that if a sheet is not well designed and fit, a tail flap can prevent the horse from lifting his tail high enough to defecate without causing a mess.

Ideally, any turnout (and any piece of horse clothing for that matter) should be cut and fitted to a horse's contours. Some of this is breed-specific, but certain curves are present on all horses, and I find a poorly cut sheet causes problems for the horse and me. Poorly designed sheets make it tempting to cinch on the sheet too tightly for comfort and then, when such a sheet does slip, it stays slipped. I also like sheets that have nylon lining at the withers and shoulders, preferably all the way back to the girth area, because horses are active when turned out and the slippery nylon minimizes hair loss from shoulder movement.

FARM OFFICE

EQUINE ACTIVITY LIABILITY LAWS

Take the time to do things safely. Remember, often the slower you go, the faster you get there!

Whether you are an equine professional or just give a few lessons at your home, you should be concerned about liability. Most states have adopted equine activity liability laws, which release professionals from liability for equine-related accidents. You can purchase signs specific to your state's law to post on your premises (see Web site in the appendix).

Before deciding whether you need additional liability insurance, make sure you understand the verbiage of your state's laws thoroughly. Find out if the law, as related to equine professionals, has been tested in court. Also find out if you need also to have all persons sign a liability waiver and exactly what the wording needs to be to release you from liability. Even with the state laws, if you give lessons at your home or run a full-service training facility, in order to be fully covered you should consider a commercial liability policy.

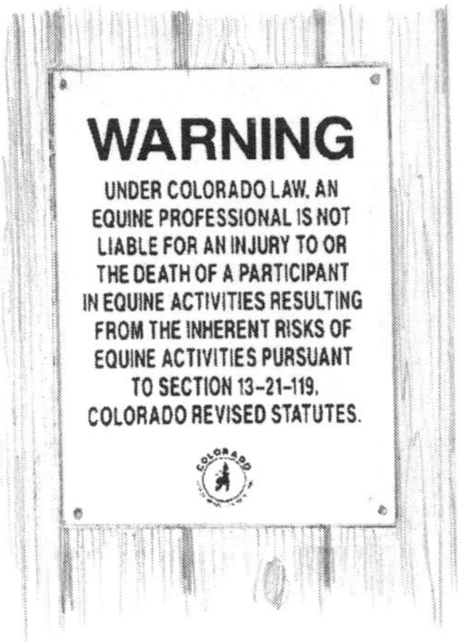

You can purchase a liability sign specific to your state's laws.

LIABILITY AND LOOSE HORSES. Each case of loose horses that cause damage, injury, or death will be evaluated in light of the laws of the state where the incident occurred. Most state laws say the owner or responsible party, such as a boarding stable owner, is negligent in letting a horse get loose. The negligence is usually due to poor fencing, gates, latches, or management.

Fencing In or Out

While most states require livestock owners to fence their animals in, some require landowners to fence animals out. Certain states, such as Colorado, have an open-range policy. This basically means that we have to fence other peoples' animals out of our property. Technically, it is legal for livestock to roam on the roadways. It is the driver's responsibility to watch out for loose cattle, horses, deer, elk, moose — you get the picture.

SAFETY

We zoom through the summer in high gear, packing in as much horse time as we can. Sometimes we are in a hurry, which can be the cause of a simple but avoidable accident. For example, when you lead a horse through a gate that opens toward you, if you don't swing it open all the way, your horse could get his ribs or hip caught on it and then pull the gate closed as he passes through. As the horse feels the gate trapping him, he could panic and try to bolt through, possibly injuring you and making his injury worse.

Horse Sense and Safety

Halters Off in Turnout

Do not leave a halter on a loose horse, as he may hook it on a post or a tree when rubbing or on his own hind shoe when scratching his head with his hoof.

Safe Handling

To be safe whenever you are handling your horse, start with a safe attitude, dress properly, use safe equipment, work in safe facilities, and use sensible horse-handling methods. Knowing the best way to handle a horse is your best insurance against injury. Learn some simple safety rules and methods, and put them to use whenever you are working with horses. The best way to gain your horse's trust is to be sensible and safe.

NOT ALWAYS TRUE

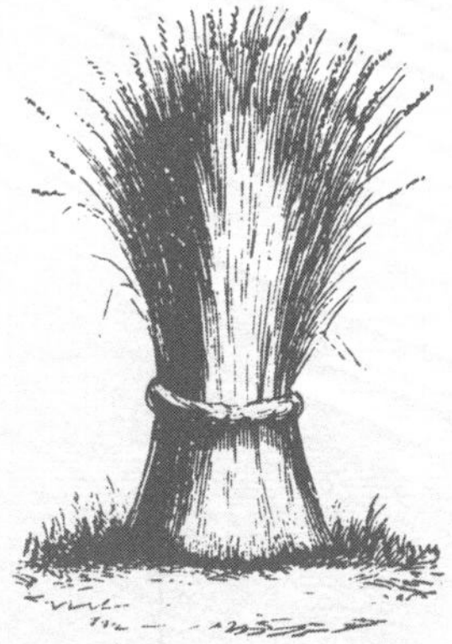

Historical Horsekeeping

"Hay tea is . . . a good stimulant. To make it — fill a bucket three-quarters full of bright, clean hay, pour over it enough boiling water to fill the pail, and cover tight, to keep in the steam. Press the hay down occasionally, let it stand fifteen minutes, turn off, and add enough water to make a bucket three-quarters full. Give to the horse when the liquid is cool enough to drink."

— Gleason's Horse Book *by Prof. Oscar R. Gleason, 1892*

Safety Dos and Don'ts

★ **Don't** be careless or take shortcuts when performing everyday chores. *Example*: You are bathing your horse and don't want to take the time to wet his head with a sponge, so you spray his head with a hose and get water in his eyes and ears. He rears up and lands on you with his front feet.

★ **Do** take the time to accustom your horse to routine procedures.

★ **Don't** lose your temper. *Example*: You are headed for an important show but your horse refuses to load in the trailer. You try to force him in using a whip and the help of two burly friends. The horse rears and falls over backwards on one of your friends.

★ **Do** make friends with experienced horsemen and -women who will be a good influence on you, help you figure out why you and your horse aren't communicating, and keep you from getting frustrated, angry, or hurt.

★ **Don't** show off or be dangerously silly. *Example*: You are showing your friend how quiet and sweet old Buck is by wrapping his lead rope around your waist. All of a sudden, some bot flies go into Buck's nose. He snorts, rears, and takes off, dragging you behind, tangled in the rope.

★ **Do** "show off" your excellent horse-handling skills and horsekeeping habits.

★ **Don't** use unsafe equipment. *Example*: You tie a horse up with a weak, old halter, and while you are cleaning his hoof, he leans backward, breaks the halter, and lands on top of you.

★ **Do** make sure all your tack is fit for the job — sturdy and safe.

★ **Don't** work in unsafe facilities. *Example*: You are riding in a pen with a barbed-wire fence. A small, yapping dog runs into the pen and nips at your horse's heels. Your horse panics and runs into the wire fence. You and your horse are severely cut.

★ **Do** think ahead and observe potential hazards. Try to fix or eliminate hazards or if not possible, postpone your ride.

★ **Don't** forget to "think like a horse." *Example*: When you try to catch your horse, you reach for his nose. He instinctively turns away, swings his hindquarters toward you, and steps on your foot.

★ **Do** learn where a horse's blind spots are and where horses like to be touched.

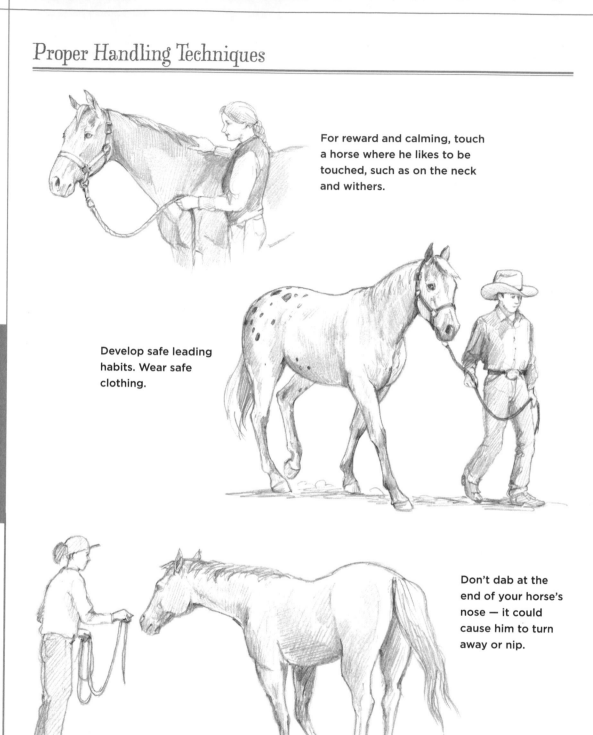

Proper Handling Techniques

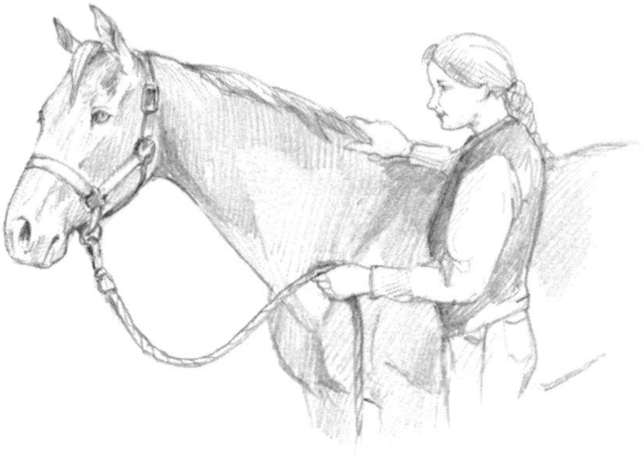

For reward and calming, touch a horse where he likes to be touched, such as on the neck and withers.

Develop safe leading habits. Wear safe clothing.

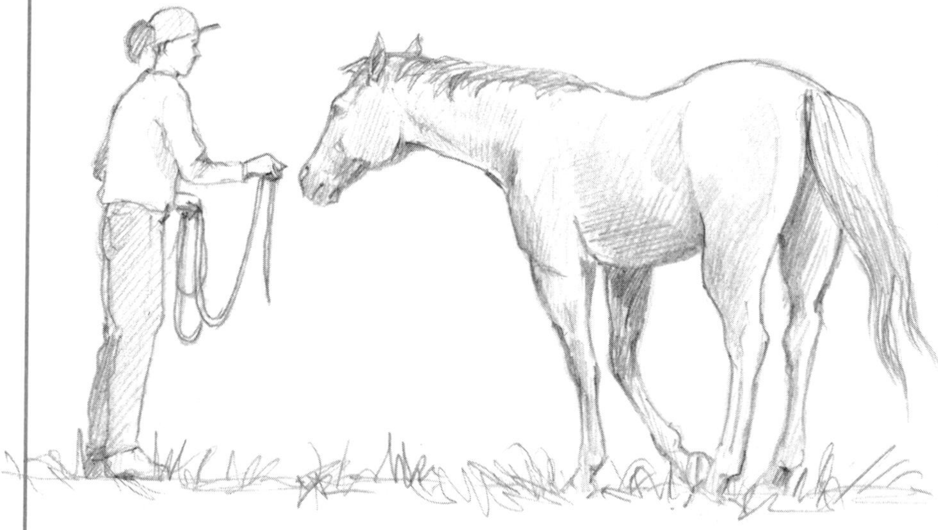

Don't dab at the end of your horse's nose — it could cause him to turn away or nip.

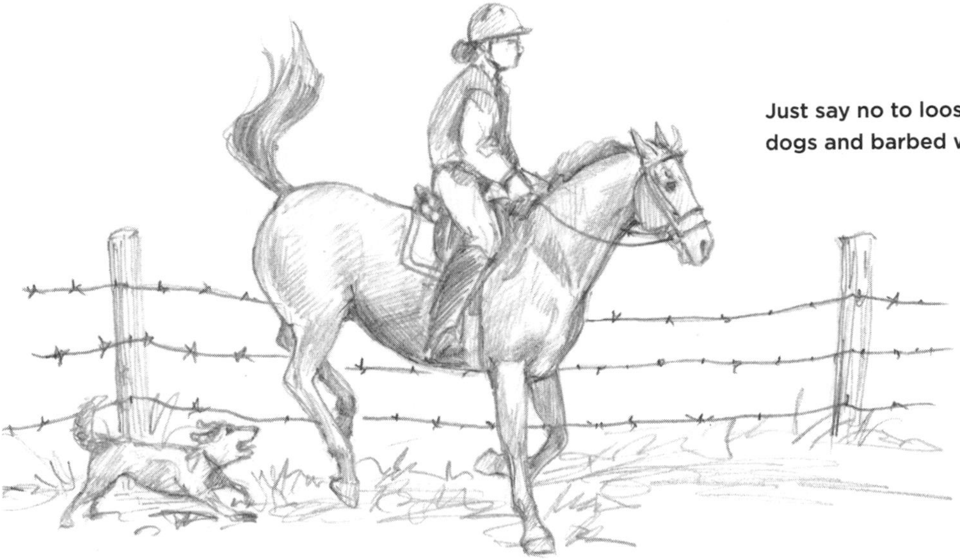

Just say no to loose dogs and barbed wire.

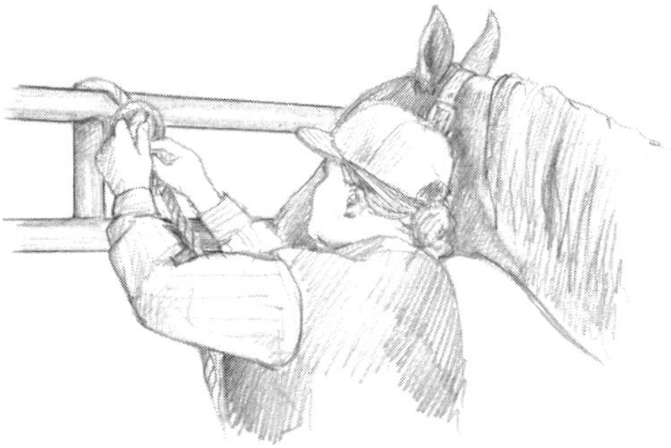

Learn how to tie your horse safely and properly.

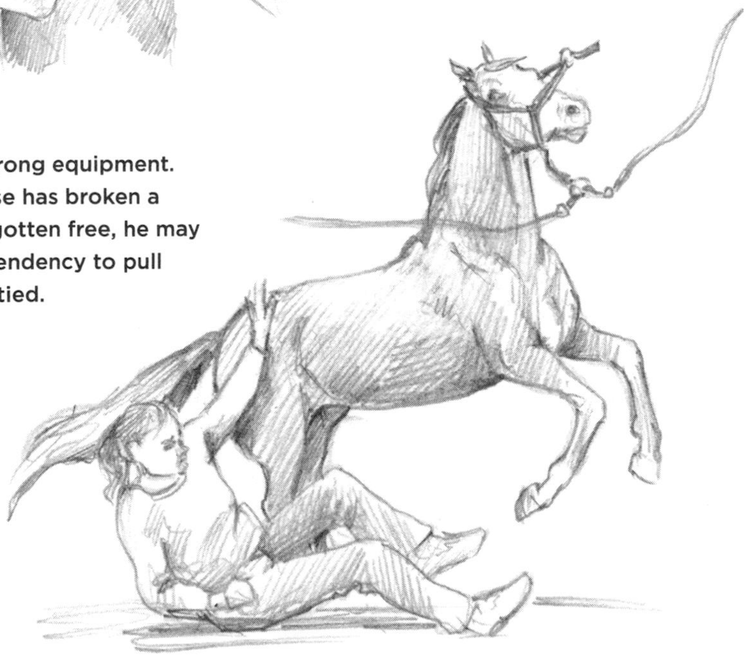

Use safe, strong equipment. Once a horse has broken a halter and gotten free, he may develop a tendency to pull back when tied.

Safe Equipment and Facilities

Use tack and equipment of the strongest type, and inspect it regularly for wear. Tack should be well stitched and constructed from durable materials. Choose a well-made rope or nylon wide-web halter for everyday leading and tying. Use a ⅝-inch-thick or ¾-inch-thick cotton lead rope with a sturdy snap on it. Be sure your tack is not so old and worn out from dirt, sweat, rain, hot sun, or long-time use that it is no longer safe.

Your training facilities should also be strong and safe. The place where you tie your horse needs to be stout, ideally the post of a specially designed tie area. If you tie to a rail or board, your horse could pull back, remove or break the board, injure himself and others, and possibly panic, dragging the board along with him. Even if this happens to your horse only once, he will be suspicious every time he is tied.

Blind Spots

When a horse is facing straight ahead and his head is at a normal level, he has four blind spots:

★ The area directly behind his tail

★ The area of his back directly behind his head

★ The area directly in front of his forehead

★ The area directly under his head on the ground and near his front legs.

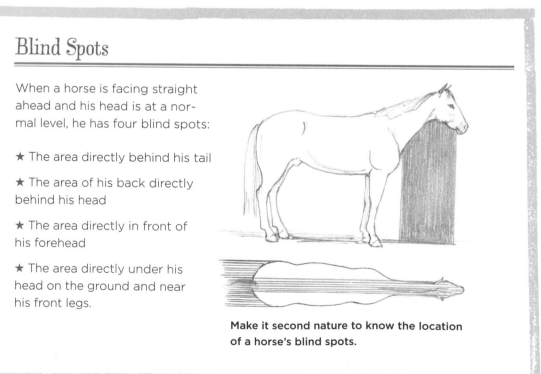

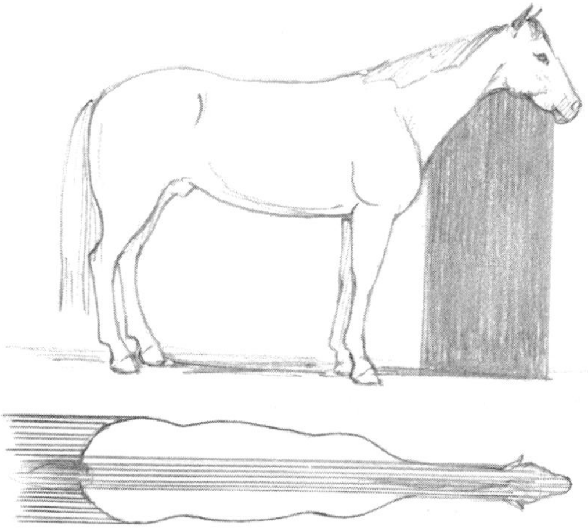

Make it second nature to know the location of a horse's blind spots.

Training pens and arenas for horses should be strong and at least 6 feet tall. When you longe or ride a horse in a training area, you want to be sure he won't try to get away. A frightened or bolting horse might try to go over or through a flimsy or low training arena fence.

REPRODUCTION ROUNDUP

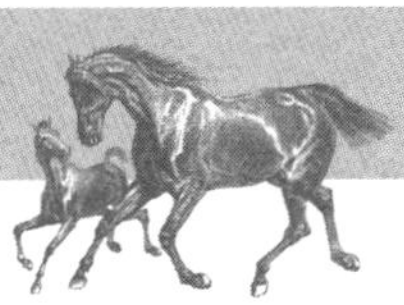

FOAL FEEDING

If you are feeding specifically designed foal feed from a trusted source, there should be a nutrient analysis on the feed tag. Otherwise, a laboratory analysis of hay and grain is the simplest, best, and most direct method to determine exactly what a horse is being fed. Your veterinarian or nutritionist can advise you on sampling procedures and can assist in interpreting results and making supplement corrections.

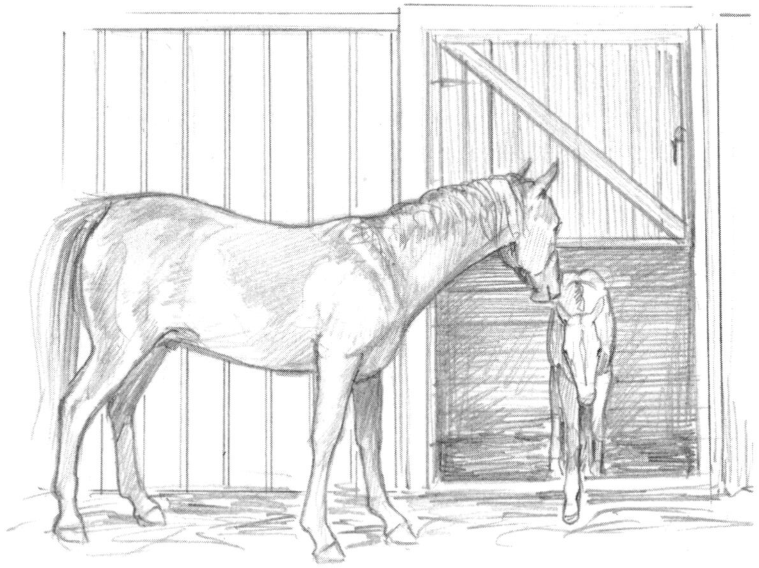

An open lower Dutch door makes an excellent creep feeder.

Feeding Time

It is best to feed most horses at least twice a day and at the same time every day, but for a foal, three or four feedings per day would be better. From birth to two years of age, the horse should have access to free-choice trace mineralized salt, water, and high quality forage. Determine the need for the addition of concentrate and mineral supplement by analyzing hay and then referring to requirement charts.

Be conservative about offering creep feed to nursing foals. By two months of age, the foal will be nibbling out of the dam's feed box. Begin offering small amounts of high quality food in a creep feeder at about three months. Feed measured amounts rather than free-choice creep feed. Be sure the feed is fresh each day. For optimal results, feed each young horse his concentrate ration separately. Group forage feeding is acceptable as long as there is enough feed for the level of competition in the group. Monitor the calcium:phosphorus ratio closely.

FINE FACILITIES

INDOOR HAY STORAGE

Due to increased fire danger and the health hazard from dust continually falling into stalls, the traditional hayloft over the stalls is no longer recommended. It is best to separate housing for horses from storage of feed and bedding. The hay barn should be located at least 75 feet from the horse barn for fire safety, yet close enough for convenience in transporting weekly supplies of hay, grain, and bedding to the feed room in the barn.

Due to increased fire danger and the health hazard from dust continually falling into stalls, the traditional hayloft over the stalls is no longer recommended.

To determine your hay storage needs, figure you will need between 3 and 4 tons per horse per year if you feed hay year-round and do not supplement it with pasture. A

Hay and Bedding

Material	Volume
Baled alfalfa hay	200–150 cubic feet per ton
Baled grass hay	200–300 cubic feet per ton
Straw	300–400 cubic feet per ton
Shavings	300–350 cubic feet per ton

ton (2,000 pounds) of hay usually comprises about thirty 65-pound bales; thirty-six 55-pound bales; or forty-four 45-pound bales. A ton of hay requires approximately 200 cubic feet of storage space, but fluffy, lighter grass bales require more space per ton than tight, heavy alfalfa bricks. This amount of storage space would be a space 10 feet by 10 feet and 2 feet high; or 5 feet by 5 feet and 8 feet high; or 6 feet by 6 feet and 6 feet high.

The hay barn or open shed should be located on a well-drained site. Because of the labor involved and the cost of hay, you simply cannot afford to have moisture get into your hay barn. For added insurance, stack your hay on pallets inside the building. You may have to incorporate ditches, berms, or retaining walls to prevent water from collecting around or moving through your hay barn or shed. In addition, the roof must be leak-free and there must be adequate ventilation in the hay barn. Build the hay barn large enough so you have room to park your tractor inside, too.

How It All Stacks Up

Hay barns can be low-profile for hand stacking, but need to be at least 17 feet, 6 inches tall to allow whole stacks to be delivered and loaded right into the barn. If you are building, ask your deliveryman what clearance he needs. For aesthetic reasons, we chose a low-profile hay barn and hand stacking. Ask me in 20 years if I still think that is a good choice!

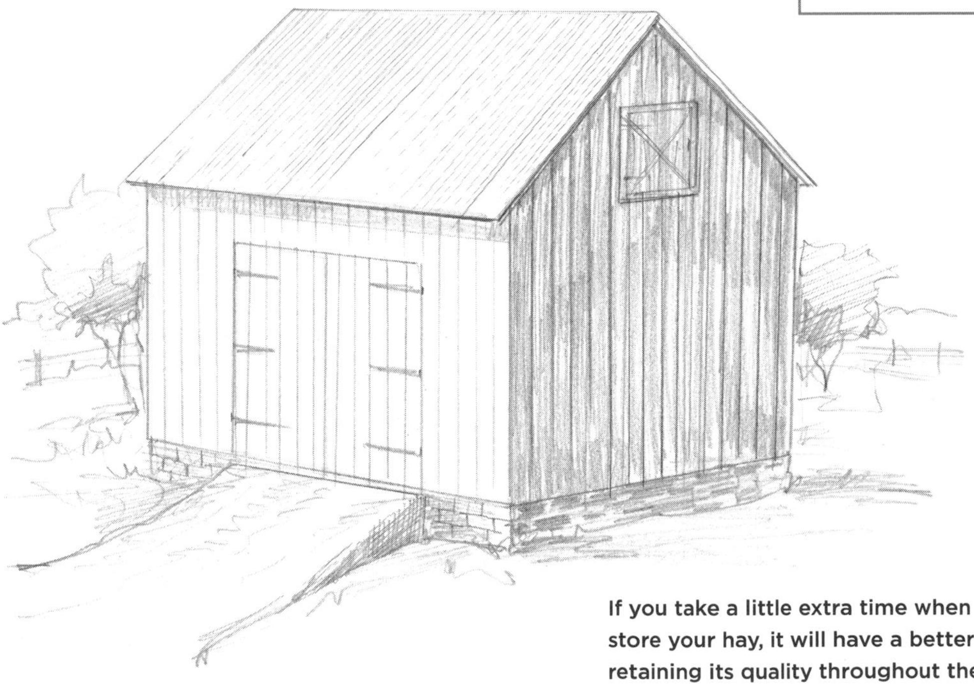

If you take a little extra time when you stack and store your hay, it will have a better chance of retaining its quality throughout the year.

Needs to Cure

Newly baled hay should be allowed to cure outdoors in a stack for a week or two before loading into the barn. If you walk into a hay barn and detect a damp, fruity, moldy, or caramel aroma, the barn probably contains spoiled or heating hay. Grain and bedding should also be well cured and dry to prevent spoilage or heating.

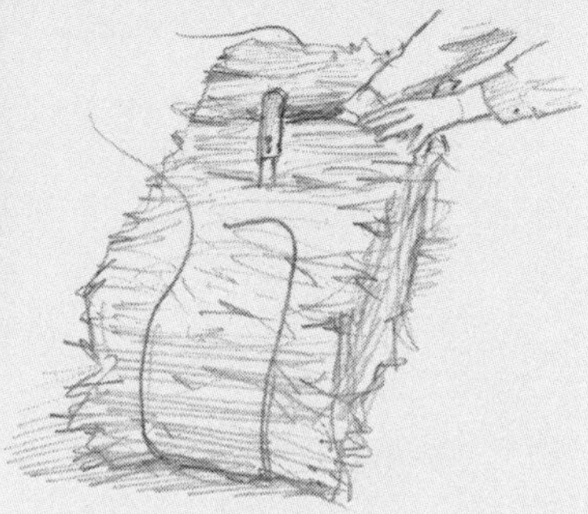

Using your hand or a hay probe, gauge the moisture content of a bale.

OUTDOOR HAY STORAGE

Although the best way to store a supply of hay is in a separate building, your budget might dictate outdoor storage, at least until a hay barn is completed. Select a level, well-drained site in a convenient location to distribute the hay for feeding. The stack can be placed to offer some wind protection for animals, but in cold-winter regions the protected side may end up covered with deep snow from drifting.

Rather than stacking hay on bare ground, place it on pallets, so the bottom layer will remain dry. Used palettes are often available free or very inexpensively from feed mills, lumber yards, or cement plants. Or, 2x4s or 4x4s can be set up side by side with the bales placed to span them.

STACKING. Stack the bales tightly together, alternating the direction of the bales every two or three layers so that the stack is more stable. If you are planning to cover the hay, finish the stack with a ridge of bales on the top rather than with a flat top. The resulting peak will help water and snow run off rather than accumulating on top and possibly leaking through.

In some geographical areas, an uncovered stack fares well with very little nutritional loss from sun or precipitation. In places with snowy, freeze-and-thaw, or rainy winters, however, it is best to cover the stack with a good tarp.

It is better not to cover a stack, however, than to cover it with a tarp that is full of holes. Water entering a covered stack will make a column of mold from the top bales all the way down to the bottom bale.

COVER-UPS. The best cover for a stack is a canvas tarp, because it is waterproof yet allows for some air exchange to minimize condensation. Although new tarps are expensive, they will last a long time. You might be able to find a used truck or machinery tarp for sale at an auction. Avoid black agricultural plastic because it can tear or be punctured by the hay stems, it is difficult to tie down, and it can result in condensation under the plastic, causing hay spoilage. Blue polyethylene tarps may be initially inexpensive, but they have very low resistance to sunshine and often deteriorate in one season. Holes in most coverings can be patched with a daub of silicone and a scrap of plastic or canvas.

TIE-DOWNS. Coverings should be secured with twine, rope, or bungee cords at all edges as well as over the top of the stack. Canvas tarps and some polyethylene tarps have sturdy grommets that are useful for tying down the edges of the cover. You can improvise by placing a pebble or marble slightly in from the tarp's edge to create a lump to which to attach your twine. It is also advisable to run several ropes across the length and width of the stack to prevent billowing by the wind, which can loosen and tear a covering. Cut up an old inner tube and use the rubber scraps under the rope or twine wherever it looks like it may cut into the covering when you tighten the rope.

PALLETS

Whether you are storing hay indoors or outdoors, it is best to put the stack on wooden pallets so that the bottom bales do not absorb moisture from the ground and get ruined by mold. Check for pallets at local lumberyards, feed mills, or warehouses. They are often free for the asking.

Wooden pallets keep hay several inches off the ground and allow air to circulate under the stack.

Calling All Mousers

It's important, of course, to keep all grain in rodent-proof containers. In addition, a feline rodent patrol can help reduce the mouse population around the barn.

SUMMER: *JULY*

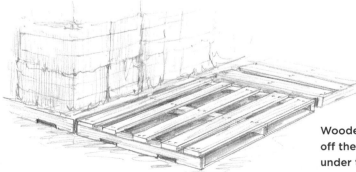

HAY ELEVATOR

A hay elevator makes it much easier to move bales from point A to B. Set at about a 30-degree angle, our elevator is 25 feet long, made of 1-inch square tubing, and has a conveyor chain with 55 finger links to grab the bales. It is powered with a totally enclosed ½-horsepower electric motor. The on/off switch is located at the low end, where I can stop it in an instant.

I place the bales at the lower end, and they travel upward and drop off the elevated end onto or near the place where Richard is stacking. Pacing is the key between the person loading the elevator and the one receiving. When harmony is reached it is a beautiful thing!

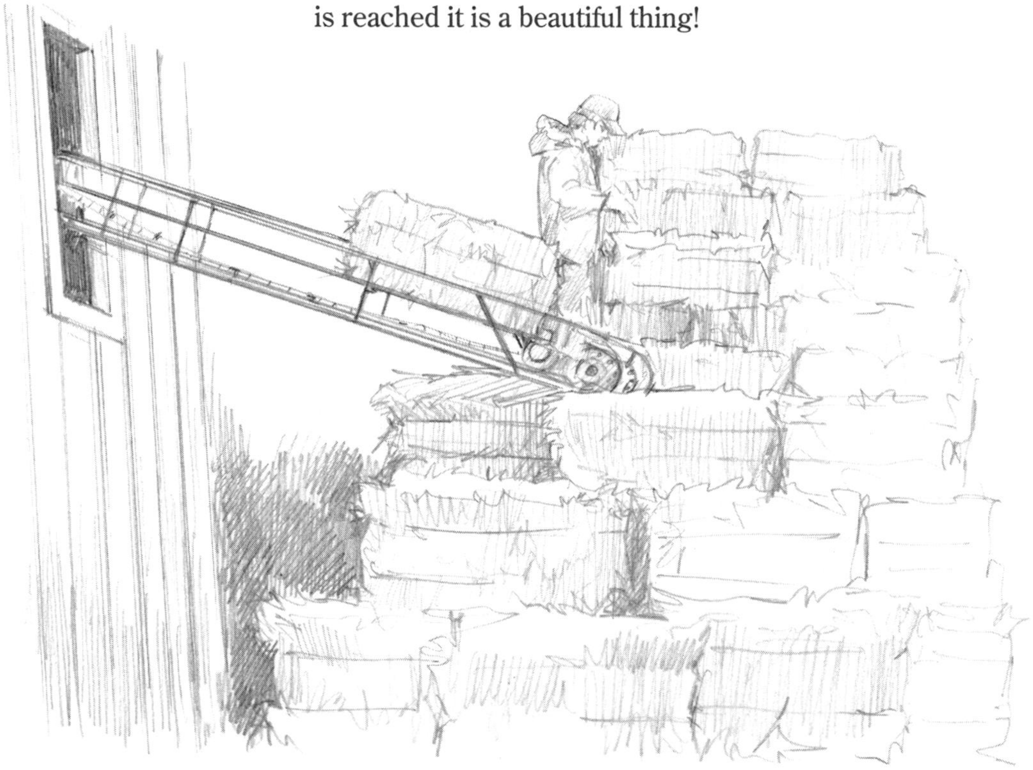

A hay elevator makes it easier to move bales.

Hay Handling by the Numbers

One day Richard, who does most of the bale hefting, wondered how many times he handles each bale of hay. So we made comparative lists and then went out and bought a hay elevator! (Note that if you have a tall hay shed that accommodates a retriever to unload a stack inside the barn, you have already eliminated the first four steps.)

The number of times a bale of hay is handled when we pick up the hay on a flatbed:

1. Throw down from the grower's stack onto the trailer.
2. Stack on trailer.
3. Throw off trailer into hay barn.
4. Stack in hay barn.
5. Carry from stack in hay barn to bucket of tractor.
6. Carry from bucket to small storage area in horse barn.
7. Carry from storage area to cart.
8. Carry from cart to horse to feed.

The number of times a bale of hay is handled when it is delivered in a stacker load:

1. Throw down from the delivered stack onto the ground.
2. Lift onto hand cart and push cart to hay barn or carry each bale to stack (a time- and labor-intensive step).
3. Stack in hay barn (lift from ground level to stack, often two steps).
4. Carry from stack in hay barn to bucket of tractor.
5. Carry from bucket to small storage area in horse barn.
6. Carry from storage area to cart.
7. Carry from cart to horse to feed.

The number of times a bale of hay is handled when the hay is delivered in a stacker load with use of elevator:

1. Throw down from the delivered stack onto the ground.
2. Place on elevator (simple and quick).
3. Stack in hay barn (bale falls right on stack, so easy to stack).
4. Carry from stack in hay barn to bucket of tractor.
5. Carry from bucket to small storage area in horse barn.
6. Carry from storage area to cart.
7. Carry from cart to horse to feed.

RANCH RECIPES

Body Wipe

Fill a gallon plastic milk container with water, adding 1 to 2 tablespoons of Calgon water softener, 2 tablespoons of baby oil, and 1 ounce of your favorite liniment. Shake or stir to mix.

Note: Calgon water softener is not the same as Calgonite automatic dishwasher detergent. Don't let the names confuse you when you are shopping.

How much Calgon to use depends on the hardness of your water. One teaspoon per gallon of water would be adequate for naturally soft water with a hardness of 5 grains or less per gallon. Two tablespoons per gallon would be more appropriate for very hard water with a hardness score of 15 grains or more per gallon.

EQUINE BODY WASH

I like to use this body wash to clean a sweaty horse after working instead of just letting the sweat dry or hosing the horse every day. Using water to hose down your horse every day is not a good long-term management practice. It results in more problems than benefits. Cold water can actually stiffen your horse's muscles. Also, the daily wet/dry cycle can be extremely damaging to the structure of the hooves, and fungus and skin problems can occur when horses are frequently wet and aren't allowed to dry thoroughly.

My solution (pun intended!) to cleaning a sweaty horse without hosing him down is to use this body wipe in specific areas, such as the head, saddle area, the underside of the neck, and between the hind legs. I also use it on the crest and dock to prevent rubbing. I keep a spray bottle near my grooming area and spritz some on a cloth for the final wipe of grooming.

This mixture lifts dirt and sweat off the horse's hair, conditions it, and stimulates the skin. If your horse is very sensitive, you may need to decrease or eliminate the liniment from the formula. For any horse, do not use liniment near the eyes, nostrils, or on the anus. You can substitute cider vinegar for the liniment.

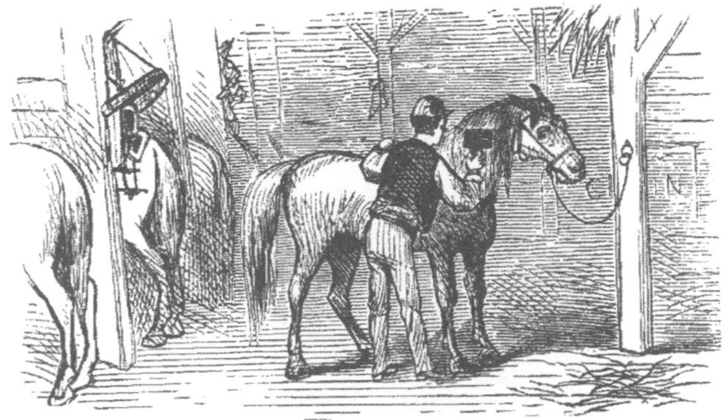

MORE IN DEPTH

CHOOSING GOOD HAY

Good-quality horse hay should be leafy, fine-stemmed, and adequately but not overly dry. Since two-thirds of the plant nutrients are in the leaves, the leaf-to-stem ratio should be high. The hay should not be brittle but instead soft to the touch, with little shattering of the leaves, since lost leaves mean lost nutrition. There should be no excessive moisture that could cause overheating and spoilage.

Dusty, moldy, or musty-smelling hay is not suitable for horses. Not only is it unpalatable, but it can also contribute to respiratory diseases. Moldy hay can also be toxic to horses and may cause colic or abortion.

Bales should not contain undesirable objects or noxious weeds. Check for sticks, wire, blister beetles, poisonous plants, thistle, or plants with barbed awns such as foxtail or cheat grass.

PURCHASING HAY

You can purchase hay by the bale at your local feed store, which is okay in a pinch but is the most expensive option. If you purchase your hay directly from the hay grower, you may be able to develop a regular account and place your order for the next year. You can also purchase your year's supply of hay at auction where you will find a variety of hay types, bale sizes, quality, and prices.

Good quality, barn-stored hay doesn't lose a great amount of its nutritive value when stored for a year. However, buy the current year's crop of hay if it has been stored outdoors. Depending on how many horses you feed, it is usually most economical to buy the largest quantity of good hay that you can store. Instead of buying a pickup load at a time, if you buy a semi load you'll probably not only get

Hay Color

Good-quality hay is free of mold, dust, and weeds and has a bright green color and a fresh smell. In some instances, however, too much emphasis on color may be misleading in hay selection. Although the bright green color indicates a high vitamin A (betacarotene) content, some hays might be bleached pale green to almost tan, yet still of good quality. The interaction of dew or other moisture, the rays of the sun, and high ambient temperatures cause bleaching. Brown hay, however, indicates a loss of nutrients due to excess water or heat damage and should be avoided.

Good-quality horse hay should be leafy, fine-stemmed, and adequately but not overly dry.

Hay Varieties & Characteristics

Hay Varieties	When Commonly Cut	Positive Attributes	Potential Problems
Alfalfa	first flower	High-quality protein especially for growth and generally a desirable calcium to phosphorus ratio, highly palatable	Needs well-drained soil; will shatter if too dry; can contain too much crude protein for some classes of horses, possibility of blister beetles; excess calcium to phosphorus
Birdsfoot trefoil	early bloom	Does well in poorly drained soils	Low yield; may have lower palatability
Red clover	early to midbloom	Does well in poorly drained soils, high-quality protein	Difficult to put up well, notoriously dusty and possible toxicity from mold
Orchardgrass	boot	Early start, high yield, safe feed	Can get tough and unpalatable after early bloom
Timothy	boot	Does well in poorly drained soils, safe for idle adult	Not drought resistant; when only hay fed, not enough energy for working horse and marginal in crude protein, calcium, and phosphorus for working horse
Brome	early to midbloom	Drought resistant, high yield	May be unpalatable if too mature and fed alone; low in protein, calcium, and phosphorus

a better price per ton, but the transportation costs will be greatly reduced as well.

Since the nutritive quality of hay can vary so greatly, it is best to test hay before a large purchase, especially if it is to be used for young or lactating horses. Your extension agent will instruct you on sampling techniques; the test results will reveal moisture content as well as crude protein, fiber, energy, and mineral content.

Depending on how many horses you feed, it is usually most economical to buy the largest quantity of good hay that you can store.

SIZE AND SHAPE OF BALES. Should you buy large round, large square, or small square bales? Large round bales can range from 4 feet wide by 4 feet in diameter to 8 feet wide by 6 feet in diameter and weigh from 500 to 2,500 pounds. Large square bales come in sizes from 3 by 3 by 8 feet to 4 by 4 by 8 feet. The smaller bales weigh from 600 to 800 pounds. Small square bales are 3 by 1½ by 1¼ feet and weigh 40 to 70 pounds.

Odd Words

flake. A section of a bale of hay; also called a flek, slab, slice, or biscuit.

bang. To cut a horse's tail straight across at the bottom; blunt cut.

Large Bales: Pros and Cons

★ Usually less expensive per ton, in some parts of the country large bales are also much more available than small square bales.

★ If you put a large bale out in a pasture to feed a group of horses, they tend to waste, trample, and foul the hay and then won't eat it. Hay lying at the base of the bale will be used for bedding, defecation, and / or urination or as breeding grounds for insects and rodents.

★ If you try to feed portions from a large bale to individual horses, it can be difficult and messy to move each ration from the bale to the feeders. And the open bale needs to be stored and protected while it is being used.

★ Bales stored outdoors need to be protected from other animals eating them, such as deer and elk.

★ Large bales require special equipment to transport to your farm and move around once on your farm.

Horse Sense and Safety

Plan a Quick Getaway
When working in an enclosed space, always take time to plan an escape route in the event of an emergency.

Large round bales typically have a higher storage loss than small rectangular bales, especially when stored outdoors. To minimize outdoor storage loss, choose dense bales. A dense bale sheds water best and sags less, putting less surface area in contact with the ground.

WRAPS AND TWINE. Choose bales covered with plastic wrap, net wrap, or plastic twine. Plastic twine spaced 6 to 10 inches apart holds the bale tight and resists damage from weather, insects, and rodents better than natural fiber twine. Net wraps are porous materials designed to shed water and permit greater airflow at the bale surface. Solid plastic covers shed water, and if they are of ultraviolet (UV) light-stabilized plastic, they result in the least storage loss.

STORING BALES. Store bales on a high, dry location (or indoors if possible). A coarse gravel base will minimize bottom spoilage. Placing the bales across heavy poles or pallets provides air space between the bales and the soil to keep the bales dry but could make a perfect home for rodents. Pack the bales tightly end to end in long row. Stacking large round bales usually traps moisture, limits drying from sun and wind, and results in more loss. Consider covering the entire stack with a large cover.

For more on hay storage, see page 344.

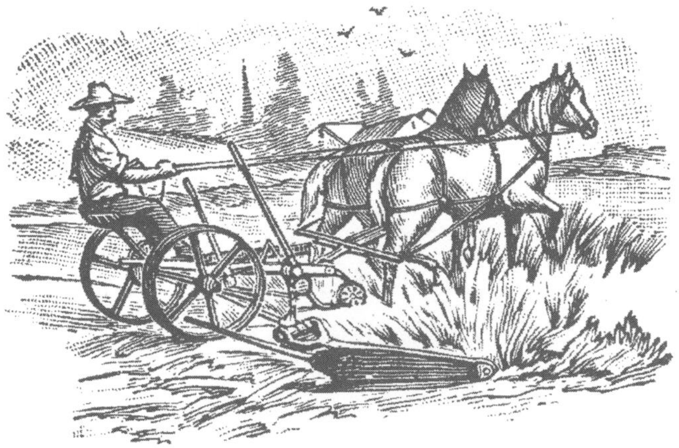

EXTREME HEAT IN THE SOUTHWEST

It seems that, lately, many parts of the country suffer periods of extreme heat. While it is expected in the Desert Southwest, over the last few years we in Colorado, along with the Dakotas and Minnesota, have experienced days with temperatures over 100 degrees and strings of days in the high 90s. During such heat, we can pare down our clothing and sneak into our air-conditioned offices, but what can we do to make our horses safe and more comfortable?

- When it is over 90 degrees, I rarely work my horses. I don't like working up a sweat in that kind of heat, so I imagine my horses wouldn't either.
- They do seem to enjoy a bath, however, and I sure don't mind getting a little wet myself, so bathing is always an option on those lazy, hot summer days.
- If you have a place to go swimming with your horse, such as a pond, stream, or river, this would be the time to do it!
- A place to get out of the sun is essential, which can be provided by trees, man-made sun screens and roofs, or the bona-fide shelter of barn overhangs or stalls.
- If you must haul your horse, try to do so in the very cool hours of early morning.
- If your horse suffers anhydrosis (inability to sweat) this means his thermoregulatory mechanisms have malfunctioned and he cannot cool himself. He will also probably not drink when in this state. This is often a red alert situation that requires a veterinarian. Sometimes you can dose a horse with electrolytes, which may put things back in balance and also get his thirst reflex going again.

Helping Horses Cope with Heat

★ As always, water must be fresh, pure, and available 24 hours a day during hot weather.

★ Salt and minerals should also be available free choice, so that horses can replenish needed micronutrients essential to body functions like thermoregulation, digestion, and hydration.

★ As indicated earlier (see January), know your horse's normal vital signs, including the pinch test, which is so vital during hot weather.

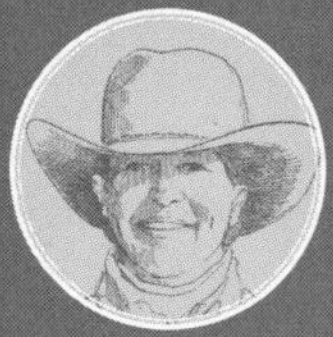

Ask Cherry

Tail Health and Beauty

Q My mare has short, dry hairs at the base of her tail. I want them long and lovely like the rest of her tail. I have her tail braided and bagged. She is on an 11-percent protein grain product, grass pasture in the summer, and quality hay in fall and winter. What else can I do to protect the hairs at the base of the tail from sun damage and keep them growing?

A It's normal for the hairs at the base of the tail to be shorter than the rest of the tail. But if they are as short as bristles and dry, you can improve the situation and get them to grow out and lie down. Here are some things to think about:

- Minimize brushing and combing.
- Remove any reason for the horse to be rubbing her tail against a tree, post, or building. This includes making sure the skin of the dock is absolutely clean and rinsed well; then I use a leave-in conditioner. Wash the udder (or sheath) so the horse is not trying to "scratch" it by rubbing.
- Inspect the area around the tailhead, anus, hindquarters and be sure there are no lice, ticks, fungus, awns from dry grass, or anything else that could be causing the horse to rub. Mares often rub when they are in heat.
- Be sure the horse is currently in a deworming program that targets pinworms.
- Consider whether the ingredients in your fly spray could be drying out the hair or causing rubbing.
- A textilene fly sheet would protect against UV rays and cover the top portion of the tail. All of my horses wear textilene fly sheets all summer, and their coats don't bleach and the tops of their tails are always in great shape.
- There are also fly sprays and grooming products that contain sunscreen that you could consider using but I don't find them necessary.

AUGUST

After a busy spring and summer, August is the gateway to my favorite riding seasons: fall and winter. In August, therefore, I regroup. It is the month when I schedule my veterinarian to do annual dental work. Also, I reorganize my tack room, making sure all of our trail-riding gear is in good order. Ever vigilant for the smell of forest fire, Richard and I rehearse our emergency plans.

Day Length in Hours

Latitude	Aug 1	Aug 16	Sept 1
60°N	16.62	15.36	13.91
55°N	15.73	14.74	13.57
50°N	15.07	14.27	13.31
45°N	14.56	13.9	13.1
40°N	14.13	13.59	12.92
35°N	13.77	13.32	12.77
30°N	13.46	13.09	12.63

See page 22 to find your latitude.

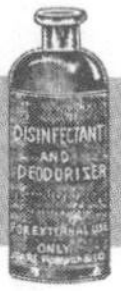

VET CLINIC

To Do

- ❑ Hoof trim and shoe
- ❑ Work arena
- ❑ Scrub feed tubs and buckets
- ❑ Move hay to barns
- ❑ Dental exam
- ❑ Clean sheaths
- ❑ Fire plan

To Buy

- ❑ Pasture seed
- ❑ Gravel stash for winter
- ❑ Complete feed wafers
- ❑ Grain
- ❑ Dewormer
- ❑ Senior feed
- ❑ Corn oil
- ❑ Beet pulp pellets
- ❑ Salt and mineral blocks
- ❑ Fly masks

INSIDE A HORSE'S MOUTH

A horse's upper jaw is wider than the lower jaw, and horses chew from side to side. As their molars wear, they form sharp points on the outside of the upper molars and the inside of the lower molars. To keep these sharp points from cutting your horse's tongue or cheeks as he eats, they should be floated (filed) regularly with a special file, called a float, attached to a long handle.

At the same time, your vet can remove caps or wolf teeth. Caps are temporary premolars (baby teeth) and molars that have not completely dislodged, even though the permanent ones have erupted.

DENTAL CLINIC

Summer is a good time to have routine dental work completed: floating sharp points on teeth, removing wolf teeth if necessary, and removing retained caps.

SHARP POINTS. Here's how to see if your horse has sharp points that need floating.

1. With his mouth closed, try to move his upper jaw to the left while moving his bottom jaw to the right and vice versa. Since a horse moves his jaw from side to side as he chews, if you find there is something blocking this movement, it is likely to be points.
2. Then run your fingertips down the sides of his face on the outside, pressing his skin against his cheek teeth. If he has points there, it will likely be painful when you do this and he will raise his head. If you are confident about the anatomy of a horse's mouth, you can insert your fingers in the area between the cheek and the molars to feel for upper points.

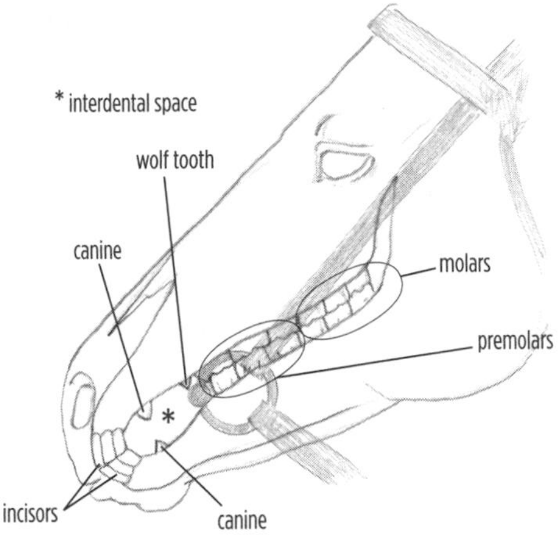

At the front of your horse's mouth are the incisors; at the back are the premolars and the molars. In between is the interdental space, also called the bars, where the bit rests. Wolf teeth can interfere with the action of a snaffle bit and could cause painful pinching.

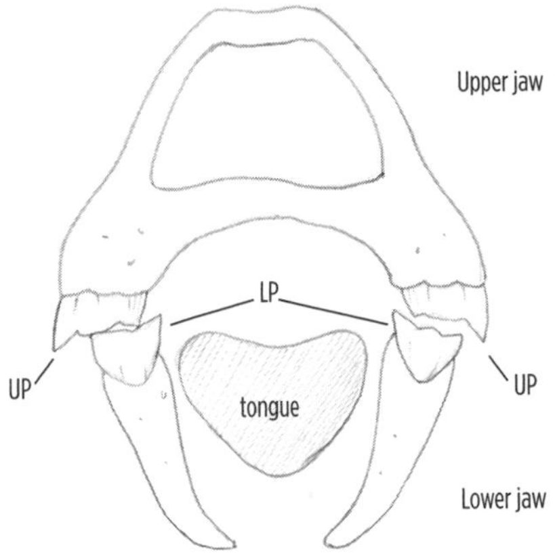

The sharp points that form on the inside of the lower molars (LP) and the outside of the upper molars (UP) can make chewing painful for your horse.

WOLF TEETH. In the interdental space of a horse's mouth there might be certain additional teeth. Most male horses five years of age and older have four canine teeth in the interdental space, located about an inch or two behind the incisors. Some mares (about 20 percent) have small canines or canine buds, usually on the lower jaw.

Most, but not all, horses have wolf teeth, and both male and female horses can have them. Appearing more often in the upper jaw, they start emerging at about 6 months of age and are fully visible by 12 to 18 months. Some wolf teeth fall out at about three years of age when the horse sheds the temporary second premolar.

Tooth Trouble

Monitor your horse to determine if he needs more frequent visits. Here are some signs that a horse needs dental work:

- ★ Bad breath
- ★ Quids (food wads in feeding area)
- ★ Feed falling from mouth while eating
- ★ Weight loss
- ★ Sharp points on teeth

Removal of Wolf Teeth

Many wolf teeth are fine left undisturbed, but they are surgically removed if their size or location could cause painful bumping by the snaffle bit or pinching of the horse's skin between tooth and bit. If a wolf tooth is small and fits tightly

Prehistoric Teeth

True first premolars, wolf teeth are smaller than the other premolars. They are remnants of teeth from prehistoric horses and through evolution have decreased in size and frequency of appearance.

up against the second premolar, it might be fine. The problem occurs when the tooth is standing alone and large.

Wolf teeth are usually removed when a yearling colt is gelded, when he is already sedated. With fillies, wolf teeth can be removed any time after about 12 months of age and before snaffle-bit training begins. Your veterinarian will likely use a sedative and a local anesthetic to perform the extraction. The root of a wolf tooth is shallow, about half an inch in young horses. These teeth are relatively soft and can be easily crushed during removal. If a tooth splinters during removal and small pieces are left in the jaw, an abscess can result. However, if a small portion of the root breaks off below the gum line, often the remaining root tip will be absorbed and cause no problem.

Have your veterinarian examine your horse and advise you as to whether the wolf teeth should be removed. If your horse has become more difficult to turn or stop, or if he throws his head up when you make contact with the rein, then he might be having dental problems, and one explanation could be wolf teeth. A thorough dental examination can reveal any problems.

NOT ALWAYS TRUE

Historical Horsekeeping

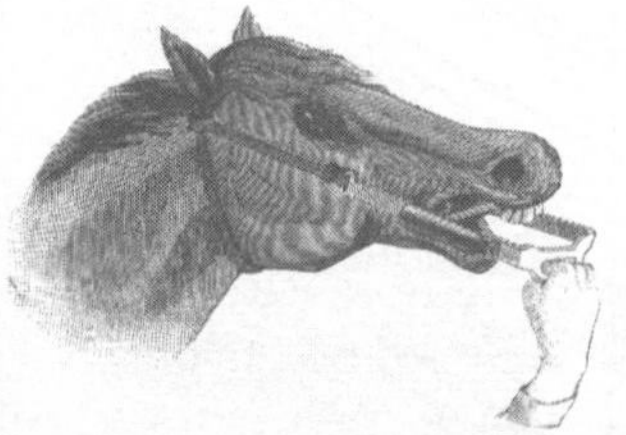

"These rudimentary teeth [wolf teeth] . . . which have been supposed by ignorant persons to produce blindness, and other diseases, are entirely harmless except for the abrasion they occasion to the tongue and cheeks. If they do, they are taken out by any sensible blacksmith."

— Gleason's Horse Book *by Prof. Oscar R. Gleason, 1892*

FOOT NOTES

LOST SHOES

One of the main reasons for loose or lost shoes is that the hooves overgrow the edges of the shoes, which causes the nails to loosen. The shoe on a freshly shod hoof should be slightly wider than the hoof to allow the hoof room to expand as it grows. When the hoof is flush with the edge of the shoe, usually five to eight weeks after shoeing, it is ready to be reshod. When a hoof has started to grow over the edge of the shoe, it is past time to get the horse shod. To prevent lost shoes, regularly check how close the hoof wall is to the edge of the shoe.

PROTECTING A BARE HOOF

An unshod hoof should have rounded, smooth edges that resist chipping and cracking. When a hoof is prepared for shoeing, however, the edges are left sharp and are protected by the shoe. When a horse loses a shoe, the sharp edge can easily break. There are several ways to protect the bare hoof until your farrier can replace the shoe.

Hoof boots come in various sizes and styles, so look for one that will fit your horse's hooves. Hind hooves usually take a smaller boot than the front hooves. The boot should fit snugly and not rub the skin of the coronary band or pastern.

If you do not have a hoof boot, you can use several layers of duct tape to protect the edge of the hoof from chipping. If your horse has a tender sole, you can tape a cloth over the bottom of the sole to protect it.

Movie of the Month

CLOUD: WILD STALLION OF THE ROCKIES **(1982)**
A dedicated filmmaker, Ginger Kathrens, documents the life of a band of wild horses in the Arrowhead Mountains in Montana over a period of nine years. She focuses on a pale Palomino colt that she names Cloud. The story pivots around him from the day he was born and throughout his role as a band stallion. Upclose behavior of foals, stallion fighting, bachelor bands, and more. An excellent production with a sequel, *Cloud's Legacy*.

One of the main reasons for loose or lost shoes is that the hooves overgrow the edges of the shoes, which causes the nails to loosen.

Removing a Loose Shoe

Use the following procedure to remove a shoe that has become bent or dangerously loose, or has rotated on your horse's hoof.

PULLING OUT THE NAILS

A clinch is the end of the nail folded over; this needs to be opened so that the nail can slide straight through the hoof wall when pulled without taking large hunks of hoof with it.

1. Using the chisel end of the clinch cutter, open the clinches by tapping the spine of the clinch cutter with the hammer.
2. If the shoe has a crease on the bottom, you may be able to use the crease nail puller to extract each nail individually, allowing the shoe to come off.
3. Nails with protruding heads can be pulled out using the pull-offs.
4. If you can't pull the nails out individually, then you will have to remove the shoe with the pull-offs.

PRYING OFF THE SHOE

1. After the clinches have been opened, grab a shoe heel and pry toward the tip of the frog.
2. Repeat with the other shoe heel.
3. When both heels are loose, grab one side of the shoe at the toe and pry toward the tip of the frog.
4. Repeat around the shoe until it is removed. Never pry toward the outside of the hoof or you risk ripping out big chunks of the hoof wall.
5. As the nail heads protrude due to the loosening of the shoe, you can pull them out individually with the pull-offs. Pull any nails that may remain in the hoof.

To protect the bare hoof, keep the horse confined in soft bedding and follow the advice on page 361.

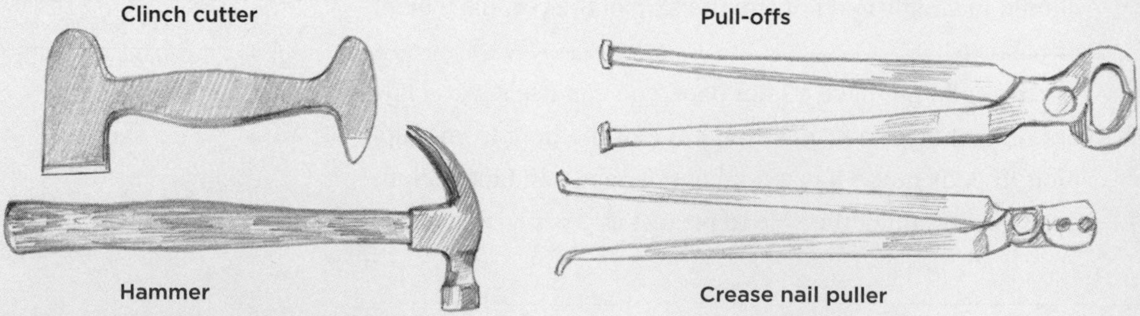

Necessary tools include clinch cutter, hammer, pull-offs, and crease nail puller.

WILD LIFE

WILD HORSES

In some parts of the United States, wild horses and burros roam with other wildlife and with domestic range animals. The management of wild horses on public rangelands is under the jurisdiction of the Bureau of Land Management (BLM), which is responsible for managing the nation's public lands. The BLM also takes into consideration the other natural resources (wildlife and vegetation) and other uses such as by livestock owners and recreational users.

ADOPTION POLICIES. Currently you can adopt wild horses by visiting adoption sites in person at scheduled

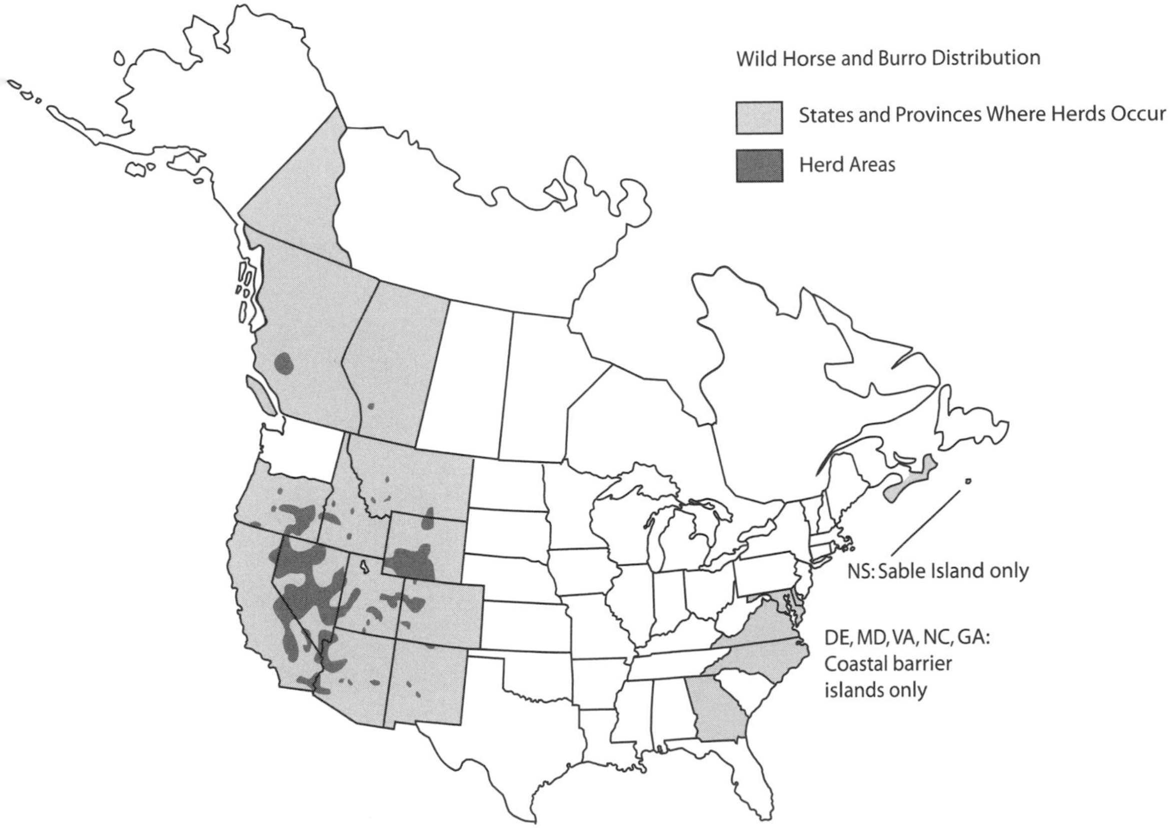

SUMMER: AUGUST

Feed Bag

Salt and Minerals

Horses need access to salt at all times. I offer each horse two salt blocks: a plain white salt block (simply table salt or sodium chloride) and a calcium/phosphorus trace-mineral salt block. Sometimes called a 12:12 block because it contains 12 percent calcium and 12 percent phosphorus, or an equal ratio of calcium to phosphorus, it is good for most adult horses. All my horses prefer one block or the other, but choose different blocks at different times.

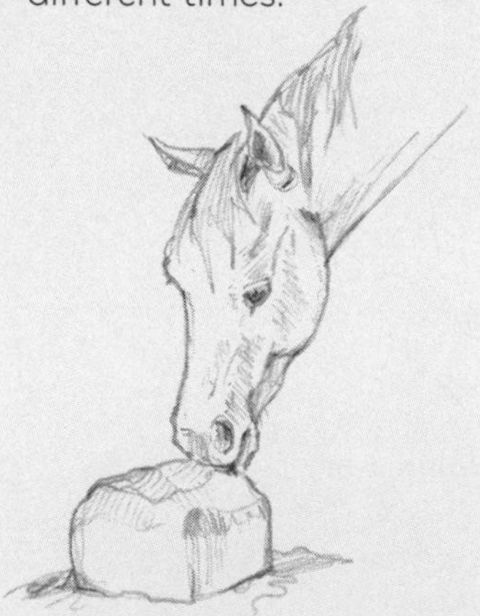

Free choice trace-mineral salt is a must.

times or by using the BLM's online adoption system (see the appendix for Web sites). Seventeen states also have state wild horse adoption programs. For example, in Colorado you can adopt a wild horse year-round. The BLM holds adoptions at the East Cañon Correctional Complex outside Cañon City two Fridays per month, where you can usually choose from more than 400 wild horses and burros. There is a minimum adoption fee per animal, and you must be a preapproved adopter in order to make an appointment.

The program appears to be working. When the 1971 legislation was passed, it was estimated that there were 17,300 wild horses and 8,045 wild burros, for a total of 25,345 wild horses and burros. Since 1977, between 2,500 and 11,600 wild horses and burros have been adopted each year, with an average of about 5,000 per year. There have been 177,832 wild horses and burros adopted since 1971. In 2005, there were 27,369 wild horses and 4,391 wild burros, for a total of 31,760 wild horses and burros roaming the rangelands of the United States.

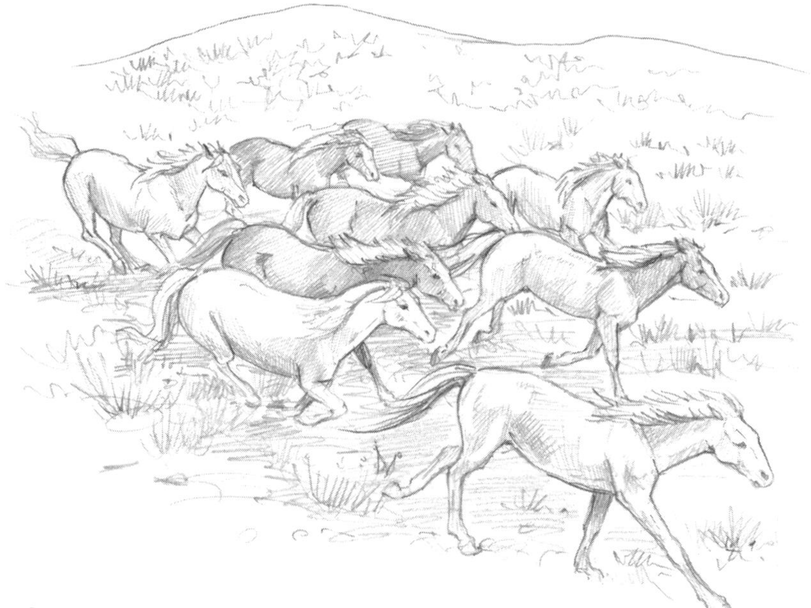

Seventeen states have wild horse adoption programs.

A Complicated History

In response to widespread slaughter of wild horses, a federal bill (Public Law 92-195, the Wild Free-Roaming Horses and Burros Act) was passed in 1971 to manage, protect, and control wild horses and burros. In 1976 it was amended to authorize use of helicopters and motorized vehicles to manage wild horses and burros on public lands.

In 1978, Public Law 95-514, the Public Rangelands Improvement Act of 1978, further refined the program to emphasize the need for inventory, identification of animals, the monitoring of rangeland conditions, and further protection of wild horses, along with the removal of excess horses that posed a threat to themselves and their habitat. It also established the transfer of title of ownership to those who adopted wild horses, provided the animals had received proper and humane care and treatment for one year.

Toxic Cherries

Chokecherries are ripe during August. Although horses don't eat the berries, the leaves are poisonous to horses and the berries attract bears.

CLEAN-UP CREW

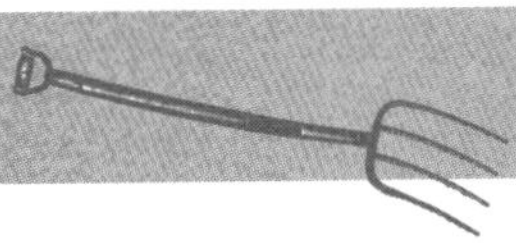

TEN STEPS TO A CLEAN STALL

Here's how I clean a stall.

1. I turn the horse out.
2. I pick up any good hay on top of the bedding and put it in a tub to feed later.
3. I then remove all manure using a stall fork that catches fecal balls but lets sawdust bedding fall through.
4. Next, I locate wet spots from urine and pull all the clean dry bedding away from them. I heap the dry bedding along the walls to reuse later.
5. I pile all the wet and dirty bedding in the center of the stall, and use a scoop shovel to load it into the cart.

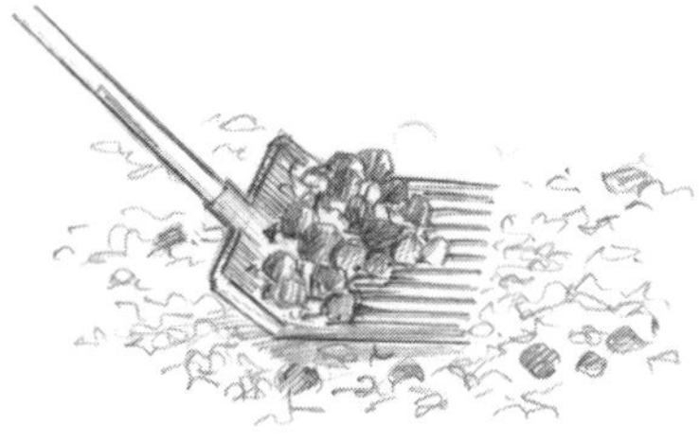

Remove manure.

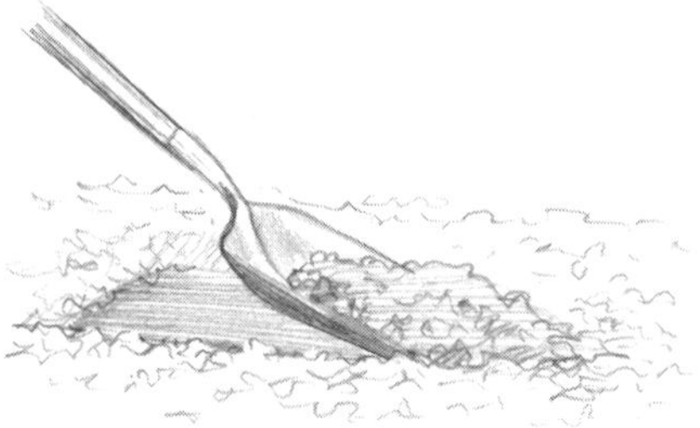

Pick up bedding.

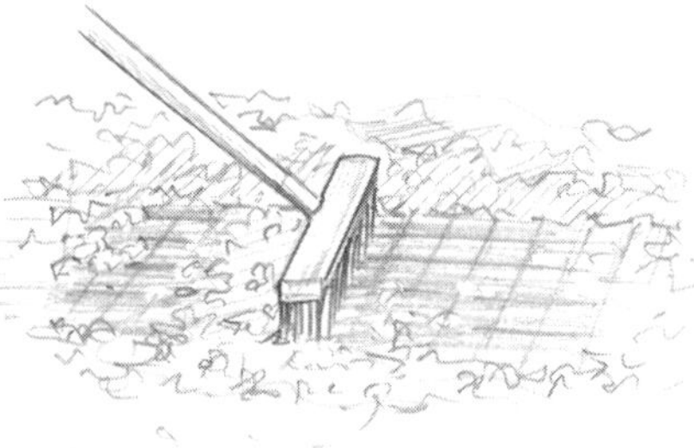

Sweep.

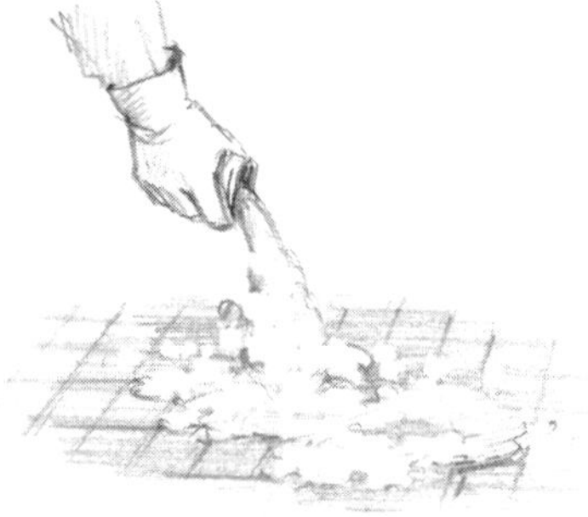

Sprinkle wet spots if needed.

6. I use a push broom to sweep a small amount of dry bedding back and forth over the wet spots to further dry the floor, and then discard this bedding.
7. If needed, I sprinkle an absorbent stall freshener on the wet spots.
8. To finish, I sweep all bedding away from the feed area, and sweep any bedding that has been dragged into the barn aisle back into the stall.
9. After the floor has dried with the windows and doors open, I spread the clean, old bedding on the floor where the horse tends to urinate and add fresh bedding where the horse tends to lie down.
10. Finally, I return the horse to the stall.

AUGUST
Manure Pile Maintenance

PILE A
Turn once, water as needed.

PILE B
Turn twice, water as needed.

PILE C
Sell, store, or spread.

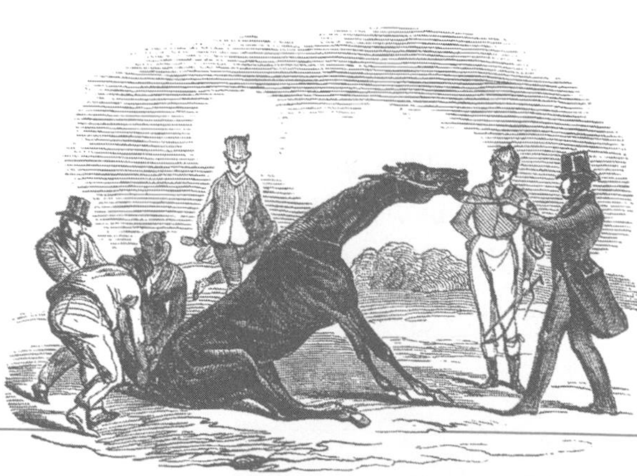

Pasture Perfect

Protect Riparian Areas

Horses can easily damage precious riparian areas. "Riparian" refers to the vegetation and soils alongside streams, creeks, rivers, and ponds. Manure, urine, overgrazing, destruction of trees, and the creation of muddy banks all can lead to less vegetation, warmer water temperatures, more algae, fewer fish, and decreased wildlife habitat. Monitor and limit horses' access to natural water sources so that a natural buffer zone of grasses, brush, and trees is preserved around the edges of ponds and creeks. This buffer zone is essential for filtering nutrients from excess runoff before it enters the water.

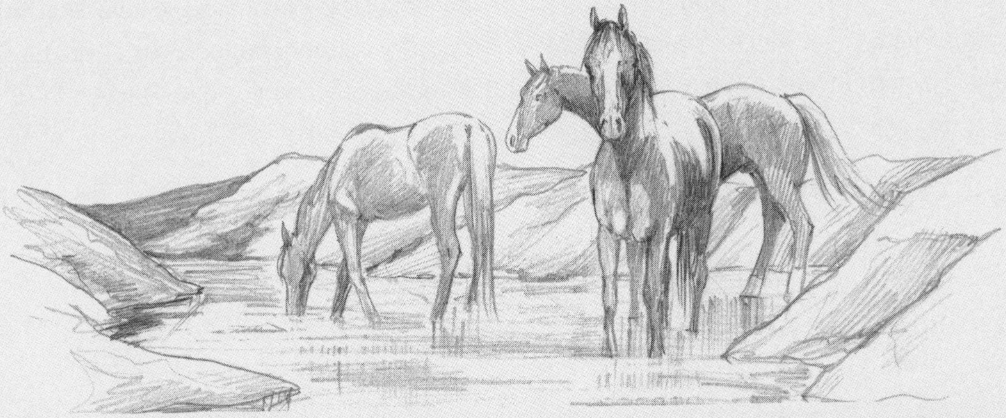

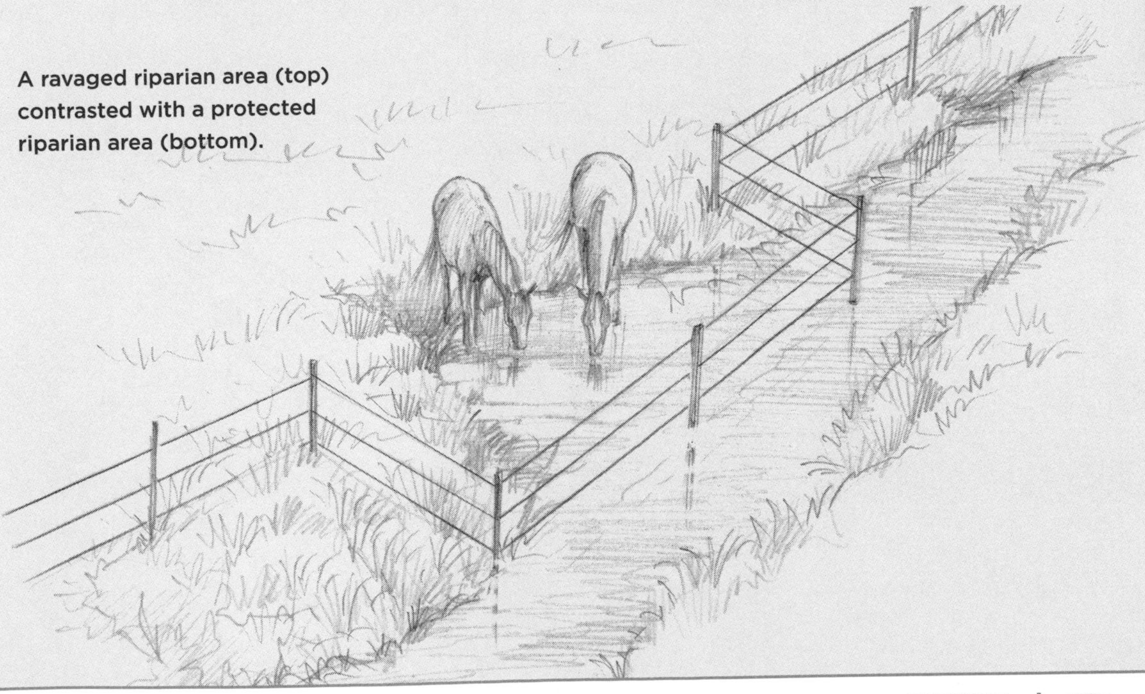

A ravaged riparian area (top) contrasted with a protected riparian area (bottom).

Pest Patrol

Blister Beetles

Four to 6 grams of blister beetles (whole or part, fresh or dried) can kill a 1,100-pound horse. That's because they contain cantharidin, a toxic and caustic poison. There is no antidote. Research has shown that the striped blister beetle is the source of cantharidin. Typically, blister beetles appear after the first cut of hay (mid-June or later) and disappear by October, so usually first cut and last (late fourth) cut hay is safer than second or third cut. Blister beetles tend to cluster in large groups, often in the area of one or two bales, but hay growers know that if left alone after cutting, most blister beetles evacuate the field.

This is why it's important to know your alfalfa hay grower. Ask him what he did to eliminate blister beetles in the field. Buy only first cut or October hay. Inspect alfalfa hay before you buy and again before you feed.

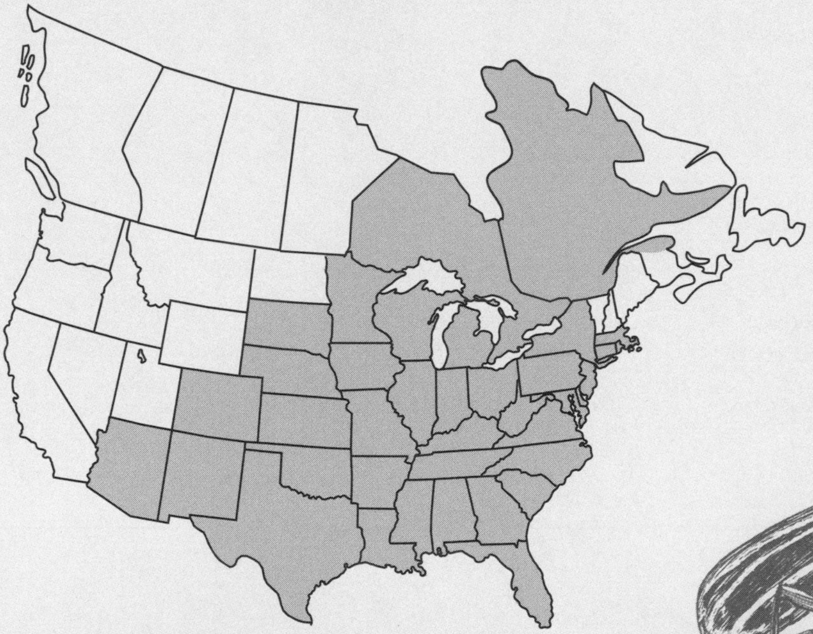

Striped Blister Beetle Occurrence

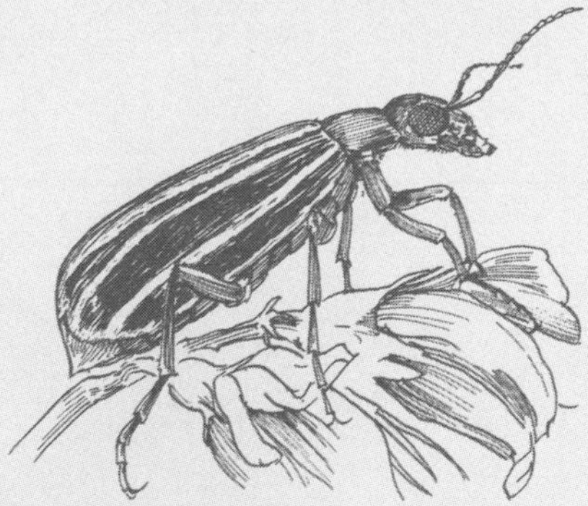

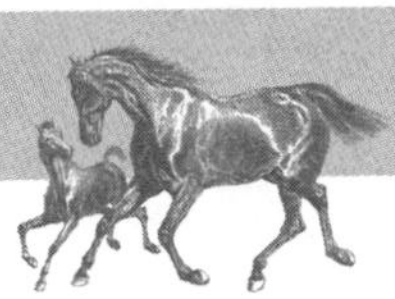

GELDING YEARLINGS

The castration of a male horse is a simple surgical procedure with few risks. Sperm cells are produced in the testicles, matured and stored in the epididymus, and transported via the vas deferens to the ejaculatory site. Gelding removes the testicles, epididymus, part of the spermatic cord, and the covering of the testicles.

With gelding the production of sperm cells stops, yet newly gelded horses can impregnate mares. This is due to the ampulla, a sperm reservoir at the end of the vas deferens. Because the ampulla is not removed, a gelding can potentially settle a mare for up to one month after castration. After one month, the sperm that were stored in the ampulla at the time of castration are no longer viable.

WHY GELD? Improvement in quality and performance in the equine gene pool begins with selection of only the best individuals for breeding purposes. Up to 90 percent of male horses are not of breeding-stallion potential, so gelding is very common. Due to a decrease in the production of androgens (the male hormones) after castration, geldings generally have a more stable disposition than stallions.

Gelding makes a male horse suitable for a greater range of uses. Male hormones are responsible for much more than the desire and capability to breed mares. Athletic performance can be helped or hindered by testosterone. It can make a stallion perform with more energy and brilliance than a gelding, yet it can also distract a stallion from the work at hand. Similarly, secondary sex characteristics, such as muscle bulk, that are influenced by testosterone production can manifest as desirable muscle definition and strength or as an undesirable cresty, thick, and inflexible neck.

Behavior Modification

Although sexual interest is desirable in a stud, sexual aggressiveness is dangerous in a performance animal.

The urge to copulate is just one part of the breeding ritual; related breeding behaviors include whinnying, squealing, pushing, rearing, striking, and biting — all socially acceptable behaviors among horses but not between people and horses. A small percentage of young male horses exhibit sexual frustration or self-mutilation tendencies. Avoid such behaviors by gelding horses without breeding potential early.

Although gelding will remove the underlying cause for such behaviors, it will not change poor manners and bad habits. This must be accomplished by proper training.

BEAUTY SHOP

SHEATH CLEANING

Male horses might have difficulty urinating or might rub their tails because of a dirty sheath. The sheath is the protective envelope of skin around the penis. Fatty secretions, dead skin cells, and dirt accumulate in the folds of the sheath.

In addition, a "bean" of material can accumulate in the diverticulum adjacent to the urethral opening. This black, foul-smelling, somewhat waxy substance is called smegma. Depending on the individual horse's smegma production, the sheath should be cleaned about once or twice a year.

You can clean the sheath somewhat with the penis retracted into the sheath, but you can do a more thorough job if the penis is down. Once a horse is accustomed to the procedure, he will likely relax and let his penis down for cleaning. Usually the best time for this is on a warm day after a workout when the horse is somewhat tired and relaxed. If the horse is very touchy in his genital area, you could have your veterinarian tranquilize the horse so your horse will be more manageable.

PREPARATION. To clean a sheath, you will need warm water, a hose, a small bucket, mild soap, rubber gloves, a tube sock, and hand towels. Because smegma has a strong, offensive odor, first put a rubber glove on your right hand and then cover it with a large tube sock. Use a safe handling position with your left hand up on the horse's back. Do not lower your head to see what you are doing or you could be kicked.

WASHING. Soak the sock in warm water and wet the sheath area with handfuls of water. Add a very small amount

The Udder Side

Udder cleaning is a snap compared to sheath cleaning. Use the same supplies, techniques, and safety principles.

Odd Words

smegma. A black, sticky substance composed of fatty secretions, dead skin cells, and dirt found in the sheath.

bean. A ball of smegma that accumulates in a flap of skin near the urethral opening; can interfere with urination and must be regularly removed.

of liquid soap (such as Ivory) to the tube sock and begin washing the sheath inside and out. There are also several commercial products designed especially for sheath cleaning. You will be able to remove large chunks and sheets of smegma as you work.

RINSE WELL. The best way I have found to rinse the sheath thoroughly is to use a hose with warm water and low to moderate pressure. Most horses learn to tolerate and then enjoy this after one session. You can insert the hose 2 to 3 inches into the sheath to rinse. However, until accustomed, a horse's natural reaction is to kick upward with one of the hind legs. A horse can easily reach a fly on his belly this way, so your hand and arm could be in danger. Hold them as high and as close to the horse's belly as possible until the horse gets used to the sensation of the water.

Older horses that are quite used to the process will lower the penis so you can clean it also. Use only warm water on the penis, no soap.

> **TIPS & TECHNIQUES**
>
> **Removing a Bean**
>
> Often a ball of smegma, called a "bean," will accumulate in the diverticulum near the urethral opening. The bean can build up to a size that could interfere with urination. Sometimes the "bean" material is white, but usually it is black.
>
> To remove it, move the skin at the end of the penis near the urethral opening until you find a blind pouch. This part of sheath cleaning is the time when your horse is most likely to kick. Usually once you find the bean, you can roll it out quite easily.

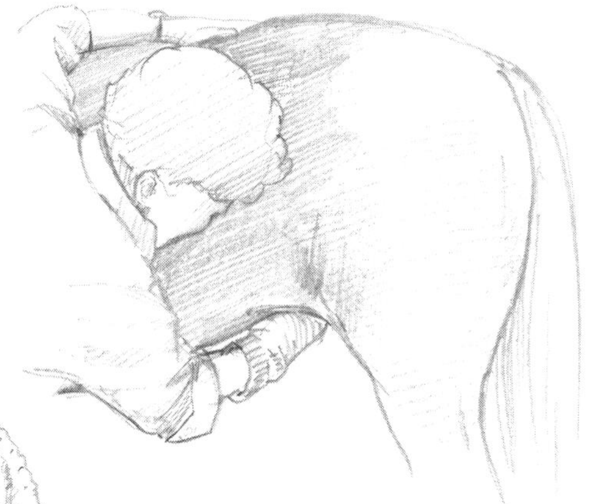

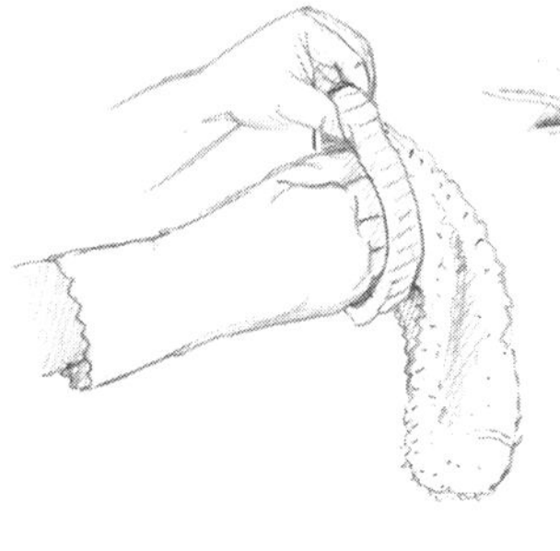

A thin Latex glove covered by an inside-out terry sock makes a great sheath-cleaning mitt.

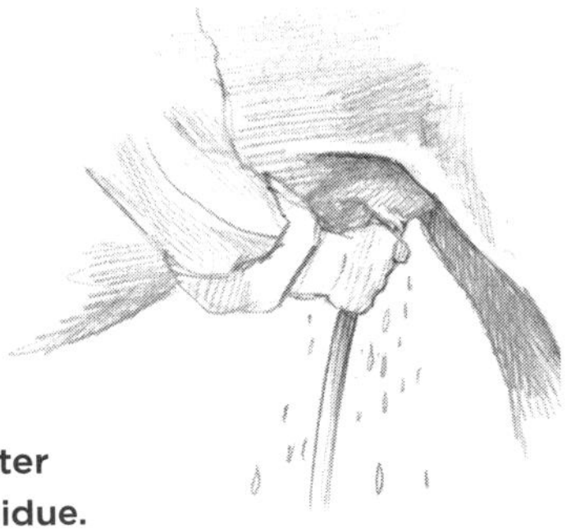

Hosing with warm water removes any soap residue.

TACK ROOM

GETTING ORGANIZED

If you set your tack room up to fit your specific needs, it'll be easier to do a better job taking care of your horse and your tack. I divide things into three categories: things I use daily, seasonally, and only occasionally. I make sure my daily items are close to where I'll use them. I further sort items into categories (see ID Required), so when I need something I know where to look. I continually go through my gear and supplies, tossing empties, recycling broken tack, or giving away or selling things I no longer use. Otherwise, a tack room can be overwhelming.

To cluster things, I use transparent containers or small cardboard boxes with the ends clearly labeled. I'll usually use the latter for seldom-used items in storage on the highest shelf. I store dewormer tubes in a covered clear plastic box with a label. Likewise, I group wound-care products and vet supplies so at a glance I can see what is where.

I also use new muck buckets to gather groups of things like leg boots or saddlebags and canteens. I try to locate supplies near where I will use them. For example, I have a tack-cleaning hook above my sink, and my favorite tack-cleaning products handy on a shelf behind the sink. Over my washer and dryer, I have shelves and cabinets for storing laundry supplies, towels, and rags.

Items that I use seasonally or rarely are up on very high shelves, out of the way, but things I use frequently are at hand: freestanding saddle racks are close to the door for easy access; bridles hang just inside the tack room door. You can never have too many hooks for storing tack — from bits and extra reins to lunge lines, surcingles, cavessons, blanket straps, spare halters and lead ropes, and more.

ID Required

I try to label most things, because there are two of us using the equipment. Having labels helps things get back to their proper places. I use plastic cattle ear tags to designate which blanket is for which horse. I write the name of the horse and blanket size in permanent marker on the ear tag, and then attach the tag to one of the blanket buckles with a shower curtain rod ring.

If you set your tack room up to fit your specific needs, it'll be easier to do a better job taking care of your horse and your tack.

Necessities in Your Tack Room

- ❑ Items used daily, such as grooming tools
- ❑ Year-round products, such as grooming supplies
- ❑ Seasonal horse-care products, such as fly products
- ❑ First-aid supplies
- ❑ Extra bandages, gauze, and wraps for continued follow-up treatment
- ❑ Medicines
- ❑ Shampoos and other items you use in the wash rack
- ❑ Tack-cleaning supplies
- ❑ Towels and rags
- ❑ Dewormers
- ❑ Veterinary equipment (needles, syringes, stethoscope)
- ❑ Clippers, blades, oil, and supplies
- ❑ Specialized mane care tools and supplies, such as mane banders, pullers, and thinning shears, which you use only occasionally
- ❑ Travel-related items such as leg boots and tail wrap
- ❑ Blankets and sheets organized by season and size
- ❑ Tack for riding and training
- ❑ Horse records, equipment warranties, phone numbers, and office materials

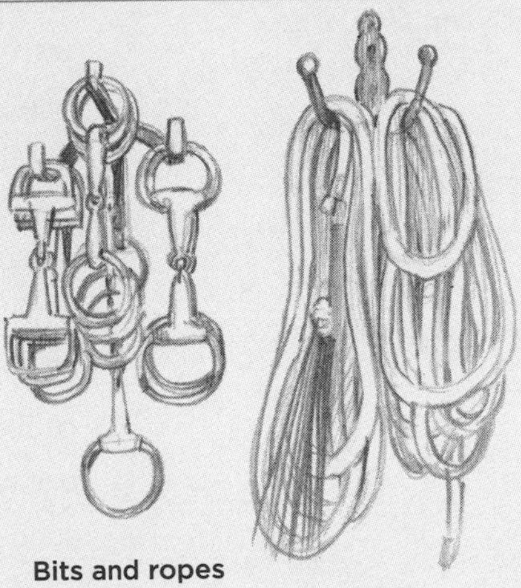

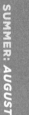

Bits and ropes

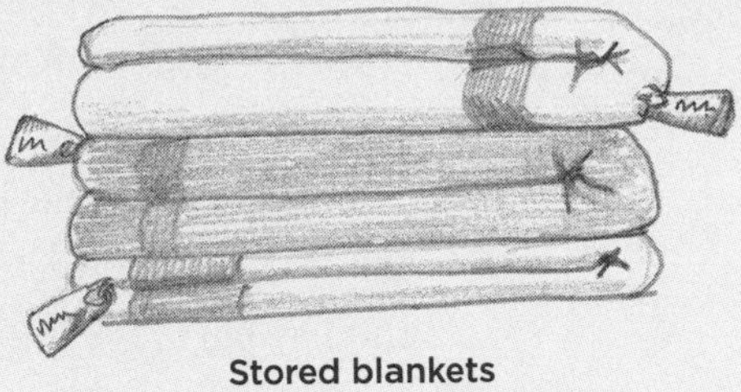

Stored blankets

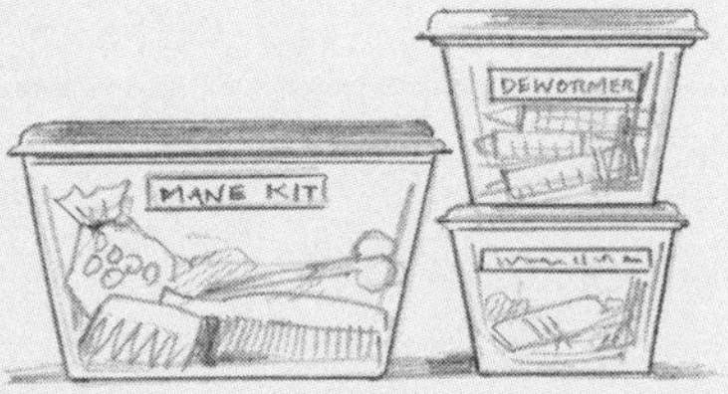

Grooming and vet supplies

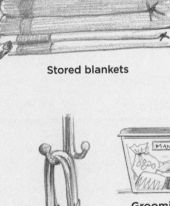

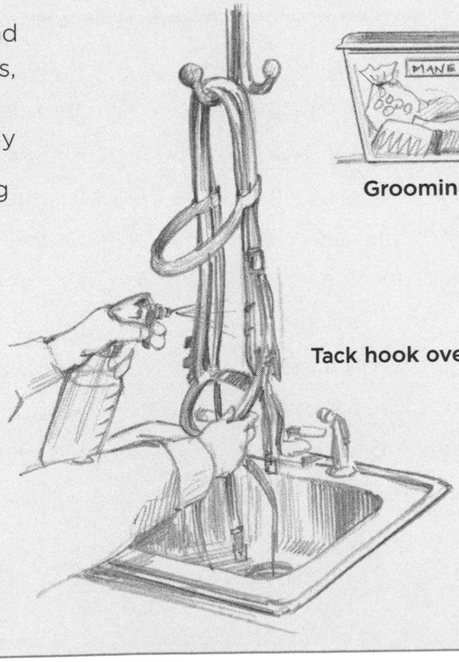

Tack hook over sink

TIPS & TECHNIQUES

Extra Storage

For extras or stored items, I use a large wooden trunk (originally made to hold deck items). The trunk lid doubles as a worktable and seat. In the barn aisle, I have two tall, rodent-proof metal cabinets with shelves where I store more seasonal items like fly sheets.

For small items, I have a wall-mounted set of small transparent bins (found at a home improvement or hardware store) that help me find something at a glance. I store blankets, saddle pads, sheets, and other bulky horse clothing that I am currently using on blanket rods.

For certain items, you can't beat a chest of drawers. I chose an old-fashioned, five-drawer bureau at a furniture store and use it for small things that don't store well on shelves. In one drawer there are syringes, gauze, medicines, rubber gloves, and a stethoscope; in another, spare clipper parts; in a third, extra bandages. I use small trays and boxes, such as old silverware trays, to keep things organized.

A two-drawer file cabinet works great for the paperwork I store in my tack room: vet records, receipts, horse information, equipment warranties, and other important information. I also have a "Where Is It?" file, a 4-inch by 8-inch index card box that lists, for example, the whereabouts of that extra foal creep feeder. It tells me at a glance if it's in the hay barn, the loft of the horse barn, or the shop.

Grab & Go Kits

I like to make grab-and-go kits. I have one for deworming, one for mane overhauls, one for shoe pulling, and one for pasture visits (see 279).

- ★ **Deworming Kit.** I fill the four pockets across the front of a waiter's waist-pouch apron with these items, from left to right: new dewormer; toothbrushes; cloth; used dewormer tubes.
- ★ **Mane Kit.** In a tote, I have a brush, several types of combs, a mane puller, a mane thinner, a mane trimmer, and scissors. A separate kit has all the supplies for mane banding.
- ★ **Shoe-Pulling Kit.** In a wooden box, I store a clinch cutter, hammer, pull-offs, and a crease nail puller, along with either a hoof boot or a cloth and duct tape. (See this month's Foot Notes for a shoe-pulling technique.)

CLOTHES HORSE

FLY GEAR

I do not like to use fly spray unless it is absolutely necessary, partly because most fly sprays do not smell that great, but mainly because they make my eyes and my skin burn. Therefore, to reduce the amount of chemicals that we use while maximizing the comfort of our horses during fly season, we keep our facilities clean and dry and use lots of fly gear. When a quiet horse is hanging out in a stall, a fly scrim makes a suitable sheet. (Scrim is a thin, durable, open-weave fabric of nylon, cotton, or linen.) But for turnout, I choose sheets made of PVC-coated mesh fabric. It is tough and provides UV protection as well.

I use fly masks on certain horses to provide them with protection from flies and sun. There are plain masks, masks with ears, and masks with nose shields. To reduce stomping, you can use leg boots made out of a similar material. For pasture horses that are bothered by flies or gnats under the jaw or on the chest we use browband/neckbands that have dangling strips impregnated with insecticides.

FYI

The Cycle of Conjunctivitis

Conjunctivitis is often a self-perpetuating cycle. First, the flies feed on the watery secretion of the eyes, bringing filth and bacteria with them, and soon the exudate is a bacteria-laden mucopurulent (pussy) discharge. This in turn causes the horse to rub its eye, resulting in more inflammation, attracting more flies, and so on.

Fly Masks

The idea behind fly masks is to provide your horse with protection from face flies while minimizing the use of fly repellents in and around the sensitive areas of his face, namely his eyes. Flies are attracted to the moisture around a horse's eyes and can cause conjunctivitis, an inflammation of the conjunctiva (the membrane that lines the eyelid) of the eye.

Fly masks especially help for the pasture horse that is out munching grass where flies thrive. Some masks have the additional benefit of protecting the horse's eyes from a constant dose of bright sunlight. Such masks occlude the light while still allowing the horse to see.

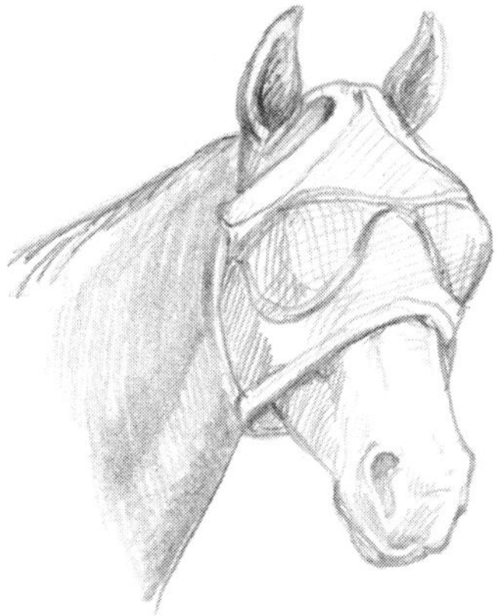

For some horses during some seasons, a fly mask is essential.

Choosing a Fly Mask

A fly mask's primary purpose is to prevent flies from sponging fluids from the horse's eyes and from biting and sucking blood from the vessel-rich head. Here is what to look for when selecting one.

- ★ A fly mask should fit well and be comfortable so the horse does not want to rub it off.
- ★ Flies should not be able to enter the mask, because that would be worse than no mask at all.
- ★ The mask should be durable so that it survives the horse's natural rubbing of his eye on his cannon bone.
- ★ It would be economically good if a mask could last more than one season.
- ★ Last but not least, a mask should be made of a washable, breathable fabric that allows the horse to see!

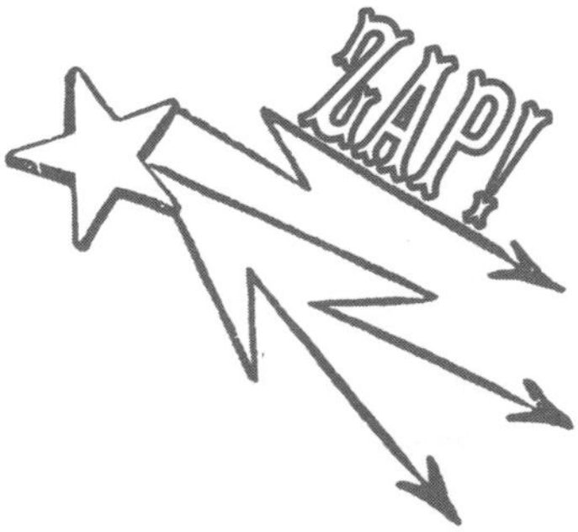

FLY MASKS FOR THERAPY. Horses that are sensitive to sunlight, dust, and dirt or those that have chronic eye problems such as conjunctivitis or periodic opthalmia (also called uveitis or moon blindness) can benefit from the use of masks year-round. Horses that suffer from uveitis are extremely sensitive to bright light, especially during periodic attacks, and suffer excessive tearing, which attracts flies. When choosing

Avoiding Blanket Zap

During dry weather, when you remove a blanket from a horse, static electricity can create a loud zap and a stinging shock that can make a horse blanket-shy. When a horse's hair coat is very dry and fluffy, it is more likely to zap. Natural oils insulate the hair shafts and cut down on zapping. That is one reason I minimize bathing, which removes natural oils, and emphasize currying and brushing, which distribute the oils to the ends of the hair.

Nylon and fleece linings seem to generate more static electricity than cotton or wool linings. Another influence on the zap factor is the temperature and humidity in your particular barn.

When I remove a horse blanket, I do not just grab the blanket and slide it across the horse's body. If I did, I would create a lot of friction, and friction creates electricity, and we do not want that. Instead, I fold the blanket in half from front to rear. Then I lift the blanket up and away from the horse's body, and when I remove it I do it one-handed. I use my left hand to remove the blanket and I leave my right hand free. That way, I don't complete an electrical circuit and the horse does not get zapped.

a mask for therapeutic purposes, it's important to take into consideration the ease of use for daily treatment because horses with chronic eye problems require a daily check, cleaning, and possibly the application of an ointment.

ANTISWEAT SHEET

An antisweat sheet is hot-weather horse clothing with two uses in our barn. We use it to prevent stalled horses from breaking into a sweat on very hot days. And we use it after a workout and cool-down or after a bath to allow a horse to dry. We tend to use antisweat sheets in our cool-down procedure in the summer and wool or synthetic fleece coolers in the winter.

Antisweat sheets are generally not used on turned-out horses, as conventional knit antisweat sheets are too easily snagged and ultra-light sheets tear if a horse rolls.

> ## Reproduction Roundup
>
> **Foal Immunization and Deworming Plan**
>
> Refer to the current recommendations of the American Association of Equine Practitioners (AAEP) or confer with your veterinarian for advice about when to begin foal immunizations. (See the Appendix for the AAEP Web site.) Opinions will vary.

FARM OFFICE

REGISTRATION AND TRANSFER OF OWNERSHIP

When buying or selling a horse, be sure that all the necessary paperwork is taken care of before money changes hands. This is especially important if you are the buyer. If you are not experienced in paperwork matters, bring along someone who is. Registration papers should bear clear title from the seller to the new buyer. Be sure the description of the horse on the papers matches the horse being sold exactly. Brand clearance and ID certification papers should unmistakably be for the horse being sold or bought. If there is a shadow of a doubt, clear it up before the final sale.

Brand clearance and ID certification papers should unmistakably be for the horse being sold or bought.

If you are a seller, the registration papers must be in your name if you are the current owner. If a previous transfer of ownership was not registered with the breed association, it could make the current sales transaction sticky. It would be as if you were trying to sell a car in San Clemente, but the title is still in Joe Brown's name and he lived in Buffalo a while back but is now deceased. This type of situation pops up quite frequently when horses change hands.

Each breed association has its own specific rules on the transfer of ownership. Often, the seller is responsible for sending in the correctly completed transfer form, the transfer fee, and the horse's current (original) registration papers. The time to find out about the required regulations is well ahead of the day you sell the horse.

RISK OF LOSS As soon as the purchase contract or transfer form is signed by the seller and the name of the buyer is entered as new owner, in most instances the risk of loss passes from the seller to the buyer. That's why a buyer can "legally" take possession of a horse before he or she actually receives "title" (the return of the papers from the breed association).

In certain transactions, instead of relying solely on this inference, it might be wise to state in the purchase agreement exactly when the risk of loss is transferred. If a buyer pays cash, the papers can be picked up on the day of sale. Otherwise, papers are held until the check clears at the bank. The buyer is usually responsible for all transfer and association fees (unless the seller has not kept the papers up to date as previously stated).

INSPECTIONS. Many states require a brand inspection each time a horse is sold or purchased. The state livestock boards are charged with protecting livestock owners. They certify that the seller or shipper is the legal owner prior to issuing a brand certificate, so inspection is usually required at the point of origin. Inspection is required on all horses

Ranch Recipes

Homemade Citronella Fly Spray

In an effort to stay away from harsh chemicals and save costs, horse owners have come up with all sorts of homemade fly spray recipes. Here is my favorite. Combine:

- ★ 2 cups water
- ★ ½ cup cider vinegar
- ★ ¼ teaspoon citronella oil

Some people prefer to use white wine vinegar.

To this mixture you can add, for your own pleasure, a few drops to ½ teaspoon of any of the following essential oils: lavender, sandalwood, cedar, tea tree, or eucalyptus.

The time to find out about the required regulations is well ahead of the day you sell the horse.

in states with brand boards, whether or not the horse is registered or branded. All horses being transported within and outside the state of origin must have a brand inspection and current health certificate (contact a local veterinarian or the state veterinarian for current information, or see the appendix). If you are selling or buying in a state that does not have an inspection law and therefore you cannot obtain a certified inspection, be sure you obtain a bill of sale and a health certificate.

Brand Awareness

Most states have brand boards that are designed to protect livestock owners by providing inspection of animals before and during transport. A "brand" inspection does not necessarily mean that the horse has been hot-branded. Even horses that have no identification markings must be inspected.

Usually any time a horse changes ownership, crosses a state line, or is transported more than 75 miles within the state, a brand inspector must physically inspect the horse and the paperwork and issue a brand clearance. In states without an inspection law, during a sale transaction you must get a bill of sale and health certificate from the seller before you transport the horse. The bill of sale must have the seller's name and signature, the buyer's name and signature, and a description of the horse (color, sex, breed, markings, registration number, brands, and so on). A witness should sign the bill of sale; notary is optional.

A Bill of Sale

Unregistered horses, those with no official papers, can be sold with or without paperwork. Inexpensive horses often change hands without a sales contract. But every transaction should be at least documented with a bill of sale.

FYI

Proof of Ownership

Horse ownership can be proven using state brand board paperwork, brands, tattoos, microchips, registration papers, and bills of sale. Each state is different, so check the laws in your state.

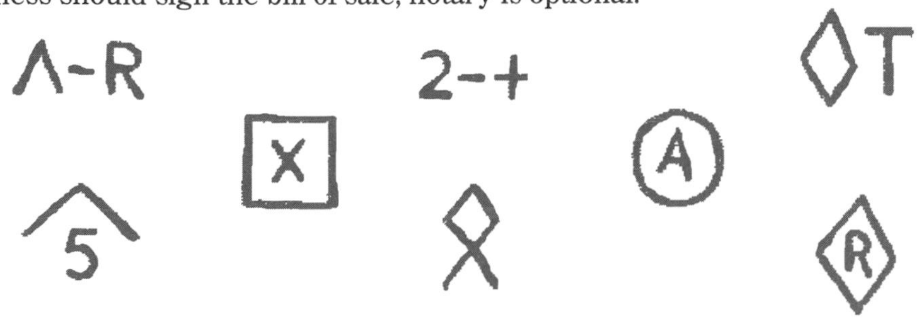

Historic brands from Wyoming

ROAD-PROOFING

Riding on the wide shoulder of a safe roadway can provide you with all sorts of opportunities to extend your horse's training. As you encounter new sights and sounds, use these opportunities to continue building the horse's confidence. Work on lengthening gaits as you head away from home, and shortening gaits on the way home. Use the edge of the road as a guide for your lateral work. But before a horse can concentrate on performing any specific maneuvers along a road, he must be relaxed and familiar with the surroundings.

Road-Riding Safety Tips

- ★ Be sure your horse is absolutely solid at all mounted work in the arena before you venture along a roadway.
- ★ Wear bright, reflective clothing.
- ★ Know the laws in your state regarding whether you should ride with or against the traffic.
- ★ If you are not completely comfortable with the idea of road riding, don't do it.

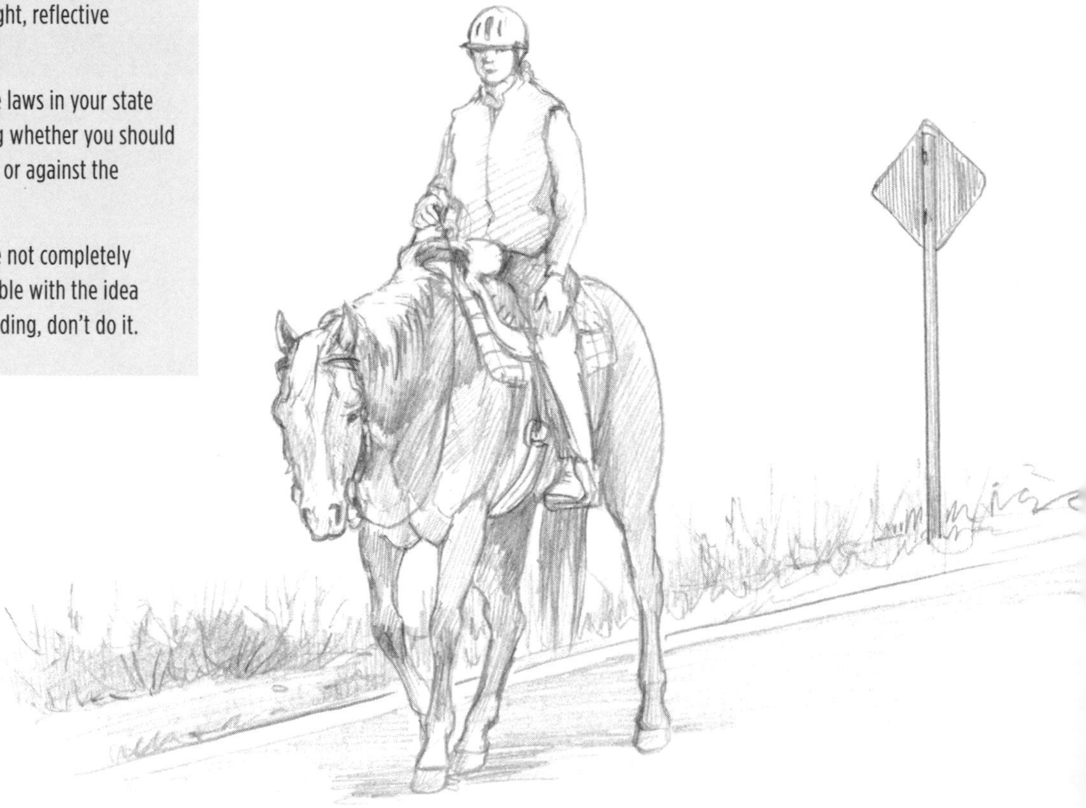

Especially if you live on a rural road, riding on the shoulder could prove to be a good change of pace from arena riding.

PREPARING FOR THE UNEXPECTED. It is impossible to predict what you will encounter on a road ride, so it will help if you can allow your horse to inspect, ahead of time, the unusual things that are commonly seen along a roadway: culverts and manholes, road signs, pieces of flapping plastic on poles or wire fences, mail boxes, and cattle guards, to mention just a few.

Approach a new object at a walk, with a relatively soft contact on the reins so that the horse can stretch his neck. This relaxes his back and allows him to reach forward to smell the new object and hopefully allay his fears. Be ready, however, to ride a sudden reaction calmly. If your body language and voice truly convince your horse that there is nothing to fear, he may pass a potentially frightening object with just a sideways glance. If you anticipate a strong reaction to a new object, the horse may sense your apprehension through his back, on his sides, and in his mouth, and you may make him unnecessarily suspicious and tense.

STAGING THE SCENE. It is often beneficial to stage some roadside scenarios in which you know what's coming and can concentrate on your horse. For example, you will inevitably encounter large and noisy vehicles and machinery on a road ride. Tractors, school buses, road graders, and the like tend to overload a horse's sensory apparatus and can cause panic. Don't expect drivers to be safety-conscious or considerate.

Horses that are pastured alongside a busy highway may have no fear of large vehicles, but a horse not so broad in his experiences may become terrified if a stock trailer comes rattling up behind him or the driver of a large truck applies the air brake just as he passes you. Therefore, familiarize your young horse first with parked cars, pickup trucks, and tractors, then with vehicles that are idling, and finally with vehicles that are moving. Arrange for someone to pass

Horse Sense and Safety

Leading a Horse

★ Make the horse walk beside you. You should be next to his neck or shoulder. He should not lag behind or pull ahead of you.

★ Turn the horse away from you and walk around him rather than having him walk around you. Turning away is the safest way to turn. Once you know your horse, you will want to be able to turn him toward yourself, too.

I've spent most of my life riding horses. The rest I've wasted.

— Anonymous

repeatedly on the road in a vehicle until your horse is no longer afraid. Initially, a horse may veer sideways as the vehicle passes, but by the fourth or fifth pass, his reaction will probably be reduced to just a shudder of concern.

A horse may be reassured if he realizes that there is a human associated with the vehicle. The sound of a human voice allows the horse to relate the vehicle to something he already has experience with and trusts — humans. Exchange verbal greetings with the driver to set a horse at ease. Some horses need further reassurance: allow the horse to approach the stopped vehicle and smell it or even sniff the driver's outstretched hand.

> *It is not best* to swap horses while crossing the river.
> — Abraham Lincoln, 1864

Although it is generally best not to dismount in order to encourage a horse to move near or over an object, there are no absolutes in horse training. There are occasions where it might be beneficial to lead a horse up to an object. This is where your thorough in-hand work will prove its worth.

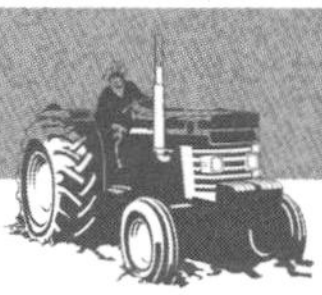

RPMS & PTOS

MANURE SPREADERS

Manure spreaders are wagons with a mechanical apparatus designed to distribute manure as the tractor is driven through a pasture or field. Smaller spreaders are friction-driven; larger spreaders are powered by the tractor's power take-off (PTO).

Friction-drive spreaders (also called ground-drive spreaders) are ground driven, that is, the power for unloading and spreading is generated by the tires of the spreader rolling on the ground. A ground-drive spreader is usually a simple setup with just two levers: one to control the speed of the apron chain, which moves the load toward the rear of the spreader, and one to activate the beater bars at the

Friction-drive spreader

PTO-drive spreader

back of the spreader. The beater bars break up the manure and fling it into the air. You can drive to your pasture without spreading manure along the way, and then activate the apron chain and beater bar to start spreading. Since these spreaders don't have a rotating driveline, they are potentially safer than a PTO-driven spreader.

The drawback to this type of spreader is that the tow vehicle must be moving for the spreading mechanism to be activated. A friction spreader can be operated behind a tractor, pickup, or even a team of horses, though in order to use a spreader with a team, you must purchase a conversion kit.

Spreaders powered by a PTO are usually bigger, heavy-duty machines, suitable for a horse farm or ranch as opposed to a small acreage. The PTO can make them more difficult to hook up, but they have several advantages, one being larger capacity. Another advantage is that because the spreader speed can be controlled separately from the ground speed, the manure can be spread heavily or lightly or even piled in one spot if desired.

en español

bronc, bronco. Comes from *el bronco*, meaning 'wild horse'.

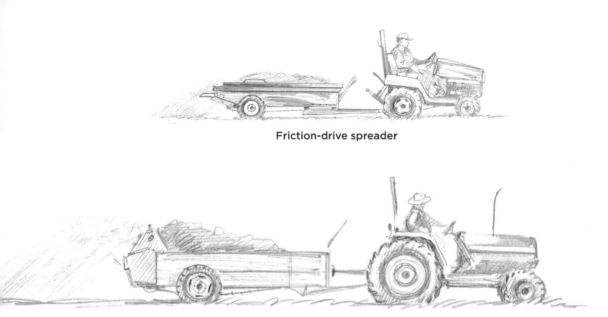

What to Look For in a Spreader

With any spreader, look for one with up-front controls that you can operate from the tractor seat. A hydraulic gear case selector is more desirable than a rope pull. Some spreaders have as many as five apron chain speeds. There can be as many as three sets of beater bars (with ripper teeth) or paddles at the rear of the spreader.

Spreaders are most commonly available with rubber tires, but flotation tires are available for soft ground. Steel wheels (rims only) are seen on older spreaders. A separate brake system on the spreader is appropriate for heavy loads.

An end gate is an option that comes in handy if you will be hauling wet loads or if you want to heap the spreader to capacity. End gates are either manual or hydraulic. A front box extension builds up the front of the spreader to allow more heaping and to prevent manure from dropping onto the drive mechanism.

Spreader floors are made of ¾-inch tongue-and-groove polyethylene, marine plywood, or steel. Some spreader boxes are lined with recycled high-density plastic. A slick surface is preferable, because manure doesn't freeze to it and it is easy to clean. Choose a floor material that doesn't warp, bulge, or bow, which could hamper the movement of the conveyor bar.

A slip clutch can protect your chain and beaters. A large, frozen clump of manure wedged in the beater can break shear bolts, snap the chain, or damage bars or paddles. With a slip clutch feature, the spreader mechanism stops operating when it gets clogged.

To comply with regulations requiring thin application to reduce contamination from runoff, you can purchase optional equipment to further reduce the conveyor speed. This is especially good if you spread fresh manure or manure without bedding.

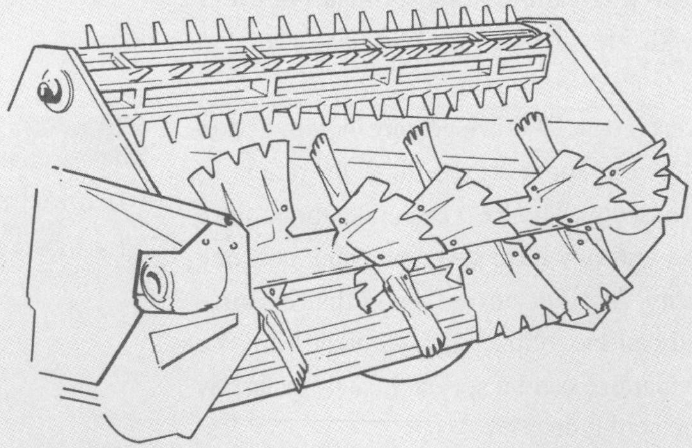

WHAT SIZE SHOULD IT BE? Spreader capacity is measured in cubic feet. You will see two figures in spreader capacity stats — struck and heaped. Struck refers to a level load, and heaped is a mounded load. What size spreader you choose will depend on whether you spread manure daily on cropland or non-horse pasture. If you do, you may prefer a smaller spreader that can be pulled by a garden tractor, ATV, or UV and that is narrow enough to fit in pens and barn aisles or can back into a stall. If you compost manure (the most environmentally responsible method) and spread it months later as humus, your annual or semiannual spreading will go faster with a larger-capacity spreader, especially if the distance from the pile to the field is far. For five or more horses, figure on a 75-cubic-foot manure spreader or larger. For operations with very large manure-hauling needs, truck-mounted spreaders are available and would be warranted if you need to drive far on highways to spread.

If you spread daily, refer to the chart below to evaluate spreader capacity.

Odd Word

"Long in the tooth." This phrase means "old," although it is not completely accurate in our modern context. It has its origin in the early 1900s. Back in those days, horses didn't live as long as they do now. When a horse's teeth became elongated and angled, he was termed "long in the tooth" and was considered old. Today, horses live until their 30s and even 40s, and because horse teeth quit growing, they wear their teeth short or lose them. Thus, an equivalent phrase today might be "short in the tooth" or even "gummin' it"!

Choosing Your Spreader Capacity

Number of stalls or pens	Spreader Capacity (in cubic feet)	Type of tractor	Wheelbarrow equivalent
1	10	Garden tractor, ATV, or UV	2
2–4	25	Garden tractor, ATV, or UV	5
4–6	35	Garden tractor, ATV, or UV	7
5–10	55	Compact	11
12–20	75	Compact	15
More than 20	100	Utility or standard	20
Commercial stable	125 or larger	Utility or standard	25

WHAT WE DO AT LONG TAIL RANCH. We have seven horses. We collect manure every day, compost it, and spread the humus once a year. We have an International Harvester 540 PTO-driven manure spreader that has a 90-cubic-foot capacity struck and 135-cubic-foot capacity heaped. It takes seven tractor bucket loads to fill the spreader to heaped capacity. We have 70 acres divided into nine pastures. We spread approximately 10 to 15 manure spreader loads of humus on our pastures per year, rotating between pastures from year to year.

FINE FACILITIES

FIRE PREVENTION

Fire is the most common disaster on a horse farm or ranch. Preventing fires and being prepared in the event of a fire can mean the difference between life and death for your livestock. Fire prevention and safety practices are essential.

Prohibit smoking in or around barns, hay and bedding storage, and machinery storage buildings. A discarded cigarette can ignite dry bedding or hay in seconds.

Avoid parking tractors and vehicles in or near the barn. Engine heat and backfires can spark a flame. Also, store other machinery and flammable materials outside the barn.

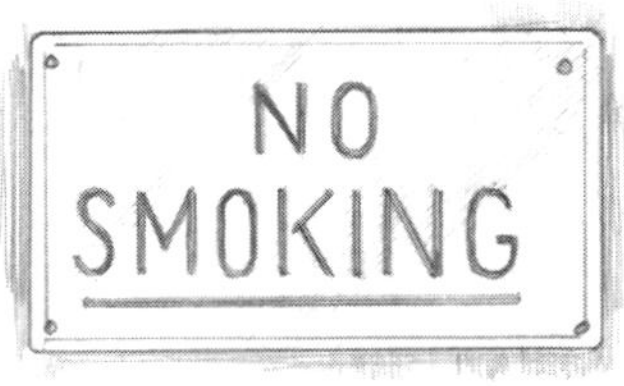

Inspect electrical systems regularly. Immediately correct any problems. Rodents can chew on electrical wiring and cause damage that quickly becomes a fire hazard.

Keep appliances to a minimum in the barn, and use them only when someone is in the barn.

Be sure hay is dry before storing it. Hay that is too moist may spontaneously combust. Store hay outside of the barn in a dry, covered area when possible.

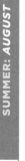

Fire Prevention Checklist

1. Store the majority of your hay in a building separate from the barn.

2. Keep grass and weeds mowed for 20 to 30 feet around the barn, pens, and storage buildings, and keep this area free of brush and debris.

3. Clearly post phone numbers of the fire department and police next to phone, along with your address and directions to your barn.

4. Make sure electrical wiring complies with the National Electrical Code; run wire in conduit; protect outlets and switch boxes from dust and moisture with spring-loaded weather-proof covers and replace broken faceplates; keep panel boxes covered, dry, and dust-free.

5. Maintain a serious rodent control program: most barn fires are caused by electrical system malfunctions, and rodents can chew through the plastic insulation on wires, causing them to spark (see September Pest Patrol).

6. Keep a garden hose hanging next to each hydrant; in freezing weather, keep the hose drained and free of ice. Buckets of sand are also useful for smothering a fire.

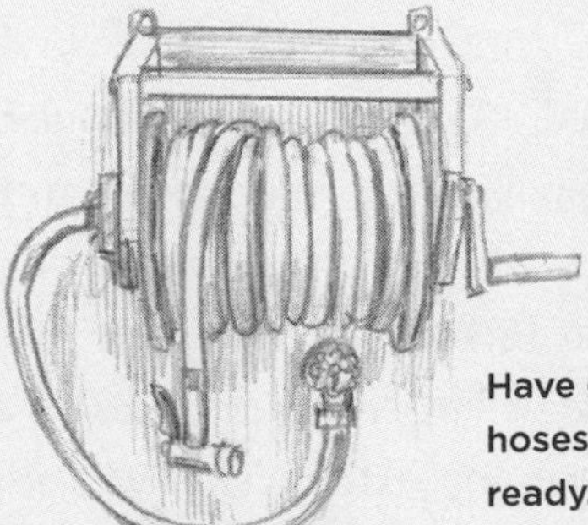

Have garden hoses at the ready.

7. Post "No Smoking" signs throughout your property and strictly enforce them.

8. Keep your barn clean, well organized, and free of combustible trash.

9. Locate fully charged fire extinguishers, at least one by each entrance, so a person doesn't have to travel more than 50 feet from anywhere in the barn to reach one. Clean and inspect each unit once a month.

10. Install appropriate smoke detectors inside the barn and hook them to a siren or bell on the outside.

11. Install a system of 12-foot-tall lightning rods, no more than 20 feet apart, connected by a braided aluminum or copper cable to at least two 10-foot-long ground rods.

12. Keep dust and moisture off light bulbs with protective covers.

13. Consider installing a sprinkler system if your water supply can support one.

14. Remove cobwebs and dust periodically; a vacuum works well.

15. Clean the barn thoroughly at least once a year.

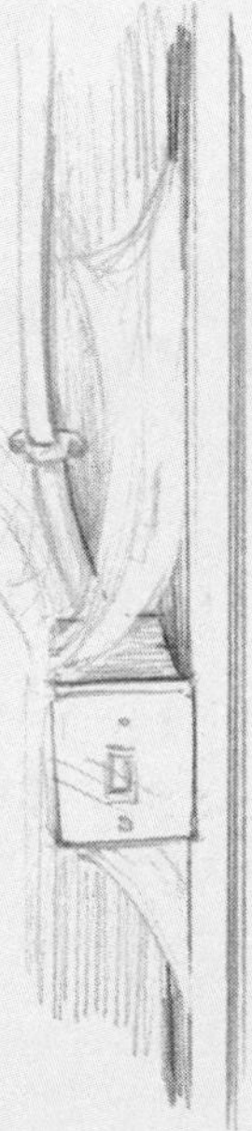

Keep all light switches and plugs free of dust and spiderwebs.

BE PREPARED FOR A FIRE. Mount fire extinguishers in all buildings, especially at all entrances. Make sure they are current and that your family, boarders, and employees know how to use them. Keep aisles, stall doors, and barn doors free of debris and equipment. Have a planned evacuation route for every area of your farm, and familiarize all family members and employees with your evacuation plans. Consider installing a sprinkler system if you have the water supply and water pressure to run one.

If you have a large breeding or boarding farm, host an open house for emergency services personnel in your area to familiarize them with the layout of your property. Provide them with tips on handling your animals or present a mini-seminar with hands-on training. Familiarize your animals with emergency procedures and common things they would encounter during a disaster. Try to desensitize them to flashlights and flashing lights.

FIRE EXTINGUISHERS. Fires are classified A, B, or C according to what substance is burning, and fire extinguishers are likewise rated by which type of fire the unit is designed to extinguish. Class A fires involve solids such as paper, wood, and hay. Class B fires involve liquids such as solvents and paint. Class C fires are class A or B fires that also involve electrical wiring or equipment that is plugged in, such as vacuums, clippers, and heaters. A fire extinguisher rated A:B:C is best for a barn, because it will work on all three types of fire.

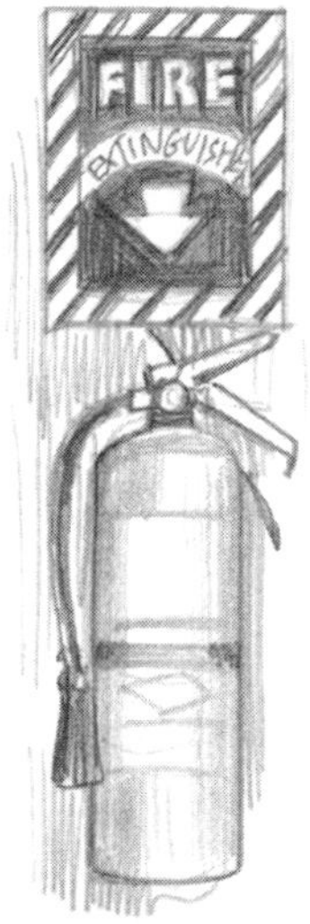

Make sure all fire extinguishers are current and that everyone who uses your barn knows how to operate them.

An extinguisher rated 3A:40B:C weighs about 8 to 10 pounds, which is light enough for most people to handle easily. Units of this size will project a stream of chemical about 15 feet for 8 to 15 seconds. Have one fire extinguisher, at least this size or larger, for every 3,000 square feet of barn space. Locate one extinguisher at each door, and have enough units so a person doesn't have to travel more than 50 feet from anywhere in the barn to reach one. Each fire extinguisher should be mounted in plain view and should not double as a blanket or tack hanger.

IN THE EVENT OF A BARN FIRE

- Immediately call 911 or your local emergency services.
- Do not enter any building if it is already engulfed in flames.
- If it is safe for you to enter the barn, evacuate animals starting with the most accessible ones.
- Move animals quickly to a fenced area far enough from the fire and smoke. Never let animals loose in an area where they are able to return to a burning building.

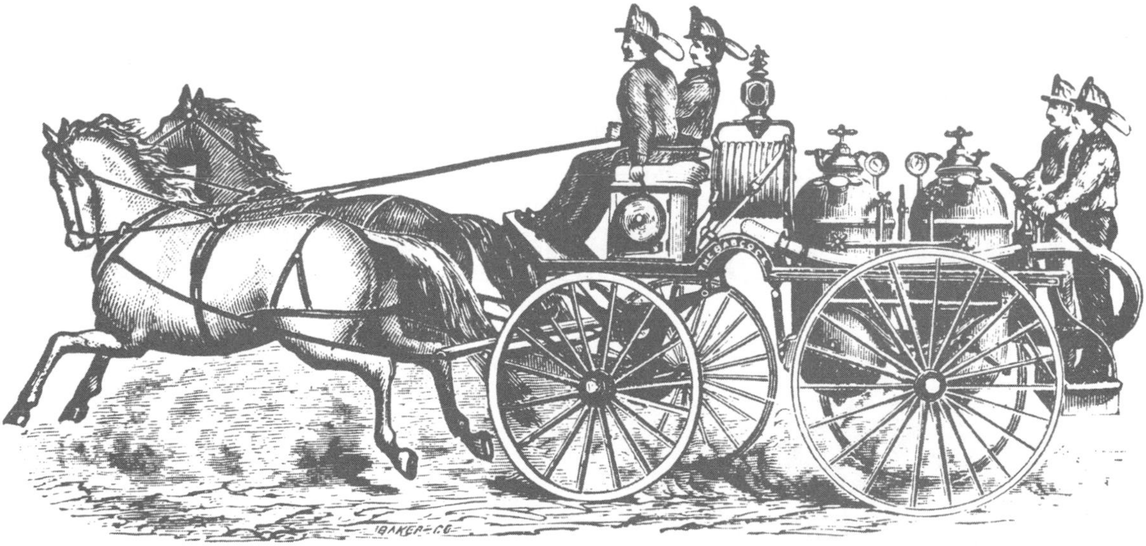

MORE IN DEPTH

Fire Bans

Fire bans during the summer can include any or all of the following, so check with your local authorities: no open fires, fireworks, or explosives, and during extreme conditions, no grills, outdoor welding, or smoking outdoors.

FOREST FIRES

Often during August there will be one or two forest fires raging within 100 miles of our ranch, and sometimes as many as five in the state at one time. They range in size from a few acres quickly brought under control to forest fires that burn more than 10,000 acres. Sometimes they are caused by dry lightning, the kind that rumbles and cracks and produces ghost rain. Other times they have been caused by an irresponsible camper, a transient, an arsonist, or a homeowner burning leaves or trash during a drought.

One day as Richard and I were coming home from town we came upon a scorched SUV with a black patch radiating out from it for hundreds of acres. Apparently, the brakes caught fire and the folks pulled over and abandoned their vehicle. The grass fire quickly whipped up the mountainside, where the timber provided more fuel. By the next evening, there were about a dozen hot spots left, but firefighters had it 90 percent contained and were able to stop the fire about a mile and a half from our southernmost pasture fence. All the while, we were rehearsing our fire plan. Be sure you have one.

Estimating Water Use

I estimate that during 90° to 100°F drought weather, with 20 to 30 percent humidity, my adult horses drink between 15 to 20 gallons per day depending on their level of activity. Horses in work might consume even more than that (but who would work in such heat!), and a lactating broodmare certainly requires more water.

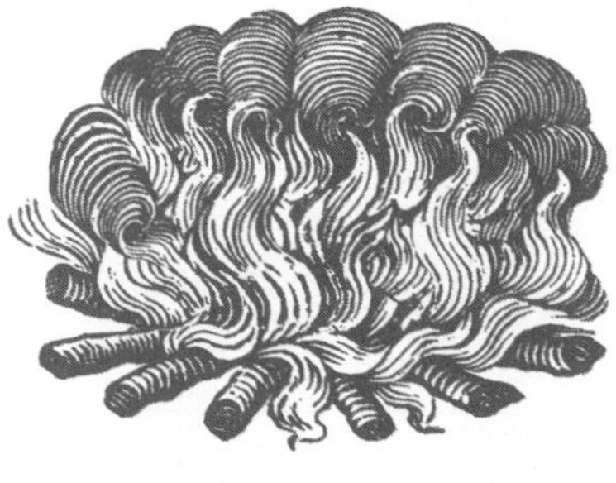

Horse owners in fire areas that have to evacuate their stock do so either by making several trips with horse trailers or by turning their animals loose with phone numbers painted (with a livestock grease pencil) on the animals' sides. Although many area residents volunteer their trucks and trailers to help fire victims evacuate their horses, it is not as simple as that. Often the normal roads are closed or traffic is limited to fire-fighting equipment only. All horse owners should have a fire plan in place, whether you live in a forested area or not.

———————— ★ ————————

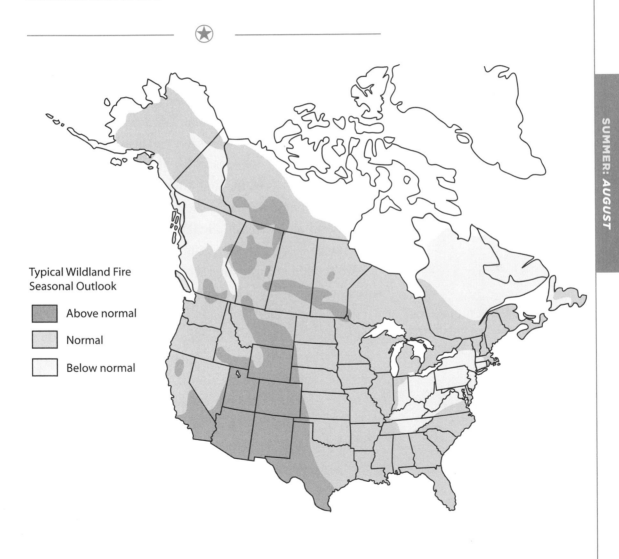

Typical Wildland Fire
Seasonal Outlook

■ Above normal

▨ Normal

□ Below normal

DROUGHT

When water is plentiful, I take for granted being able to spray off a horse after a workout, being able to do weekly horse laundry, or, for that matter, being able to water my flower barrels up at the barn. A drought can change all that.

If you are relying on natural water sources for your horse, check daily to be sure water is flowing, because stagnant water is not good for horses and no water at all is really not good.

DRINKING WATER. When our creek goes dry, we know we are in a drought. If you are relying on natural water sources for your horse, check daily to be sure water is flowing, because stagnant water is not good for horses and no water at all is really not good.

When you estimate your water usage you might find that you need to have supplementary water on hand in case of well problems. Extra water can also come in handy for fire control if necessary. We have two 1,000-gallon underground cisterns for such water emergencies, but we recently bought a 425-gallon pickup water tank, a popular item in arid and semiarid climates. They are available at farm supply stores. The tank fits into the back of a pickup truck. When filled with water it weighs 3,400 pounds, so be sure to haul it with a vehicle can tow that weight.

We prefer to haul our water tank on a flatbed trailer so the pickup is not "tied up" being a water tank carrier. Alternatively, you could empty the pickup tank as soon as you get the water home. Our tank has a hose bib at the bottom, and we leave the tank on the trailer parked uphill from the horse pens to gravity-feed water to the horse tubs as needed. We use the tank to haul water out to pasture horses and deer or other wildlife.

A water tank that fits into your truck is a great advantage in a drought- or fire-prone area.

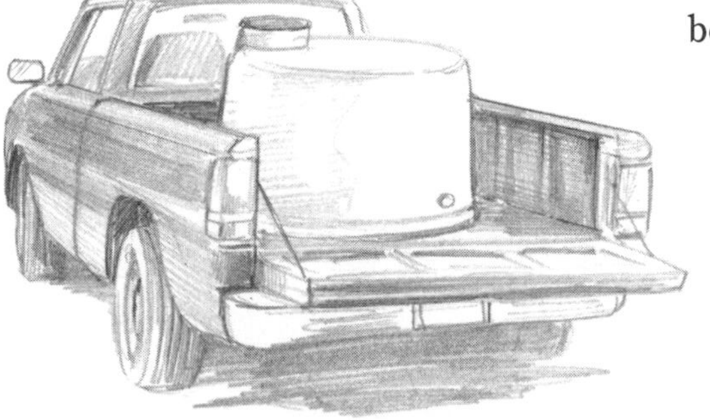

SHADE. Provide natural or man-made shade areas for horses on pasture or in pens. Trees, run-in sheds, or lean-to shelters will give your horse a place to get out of the direct rays of the sun and escape the flies as well.

HORSE EXERCISE. Reduce your riding and training program during abnormally hot and dry weather. When bringing a horse back to work that has been standing for even just a few weeks, be careful. The extra pounds of fat that the horse might have gained will make it more difficult for him to cool his body. Heat dissipates slowly and fatigue sets in more quickly when a horse is fat or out of condition. When a horse is fatigued, and especially when his tendons and muscles are not in condition, he is more likely to injure himself. So start back slowly.

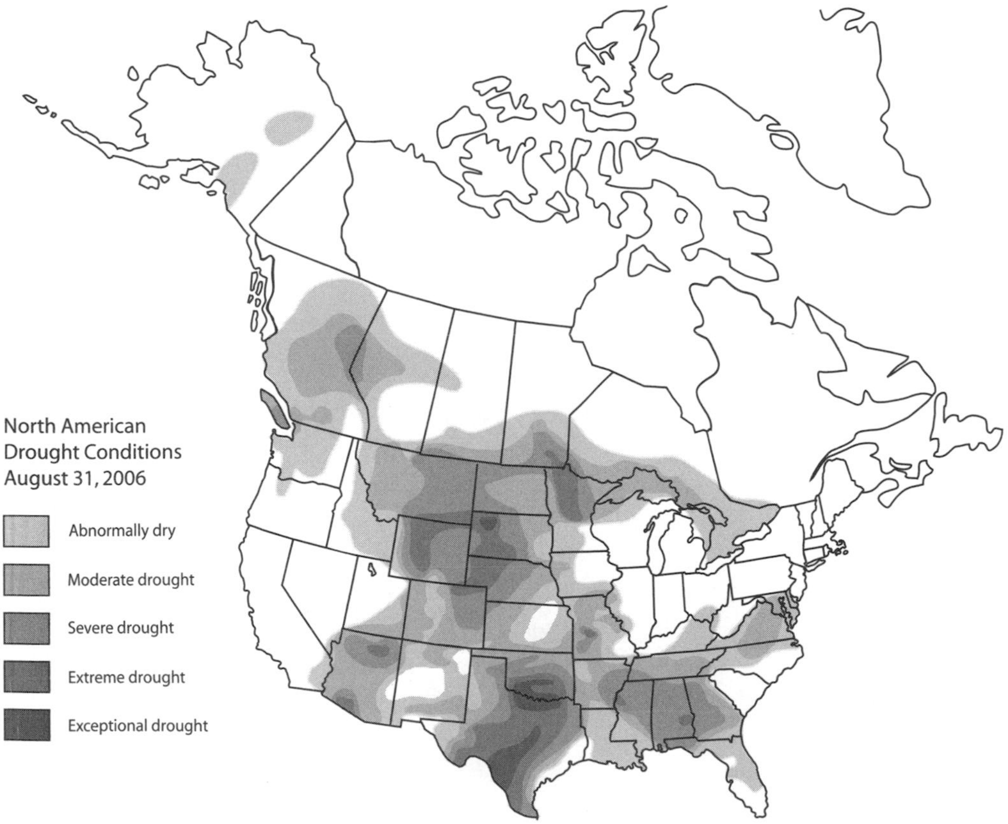

Drought and the Diet

Feed

I'm not a big fan of feeding alfalfa to horses anyway, but legume hays such as alfalfa increase water intake so it is best to eliminate feeding alfalfa during hot weather and focus on grass hay. Also, grains that are quickly digested actually keep the horse "cooler" than those that take longer to digest. That is why corn is a better summer feed and oats (which take longer to digest because of their hulls) make a better winter feed.

Salt

Be sure each of your horses has access to salt 24 hours a day. I provide each of my horses with a plain white salt block (NaCl, sodium chloride) plus a 1:1 Ca:P (that's one part calcium to one part phosphorus) trace-mineral salt block.

Fiber Alternatives

Remember that your horse should receive 1½ to 2 percent of his body weight per day in hay or an equivalent in another fiber. Some options include:

- **Hay cubes.** Most are alfalfa, which might not suit many horse's dietary requirements. Grass cubes are less common.
- **Pellets or wafers.** Again, the base is mostly alfalfa and some horses can gobble pellets, meaning less satiation, less chewing, and more choke.
- **Beet pulp.** Can be used for up to half the fiber requirements (see January Ranch Recipes and March Feed Bag).

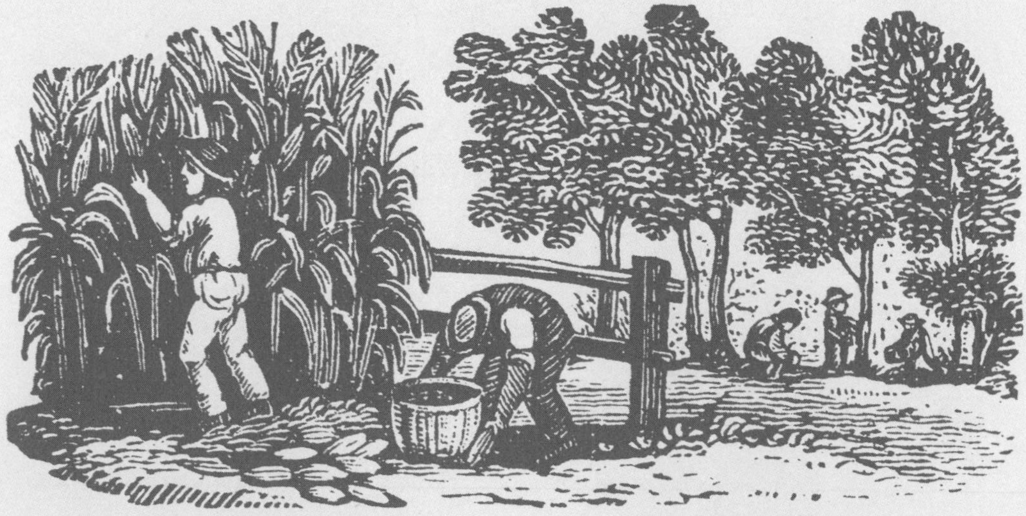

PASTURE MANAGEMENT. During extreme drought, pasture management is simple: no grazing. We take all of our horses off pasture and keep them on dry lots. All pastures are empty (except for our resident deer population). When it is abnormally dry, many pasture grasses are stunted, but the opportunistic drought-resistant weeds thrive, especially without the competition from the pasture grasses. Often during a drought, the toxic substances in poisonous plants can become concentrated and problems can even occur with grasses and nonpoisonous weeds that tend to concentrate their nutrients during a drought. Hay grown and harvested during a drought can be similarly affected.

Our weed control during a drought consists of:

- Hand-pulling, boot-kicking, and hoeing of large-stem weeds that have cropped up in small concentrated patches
- Spot spraying using a shoulder-mounted tank and walking through pastures for those loner weeds that don't group
- Mowing large areas of weeds with tractor mower set just above the grasses but low enough to lop off seed-forming weed tops

> *en español*
>
> **mustang.** Comes from *el mestengo* or *el mesteño*, 'a stray animal'.

> *Often during a drought, the toxic substances in poisonous plants can become concentrated.*

Disaster Preparedness

Disaster preparedness is important for horses, due to their size and their shelter and transportation needs. While it is true that disasters might be more likely in a flood plain, near an earthquake fault line, or in a coastal area, disasters can include barn fires, flash floods, hazardous spills, and explosions. Have one plan for evacuation and one plan for sheltering in place. Create a list of emergency telephone numbers, including those of your employees, neighbors, veterinarian, state veterinarian, poison control, local animal shelter, animal care and control, county extension service,

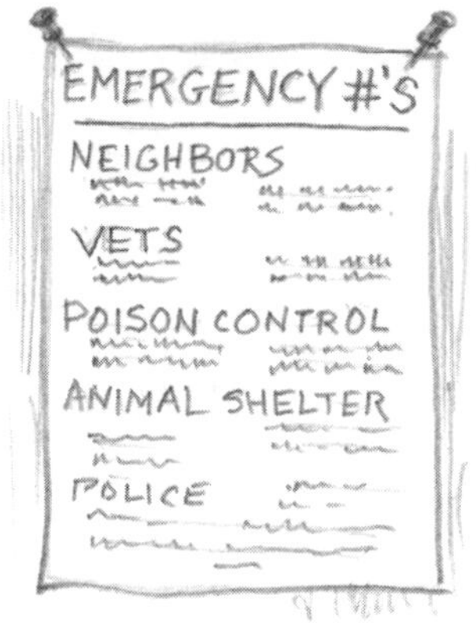

local agricultural schools, trailering resources, and local volunteers. Include a contact person outside the disaster area. Make sure all this information is written down and that key people in your group have a copy. Make sure every animal has durable and visible identification.

DISASTER-PROOF YOUR PROPERTY

If you are in a wind- or hurricane-prone area, install hurricane straps and other measures. Secure or remove anything that could become blowing debris; make a habit of securing trailers, propane tanks, and other large objects. Perform regular safety checks on all utilities, buildings, and facilities on your farm. Use only native and deep-rooted plants and trees in landscaping (nonnative plants are less durable and hardy in your climate and may become dislodged by high winds or broken by ice and snow).

Barbed wire should not be used on a horse farm or ranch, but if you've inherited an older place, remove all

Farm Disaster Kit

Gather the items you will need in one safe, central location where everyone at your site can access them. Include the following items:

- ❑ Current list of all animals and their locations
- ❑ Proof of ownership and ID papers
- ❑ Supplies for temporary identification of your animals, such as plastic neckbands and/or grease pencils to label animals with your name, address, and telephone number
- ❑ All contact information
- ❑ Basic first-aid kit
- ❑ Halters and lead ropes
- ❑ Water, feed, and buckets
- ❑ Extra flashlights and batteries
- ❑ Other safety and emergency items for your truck and trailer

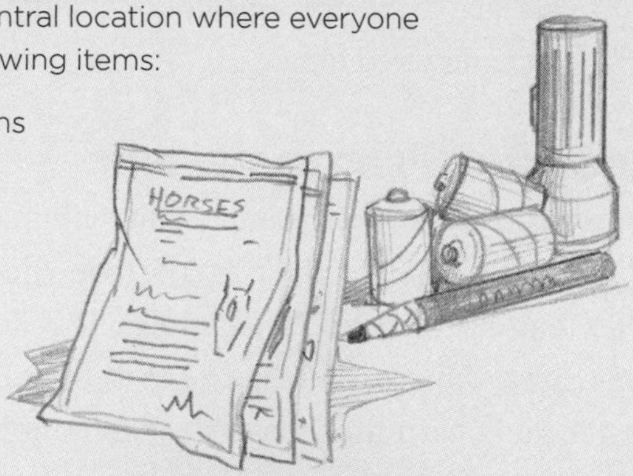

barbed wire, and consider rerouting permanent fencing so that animals may move to high ground in a flood and to low-lying areas during high winds.

Install a cistern or other container for water storage. If you have large feed and water troughs, fill them up ahead of time with water. You can even fill up a boat — this will not only keep it from blowing away but can provide you with needed water. Set up the water supply for gravity feed, hand pump, or generator so you can pump the water in the event of a power outage or water contamination. A generator with a safely stored supply of fuel can help you operate some necessary electrical equipment.

EVACUATION PLANNING

The leading causes of death of large animals in hurricanes and similar events are collapsed barns, dehydration, electrocution, and accidents resulting from fencing failure. Be ready to leave once an evacuation is ordered. In a slowly evolving disaster, such as a hurricane, leave no later than 72 hours before anticipated landfall, especially if you will be hauling a high-profile trailer such as a horse trailer. Even a fire truck fully loaded with water is considered "out of service" in winds exceeding 40 miles per hour. If there are already high winds, it may not be possible to evacuate safely.

Arrange for a place to shelter your animals. Plan ahead and work within your community to establish safe shelters for your horses. Potential facilities include fairgrounds, other farms, racetracks, humane societies, convention centers, and any other safe and appropriate facilities you can find. Survey your community and potential host communities along your planned evacuation route ahead of time. Contact your local emergency management authority and become familiar with at least two possible evacuation routes well in advance.

Ready for Anything

Post emergency telephone numbers at each telephone and at each entrance. Emergency telephone numbers should include those of the veterinarian, emergency response personnel, and qualified livestock handlers.

Keep your barn's street address clearly posted to relay to the 911 operator or your community's emergency services. Be sure your address and the entrance to your farm are clearly visible from the main road.

Install smoke alarms and heat detectors in all buildings. New heat sensors can detect rapidly changing temperatures in buildings. Smoke detectors and heat sensors should be hooked up to sirens that will quickly alert you and your neighbors to a possible fire.

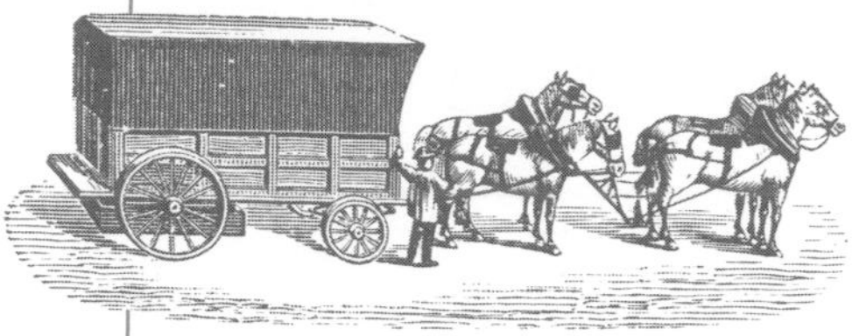

Set up safe transportation. Trucks, trailers, and other vehicles suitable for transporting livestock (appropriate for each specific type of animal) should be available, along with experienced handlers and drivers.

Take all your disaster supplies with you or make sure they will be available at your evacuation site. Have or be able to readily obtain feed, water, veterinary supplies, handling equipment, tools, and generators if necessary.

If your animals are sheltered off your property, make sure they remain in the groupings they are used to. Also, be sure they are securely contained and sheltered from the elements if necessary, whether in cages or kennels, fenced-in areas, or buildings.

Although summer seems to be the jewel in the crown, truth be told, I'm looking forward to my favorite season, fall.

Sheltering in Place

Depending on the lay of your land, the particular disaster, and your capabilities, you might be better off sheltering in place. First, decide whether to confine large animals in an available shelter on your farm or leave them out on pasture. While you might think that your horses would be safer inside the barn, in some circumstances, they would be better off fending for themselves, avoiding danger. If your pastures pass the following list of criteria, your horses might fare best on pasture.

★ No exotic (nonnative) trees, which uproot easily

★ No overhead power lines or poles

★ No debris or sources of blowing debris

★ No barbed-wire fencing

★ Not smaller than 1 acre (smaller pastures make it more difficult for horses to avoid debris)

Buddy-Sour Solutions

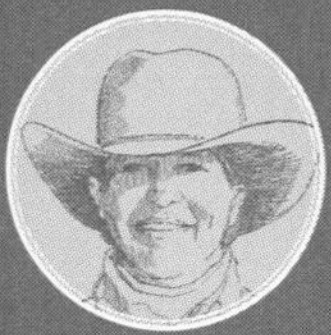

Ask Cherry

Q

After 20 years away from riding, I purchased a four-year-old Quarter Horse/Arab. She's about 14.2 hands. I feel comfortable on her but she is buddy-sour and that is why she was sold. When I rode her alone, she tested me to see if I'd let her return to the barn, but she responded to my cues for turning and moving forward. I used a hollow O-ring snaffle; they had used a Tom Thumb curb. I felt I could manage her.

The second time I rode her for two hours along with her buddy. She was very relaxed until I moved her away from her buddy. Then she "pretended" to shy, pranced, rose up slightly on her back legs, and held her head up high. I made her stand still, facing away, for about two seconds, then cued her to turn and walk back to her buddy.

When I bring her home, she'll be alone except for some chickens beside her 15 x 9 stall, a dog, and my horse-crazy 12-year-old daughter. I worried she'd be stressed being alone, but I've heard this might be good for her and help her become bonded to me easier. I plan to leave her in her stall and work around her a lot until she settles down. Then I will hand-walk her around our pasture and property until she is familiar with the surroundings. Do you have any other advice about managing her stress level when I bring her home? Thank you so much!

A

It sounds as though you have connected well with this horse and have a good handle on things. And I agree that having the mare alone at your new home will be a good thing. You will be able to continue building your horse–human bond while she adapts to her new home. This really is ideal and is actually the "treatment" I recommend to people who have buddy-sour horses. I often suggest they try to find a neighbor who will take the buddy for a while to help break the bond and allow for the formation of a better human–horse bond with the horse that remains at home.

My suggestions are: make sure the horse gets plenty of exercise, including turnout, in-hand work (as you suggested around your property), some ground work (such as longeing and ground driving), and riding in various places and at various times of the day. The more varied you can make your interactions, the more solid and strong your bond will become. Don't overfeed your horse or it could create excess energy and don't leave her in the stall for too long as that can tip the anxiety scale as well.

Dealing with Rearing

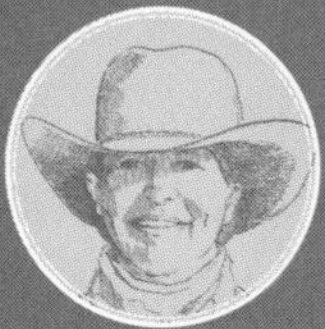

Ask Cherry

Q

I'm leasing a horse that rears when she doesn't want to go — not very high, but enough to be annoying. I've tried her with other riders, saddles, bits, and bridles, and with and without splint boots. I was wondering if I should find another horse to lease and give up on Scooter or if I should keep looking for the root of the problem?

A

It is admirable that you are trying to solve this horse's problem, but there are two habits that often require the assistance of a qualified professional horse trainer — rearing and kicking. Work with an experienced instructor who can diagnose this horse's problem in person. Although the mare isn't rearing very high now, such behavior often gets worse rather than better. When a horse rears, you can easily fall off, and when a horse really gets into rearing high, he can fall over backwards, which can be deadly.

What causes rearing? Rearing is an "avoidance behavior." The horse is trying to avoid going forward. She has not learned that when you say go forward, she must go forward, so she is confused and needs progressive training and a review of the basics. It could be a horse that is becoming herd-bound or barn-sour and does not want to leave the barn or her buddies. She is saying, "No." The horse needs to develop security and confidence in the rider. It could be that at one time this horse received a sharp jerk or rough handling when she did go forward, so now she is afraid to go forward. When a horse that rears is switched from a curb bit to a snaffle and the rider is very good with her hands (following the horse's movement), the horse can learn to move out (forward) rather than up (rearing). It is important that when you apply the leg cue for the horse to go forward, you don't pull on the bit, as those would be conflicting, confusing signals. (You should rule out dental and spinal causes by having a veterinarian check the horse's mouth and back.)

You can also review forward lessons with in-hand work (walk out and trot out promptly when leading) and longeing, concentrating on the horse working in a long, low frame with lots of extended trot-type work, rather than collected work. Collecting a horse too soon or improperly can lead to rearing. Since you are leasing this horse, ask the owner for insights into this behavior. If you are unable to resolve the problem, then yes, you should find another horse to lease. It is not worth the risk.

FALL

SEPTEMBER TO OCTOBER

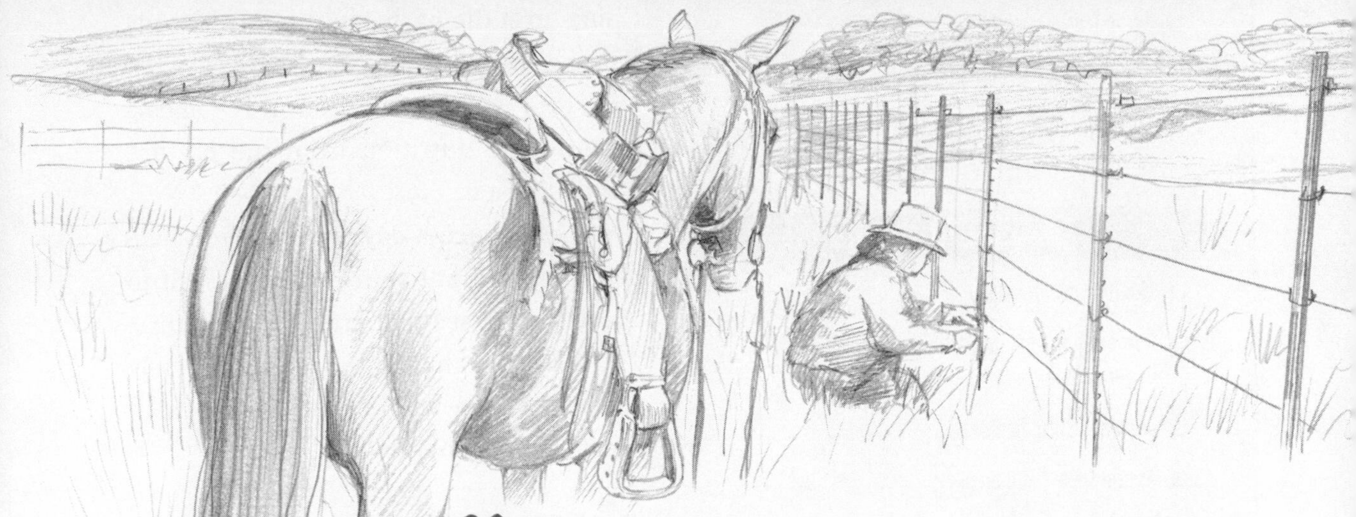

It doesn't get any better than this. Fall in the foothills of the Rockies: my favorite temperatures, the sun's rays not so harsh, beautiful foliage, and the worst of the fire season behind us. With the hay barn full and less mowing to do, the days are getting shorter but there is plenty of time for trail riding. Of course winter is just around the corner and can come early, so in between moseying down those trails and listening to those leaves crunch underfoot, we have to get things ready for winter.

Weekly Tasks

- ❑ Restock the hay supply in horse barns
- ❑ Check grain supply
- ❑ Check bedding supply
- ❑ Dump and scrub all waterers, troughs, tanks, tubs, and buckets
- ❑ Scrub feed dishes
- ❑ Check veterinary and grooming supply needs
- ❑ Check upcoming farrier and veterinarian appointments and prepare for them

Seasonal Tasks

- ❑ Monitor pastures daily
- ❑ Remove horses from pasture while there is still vegetation in the field
- ❑ Final mow of pasture
- ❑ Assign sheets and blankets
- ❑ Harrow manure on pastures that will be vacant over the winter
- ❑ Remove bot eggs
- ❑ Allow horses to gain about 5 percent body weight to prepare for winter
- ❑ Wash fly sheets and store
- ❑ Winterize tractor and truck
- ❑ Get snow removal equipment ready
- ❑ Winterize barn water pipes
- ❑ Oil hinges and latches to prevent freezing
- ❑ Give manure spreader a checkup
- ❑ Install snow fence as needed

Almost any time of the day is great riding weather, so we take our longer rides during this time of year and fit the indoor work in where there is room. Some horses are still out on pasture full time (depending on the year), but most are on short turnouts. I still keep the horses we are riding up at the barn and they are already hairing up for winter. I've increased the feed they receive at their three meals because the nutrition from the pasture has decreased.

At least once a day, frequently in midmorning, I go out with my pasture kit to check the horses that are still on pasture. The horses might still be wearing their fly sheets, or some might now wear turnout sheets or no blankets.

Fall Visual Exam

OVERALL STANCE AND ATTITUDE. As I approach the horse, does he have his head up, are his eyes bright, and is he eager for feed, or is he lethargic, inattentive, or anxious? Does he need to gain weight before winter?

LEGS. I look thoroughly at the horse from both sides so I will quickly spot any wounds, swelling, or puffiness.

APPETITE. Has the horse finished all of his feed from the previous feeding?

WATER. Is there evidence that he has taken in a sufficient amount of water?

MANURE. Is the fecal material well formed, or is it hard and dry, loose and sloppy, covered with mucus or parasites, or filled with whole grains? Are there at least three or four manure piles since I last fed?

PEN, SHELTER, OR STALL. Are there signs of pawing, rubbing, rolling, thrashing, or wood chewing?

✷	My Day	A Horse's Day
6:00 AM	Rise.	
6:30 AM	Chores, visual exam, feed barn horses.	Eat.
7:00 AM	Breakfast.	
8:00 AM	Work in office.	Walk over to the water tub for a drink.
8:15 AM		Return to the feed area or pasture to vacuum up the dregs or continue grazing.
9:00 AM	Walk out to pasture horses and give visual exam.	
10:00 AM	Head to the barn.	Exercise and training (this varies for each horse), doze, or lie down.
12:00 PM	Chores, then lunch.	Eat.
1:00 PM	Work in office or barn, do domestic duties.	
2:00 PM		Drink.
2:15 PM		Doze, lie down.
2:30 PM	Back to the barn. Train, ride, turnout.	Exercise or training if on trail ride; otherwise a lesson or a few hours of turnout.
7:00 PM	Bring horses in, light feed to those that need it; light supper for horsekeepers.	Return to pen and eat small meal or nothing, depending on individual.
8:15 PM		Mosey until dawn, keeping alert for unusual sights or sounds.
8:30 PM	Nightly movie.	
10:30 PM	Go to bed.	

SEPTEMBER

The fall equinox, also called the autumnal equinox, occurs between September 22 and 24 in the Northern Hemisphere. This is when the sun is observed to be directly above the earth's equator, so at the equinox, night and day are of approximately equal length. At the equinox, the sun rises directly to the east and sets directly to the west. After the September equinox, the sun rises and sets more to the south.

Day Length in Hours

	Date		
Latitude	Sept 1	Sept 16	Oct 1
60°N	13.91	12.52	11.13
55°N	13.57	12.43	11.28
50°N	13.31	12.36	11.4
45°N	13.1	12.3	11.5
40°N	12.92	12.25	11.58
35°N	12.77	12.21	11.65
30°N	12.63	12.17	11.71

See page 22 to find your latitude.

WACKY WONDERFUL WEATHER

PERFECT FALL WEATHER

All around the country, fall seems to be a time when nothing extreme happens anywhere. The weather patterns are often mild with no extreme heat, precipitation, or wind. (The calm before the storm?) The exception might be that the hurricane season officially continues till November 1, and some big hurricanes have occurred in September.

To Do

- ❑ Deworm
- ❑ Work arena
- ❑ Scrub feed tubs and buckets
- ❑ Move hay to horse barns
- ❑ Remove bot eggs
- ❑ Fall boosters
- ❑ Weaning
- ❑ Prepare for winter

To Buy

- ❑ Beet pulp pellets
- ❑ Senior feed
- ❑ Antioxidant
- ❑ Stall odor absorbent
- ❑ Corn oil
- ❑ Vaccines
- ❑ Horse blankets

VET CLINIC

TIME TO REMOVE BOT EGGS

When mature bot larvae migrate out of a horse's stomach in the late spring (May), they fall to the ground and pupate, then hatch into adult flies in the late summer or early fall. The bot fly then lays sticky eggs on the hair of the horse's lower limbs and flanks. When the horse rubs his mouth on these areas (which happens quite often — that's why the flies strategically lay the eggs there), it stimulates the eggs to hatch. The immature larvae end up in his stomach where they turn into mature larvae and start the cycle all over again. Two ways to break this cycle are to deworm for bots (see January Pest Patrol) and to regularly remove bot eggs from the horse.

You can remove bot eggs with a bot knife or block. A bot knife has serrated, not sharp, edges and a specially shaped tip that is designed to be safe yet allow you to get into small nooks and crannies. Bot eggs are easily removed with a simple scraping motion. Do this in a place where the horse does not eat; otherwise the horse might ingest the eggs you scrape off.

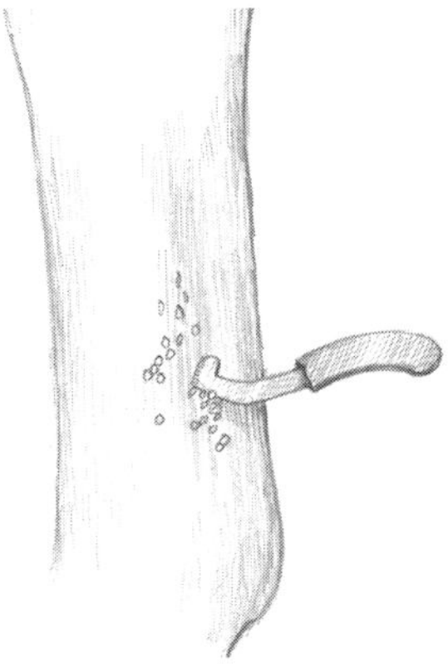

Bot eggs can be removed with a knife or block.

A bot block is a rough, porous stone that rubs the eggs off the hair. As it does, however, the pores of the block fill up with hair and dirt and the edges become rounded, so the block becomes less effective. To renew the block, run it across a sharp edge such as a board. This will clean and sharpen the edge of the block, and it will be ready to use again.

A Personal Decision

One of the responsibilities of animal ownership is to know when an animal's life is no longer comfortable for him. This is a very personal decision and I would not presume to make it for you. But I will say that if performed properly, euthanasia is very easy on the horse. A horse does not anticipate death as humans do, so has no idea that one second he might be munching some soft leafy alfalfa hay, and the next second he will be dead.

DEALING WITH THE DEATH OF A HORSE

Although many of us picture our horses grazing peacefully at pasture during retirement, the fact is that many very old horses aren't that comfortable as they get old, and especially on pasture, whether it is winter or summer. Although the free exercise of a pasture retirement can be ideal for a horse, harsh elements of pasture life can include weather, bugs, and living with other horses. Stall or pen life, on the other hand, is not ideal either for a decrepit horse. Once a horse becomes toothless, blind, chronically lame or ill, has some other debilitating condition, or is just plain worn out, it is time to consider euthanasia.

KNOW YOUR OPTIONS. Before the time comes to release the body of one of your horses, it helps to know your alternatives. Speak with your veterinarian about the options in your area for euthanasia. Even if you plan to use the services of your veterinarian to put down your horse using chemical means, you should know how to humanely destroy an animal that is severely injured or near death and has no hope of recovery. Shooting a horse is quick and painless when carried out correctly. If you are competent with the use of a firearm and know the legal considerations in using it, I recommend you consult instructions developed in Australia (See Web site information in the appendix).

Barn Cats

Although poisons and baits can be used to control rodents, good sanitation and cleanliness, with the help of a few cats, work best. Take good care of your barn cats, as they are worth their weight in gold. Make sure they get their annual vaccinations according to your veterinarian's recommendations. In addition, especially since cats eat rodents, be sure they are dewormed frequently, including for tapeworms.

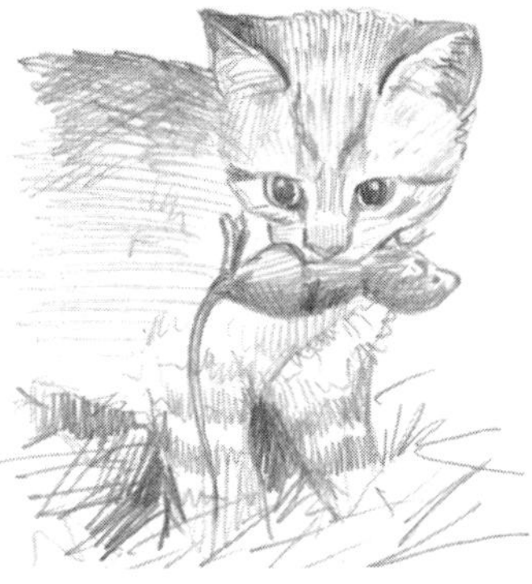

FOOT NOTES

HOOF PADS

Your farrier might suggest using pads with your horse's shoes. There are four main reasons to use hoof pads: to change the angle of the hoof, to protect the hoof, to reduce concussion, and to prevent snowballing. There are six general types of pads: full flat pads, shock-absorbing pads, wedge pads, bubble pads, rim pads, and tube-type rim pads.

There are four main reasons to use hoof pads: to change the angle of the hoof, to protect the hoof, to reduce concussion, and to prevent snowballing.

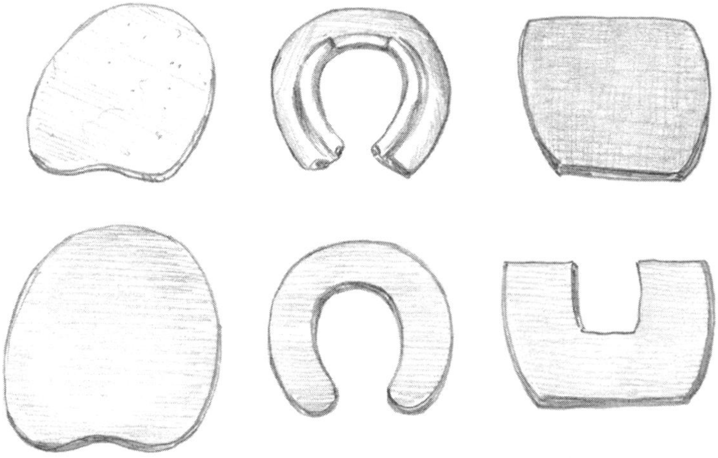

Hoof pads come in many shapes and sizes for a variety of purposes.

FYI

Hoof Pads at Shows

Some breed and performance associations have rules specifically related to the use of hoof pads at horse competitions. It is the horse owner's and exhibitor's responsibility to know and abide by any regulations related to shoes or pads.

FULL FLAT PADS. These come in leather, plastic, or metal and cover the entire sole. They protect the sole and keep it clean. Leather pads compress between the shoe and the hoof and conform to the sole, and while they allow more normal hoof respiration than plastic pads, they absorb water and will deteriorate. Plastic pads are available in a variety of thicknesses, hardness, colors, and durability. They do not allow the hoof to respire and may or may not conform to the sole. Metal pads (usually for therapeutic purposes) are made of thin steel or aluminum. They provide positive protection to the sole and frog but greatly reduce traction.

A full pad covers the entire bottom of the horse's foot and is installed between the hoof and the shoe with or without hoof packing. Horses with thin, sensitive soles may benefit from wearing full pads, as would a horse worked on gravel or rocky terrain.

With the use of full pads comes an interruption in natural hoof respiration. As hooves "breathe" they release moisture. You can see evidence of this if your horse is barefoot or shod without pads and is standing on a rubber mat. When you pick up his foot, you will likely see a circular patch of hoof fog on the mat. When a full pad covers the sole of a hoof, this outward moisture migration is halted, the moisture collects under the pad, and the hoof structures can become softened and weakened. In addition, full pads tend to trap invading slush, mud, and snow, providing a suitable environment for growth of bacteria, fungus, and yeast.

Some horses seem to develop an even thinner and more vulnerable sole from wearing pads full time, and therefore become "pad dependent." However, some horses with weak soles develop a thick normal sole with the use of full pads and proper hoof packing (see hoof packing later).

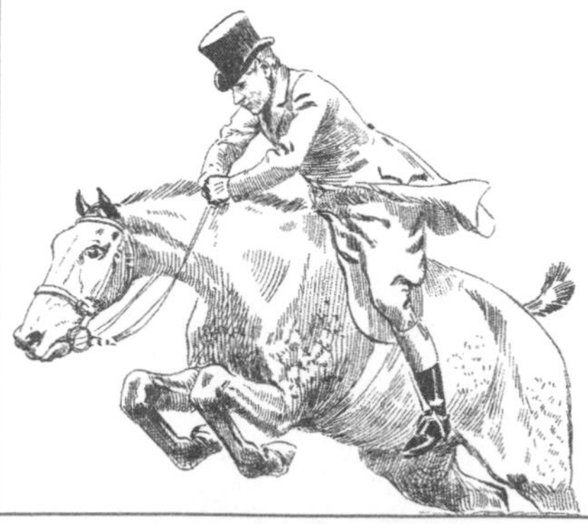

SHOCK-ABSORBING PADS. These are designed to reduce concussion and vibration to the structures of the hoof and limb. A healthy, properly shod foot provides all the shock absorption necessary for normal work by transferring the energy of the hoof's impact to the shock-absorbing structures: the hoof wall, the laminae, the frog, the digital cushion, and the blood vessels. If the hoof structures are abnormal or the work is excessive, concussion-reducing pads are sometimes prescribed.

WEDGE PADS. Usually plastic, these tapered pieces of material are placed between the shoe and the hoof, generally to raise the heels of a low-heeled hoof. Wedge pads are also called degree pads because they are manufactured in various thicknesses or degrees. They are available as a full pad or bar pad. A bar pad is solid across the thick end and open in the middle. Thicker wedge pads are often stiff enough across the heels to protect the frog and underlying navicular area from direct ground pressure.

BUBBLE PADS. These full, hard plastic pads have a 2-inch-diameter dome molded into the center of the ground surface. Originally designed for antisnowballing, they can also be used to relieve pressure over the navicular region or

Fall Boosters for Influenza and Rhino

Depending on your locale and schedule, your veterinarian might recommend fall boosters for the respiratory diseases. See the main immunization program outlined in March.

NO WAY!

Historical Horsekeeping

"Take three hen's eggs and break them into a quart of clear, cold rain-water. Stir until a thorough mixture is effected. Boil over a slow fire, stirring every few minutes. Add half an ounce of sulphate of zinc. In this preparation a solid substance or curd is precipitated or thrown down, and a liquid solution rests upon the top. This liquid is the best wash for the sore eyes of either man or beast that was ever made."

— American Farmer's Horse Book, *1868*

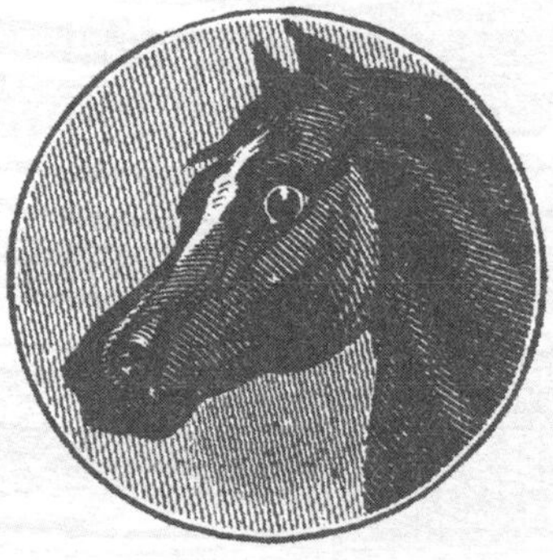

FALL: SEPTEMBER

another sole area. With bubble pads, traction is reduced and a thick shoe is required to prevent the bubble from bearing the horse's weight.

RIM PADS. These fit between the shoe and the hoof wall; the sole and frog are open. They are used to put more distance between the sole and the ground.

TUBE-TYPE RIM PADS. These are composed of a small rubber tube that lines the inside rim of the shoe and is held in place by an attached flat, thin tab (flange) that lies between the shoe and the hoof. They are designed to eliminate snowballing. For a discussion of antisnowballing pads, see October Foot Notes.

Hoof Packing

The space between the pad and the hoof can be left empty (such as with a bubble pad) or packed with various materials. Traditional packing was pine tar with oakum, but that has drawbacks. Oakum is a loose, stringy hemp fiber that retains water, disintegrates, and shifts beneath the pad, often working out between the heels.

Silicone caulking can be either squirted into the sole space from a caulking gun after the shoe and pad are in place or mixed with a catalyst to speed curing and applied to the sole before the shoe and pad are nailed on. However, there are several significant drawbacks to using silicone. It tends to concentrate moisture and heat against the sole, and if too large an amount is used, it puts pressure on the sole and prevents the sole from descending as part of its normal shock-absorbing function. Also, silicone allows sand and mud to accumulate between the pad and the sole, causing sole pressure.

Movie of the Month

***SEABISCUIT* (2003)** The true story of a small, ornery racehorse that was deemed uncontrollable but was saved by a legendary trio: a trainer with insight, an owner with an emotional scar, and a feisty jockey full of hope and determination. Seabiscuit lifted the spirit of Americans during the Depression and won Horse of the Year in 1938.

FYI

Commercial hoof-packing preparations can be used with varying degrees of success. A healthy alternative is the CVP Gasket Pad. (See the appendix for the CVP Gasket Pad Web site.)

WEIGHT GAIN FOR WINTER

If you live where there is winter cold, allow your horse to gain 5 to 10 percent of his body weight. A 1,200-pound adult horse should gain 60 to 120 pounds in the early fall. This extra flesh and fat will provide added insulation and an energy reserve for heat when weather is particularly bad.

COLD WEATHER FEEDING RULE. For every 10°F below freezing (32°F), increase the hay portion of your horse's ration by 10 percent.

HAY TRICKS

HAY, WHERE'S THE KNIFE? For safety and so that the knife is there when I need it, my barn knife has a brightly colored handle. I park the knife in one of the next bales I'll be opening. If the knife does happen to get knocked to the floor, the handle makes it easy to spot.

When a hay knife has been borrowed for another job and not returned (which, of course, never happens at our barn) and I have to open a bale, I use a piece of baling twine.

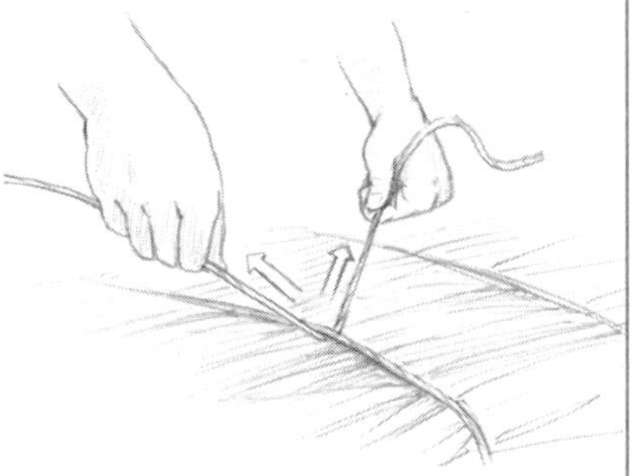

I thread a piece of twine through one of the strings of the bale I want to open, saw back and forth, and *voilà*! The friction cuts the twine. I do the same with the other bale string. Hay — who even needs a knife?

A HOMEMADE HAY CARRIER. When we carry hay out to pasture horses, a hay carrier makes the job easier and keeps the flakes from falling apart on the way. We have a homemade hay carrier that is 19 inches wide by 45 inches long, made from heavy denim, with a wooden handle on each end. The handles are 1-inch-diameter dowels, 24 inches long. The carrier holds about 20 pounds of hay and when bundled up, it becomes a neat and efficient hay suitcase. A 36-inch-long, 2-inch-wide web strap is attached to one handle to allow us to carry more hay if necessary. Alternatively, you can buy a commercially made hay carrier.

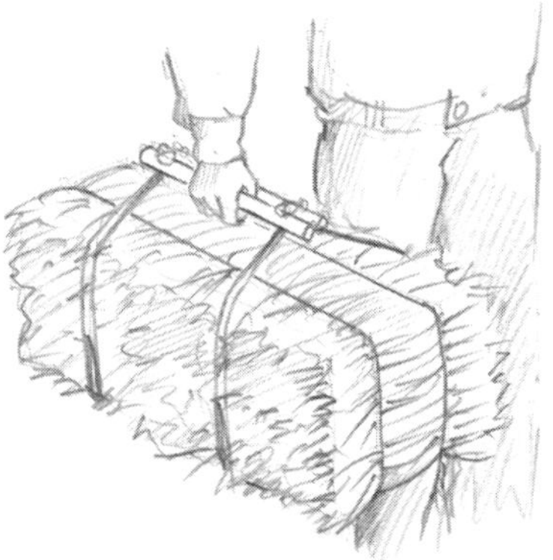

With a hay carrier, you can transport feed to pasture horses.

FYI

Bear Grub

Bears are omnivores, eating plants and animals. Their typical diet could consist of berries, nuts, grubs, insects, carrion, and field crops like corn. They might visit orchards, beehives, garbage cans, bird feeders, hummingbird feeders, or pet-food dishes.

BLACK BEARS

Black bears can be black, honey-colored, brown, or blond overall with a tan muzzle. They have large, well-padded feet with large claws. Males average 275 pounds and can weigh up to 600 pounds; females average 175 pounds and can weigh up to 400. (Most black bears that are sighted, however, are 150 to 250 pounds.) They are 3½ to 6 feet long and stand 2½ to 3½ feet at the shoulder; 4 to 5 feet when standing upright.

With an exceptional sense of smell and good eyesight and hearing, black bears can live to be 20 years old in the wild. They are skilled at climbing and loping.

Hibernating in the winter, bears tend to be most active during the day in the spring and fall. In summer they rest during the heat of the day and roam during dawn and dusk. They mate in midsummer, and cubs are born in a den in midwinter. Mother and cubs exit the den in early April, although females without cubs might exit earlier.

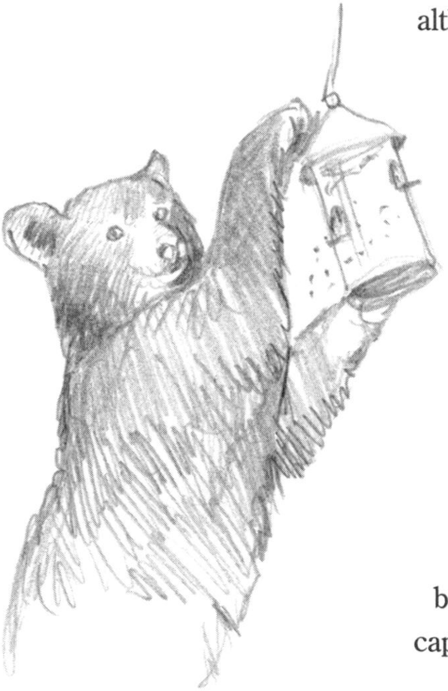

ENCOUNTERING A BEAR. Normally wary of people, bears will usually move out of the area before they are seen. However, if you do happen upon a bear, you should make it aware of you by clapping, talking, or making some other noise. I click my aluminum trekking poles together when I see our resident bear. The "clank, clank" alerts the bear to my presence and sends it away.

If a bear seems agitated, it might be a female, and you might be between her and her cub. Do not approach bears, even cubs, or you are asking for trouble. They are good climbers and swimmers, agile and fast, capable of running up to 35 miles per hour.

KEEPING BEARS AWAY. It is best to leave wildlife wild. Here are some reminders.

- ★ Don't feed bears or set out feed where you know a bear frequents.
- ★ Keep trash in a closed garage or another outbuilding.
- ★ Put away pet food, and clean grease off your barbecue grill or store it indoors.
- ★ Take bird feeders down when winter is over.
- ★ Locate your house compost pile well away from your home.
- ★ If you have young foals or other small livestock, keep them near the barn at night.

Coyotes and their pups might appear this time of year at your place, as they do here at Long Tail Ranch. *(See Coyotes in February Wild Life, page 87–89.)*

PASTURE PERFECT

HUNTING SEASON SAFETY FOR PASTURE HORSES

If your area has hunting seasons, mark all property boundaries clearly with "No Hunting" signs. When possible, keep your horses off pasture between dawn and dusk. Use highly reflective bright orange fly sheets or turnout sheets when you do turn the horses out.

If you are on a twice-a-year spreading regimen, now is the time to vacate some of your pastures and spread manure. Plan to keep those pastures vacant until late spring or early summer.

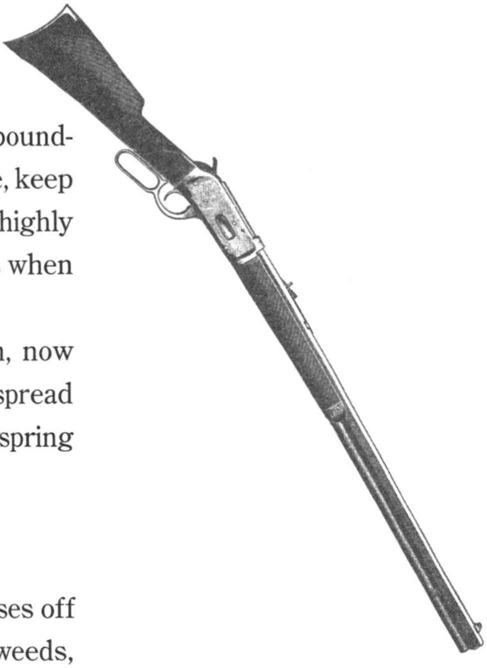

PASTURE PRIORITIES

Pasture is waning, so monitor it closely and pull horses off or rotate them. Touch up the last of the broad-leaved weeds, with the mower set on high.

Pest Patrol

Rodents

Rodents that can create problems in and around a horse barn or pasture include mice, rats, gophers, prairie dogs, marmots, pack rats, moles, and shrews. Not only are they hosts for disease-causing parasites, but they can also cause damage and health problems themselves. They can carry hantavirus (see this month's Horsekeeping Across America), bubonic plague, typhus, and rabies and are reservoirs for salmonella, Lyme disease, and sleeping sickness. They can damage tack and make a mess in a feed room.

PB TO THE RESCUE. Ideally, your feed room should be rodent-proof, and all feed stored in rodent-proof containers. If a mouse or two sneaks into a tightly enclosed area (such as a tack room) where cats are not allowed free access, simple traps baited with a dab of peanut butter will eliminate the population before breeding begins.

Rodents need to gnaw to keep their incisors worn down, so they chew inedible things such as electrical wires and tack. Gophers and prairie dogs create burrows in pastures and subsist on the pasture vegetation; this destroys plants and results in holes dangerous for horses and people. Marmots dig under buildings and wreak havoc with gardens. Having a few of any of these rodents on a farm or ranch is just a natural part of the ecosystem, but when a population grows so large that it renders a pasture unusable or begins to damage buildings and utilities, then it is past time to do something about it.

CONTROLLING RODENTS. Natural predators of rodents include hawks, owls, and snakes. Providing desirable habitats on your property may encourage predators to take up residence. Terriers are good rodent deterrents, but are more prone to digging than cats are.

Rodent-control measures for pastures range from trapping live for relocation, to sonic deterrents, to poison and kill traps. Choose the method that you are most comfortable with.

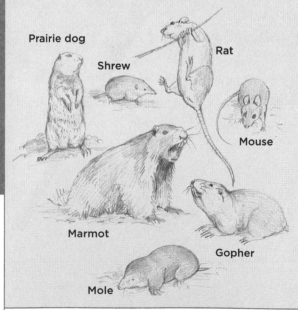

DISPOSAL OF A HORSE'S BODY

You may have to decide what to do with a horse's remains. The options for disposing of a 1,200-pound carcass are limited. If you have a large animal disposal service in your area, get a phone number and keep it current and available. Your veterinarian or farrier or agricultural extension agent should be able to provide you with contact information. And in fact, if you live in a suburban area, your best option might be to have your veterinarian arrange for euthanasia and disposal of your horse's body.

If your farm or ranch is large enough and your local ordinances allow, you might want to consider preparing a final resting place for your horse on your own property. Check local zoning and health regulations ahead of time. Burial of dead animals should not result in contamination of ground water, and the grave needs to be deep enough so as not encourage or permit access by vermin, scavengers, or other potential vectors of disease.

If it is legal to bury a horse on your property, you will likely need to hire a backhoe operator to dig an 8-foot-deep hole that is approximately 6 feet by 10 feet. This will ensure that there will be 3–4 feet of earth on top of the horse's body. Locate the hole at least 100 feet from any water source and on high enough ground so that the bottom of the hole does not contact ground water.

SEPTEMBER Manure Pile Maintenance

PILE A
Turn once, water as needed.

PILE B
Turn twice, water as needed.

PILE C
Sell, store, or spread.

No hour of life is lost that is spent in the saddle.

— Sir Winston Churchill

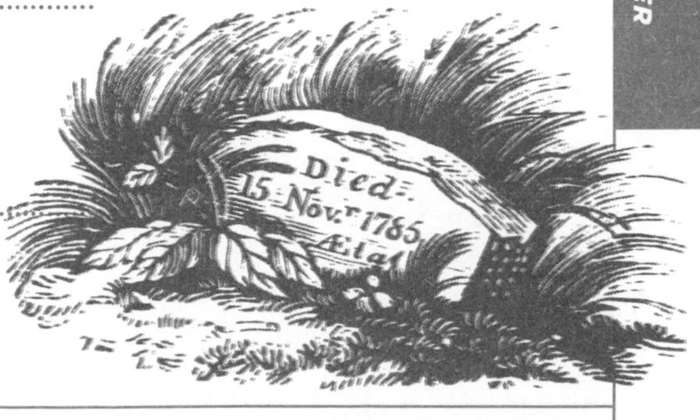

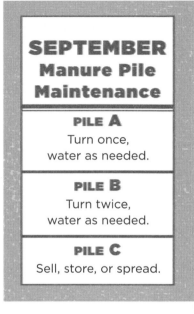

BEAUTY SHOP

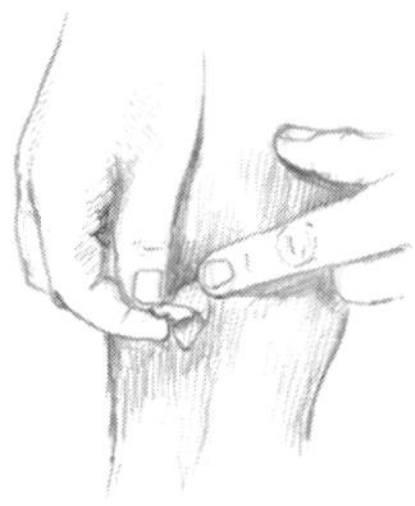

Chestnuts are easy to peel after a bath.

FALL SHEDDING

Horses shed their hair coats twice a year — once in the spring when they lose their long winter coats and once in the fall when they start replacing their short summer coats with long hair. Here at 7,000 feet in the Colorado Rockies, the fall shed occurs in September, so I often give the horses a bath during this month. See all about bathing in May Beauty Shop.

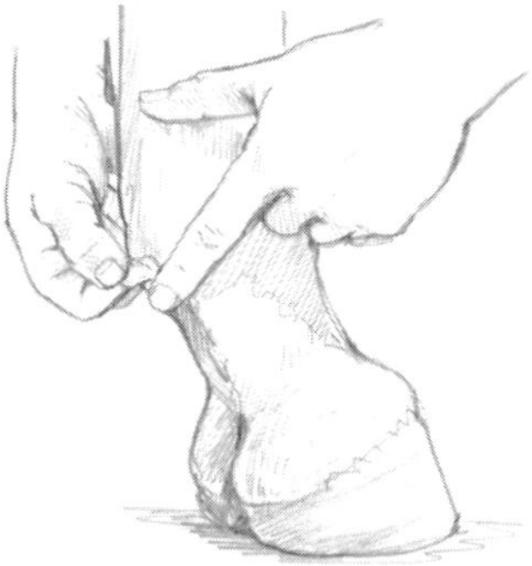

Ergots can be peeled or snipped off.

ERGOTS AND CHESTNUTS

Chestnuts are evolutionary remnants from when the horse had more than one toe. Today they serve no purpose, so they can be removed.

During moist weather or after a bath, when they are softened, remove long chestnuts and ergots by peeling or cutting them off carefully with a sharp knife. Remove the horny material in layers until the chestnut area is level with the hair coat. A flush chestnut will make it easier for you to do a neat job of clipping the legs. Removal will also prevent a long chestnut from being caught and ripping the skin.

LOOKING AT HORSES

Neck Conformation

The horse's neck should attach smoothly to the shoulder without an abnormal dip. The upper neck length (poll to withers) should be at least twice the lower neck length (throatlatch to chest). This largely depends on the slope of the shoulder. A horse with a very steep shoulder has an upper neck length almost equal to the lower neck length. The more sloping the shoulder, the longer the neck's topline becomes and the shorter the underline. The topline muscling should be more developed than the underside muscling. A thick underside to the neck is associated with a horse that braces against the bit and hollows the neck's topline.

QUARTER SHEETS

Quarter sheets, also called exercise rugs, are used while longeing or riding during cold weather. They keep the horse's hindquarters warm during warm-up, and during active work they prevent rapid muscle cooling, which can lead to chilling and cramping. Wet heat loss is 23 times faster than dry heat loss. If a sweaty horse is allowed to become cold during a cooling-out period, he will likely lose so much heat as to experience muscle chill.

Blanketed, stabled horses with very short or clipped coats are prime candidates for quarter sheets. The sheets are placed under the saddle or affixed around the saddle, depending on the style.

MATERIALS. Quarter sheets perform different functions depending on what material is used in their construction. They can keep a horse warm, prevent him from cooling out too rapidly during strenuous work, minimize moisture buildup under the sheet by wicking it away from his body, and/or keep him dry when being worked in wet weather.

Wool, the traditional fiber from sheep fleece, absorbs moisture vapor from the hair and skin, leaving a dry layer of insulating air between the horse's body and the wool. The natural crimp of wool fibers makes them stand apart from each other, which allows air to be trapped between the fibers, further insulating and holding in body heat. Although wool can absorb moisture vapor, it cannot absorb liquid, so it has a good degree of water repellency. The scales on the outside of wool fibers cause liquids to roll off, so it takes quite a bit of moisture for wool to get wet and when it does, it tends to be comfortable rather than cold and clammy. Wool allows the body to cool down slowly, thereby reducing the chance of chills.

Beauty Shop

Winter Ears

Certain places on a horse's body have extra hair for a reason. The ears, for example, grow extra hair both inside and outside in the fall to keep them warm during the winter. If you need to tidy up your horse's ears for the winter, just clip them flush and maybe tweak the outline.

Polarfleece and Polartec are registered trademarks for the original double-faced fleece fabrics made by Malden Mills from 100 percent polyester. The warmth of Polartec is comparable to wool with less bulk and weight; it is more durable than acrylic; the double facing makes it soft on both sides. Polarfleece machine-washes well on cold without fading or losing shape. The fiber absorbs no more than one percent of its weight in water so stays very light and is a very rapid-drying fabric.

> "Then we began to ride. My soul smoothed itself out, a long-cramped scroll freshening and fluttering in the wind."
> — Robert Browning

GoreTex is windproof and waterproof, which means moisture won't penetrate even if pressure is applied to the fabric, such as from a saddle. GoreTex is also breathable, which means perspiration vapor is able to pass out through the fabric. To keep GoreTex at its maximum waterproof/breathable performance, wash and tumble dry the item and occasionally iron using a warm setting. If it is professionally dry-cleaned, request clear distilled solvent rinse and spray repellent.

SympaTex is also a windproof, waterproof, breathable fabric with the same properties as GoreTex. Wash in warm water on gentle cycle using a mild detergent but no fabric conditioner. Do not use a fast spin. Allow the garment to drip dry.

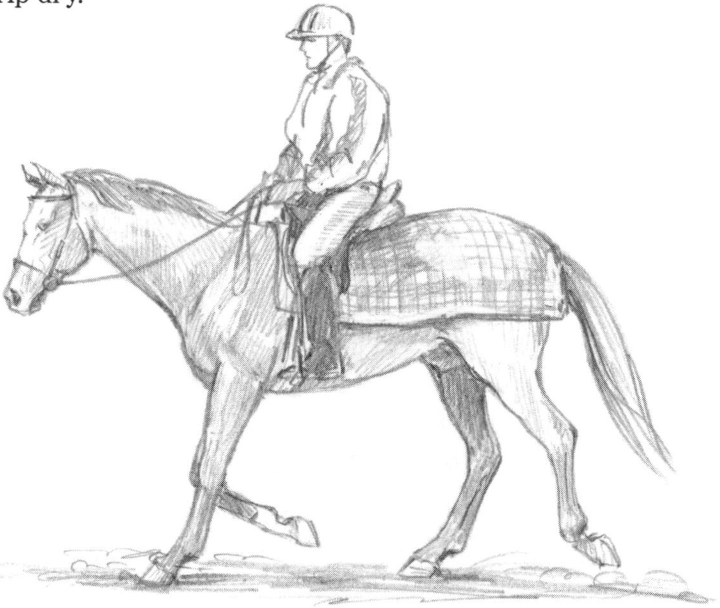

A quarter sheet keeps your horse's hindquarters warm during cold-weather riding.

Choose Your Style

Quarter sheets, originating in the military, were initially just long saddle blankets that ended at the junction of the loin and croup and had normal-length sides. Many of today's quarter sheets are cut more like a partial blanket, covering not only the entire back, loin, and croup but the entire side of the horse as well. The sheets with maximum coverage provide warmth and prevent chilling over a large area, but they can inhibit movement if too snugly fitted over the hindquarters and tail, and they can interfere with leg aids or the use of spurs if too long on the sides. Larger sheets also have a tendency to billow, necessitating a fillet string or tail cord or loop to keep the back of the sheet from flapping.

TRADITIONAL CUT. The traditional-cut quarter sheet is a large rectangle that runs from withers to tail, down the shoulders, sides, and hindquarters. The saddle sits on top of the sheet and is secured via girth loops and stabilized with a tail loop. Girth and saddle must be removed in order to remove the traditional quarter sheet. The traditional style is either sparse like the original military quarter sheet or full like a stable sheet with the front missing.

EUROPEAN CUT. With this style, a cut-away section under the girth helps prevent the sheet from gathering in that area and allows for normal use of leg aids and spurs. Tack must be removed to remove this style of quarter sheet.

EASY-ON/OFF STYLE. This version features a cut-out area for the saddle and hook-and-loop fasteners in front of saddle. The sheet is put on after the horse is saddled and can be removed without removing the girth or saddle. Usually this type of sheet does not have girth loops and goes over the fastened girth.

Close-Up on Wool

Wool has a natural elasticity: dry wool can stretch about 30 percent and wet wool between 60 and 70 percent, allowing freedom of movement. Good-quality wool should return to its natural shape when dry. Wool's flexibility also makes it durable — the coiled, crimped fibers stretch instead of snapping when stressed.

Virgin wool is 100 percent new wool that has never been processed. It has a distinctive fluffy crimp to it. Processed and reprocessed wools are usually more dense and compact. Often other fibers are added to vary the characteristics of the wool, such as acrylic for softness or nylon for wear resistance.

Fit Factors

Fit will depend on the cut of the pattern, whether there are seams and darts, and the type of material. Some materials conform and mold to the horse's contour better than others do. Sheets made of two or more pieces and with hindquarter or croup darts tend to fit the contours of a horse's topline better than a single-piece drape, thereby staying in place and providing a snug, cozy fit. However, these same well-fitted sheets could inhibit movement.

This style of sheet usually has a tail tie, which, if tied with a quick-release knot, makes the sheet easy to remove even while mounted. If it comes with a tail loop and you expect to take it off during the work, you can opt not to put the loop under the horse's tail or you can dismount to remove the sheet. In any event, you don't have to remove tack to remove the sheet.

With this style, the rider can use it under her leg as a traditional exercise rug or over her legs to keep her warm. A great bonus of this type of sheet is in temperatures where a quarter sheet is not needed during warm-up and active work but is beneficial during cool-down. This style can quickly be put on without removing any tack or even dismounting in some cases.

ENGLISH BRACE. This is a reinforced wither area that offers extra protection in the most vulnerable section of the quarter sheet, directly under the saddle where there is extreme pressure. A well-made English brace usually means a longer-lasting product.

Sizing to Fit

Although listed several ways, sizing is usually expressed as the length from the front edge of the quarter sheet to the

STILL TRUE TODAY

Historical Horsekeeping

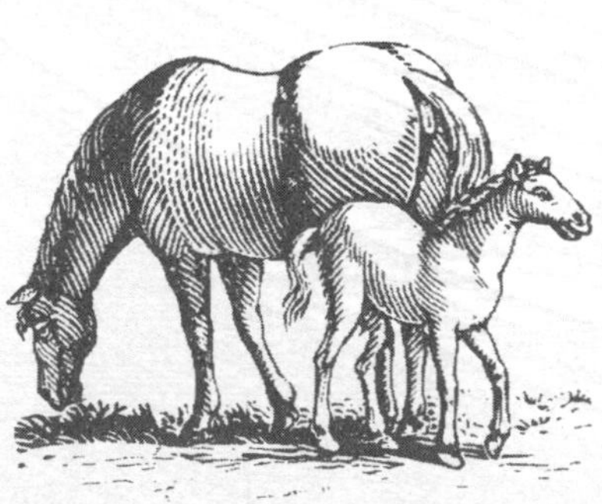

"If the colt is healthy and thriving, he should be weaning at from five to six months old. If allowed to run with the dam after this period, he is an unnecessary burden to her, since he has already learned to pick up and devote to his own use other sustenance, and he may most judiciously be taken away."

— Gleason's Horse Book *by Prof. Oscar R. Gleason, 1892*

rear edge of the sheet, in feet and inches, inches, or centimeters. Thus, a 4-foot, 6-inch sheet might also be called a 54 (inch) sheet or a 137 (cm) sheet, or it might be designated Medium or Large, depending on the manufacturer. Each manufacturer determines the actual dimension of its sizes: Large, for example, can range from 54 to 57 inches.

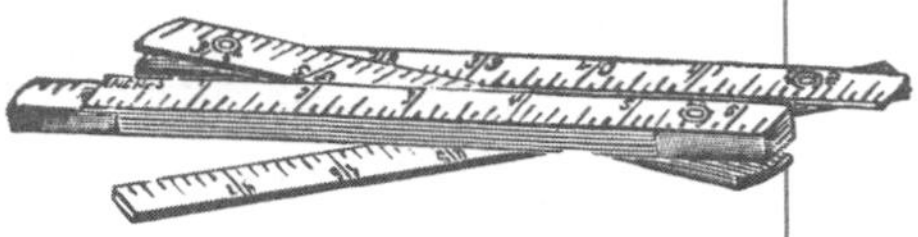

Sometimes a quarter sheet size is the horse's equivalent stable blanket size. The quarter sheet described above would fit a horse that would wear a size 78 blanket (197 cm), so sometimes the sheet is referred to as a 78, even though it is not 78 inches or 197 cm long. All of this varies greatly with sheet design, country of origin, and manufacturer.

CLOTHES HORSE

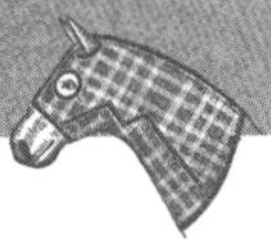

ALL ABOUT COOLERS

A cooler is a lightweight, absorbent cover designed to help a wet horse dry slowly without getting chilled. Essential during cold or cool, breezy weather, these items are also valuable in hot times. Even when he doesn't need protection from chilling, a cooler can help dry a horse more quickly by wicking moisture away from his hair and letting it evaporate from the outer surface of the cooler. Sometimes, during cold weather, frost will form on the outside of the cooler, a sure sign that it's working! In the winter, you can layer two coolers after bathing a horse and remove the inner cooler once it has absorbed most of the moisture.

The typical cooler style covers the horse from poll to tail and hangs very long on the sides. It usually has a browband, two or more light tie straps under the neck, and a tail loop, but no surcingle or leg straps. This style is good for throwing over a horse, tack and all, after a workout to allow him to cool down while walking or untacking. Small size is

TIPS & TECHNIQUES

Moth Proofing

It's essential to protect wool coolers from moths, who like wool as much as we do (but for different reasons). When coolers will not be used for a long period, store them clean in tightly sealed plastic bags or containers and use aromatic cedar or mothballs to discourage moth infestation.

Ranch Recipes

Shampoo Dilution

Most shampoos are too concentrated to use full strength on a horse's body, mane, or tail because they may never rinse out completely. That is why I dilute shampoos before I use them on the horse.

I start with a clean, empty ketchup bottle and fill it with lukewarm water to just below the neck. Then I add 3 or 4 ounces of shampoo. I invert the bottle gently to mix the shampoo solution. This makes up a perfect amount of shampoo solution to bathe one horse.

66 by 72 inches, Regular size is 84 by 90 inches, and Large is 90 by 96 inches.

Coolers also come in a more fitted stable-sheet style, with one or more belly attachments, front closures, and possibly leg straps. Because this style is more secure on the horse, it's better suited for a horse that's unattended, such as a horse turned into a stall or paddock to munch hay after a bath or workout.

Coolers used on sweaty horses need to be easily washable, since the dirt and minerals from sweat remain in the material after the moisture evaporates. Since wool coolers, even when washed cold, are more prone to shrinking than synthetic coolers, you can minimize their trips to the washing machine by double-layering them with a more washable synthetic cooler next to the horse.

A cooler comes in handy after a fall bath
or for cooling out a sweaty horse in cold weather.

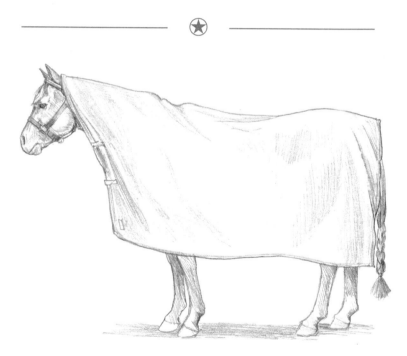

FARM OFFICE

SELLING A HORSE

If you need to sell a horse before winter (with a hay bill looming), you will discover that horse marketing is a very competitive business. Marketing requires a business plan. Advertising is just one part of it (see Equine Marketing 101 on next page).

Usually there is a good number of horses available for every prospective buyer, including a large supply of partially trained, out-of-shape, "backyard" horses for sale. It is much more difficult to sell a horse that has not been worked for some time, is overweight, is either very lazy or a little bit wild, and has not been professionally cared for or presented. It is easier to sell a horse at the beginning of a riding season (spring or early summer) than at the beginning of the feeding season (fall or winter), yet fall seems to be when the market is flooded.

Not many potential buyers will take a seller's word that "He's a wonderful pleasure horse (but he hasn't been ridden for five years)" and buy a horse without being able to test him thoroughly. If you hope to sell your horse, you must get him in shape, highlight his positive attributes, and direct your sales efforts to the specific market for which he is suitable. Don't hope to sell a horse by saying he is a hunt-seat prospect if he has never been in the show ring, let alone never had hunt-seat training.

Early in your sales efforts you must decide whether you will market your horse locally or nationally, at private treaty or auction, how you will advertise and where, and what price you will ask for him. Remember, unless you are offering a very specific age, type, color, or bloodline, there will be many other contenders in the marketplace.

What Makes a Horse Sell?

- ★ Quality
- ★ Training
- ★ Presentation
- ★ Performance
- ★ Appropriate price
- ★ Paperwork in order

If you need to sell a horse before winter, you will discover that horse marketing is a very competitive business.

If wishes were horses, beggars would ride.

— Attributed to James Halliwell and also John Ray

Sell the cow,
buy the sheep, but never be without the horse.
— Irish Proverb

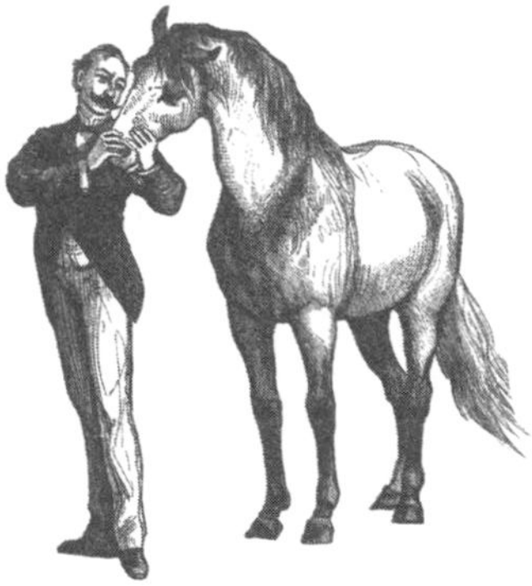

HIRING AN AGENT. If you are busy or inexperienced in the sale of horses, you may want to consider having a professional aid you in selling your horse. You can either use a private treaty agent or an auction sale company. Agents set up their sales arrangements many different ways but generally charge a flat fee and a percentage of the sale price of the horse. In addition, most agents require the horse to be boarded and in training at the agent's facility. Thus, not only will you receive a reduced price (less agent's fee) for your horse, but you may also need to invest money (for training and boarding) in order to sell him.

The advantage is that having your horse at the agent's barn makes it most efficient for the horse to be prepared and presented to prospective buyers in a professional manner. An agent does all of the advertising, promotion, and phone, mail, and video follow-up to queries and is responsible for grooming, training, showing, and presenting the

Equine Marketing 101

Marketing can include:

★ Knowing what you have

★ Knowing how to present it

★ Identifying the market niche

★ Checking out the competition (prices, products, techniques, successes)

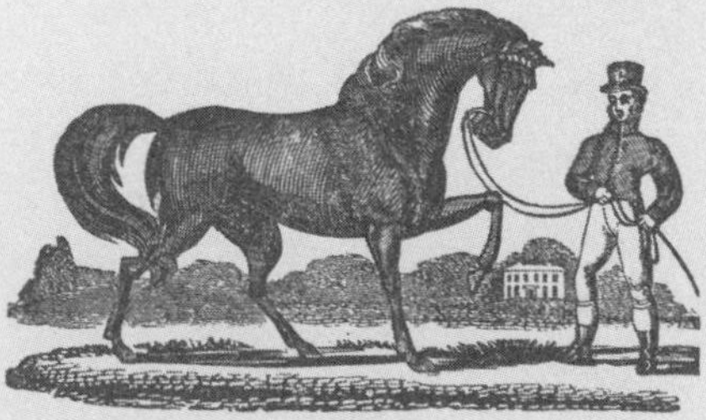

★ Showing what you have to offer that is different or better, such as
- A more thoroughly trained horse
- Lessons included in the sale
- Lower price
- Installment contract
- First month's board free

★ Setting goals and reasonable expectations regarding the horse's price, the amount of time it will take you to sell him, and the type of owner (home) the horse will go to

FALL: SEPTEMBER

horse. Most agents network with other agents, often across the country, so a horse may receive wide exposure.

SELLING THROUGH AN AUCTION. Selling a horse through an auction also has its pros and cons. Auctions are less time-consuming than private treaty sales because all the buyers are in one place at one time and the horse sells. However, you will still need to invest the time and money to prepare the horse for the auction. The horse must be fit, well groomed, and well trained. Most auctions require horses more than two or three years old to be ridden in the sales ring. Many auctions have requirements that must be met by the horse and the consignor. (See Auction Terms and Conditions on page 426).

The fees involved in selling a horse at auction vary greatly. Most charge a nonrefundable consignment fee. If the horse does not sell (if you exercise your right to reject the highest bid and retain title to the horse), the consignment fee compensates the auction company for the catalog listing, the stall space at the sale, and the exposure it received in the sale ring.

If the horse does sell, in addition to the consignment fee a commission will be charged on the sale price of the animal. This varies from 5 to 15 percent, depending on the circumstances, with averages ranging from 7 to 10 percent. Some small sales (with less expensive horses) charge only a consignment fee, and some charge only a commission, but most commonly, both are charged. Some sales stipulate a consignment fee plus either a commission (percentage) or a dollar amount, whichever is greater. (Example: $275 consignment plus 8 percent commission or $150, whichever is greater.)

Finding a Sales Agent

To locate an agent, ask for local recommendations. An agent might simply be a respected trainer or instructor with whom you have done business previously. Other sales agents will advertise "Let us sell your horse for you."

If possible, visit the agent so you can get a feel for his or her manner and view the facilities. Ask yourself how you would feel arriving at these facilities and dealing with the agent if you were a buyer.

The great thing about dealing with an honest, respected sales agent is that you have minimal time investment in the sales effort.

Auction Terms and Conditions

The following are sample terms and conditions to be considered before consigning a horse to an auction. They will vary greatly by sale and state.

★ Horse must be registered and have papers in order.

★ Consignor must have absolute title to horse.

★ Consignment fee, registration papers, and transfer must accompany application.

★ Sale screening committee will select horses for the sale and reserves the right to reject any applicant.

★ After a horse has been accepted and consigned, the seller agrees not to sell the horse through private treaty. If horse is withdrawn from the sale, a withdrawal fee will be charged in addition to the consignment fee.

★ Horse must have current (30 to 180 days) negative Coggins test.

★ Horse must be HYPP negative.

★ Horse must have health certificate dated fewer than 10 days before the sale.

★ Consignor must furnish own feed, bedding, and care for the horse until it is sold.

★ Consignor must furnish a halter and lead rope.

★ All responsibilities and guarantees lie solely between buyer and consignor.

★ A video- or audiotape will be recorded to determine what announcements or claims were made during the sale.

★ Sales management will settle with consignor not later than 10 banking days after the sale.

★ Consignor will pay transfer fee.

★ Consignor releases sales management from all responsibilities, liabilities, obligations, claims, lawsuits, or legal proceedings arising from the sale of this horse.

★ The sales management company will hold a drawing for sales order.

★ Consignor must notify sales management if the horse has been on medication or drugs within 30 days of the sale.

★ If a consignor wishes to repurchase the horse or to "no sale" the horse, it is the sole responsibility of the consignor (or his agent) to be present to do the bidding.

REPRODUCTION ROUNDUP

WEANING A FOAL

At weaning time at four to six months of age, the horse has reached the human physical equivalent of about a four- to five-year-old child, and the emotional equivalent of a two- to three-year-old. With a short attention span and unpredictable outbursts, weanlings are best left to be horses, with any necessary lessons kept safe and fun. The weanling is very impressionable and can experience deep emotional and physical trauma. Separated from his mother and uncertain about his safety, the young horse is being asked to form his own behavior patterns for the first time. Care must be taken to preserve his interest in eating and other routines so that he does not become unnecessarily depressed.

I wean my foals at four months. There is neither harm nor advantage in waiting until six months, but it is good to do it at a time when the weather doesn't add to the stress of separation. That's why I usually do it earlier in the year (like now) rather than in the winter. I use the complete separation process and have found that it's best to leave the foal in the pasture, pen, or stall where he has been living with the mother, as long as the fences and facilities are safe. The four- to six-month-old foal should be eating hay or pasture and grain well.

Various Weaning Methods

Some foals and mares wean easily, partly due to their makeup and handling, how independent and secure the foal is, and how eager the mare is to be free of her foal. Other mares and/or foals become very stressed at weaning. If you know your mare to be excitable at weaning, a more labor-intensive, less stressful method might be necessary.

COMPLETE SEPARATION IN A HERD. If you have two or

Weaning at Long Tail Ranch

Five days prior to weaning, I eliminate grain from the mare's ration to slow down milk production. On weaning day, I remove the dam from the foal and put her in a safe place, too. It's best if she is out of sight and sound of the foal and not put back with him again, or he will nurse.

It can be helpful to wean a foal with another foal or companion horse. I've done it both ways and the horses turn out fine, but I prefer solo weaning as it tends to make horses less buddy-bound. The foals are handled a lot as sucklings and also during their weaning period.

COMPLETE SEPARATION IN A HERD. If you have two or more mares with foals, you can remove one mare from the herd at a time over a period of days. Start with the mare of the oldest foal and so on. The end result is a group of foals in their original environment.

Even the greenest horse has something to teach the wisest rider.
— Anonymous

DENY NURSING. The mare and foal are separated by a Dutch door or a safe V-mesh fence, which allows them to see, hear, and smell each other, but nursing is not possible. After a few days, they are completely separated. This seems to be a low-stress method.

GRADUAL SEPARATION. Over a period of five to ten days, the mare and foal are separated for increasingly longer periods of time. This is a time- and labor-intensive method.

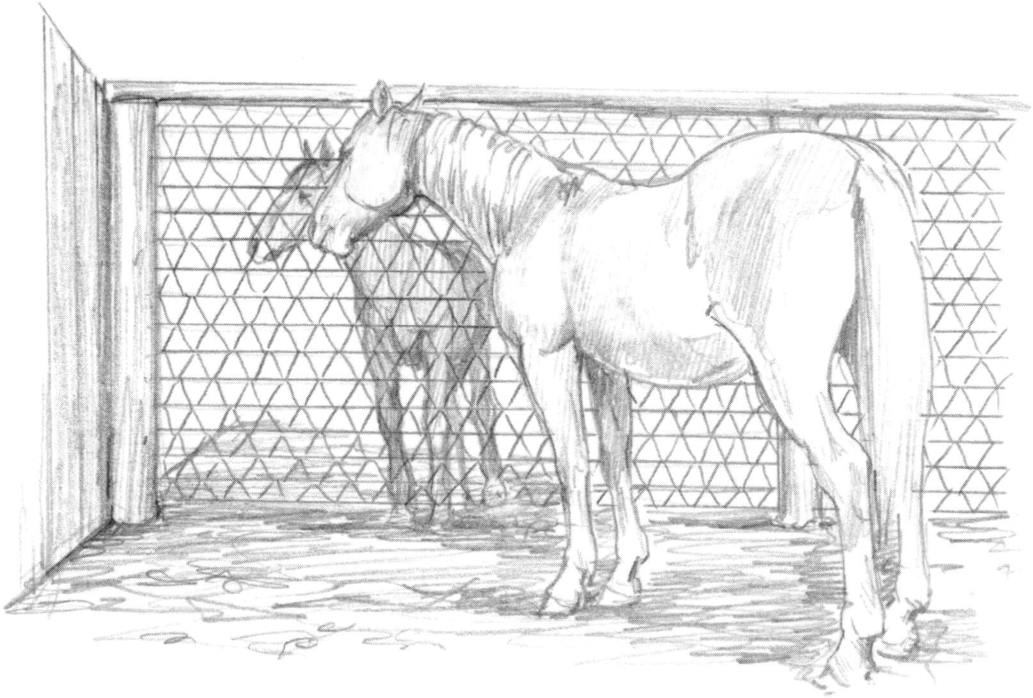

Deny nursing by means of a safe fence or a Dutch door.

FINE FACILITIES

FEEDERS

The best way to feed a horse is at ground level because it is the natural way a grazing animal eats. Eating off the ground gives the horse's topline a good stretch, which contributes to a stronger back and a neck with more desirable shape. (A shapely neck helps a horse move in balance.)

If you feed your horse at a high level, such as with an overhead feeder or high hay net, it forces his neck to work upside-down. This will cause the topline to dip and the bottom side to bulge. And if you do this over a period of time, it could lead to undesirable muscling and what looks like a ewe-neck. In addition, when a horse pulls hay down from a high feeder, flakes and dust fall in his nostrils and eyes, which can lead to tearing and coughing. And it requires a lot more grooming time to get the flakes out of his forelock and face. Not only is feeding at ground level natural, but watch your horses and you'll see that it is a very satisfying way for them to eat.

TIPS & TECHNIQUES

Trapped Food

Some feeders have nooks and crannies that trap bits of feed. This might cause a hungry, determined horse to paw the wall or pen, or bite at the feeder in frustration, both of which can turn into habits. If the trapped feed is not removed daily, it can mold and, if moist, can cause the feeder to rust.

TYPES OF FEEDERS. Although I feed all hay and grain at ground level, there are so many feeders on the market that I must discuss their pros and cons. Most horses prefer grain to hay, so if hay and grain are fed in the same container, they will pull the hay out onto the ground to get at the grain. It's best to feed hay and grain separately and to keep both feeds well away from the water supply to minimize the horse fouling the water

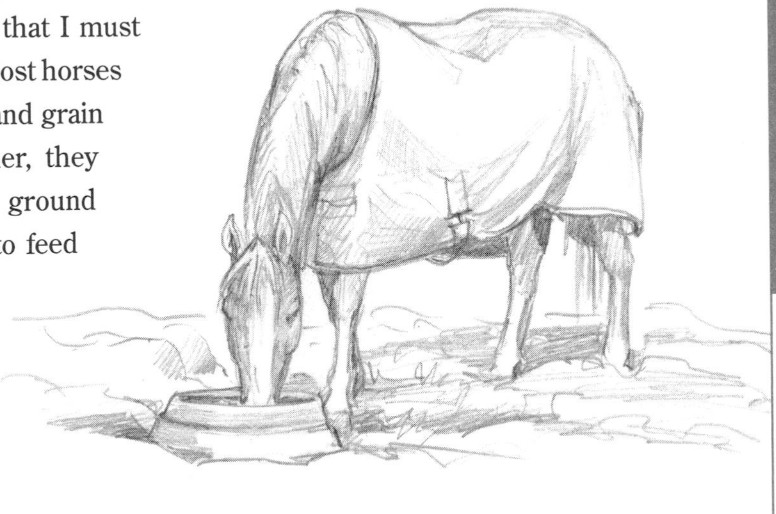

with feed. Hay and grain feeders mounted at head level might keep most of the hay from falling to the ground and being trampled, but hay stems and seeds can irritate the horse's eyes as he dives deep for tasty morsels. Also, the forelock and face get covered with hay flakes, requiring extra grooming.

TIPS & TECHNIQUES

Clean Is Good

Feed dishes and water buckets should be scrubbed with hot soapy water regularly. Be certain to rinse off every bit of soapy residue and let the buckets and feeder dry in a sunny spot.

GRAIN FEEDERS. Horses like to rub and chew on grain feeders, so choose one with no lip on the edge if possible. Some horses root around in a grain dish and push half the grain out onto the floor. When feeding a moderate to large amount of grain in a small, deep bucket, it is easy for the horse to bolt (gulp without chewing) his feed or push it out of the bucket onto the floor or ground.

A large round soft rubber tub spreads the feed over a larger area, which will slow the horse down. However, horses interpret this type of grain dish as a toy, something to pick up, throw, chew, and generally abuse. Large square hard plastic feed dishes with tapered sides are very difficult for a horse to pick up or tip over. These dishes are ideal for pen and pasture feeding and last a very long time. Wafers can be added to the grain to encourage the horse to sort, sift, and chew his feed thoroughly.

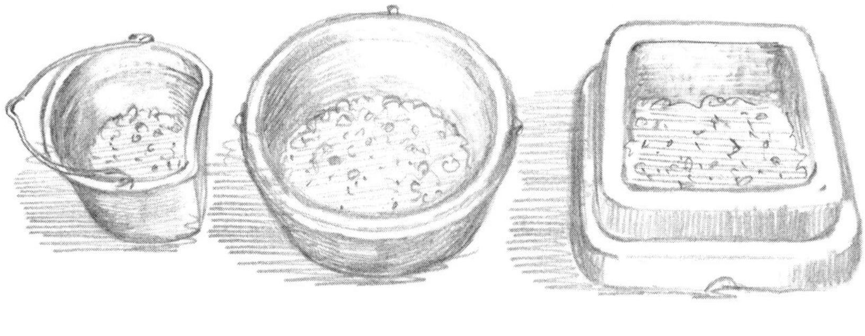

Three different feeders: too deep (left); better (center), but easily flipped; best (right).

Additional Feeder Tips

★ Because horses will almost certainly chew feeders made of wood, metal or durable plastic feeders are preferable.

★ When feeding a group of horses, a round metal feeder is a good way to prevent a bully from monopolizing all the hay.

★ Although heaping a hay rack might mean you won't have to feed the horses for a week or more, you'll likely end up wasting a large percentage of the hay that gets rained on, pulled out, or trampled.

★ With a swing-out hay and grain feeder, you don't have to enter the stall to feed.

★ Plastic corner stall feeders mounted low on the ground allow a horse to eat in a more natural position. Some horses will pull most of the hay out onto the floor anyway, so the bedding should be swept off the mats around the feeder.

★ A system that works well in stalls is to feed grain in a safe plastic corner model and feed hay on the floor.

★ A feeder should have no sharp corners or edges that might encourage rubbing.

★ A few large rocks in the grain will force him to search and browse in the grain, rather than gobble.

HAY BAGS AND NETS. Hay bags are useful when in transit or during wet or windy weather when a feeding area doesn't provide adequate shelter. A hay bag must be made of extra tough material and sturdy construction because horses are serious eaters. Secure it high so a horse can't get a foot caught in it, and fasten it to the pen at the bottom and top so he can't flip the bag over the top rail to the outside and then not be able to reach it.

Hay fed in a net, or even a double net, will occupy a horse longer than hay fed on the ground or in an open manger. For bored horses in a stall, double hay nets within a feeder will keep them busy and minimize vices caused by boredom. Make sure the hay net is tied to the feeder to prevent a horse pulling it out and getting tangled.

In outdoor situations during wet and/or windy weather, putting hay in a net within a feeder prevents a horse from pulling out huge sections of hay that can be blown away or trampled into the mud. In some cases, using a hay net in a sheltered area is better than feeding on the ground, since it prevents a horse from pushing the hay out into the wind.

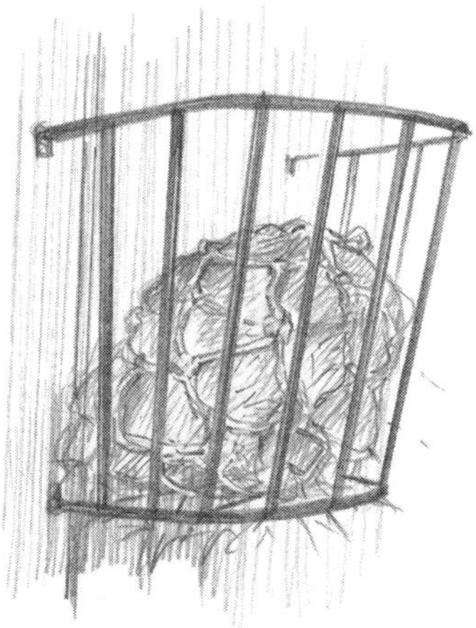

Using a hay net in a feeder.

MORE IN DEPTH

HORSE BLANKET TYPES

Here's an overview of types of blanket: fabric recommended; purpose; and care.

- **Stable sheet.** Cotton or cotton/polyester; to keep off dust or flies or to provide minimal warmth during cool weather; field wash or machine wash (cool or warm), or dry-clean, hang to dry.
- **Stable blanket.** Nylon and polyester; for moderate warmth in a stall; insulated; not waterproof; field wash, machine wash (cool or warm), or dry clean, hang to dry.
- **Turnout sheet.** Waterproof fabric, breathable; machine wash and dry.
- **Turnout blanket.** Waterproof fabric, breathable, insulated; machine wash or field wash, hang to dry.
- **Turnout fly sheet.** Textilene, for rugged conditions; machine wash or field wash, hang to dry.
- **New Zealand rug.** Canvas turnout rug often with blanket lining; for wind and water protection as well as warmth outside; field wash only and hang to dry.
- **Wool cooler.** Usually 85 to 100 percent wool; to cool out hot or sweaty horse; dry clean, hand wash cold, or machine wash cold gentle cycle; hang to dry.
- **Acrylic cooler.** Same as wool cooler, but machine wash and dry.
- **Scrim.** Stable fly sheet often made of nylon mesh; hand wash or machine wash gentle, hang to dry.
- **Antisweat sheet.** Heavy, breathable cotton mesh for stabled horses in hot, humid climates; machine wash cold, gentle, hang to dry, with stretching.

TIPS & TECHNIQUES

Soaking Hay

A hay net works well for soaking hay that is a bit dusty.

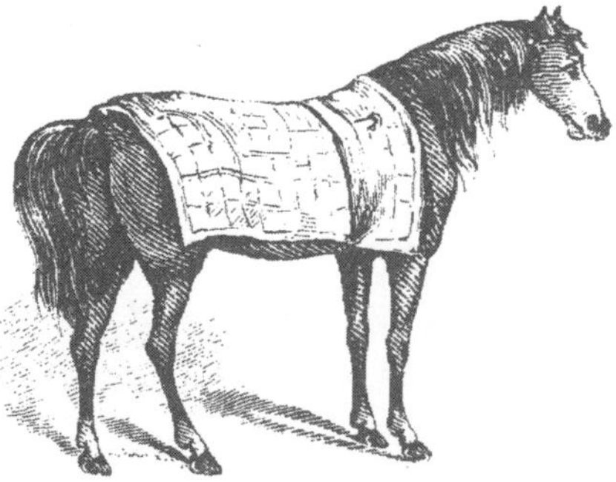

GETTING READY FOR WINTER

Richard and I have a "before the snow" list that we've been working on the last few weeks. No matter where you live, there are probably certain things you need to do before winter hits. Here are some of the things on our list:

1. **Be sure you have enough hay to last until next hay season.** You don't want to run out of hay in the middle of winter and go scrambling or pay high prices. Read how to choose good hay in July's More in Depth.

2. **Prevent wood chewing.** Research at Colorado State University has shown that wood chewing increases during cold, wet weather. If your horses have access to wooden fences, gates, or buildings, be sure the wood is protected from their destructive teeth. Not all horses are wood chewers, but even the most angelic horse can take a few bites when the weather is stressful. That's why it is important that during winter weather, horses get ample long-stem hay (as opposed to roughage in pellet or wafer form). The slow chewing associated with eating roughage is soothing and satiating to your horse.

3. **Get winter turnout sheets and blankets ready.** Any day now, I'll be putting breathable, waterproof turnout sheets or lightweight turnout blankets on my horses; they live in sheltered pens or on pasture. If your horse lives indoors, you will be shifting to a stable blanket of appropriate weight for your climate. Although you laundered and repaired all of the blankets in the spring, double-check them all now (examine buckles, Velcro, tail ties, surcingles) so they are ready to use at a moment's notice. For more on blankets, see October and November Clothes Horse.

en español

latigo. Comes from *el latigo*, 'a strap for tightening a cinch'.

RPMs & PTOs

It's time to check the antifreeze in the truck and the tractor.

Treat gas in all vehicles, including mowers and trimmers.

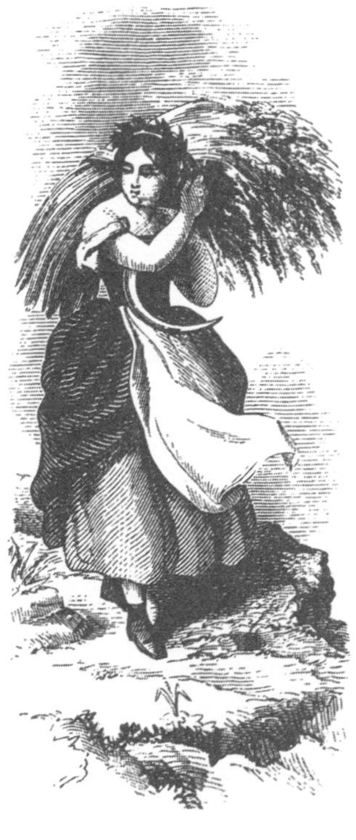

Horse Sense and Safety

Be Two-Sided

Work your horse from both the right and left sides so that he develops suppleness and obedience each way and does not become one-sided.

4. **Put tails up for the winter.** This will protect your horses' tails from accumulating ice and frozen mud and minimize breakage. See more on tail care in May and October Beauty Shop.

5. **Get any new fence posts into the ground.** Plan for this well before it freezes.

6. **Check your barn water lines, appliances, faucets, and hoses.** Be sure they are protected from freezing.

7. **Move all of your freezable items.** Store fly sprays, grooming products, and other perishables in a heated cupboard or room.

8. **Oil gate hinges and latches.** If they operate freely they will have less chance of freezing up.

9. **Plan your winter shoeing needs.** Go over these with your farrier. See more in October Foot Notes.

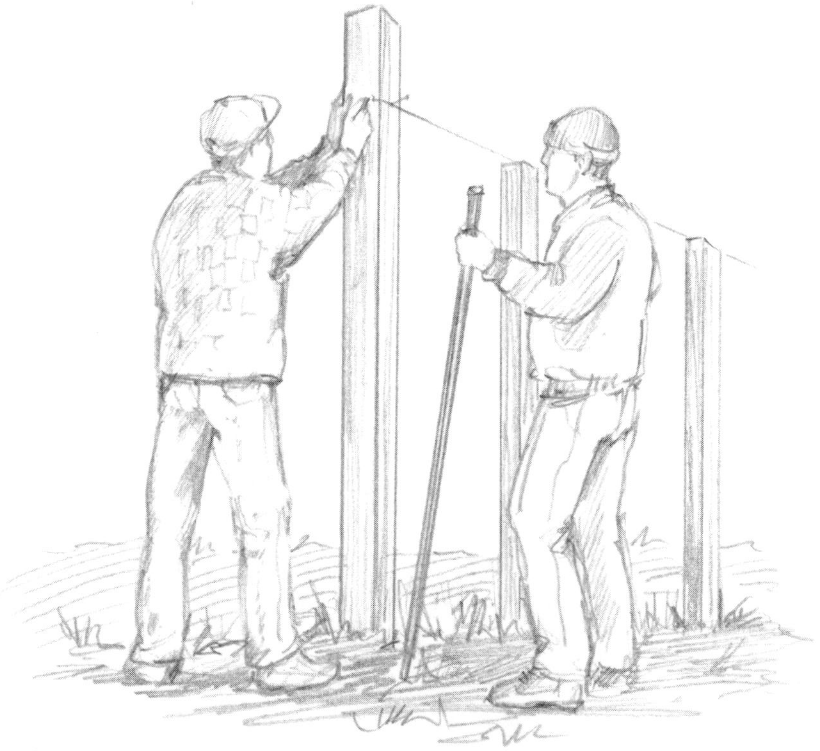

If you have fence posts to dig, do so before the ground freezes.

HANTAVIRUS

The deer mouse and the white-footed mouse carry viruses that can lead to hantavirus pulmonary syndrome. The hantavirus is a zoonose, a disease that can be transmitted from animals to humans. The virus spreads through aerosolization, when humans stir up infected rodent living quarters (such as when cleaning out a hay barn). The humans inhale infected particles that were shed with saliva, urine, and droppings. Therefore, avoid stirring up dust. If you are clearing out a suspected rodent nesting area, wear a respirator mask, wet the area with a disinfectant before you work, pick up debris, and then wet again before you mop or sweep.

FYI

Sin Nombre

Normally hantavirus has a 10 percent mortality rate, but the strain that broke out in Four Corners (Colorado, New Mexico, Arizona, and Utah) in 1993 had a 50 percent mortality rate. During that outbreak, the virus was called the '*Sin Nombre*' virus, meaning 'Without Name.'

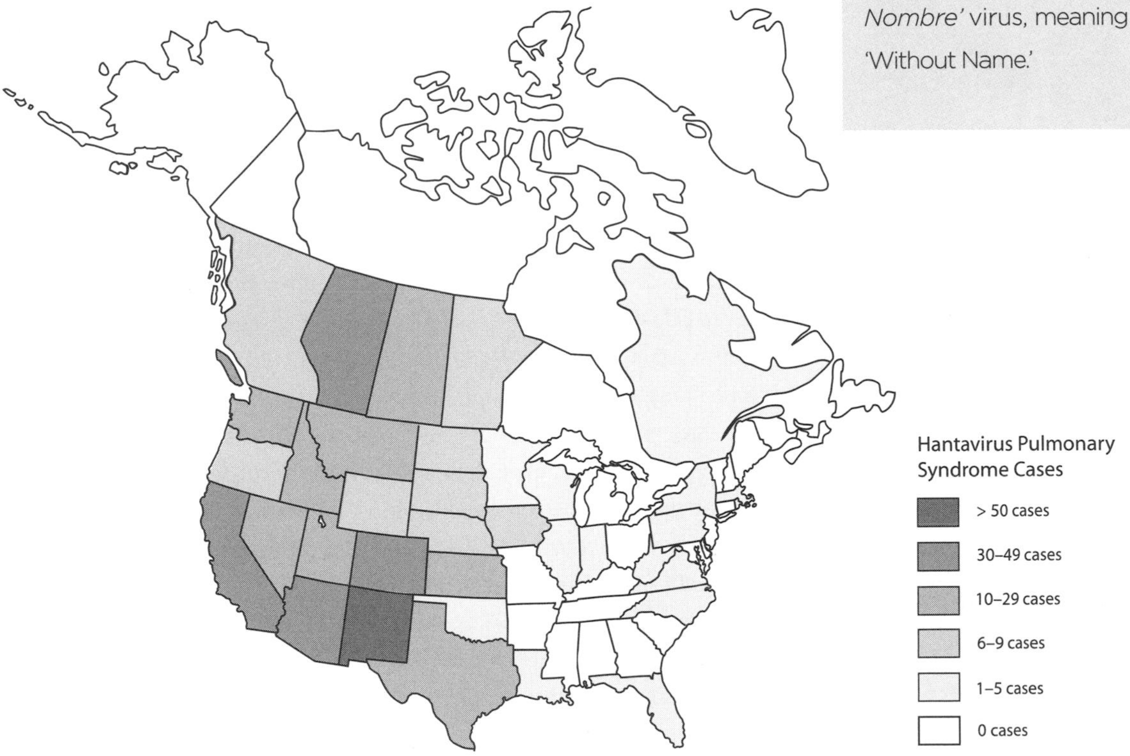

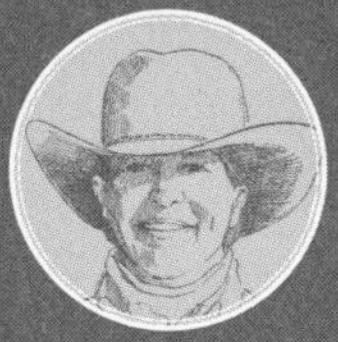

Ask Cherry

Fear of Water

Q

I recently bought a horse that is petrified of puddles. I want to trail-ride him and we have to cross a lot of small streams. I don't want to get out there and have a bad situation develop. Help !

A

Fear of water can be overcome by using a progressive training program. First, lead your horse over suspicious, but safe, obstacles such as a sturdy wooden bridge, a rubber mat placed in the middle of a grassy area, sheets of plastic or canvas, or an old horse blanket or coat. Choose the obstacles carefully. You want your horse to trust you, so don't ask him to cross anything dangerous. Your horse should approach the obstacle with his body straight, take a look at it as he approaches, and then walk straight across it without veering his hind legs off to one side as he crosses. Horses can't see things directly below their heads, so as you approach an obstacle, let him lower his head (remember this when riding) so he can get his eyes down to where he can focus. Once you can work obstacles in-hand, ride the horse over the obstacles as part of his at-home training. But don't just work on obstacles over and over and over. Instead, ride a little, come to the obstacle and work it, then take a spin around the pasture or arena and come back later. This will be more like trail conditions where you ride a while and then encounter a stream.

For the next stage, you will need puddles. Start with the largest you can find because a horse will more likely walk through a large puddle but try to sidestep or hop over a small one. Use the same technique as with the obstacles. Start by leading him across puddles. Let him take his time to inspect — let him put his head down so he can look at the puddle. Step into the puddle yourself to show him it is safe, and ask him to walk forward with you. If he veers, balks, or rushes, go back to one of the previous obstacles and work on one step at a time, proper position, moving forward at an even pace with calmness. Then return to the puddles. Let your horse stand in the puddle.

Once he is calm about being led through puddles, begin riding him across them. Use this type of progressive training to build your horse's confidence, and he will trust your judgment when you come to a stream on the trail.

OCTOBER

I love to ride in the snow, so in October I winterize my horses. Richard outfits them with winter shoes to prevent snowballing and provide good traction. Since the horses' tails aren't needed as flyswatters, I put them up for the winter. That way they won't drag through the snow and develop frozen dangle balls. Also, since the flies are gone here in Colorado, this is an ideal time for gelding.

Day Length in Hours

Latitude	Oct 1	Oct 16	Nov 1
60°N	11.13	9.74	8.31
55°N	11.28	10.15	9
50°N	11.4	10.46	9.52
45°N	11.5	10.71	9.93
40°N	11.58	10.92	10.27
35°N	11.65	11.1	10.56
30°N	11.71	11.26	10.81

See page 22 to find your latitude.

WACKY WONDERFUL WEATHER

TIME CHANGE

In the United States, we used to change back to Standard Time (ST) in October, but now that change takes place in November, so read the entry in November Wacky Wonderful Weather. In Canada (except for Saskatchewan) and Mexico, however, the change back to ST takes place on the last Sunday in October.

VET CLINIC

PIGEON FEVER

If you notice a swelling in your horse's chest that grows quickly, it could be from a kick, but it also could be pigeon fever, caused by infection from the bacterium *Corynebacterium pseudotuberculosis*. It is not known exactly how the bacterium is carried into the horse's tissues, but it enters through wounds, broken skin, or mucous membranes, possibly carried by insects such as flies. Horses that get pigeon fever can be of any age or sex and are usually in good health. Most cases occur in California and Texas in the late summer and fall, but are also seen in other western states. The infection may be internal, external, or in a limb. The most common is an external abscess, very deep under the pectoral muscle area.

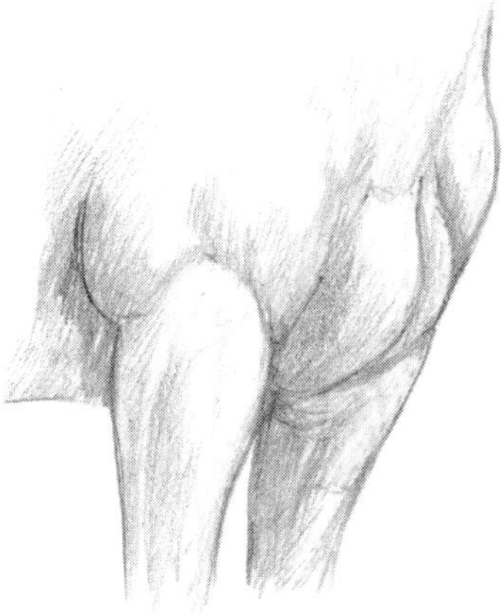

A marked swelling in your horse's pectoral muscles could be pigeon fever.

TREATMENT. All stalls, paddocks, utensils, and tack should be disinfected.

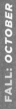

A long, large-bore needle (4-inch, 12-gauge) is used to determine when the abscess is ready to be lanced. If thick, creamy pus is aspirated, it is time to open the abscess. After the drainage incision is made, the exudate is released and carefully collected and disposed of, as it is highly contagious. Then the deep cavity is flushed thoroughly with Betadine solution. Follow-up includes hydrotherapy, a thorough cleansing with Betadine scrub, and flushing with saline or Betadine solution.

This is done once a day for a week to two weeks as tissue healing takes place. At the end of each daily treatment, the surrounding area is dried thoroughly and a film of antiseptic ointment or petroleum jelly is applied below the incision to soothe the skin and prevent the exudate from scalding the hair and skin. Full healing and complete remission of swelling and scar tissue will take two months or more.

The prognosis is good with proper care. Recovery takes 2 to 10 weeks. Some horses experience recurrence.

Use of antibiotics to treat pigeon fever is controversial. Although it is thought that antibiotics should not be administered before lancing the abscess (as that would delay formation of the abscess and prolong the disease), antibiotics (such as 30cc penicillin IM each day for four days) are often used after lancing to prevent any secondary bacterial infections from complicating healing. Confer with your veterinarian regarding his or her exact recommendations.

LOOKING AT HORSES

Hind Legs

The bone structure and muscling of a horse's hind limbs should be appropriate for the intended use. Endurance horses are characterized by longer, flatter muscles; stock horses by shorter, thicker muscles; all-around horses by moderate muscles. A line from the point of buttock to the ground should touch the hock and end slightly behind the bulbs of the heels.

To Do

- ❑ Hoof trim and winter shoes
- ❑ Tails up
- ❑ Gelding
- ❑ Work arena
- ❑ Scrub feed tubs and buckets
- ❑ Move hay to barns

To Buy

- ❑ Complete feed wafers
- ❑ Grain
- ❑ Dewormer
- ❑ Bedding

FYI

Other Names for Pigeon Fever

- ★ Pigeon breast
- ★ Colorado distemper
- ★ Breastbone fever
- ★ Dry-land strangles
- ★ Dry-land distemper
- ★ False distemper
- ★ False strangles

FOOT NOTES

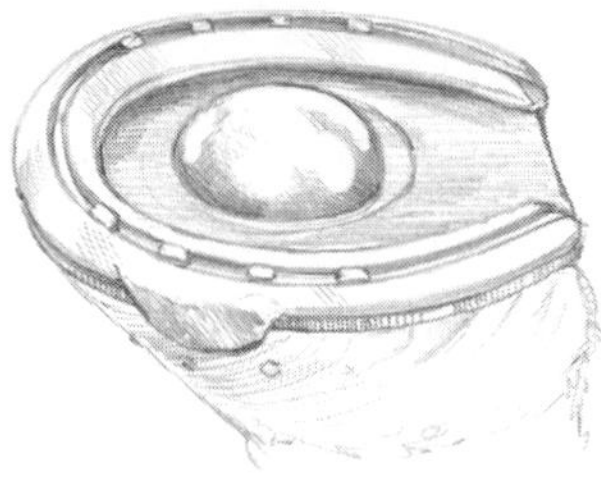

A bubble pad will help pop snowballs out of the hoof before they adhere.

WINTER SHOES

If you ride outdoors in a temperate climate in the winter, your horse will have some special shoeing requirements. One approach is to have your horse's shoes pulled for the winter. At the other end of the spectrum is having him shod with pads and traction devices so he can work in all types of footing. To design your winter hoof care program, consider the natural conformation of your horse's hooves, the level and type of his exercise during the winter months, the footing in his exercise and turnout areas, the typical weather patterns in your locale, and the expertise of your farrier.

BAREFOOT OR NOT. A barefoot horse with a naturally balanced hoof, dense hoof horn, and a well-cupped sole can often negotiate winter footings without injury or damage. A naturally concave sole sheds snow, mud, and slush well. However, a hoof with a long toe and low heel, brittle or punky horn, and a flat sole has poor traction, and the sole is vulnerable to bruising from frozen ground. During the winter, the hoof growth rate can slow to almost half its spring rate, which means the hoof cannot stand a great deal of abrasive wear.

For active winter riding, therefore, a horse often needs to be shod or booted. Shoeing offers protection for the hoof and helps to maintain proper balance. In addition, winter shoeing can serve two other purposes: providing additional traction and preventing snowballing.

TRACTION. Various amounts of traction can be utilized with shoes and boots. Here's a brief overview:

- Rim shoes provide significantly more traction than plain shoes do.

TIPS & TECHNIQUES

Winter Treads

In some combinations of snow type and temperature, it is simply impossible to provide safe traction and prevent snowballing. In most types of winter footing, however, good results can be obtained by a combination of the horse's normal shoes with an application of various traction and antisnowballing devices.

- Aluminum shoes have a slightly better grab than steel on frozen ground because the metal is softer.
- Aluminum racing plates with toe grabs and/or heel stickers could be appropriate for moderate work in relatively soft footing.
- Rubber and plastic shoes tend to provide less traction than either the bare hoof or steel shoes and can be hard and slippery in cold temperatures.
- Steel keg shoes with permanent caulks forged at the toe and/or heels sink into semi-frozen ground or "soft" ice and give good traction. However, on hard ice, such shoes are dangerously slippery.

Removable studs allow for adaptation to the constantly changing winter footing conditions. A hard surfacing material such as borium can be applied at the toe and/or heel of the horse's regular steel or aluminum shoes in smears, beads, or points. Nails with ribbed or specially hardened heads can be substituted for regular horseshoe nails to allow a horse to grab onto the ground. Although they provide good traction in snow or soft ice, when the horse is moving on uneven frozen ground, some ice nails can provide too much stick and torque, which may lead to wrenched joints and other leg problems. Also, traction devices can damage trailer and barn flooring.

ANTISNOWBALLING. Mixtures of snow, ice, mud, manure, grass, or bedding can pack densely into large, rounded ice mounds in the sole that are almost impossible to chip out. The junction of the inner edge of the shoe with the sole provides a place for the mud and ice to become securely lodged. The snow melts from the heat of the sole and freezes onto the metal horseshoe, and the snowball is born.

Applying various substances such as grease to the sole of the barefoot or shod horse or spraying it with a nonstick cooking coating may prevent snow buildup during certain

What's Wrong with Snowballs?

When a horse is forced to stand or move on the snowballs packed in his hooves, he has decreased stability in his fetlock joint. His weight is liable to suddenly roll medially, laterally, forward, or backward. It is extremely fatiguing for his muscles, tendons, and joint ligaments as he constantly must make adjustments to maintain his equilibrium. It is easy for a snowballed horse to momentarily lose his balance and wrench a fetlock.

See September for more on hoof pads.

temperatures, but only temporarily. Half-round shoes do a fair job of shedding snow because of the inside rounded edge. However, half-rounds provide poor winter traction, so ice nails or borium need to be used with them.

Full pads can help prevent snowballing in some situations. The choices include plastic of various types, synthetic rubber, and leather. Full pads with a convex bubble at the sole seem to be only marginally better than full flat pads at popping out accumulated snow. Traction, incidentally, is decreased with full pads.

BEST SOLUTION. Tube-type rim pads, which fit between the shoe and the hoof wall and leave the sole open, are the best antisnowballing option. The sole retains its cupped traction feature, can respire normally, and can descend with weight bearing. As the horse's weight descends on the hoof, the pads flex and dislodge the snow that accumulates at the junction of the shoe and sole. Tube pads with open shoes work well in most weather conditions. Bar shoes (such as egg bar shoes or full support shoes) will trap snow and not allow the tube pads to do their job as effectively.

FEED BAG

FEEDING YOUR OLDER HORSE

As a horse ages, his ability to digest certain nutrients declines. Which nutrients and how seriously the absorption is compromised vary between individuals and depend on the horse's prior parasite prevention program. In addition, a horse's ability to manufacture certain vitamins may also decline with age, so vitamin supplementation (B complex and C) is often recommended for senior horses.

Ranch Recipes

Homemade Anti-Chew

Wood chewing tends to increase as weather gets colder and wetter. To prevent it, treat wood with various "potions" to make it less palatable. Effective commercial products are available. To deter first-time nibblers, you can try rubbing a strongly scented bar of soap (such as Irish Spring) over the area.

If you try the commonly recommended home remedy of oil and chili sauce, be careful, because if you or your horse gets the substance in your eyes or nose, it will burn! And believe it or not, some horses chew more after chili oil has been applied to wood.

Senior Diet

Know the needs and eating habits of each of your senior horses and feed them individually. Individually is the operative word here — feed each senior horse separately so he gets his prescribed ration and doesn't have to compete.

Guard against anorexia, the loss of interest in eating. Once a horse gets thin, it can be a great challenge to put the weight back on. Keep a horse interested in eating by providing him with high-quality feeds in amounts he will clean up readily. Feed him two to four times per day.

HAY. The base of a senior's ration should be premium hay. Roughage is essential for proper digestive tract function, yet as a horse ages, his ability to chew and process coarse roughage decreases. Yet ultra-fine third-cut "rabbit hay" alfalfa is not the answer either. With its high leaf-to-stem ratio, such hay could lead to gaseous colic and excess weight gain. In addition, the high calcium content of alfalfa can lead to calcium oxalate kidney stones.

Ideally, look for bright green fine-stemmed grass hay or a grass/alfalfa mix containing no more than 20 percent alfalfa. To avoid respiratory problems and heaves, just say no to any hay with even a trace of dust or mold. For horses with chewing difficulty, feed chopped hay, hay cubes, or hay pellets (soaked) — all available in bags. Since choke is more common in older horses, monitor the use of cubes carefully.

GRAIN. Choose a palatable, well-balanced, easily digestible grain ration for seniors. Rolled or flaked grains are easier to digest than whole grains. Avoid whole corn and whole soybeans altogether as they are very hard and would cause excess wear and stress to the molars. Pelleted complete rations, often billed as "senior" feeds, are specially formulated for the needs of an older horse.

When a Horse Needs More

If a horse has trouble keeping on weight or needs more fat on his ribs to weather the winter, you can use a high-fat feed or top-dress the grain ration with oil. Fat has 2½ times more dietary energy than an equal weight of carbohydrates. While some horses shun oily feed, most find corn oil palatable.

Start with ¼ cup of oil per feeding; hold at that level for four feedings; then increase by ⅛ to ¼ cup at a time. The horse should clean up his grain within an hour of feeding. Also monitor the consistency of the horse's stool, as too much oil too soon can cause a loose stool.

Making Horses Last

There are many things you can do to help your horse live a long and healthy life.

1. Arrange for an annual dental exam.

2. Feed a low amount of grain.

3. Feed high-quality hay with no dust or mold.

4. Feed at ground level on clean rubber mats; use psyllium monthly if needed.

5. Give him regular exercise.

6. Arrange for regular farrier care.

7. Deworm six times a year or as advised by your veterinarian.

8. Monitor pasture grazing carefully.

Senior feeds usually have a high beet pulp content, which is a good source of calcium and contains pectin, which is very easily digestible. If you are feeding beet pulp and alfalfa hay, pay attention to the total calcium of your horse's ration, as high calcium might be detrimental to an arthritic horse or one with kidney problems.

Aim for 12 to 14 percent crude protein for the overall hay and grain ration. If you are feeding straight grass hay and the protein content of your grain mix is low, you might want to consider feeding ¼ cup or so of soybean flakes to increase the protein.

Water

If your senior horse isn't drinking, he won't eat. It's that simple, and it's that scary. Know your individual horse's water requirements (usually between 5 and 10 gallons per day) and ensure that he takes in that much during severe cold, debilitating heat, or when traveling — the times when he is most likely to go off water. Although automatic waterers are labor saving, they do not allow you to know whether your horse is drinking and how much.

Don't ever require any horse to satisfy his water requirement by eating snow; he would use precious body heat to melt enough snow to fill his needs. And similarly, don't make a senior work for a sip between icebergs in a frozen trough. Offer the geriatric horse freshly drawn water (which often comes out of the ground at about 50°F) or use a bucket heater.

DECREASE GRAIN FOR ALL HORSES

For all horses, decrease grain with work. If you are going to give your horse the winter off or greatly reduce his work load, begin decreasing his grain ration in relationship to his activity level.

WILD LIFE

DEER NEIGHBORS

Fall is a great time for viewing wildlife such as wild turkeys and our resident deer herd, which usually consists of one to three bucks and about ten does. Who wouldn't want a yearly batch of little Bambis bounding across the pastures? They are so darling. It's like Disneyland! But the fantasy has its flip side too. Some realities about a horsekeeper's life with deer (and elk and moose, for that matter) need to be considered.

TRAFFIC ACCIDENTS. Where deer are thick, it's not unusual for them to dash in front of a vehicle, day or night. When you least want to slam on the brakes (such as when pulling a horse trailer), you might have to in order to avoid smacking a deer.

LANDSCAPING. Deer will eat your favorite flowers, shrubs, and trees. It is just a fact. We have to landscape with deer-proof plants, and we protect those that aren't.

> **TIPS & TECHNIQUES**
>
> **Plague Protection**
>
> Flea powder and shampoo can protect pets from flea infestation but won't protect cats that eat infected rodents. For protection, humans should use DEET and not handle or feed wild animals.

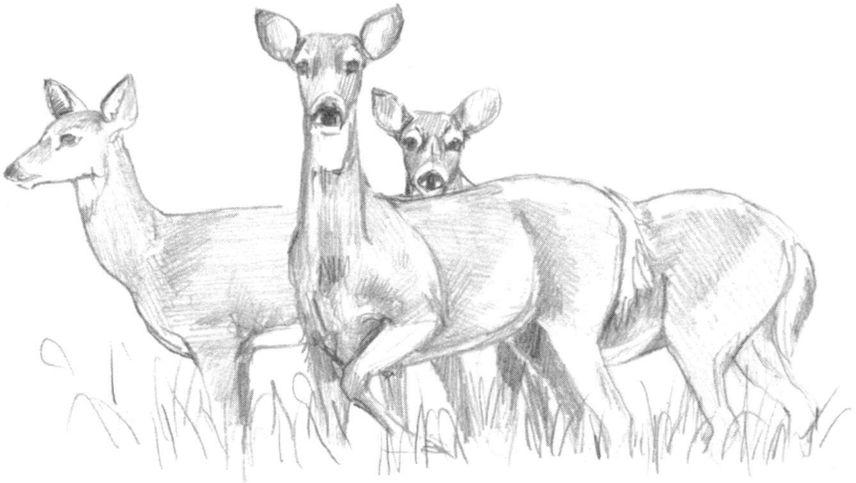

Living with resident deer herds takes some specific management.

Fleas and Plague

Because you most likely have dogs and cats on your farm or ranch, you need to know about fleas. Rodents that have bubonic plague can spread the plague through their fleas to cats. Humans can contract the plague from the bite of an infected flea or the oral or respiratory secretions of an infected animal. Cats become ill from the plague and are the most common carriers to humans. Dogs rarely get sick but can carry infected fleas into the house or barn.

Wild animals that can carry infected fleas include mice, prairie dogs, squirrels, rats, rabbits, chipmunks, marmots, and other rodents. The plague is always present but increases when conditions favor a rodent explosion.

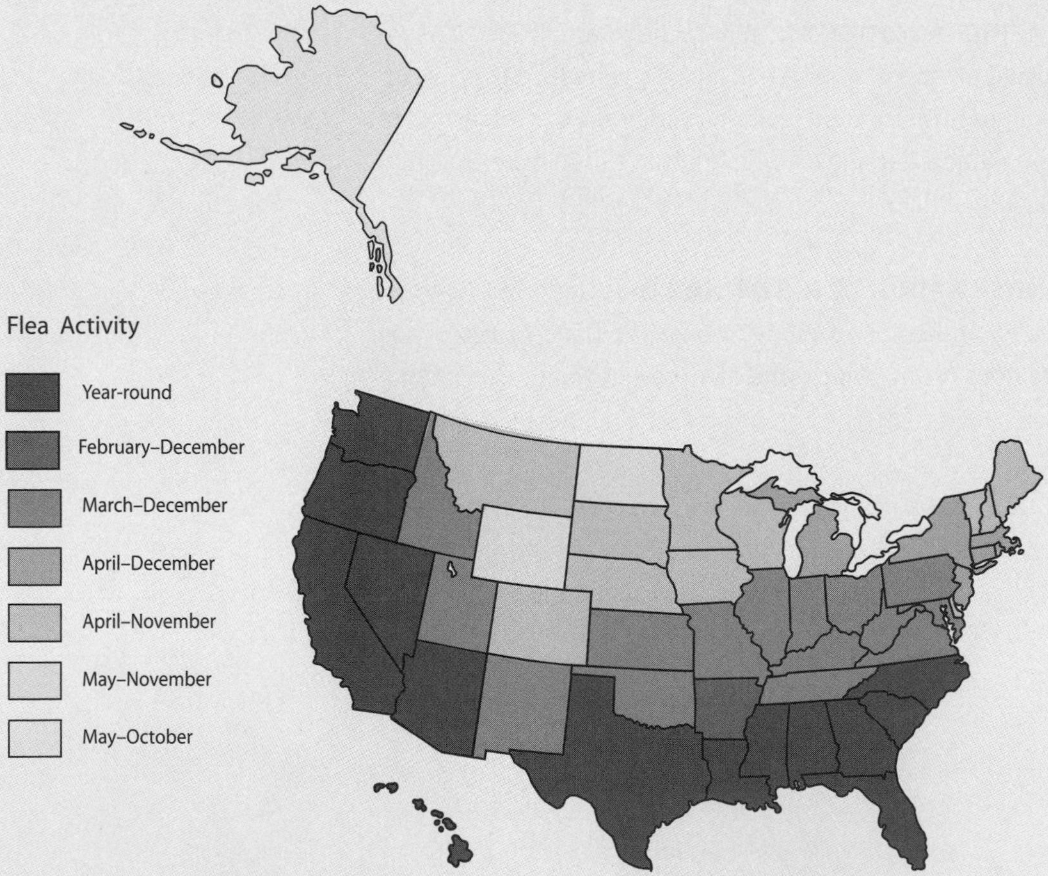

Vegetable gardens are difficult or impossible to maintain. We use a deer buster — a motion-detecting high-pressure cold-water spray — to keep the deer away from the perennial garden at the front of our house.

FENCING. Deer are hard on fences. They knock down, stretch, and break all types of fencing material, often shorting out electric fences.

If only I could train the deer to graze the roadside ditches and open lands and leave the improved pasture for my horses.

PASTURE. Our "resident herd" consumes quite a bit of pasture and some years, such as during a drought, pasture is precious. If only I could train the deer to graze the roadside ditches and open lands and leave the improved pasture for my horses.

PASTURE PERFECT

NATURAL WATER SOURCES

The Clean Water Act of 1972 requires that riparian areas (vegetation on the banks of natural water sources) be protected. We do this by limiting the grazing in our creek pastures, fencing to allow access only in certain, trample-resistant areas, and providing water troughs in the pasture when the natural streams and creeks begin to dry up. This minimizes mud, keeps water quality high, and protects the streamside vegetation from overgrazing and trample damage. The result is less erosion and contamination.

See August for more on protecting riparian areas.

WINTER PASTURES

In October I start using winter pastures — those that the horses have not grazed since about late July, so they have substantial late-season growth that has dried on the stem.

There is no secret (quite) so close as that between a rider and his horse.

— Robert Smith Surtees, *Mr. Sponge's Sporting Tour*, 1853

FALL: OCTOBER

BEDDING

Bedding should be clean, dust-free, nontoxic, absorbent, not slippery when wet, soft enough to encourage a horse to lie down without developing fetlock and hock sores, easy for you to handle, available, economical, and something that a horse won't eat. Thinking ahead about your choice of bedding will probably affect your choice of stall flooring, and vice versa. Availability greatly affects price. You'll likely find wood shavings more economical in timber areas and straw bedding less expensive in farming areas. When choosing bedding, always factor in transportation costs.

> **Minimizing Dust**
>
> All beddings, even peat moss, can be dusty. To prevent respiratory problems in your horse, be selective and don't purchase dusty bedding material.

SOFTWOOD PRODUCTS. Softwood products, such as pine sawdust, shavings, or chips, are commonly used for bedding. They are often fragrant and make a stall easy to clean. Here are the principal types:

- **Sawdust** of large particles is from logs sawn into lumber. Sawdust from smaller saws, like those in cabinet shops, may be too fine and dusty for bedding.

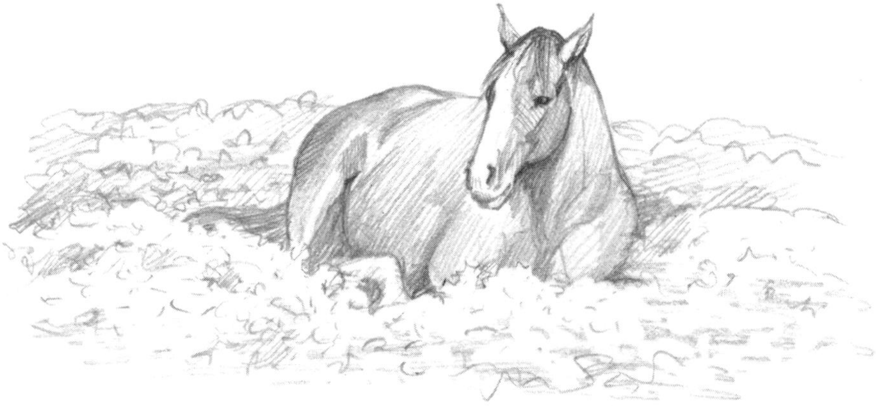

Bedding (In Order of Absorbency)

BEDDING	Lbs. of water absorbed per lb. of bedding	Cost	Comfort
Peat moss	10.0	high	thick, soft bed
Pine chips	3.0	low	rough
Oat straw	2.8	medium	good if not crushed
Pine sawdust	2.5	low	warm, soft bed
Wheat straw	2.2	high	good if not crushed
Barley straw	2.1	high	short stem, not elastic
Pine shavings	2.0	low	fluffy bed
Hardwood chips, sawdust, or shavings	1.5	low	can be rough
Sand	.2	low	soft but abrasive

- **Shavings** are very thin, small slices of wood produced by the planing or surfacing of lumber. Shavings are available at sawmills and cabinet shops.
- **Chips** are small, coarse pieces of wood produced by the drilling, shaping, turning, or molding of lumber.
- **Wood fiber and pulp** are manufactured from softwood waste, and may be more abrasive than shavings.
- **Wood pellets** are shavings and sawdust with all the oils and resins removed and compressed into granules. The pellets are placed in the stall, watered, and fluffed. Although less bedding might be used with pellets than with shavings, pellets are considerably more expensive.

Avoid Hardwood Bedding

Hardwood products are generally undesirable because of their poor absorbency and in some cases, such as with black walnut, a dangerous toxicity. Horses merely coming in contact with such shavings have experienced founder and death.

Absorbency

The bedding with the highest water-absorbing capacity is not necessarily the best bet. Extremely absorbent bedding sops up too much urine and the horse stands or lies in the soggy mess. On the other hand, bedding with very little absorbency allows too much moisture to pass through to the flooring. The ideal bedding in most cases has an absorbency of between 2.0 and 3.0 and is free from dust, mold, and injurious substances.

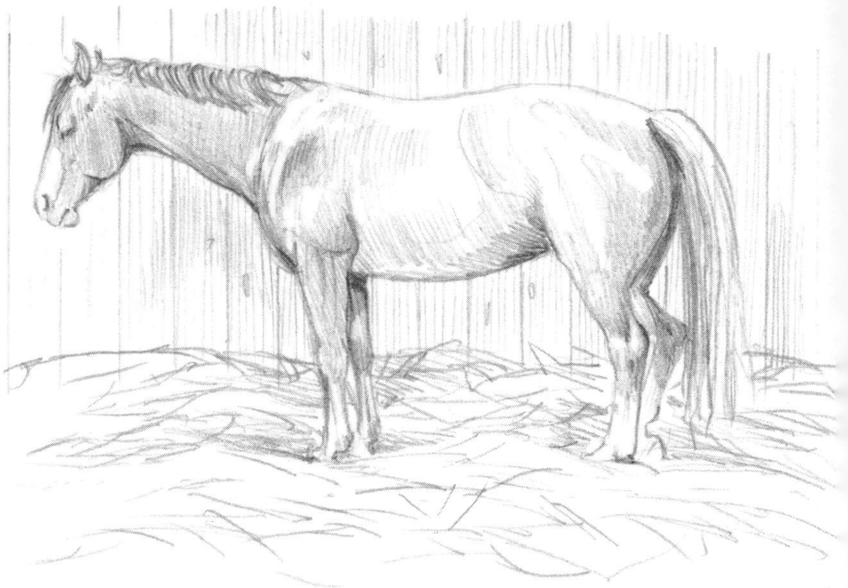

STRAW. Straw is traditional, but a stall bedded with straw is more difficult to economically clean. Straw of any kind is very slippery on wood floors. Here are some pros and cons of the different types:

- **Oat straw** is the favorite bedding for foaling, but it can be slippery and some horses eat it like there is no tomorrow.
- **Wheat straw,** because of its high glaze, does not become as slimy and sloppy as oat straw when wet. It is less palatable to horses than oat straw, so may be safer to use with the horse that overeats.
- **Avoid barley straw** because of the sharp, barbed awns that can become lodged in horses' gums.

While there are many things you can fake through in this life, pretending that you know horses when you don't isn't one of them.

— Cooky McClung, *Horsefolk Are Different*

Bedding Characteristics

BEDDING	Cleanliness	Convenience Factors	Palatability	Other
Peat moss	dusty; gets foul fast	light when dry; very heavy when wet	low	difficult to see manure; gets soggy; associated with thrush; good compost value
Pine chips	can contain foreign objects	usually hauled bulk, then must be shoveled	low	horse often gets "straw belly" from eating bedding
Oat straw	good	light bales but slimy when wet	high	can be drying to hooves
Pine sawdust	can contain foreign objects	bags OK; bulk then must be shoveled	low	can pack and be drying to hooves, can ferment when wet and heat hooves
Wheat straw	rarely dusty	light bales; heavy when wet	low; but OK if eaten	food compost value but makes large manure pile
Barley straw	often damp or dusty	light bales; heavy when wet	awns irritate eyes and mouth; can cause colic	can cause colic
Pine shavings	can contain foreign objects	very light but large volume required	low	can be drying to hooves; hang in mane and tail
Hardwood chips, sawdust, or shavings	can contain foreign objects	hauled bulk then must be shoveled	black walnut toxin can cause founder	not worth the chance of toxic effect if black walnut is present
Sand	dusty	heavy	inadvertently ingested with feed	may result in colic or hoof damage — sand particles can work their way into the bottom of the hoof wall

Odd Word

bloom. Radiance and peak health of a horse evidenced by fitness and a shiny coat; often refers to the appearance of a horse after he has been on green pasture for a few weeks.

OTHER MATERIALS. Shredded paper (from newspaper) or cardboard is heavy when wet and not as aesthetically acceptable as shavings or straw might be, especially when blowing around. Diatomaceous earth and clay are said to neutralize odors as well as absorb.

OCTOBER Manure Pile Maintenance
PILE A Turn once, water as needed.
PILE B Turn once, water as needed.
PILE C Sell, store, or spread.

STILL TRUE TODAY

Historical Horsekeeping

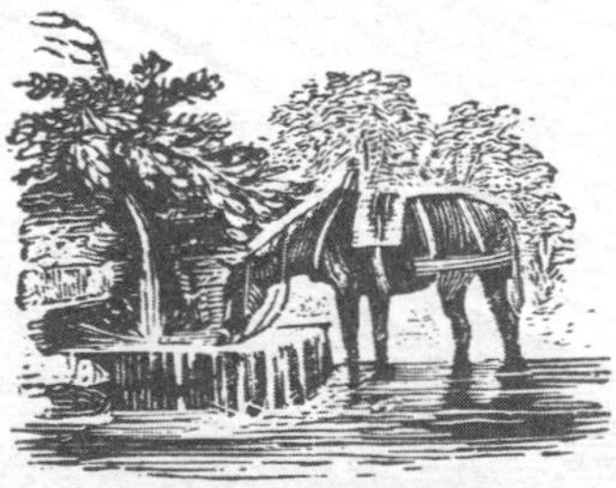

"The water of large lakes, rivers and running brooks is best and in the order named. That of ponds without outlet or inlet the worst; in fact pond water should never be used; well water is altogether better and may be given without fear, when used constantly, but as with man, the horse accustomed to lake or river water, which is always partially soft, should be given well water, when necessity requires, with care and only in small quantities, the change being gradually made."

— Gleason's Horse Book *by Prof. Oscar R. Gleason, 1892*

FALL: OCTOBER

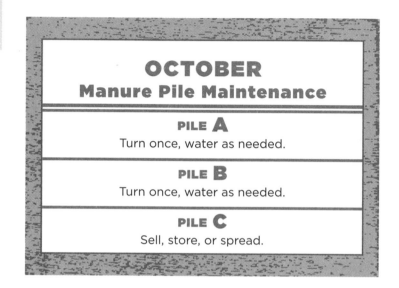

LONG TAILS

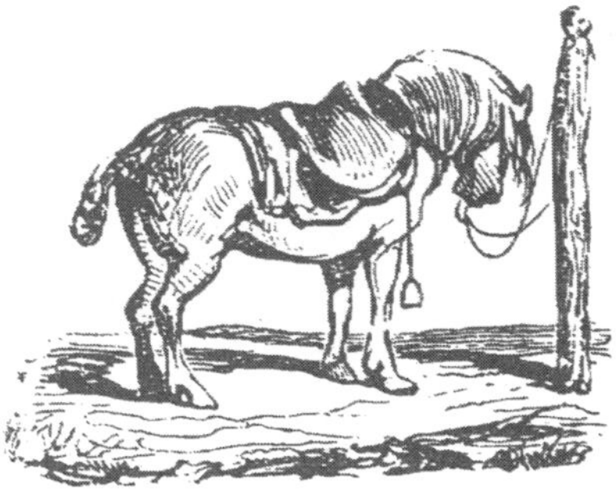

Visitors to our place marvel at the long, thick tails on every single one of our horses. To keep my horses' manes and tails long and healthy, I follow a three-part program.

First, I feed very good-quality hay. I pay particular attention to this, because hay is the mainstay of my horses' diet. Every horse also receives a hoof supplement daily. It is a high-quality, broad-spectrum nutritional supplement designed to accelerate hoof growth and improve the quality of the hoof horn. Hair and hoof are made of similar materials, so it is no surprise that it also positively affects hair growth.

Second, I follow a specific grooming protocol. I bathe, brush, and comb the manes and tails only when necessary, and I use products that I have found mane and tail friendly. I use only brushes on long manes and tails, never combs, which tend to break hairs. I keep all tails banged (cut blunt) at a level no lower than the point of the fetlock when the horse's tail is relaxed and flat and hanging the longest. (Instead of banging, you might prefer the look of a tapered tail.) When I let a tail grow longer than the fetlocks, the horse invariably steps on it when getting up from rolling and pulls out large, long hunks. When a tail is too long, I've seen horses remove large sections when backing up in a performance class or unloading from a trailer. That thins a tail in a hurry!

The world is best viewed through the ears of a horse.
— Anonymous

Third, I put the tails up for the winter (below). As soon as the last fly is gone in the fall, I braid the tails and keep them braided until the first fly appears in the spring. In March or April, because of the high level of winter nutrition and the protection of the braid, I usually cut 4 to 6 inches off the tails in order to meet my fetlock criteria. With most horses, I have to cut off an additional 4 inches in July or August.

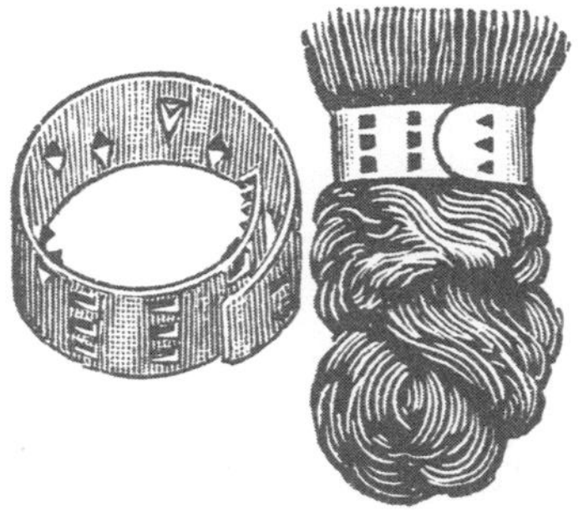

TAILS UP FOR THE WINTER

To protect my horses' tails from winter snow and mud, I put them up for the winter. When the last fly has departed in the fall, I shampoo, condition, and brush the tail. I cut a 10-foot piece of ¼-inch to 1-inch-wide gauze. Here's how to proceed.

1. Starting at the bottom of the dock (the flesh and bone part of the tail), I divide the tail into three equal sections.
2. I place the midpoint of the gauze behind the midpoint of the middle section of hair, and hold one strand of gauze with each of the other two sections.
3. I braid the tail with a three-strand braid, stopping when I am about 12 inches from the end of the tail. At this point, there are about 1 to 2 feet of gauze left on each side.
4. I tie two overhand knots in the gauze, pass the free end of the gauze through the tail where the braiding began, and pull the end of the tail through.
5. I fasten the three layers together with overhand knots in two or three places.

Now the tail is ready for winter. When I take the tails down in the spring, I usually have to cut off 2 to 6 inches to bring the tail back up to fetlock level.

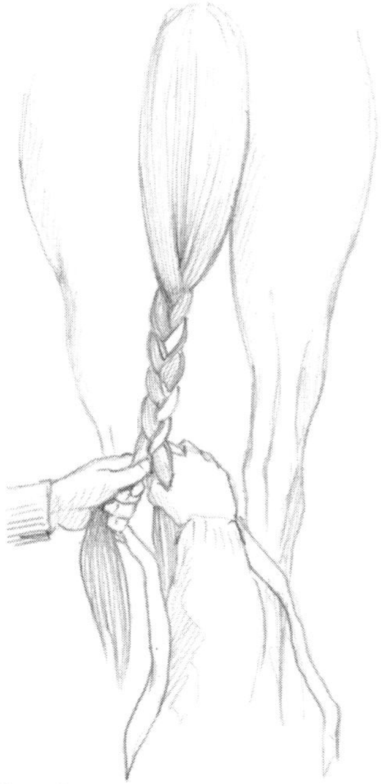

Step 3

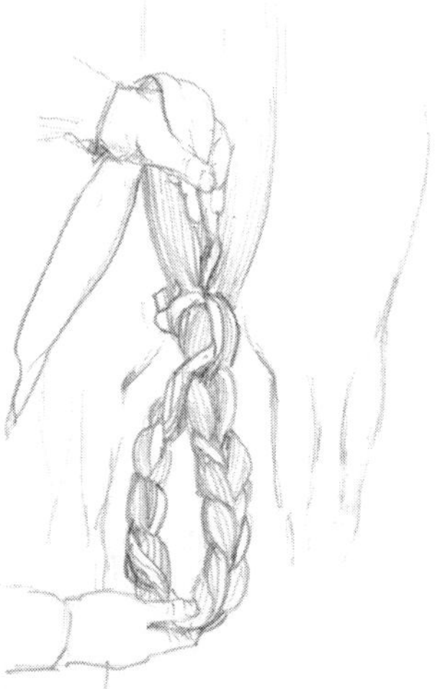

Step 4

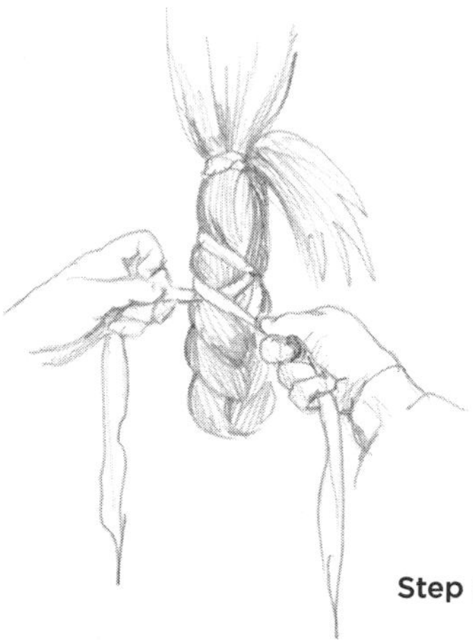

Step 5

Horse Sense and Safety

Using a Lead Rope

Use an 8- to 10-foot lead rope. When leading from the left, with your right hand, hold the lead rope about 6 inches from the snap that is attached to the halter. With your left hand, hold the balance of the rope in a safe configuration such as a figure eight. If you hold the lead rope in a coil in your left hand and your horse suddenly pulls, the rope might tighten around your left hand, which could become trapped in the tightened coil.

CLOTHES HORSE

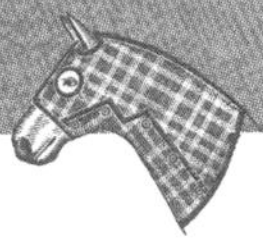

INDOOR HORSE CLOTHING

We all know what the term "clothes horse" really means when we start shelling out the bucks for our horse's wardrobe. That's because there is not one blanket for all seasons. To illustrate:

- When it is cold outside, a short-coated horse does well in a nylon-lined stable blanket; a matching hood is optional.
- A stable blanket is breathable but does not need to be waterproof, because it is used indoors. During the cool temperatures in the spring and fall, a lightweight stable blanket will suffice.
- Throughout the summer, indoor horses might switch between a light barn sheet to keep the coat clean, a fly scrim when the flies are pesky, and an antisweat sheet for those hot sticky days.

TIPS & TECHNIQUES

After-Bath Garb

After bathing, you can use a cooler (see September Clothes Horse) or a body-hugging bathrobe with straps that can be used in a stall.

The wardrobe changes sure can keep us busy, but hey, what are horsekeepers for?

Does your horse even need a blanket, you might ask? Probably not, if he is in good health and has shelter. But, if you want to keep the flies away, keep his coat from bleaching, keep him clean, or keep him dry and extra toasty, you know where to start.

> *We all know what the term "clothes horse" really means when we start shelling out the bucks for our horse's wardrobe.*

FARM OFFICE

HORSE ID

Horse identification (ID) has two purposes: to prove that a particular horse belongs to a particular person, and to prove that a particular horse is a particular horse. Registration papers for a purebred horse provide the physical description of the horse, including color, markings, and photo or drawing identification, as well as the breeder's or owner's name and address. An ID certificate or brand card might be available or required in your state as a permanent record of your horse's identifying characteristics such as age, breed, sex, color, markings, scars, brands, tattoos, microchip number, and possibly blemishes or hair whorls, too. This information might be included with your horse's yearly Coggins test paperwork or health certificate. The horse is shown either by photo or drawing from each side and from the front and back. The markings are not only indicated visually but also described in writing.

BRANDING. Branding identifies a horse as the property of a person or a farm or ranch. The brand is registered with a brand board in the horse owner's name so it serves as proof of ownership. Your personal brand must be registered; first

Movie of the Month

***BROKEN TRAIL* (2006)** A Walter Hill Western miniseries that chronicles the travels of Print Ritter and his nephew Tom Harte as they herd 500 horses from Oregon to Wyoming to sell to the British army. Stars easy rider Robert Duvall, one of my all-time favorite horsemen. Four hours of grit, hard times, some tough realities, humor, and the cowboy way. Shot in Alberta, near where I used to live. See more Duvall in the saddle in *Lonesome Dove.*

check with the state brand board as to the availability of a brand, rules of registration, and placement of a brand.

There is hot branding and freeze branding. Some breed registries also use hot-iron branding, commonly used on western ranches. An iron is heated by fire, gas, or electricity and held against the hide (on the hip, shoulder, or neck) of the animal to burn a permanent scar into the skin. Freeze branding uses cold (from liquid nitrogen) to make an indelible brand on a horse's hide. Depending on the database and how it must be accessed, finding freeze brand records can be less handy than finding hot brand records.

MICROCHIPS. Another ID method is an electronic microchip that is implanted in a horse's neck to be read with a scanner. Chips are not noticeable, which is good for the sake of appearance, but because a thief cannot see them, they don't act as a deterrent the way a visible brand does. Microchips indicate a horse's number but can identify a particular animal only if there is an appropriate scanner available and the proper paperwork to compare it to.

BLOOD TYPING. To prove definitively that a particular horse is a particular horse, you can have blood typing or DNA typing done. Although this is not a widespread option right now, some breed registries have blood-typing records and offer DNA testing.

NAIS

Although presently voluntary, it soon may be required for all horse (and other livestock) owners to register their premises and animals with the National Animal Identification System (NAIS). (See the NAIS Web site in the appendix.) Designed to safeguard U.S. animal health, the NAIS was initiated by the USDA in 2004 as a cooperative state and federal program with three components — premises

TIPS & TECHNIQUES

Keeping Track

Keep a folder on each of your horses and regularly update it with current photos from sides, the front, and the rear, with close-ups of any unusual scars, markings, or brands. Remember, a horse's hair coat changes between seasons and as he ages.

Include a detailed description of the horse along with a copy of his registration papers.

Ideally, have all of this information on one sheet of paper and have several copies so that you can distribute them to authorities if necessary. Positive ID is essential during natural disasters, and it can be used to prove a horse is a particular horse for breeding, racing, or showing. (See the appendix for microchip registries).

identification, animal identification, and animal tracking. The long-term goal of the NAIS is to provide animal health officials with the capability of identifying all livestock and premises that have had direct contact with a disease of concern within 48 hours of discovery.

TRAINING PEN

AUTUMN ARENA EXERCISES

Some of the riding trails in our area close on Labor Day and reopen on Memorial Day. This is to minimize trail damage and to allow animal species to procreate without the invasion of trail riders. So, this time of year, I brush up on arena maneuvers.

Arena exercises combine gymnastics, geometry, and mental concentration. As you practice arena exercises, remember that the quality of the work is most important. It is a much greater accomplishment to do simple things well than to stumble through advanced maneuvers in poor form and with irregular rhythm. Study the exercise, ride it in your mind, and then head out to the arena.

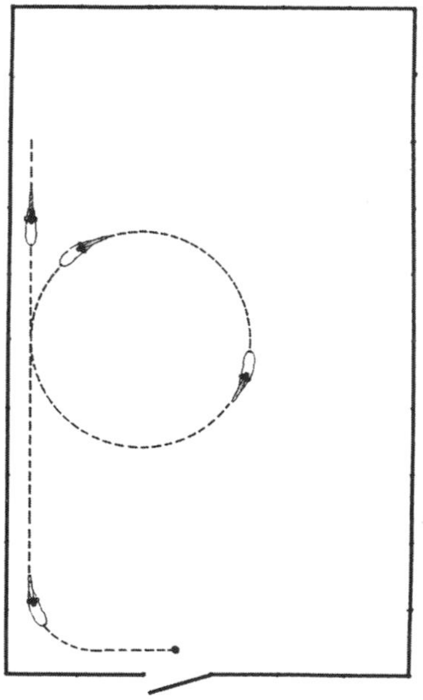

The simplest arena exercise requires concentration and balance.

Accepting Contact

In order for an exercise to produce positive, beneficial results, a horse must be ridden on contact or up in the bridle. This means that the horse readily moves forward from leg aids and accepts and responds willingly to pressures on his mouth via the bit and bridle.

How can you tell if the work is correct?

- Work regularly with a qualified instructor.
- Ask an experienced friend to watch and give you feedback, such as where the right hind was during a certain movement.

- Have someone videotape your riding. Then watch the tape thoroughly with slow motion and freeze frame.
- Watch yourself and your horse in large mirrors on the wall as you ride.
- Glance down (without moving your head) at your horse's shoulders, neck, poll, and eye during different maneuvers to determine if he is bending correctly.
- Develop a feel for when things are going right and when they are going wrong.

> TIPS & TECHNIQUES
>
> **Ride Both Ways**
>
> Be sure that you eventually perform every exercise in both directions. Whenever possible, ride off the rail so your horse is not being held in position by the rail but instead by your aids.

Developing Feel

Answer the following by feeling, not looking:

- Is there appropriate left-to-right balance on my seat bones? Can I feel them both?
- Can I feel even contact on both reins?
- Is the front-to-rear balance acceptable or is the horse heavy on the forehand, croup up, or back hollow?
- Is the rhythm regular or does the horse speed up, slow down, or break gait?
- Is my horse relaxed or is his back tense?
- Is he taking contact with the bit or is he above it or behind it?
- Is my horse loping on the correct lead?
- Can I tell when his inside hind leg is about to land?
- Can I tell when my horse is performing a four-beat lope?
- Can I tell when my horse is walking in front and trotting behind?
- Can I tell when my horse is performing a pacey walk?

Arena exercises combine gymnastics, geometry, and mental concentration. It is a much greater accomplishment to do simple things well than to stumble through advanced maneuvers in poor form and with irregular rhythm.

What to Do When Things Go Wrong

- Review each component of an exercise.
- Return to some very basic exercises to establish forward movement, acceptance of contact, or response

Checking In

Check (half halt) your horse before, during, and after every transition; before, during, and after every corner; and periodically throughout any movement to rebalance the horse.

to sideways driving aids. Often, returning to simple circle work will improve straightness and subsequent lateral work and collection.

- Ride an exercise that the horse does very well, such as the walk-jog-walk transition. Work on purity and form.
- Perform a simpler version of the pattern. If it is a lope pattern, try it at a walk or jog first.
- Perform the pattern in the opposite direction. Sometimes, because of an inherent stiffness or crookedness in a horse, you will have difficulty with a pattern to the left but no problems to the right. Capitalize on this by refining your skills and the application of your aids in the "good direction" and then return to the "hard direction" with a renewed sense of what needs to be done. Often working to the right improves work to the left.

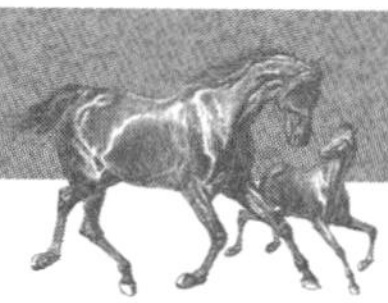

REPRODUCTION ROUNDUP

WHEN TO GELD

The testicles of the normal male horse descend from the abdomen into the scrotum around birth. Gelding can be performed soon after birth, but a delay is traditional for several reasons. First, it gives foal owners more time to determine if a young horse has stallion potential. Second, it allows desirable masculine characteristics, such as muscle definition, strength, and aggressiveness, to develop.

It is best to assess each individual to determine the optimal gelding time. Some weanlings become preoccupied with nearby mares and may go through or over fences to get near them. In other cases, a long yearling may only quietly watch the mares. Some may develop an obsession with their penises and may devise various means of masturbation or self-mutilation.

Other early gelding candidates include those that show premature signs of excess bulk such as a thick, cresty neck. Such individuals might best be gelded at eight months or earlier, while others remain very supple and moderate in musculature well into their two-year-old year. Therefore, depending on management and the tendencies of each individual, gelding usually takes place between six and 24 months of age.

> *A horse* **is worth more than riches.**
> — Spanish proverb

Proud Cut

Some horses retain sexual behaviors after gelding and are often called "proud cut." In the past this was said to be due to some testicular tissue being missed during the gelding procedure, allowing testosterone production (but not sperm production) to continue. In some cases, this may have been true, especially considering the variety of crude methods of castration practiced over the last 2,000 years. Today, however, with the availability of restraining drugs and the level of knowledge and surgical techniques, it is unlikely that missed testicular tissue is the cause for the estimated 25 percent of geldings that are said to exhibit some type of stallion behaviors.

Since the adrenal glands (located near the kidneys) also produce testosterone, it is thought that the cause of so-called "proud cut" behavior may be due to the hyperactivity of a particular horse's adrenal glands. Other stallionlike behaviors may simply be poor manners due to inadequate training.

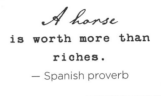

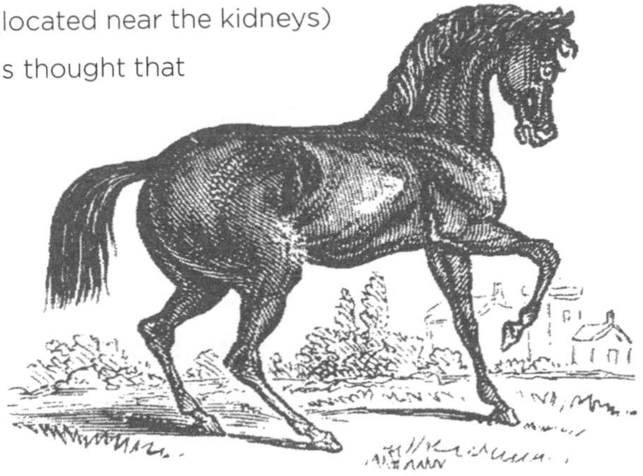

Timing Issues

When to geld is largely a management decision. Often, facilities require that young horses of both sexes be housed together, so gelding at about 12 months has become popular in order to avoid accidental breeding at puberty (18 to 24 months).

Early spring and late fall are the traditional seasons for gelding, since flies are usually not a serious problem for the healing wound site and the lower seasonal temperatures do not exaggerate swelling of the sheath. However, the mud that is characteristic of spring and fall may make dry, sanitary conditions more difficult to provide and maintain.

Research has shown that there is little difference in the behavior change toward people in horses gelded before puberty and those gelded after puberty. However, horses gelded after puberty tend to retain a greater amount of their former horse-to-horse behaviors — sexual drive, vocalization, and body language — than those gelded before puberty.

PREPARATION FOR GELDING. Proper health management practices contribute to safe and easy recovery from the minor surgery. All horses should be current in their deworming and vaccination schedules. (See January Pest Patrol and March Vet Clinic.) Yearlings should have a booster at least a month before gelding. Your veterinarian should be informed of the horse's immunization status. If the horse is not current for tetanus, the veterinarian will likely administer tetanus antitoxin at the time of surgery.

The young horse should have learned good manners for pre-tranquilizer handling. Veterinarians should not be subjected to potential injury from an unruly yearling stallion. Also, the more a horse is familiarized, in advance, with the type of handling he will receive before, during, and after gelding, the less stress he will experience.

If both testicles are not obviously visible in the scrotal pouch, it is necessary to palpate the scrotum to determine if both testicles have descended completely. Some horses are initially very reluctant to having the scrotum handled and may kick or pull away. Proper handling from birth, or at least well in advance of the gelding process, will decrease handler risk.

THE SURGERY ROUTINE. Gelding a horse that has two descended testicles is a simple on-the-farm procedure. Find a clean, level, smooth area for your veterinarian to work. A grassy spot out of the strong sun works well. The surgery is performed either under general anesthesia with the horse

Historical Horsekeeping

"If the colt is intended for farm use, castration may be performed when six months old; if, however, the withers are light, it should be postponed until the head and neck fill up to the degree required, and this may require from one to two years, or even more. If the head is large and heavy, early castration is advisable."

— Magner's Standard Horse and Stock Book *by D. Magner, 1916*

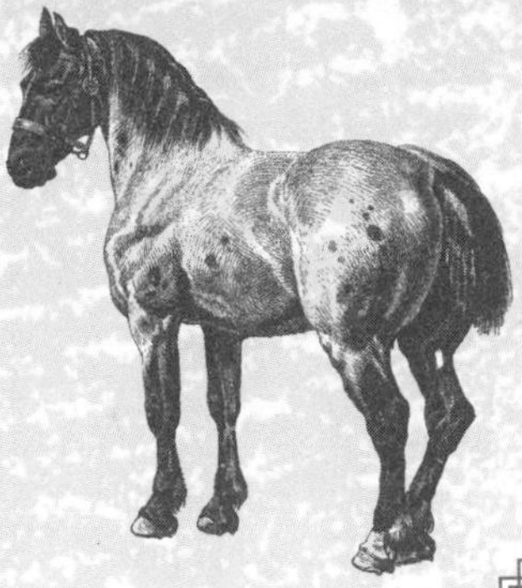

lying on one side or on his back, or with a local anesthesia with the horse standing. The veterinarian will require an accurate weight for each horse in order to determine the proper dosage of tranquilizer and anesthetic to use.

A tranquilizer is usually administered first to relax the horse. Then either a local anesthetic is administered and the surgery is performed with the horse standing, or a general anesthetic is administered, which will make the horse lose consciousness and lie down. Care must be taken as the horse collapses to ensure he does not injure his head, or lose his balance and fall backwards. As the horse is laid down and throughout the surgery, it is important to protect his eyes and head with a soft blanket to prevent injuries.

Once down, the anesthetic allows the veterinarian about 10 to 12 minutes to complete the procedure. Restraint ropes are usually applied as a safeguard because each horse reacts differently to anesthesia. The scrotal area is washed. Usually, two incisions are made in the scrotum. The testicles are pulled out of the scrotum so that about 2 inches of the spermatic cord can be removed with the testicles. The spermatic cord is made up of veins, artery, nerves, and the vas deferens, the tube that carries sperm away from the testicles. The spermatic cords are crushed with an emasculator for about 60 seconds to sever them. The veterinarian

en español

lasso. Comes from *el lazo.*

lariat and riata. Come from *la reata.* Both are 'long ropes used to catch cattle and horses'.

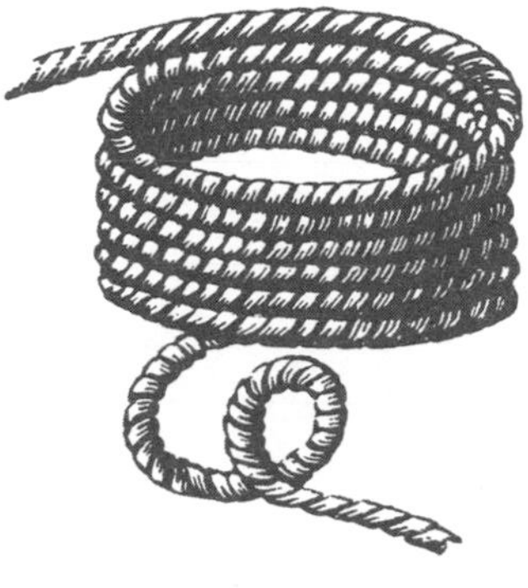

FALL: OCTOBER

enlarges the scrotal incisions and trims any excess scrotal tissues that would interfere with proper drainage.

When one or both of the testicles are not present in the scrotum, the horse is termed a unilateral or bilateral cryptorchid. The retained testicle(s) might be located high in the abdominal cavity or in the inguinal canal, the area between the abdomen and scrotum. Gelding a cryptorchid requires general anesthesia; the testicle(s) are removed via the inguinal canal, the abdominal wall, or the flank.

AFTERCARE. The gelding will get up on his own shortly after he comes out of the anesthesia, but it takes about 20 to 40 minutes for him to fully recover from the drug. It is important that he is in a safe, private place such as a round pen or arena.

Before turning him out, apply petroleum jelly to the insides of his hind legs where sticky fluids will later drip. Accumulated drainage can result in sloughed hair and chafed skin. Petroleum jelly protects the sparsely haired inner thigh and gaskin area from scalding and makes daily cleaning of the legs easier for the owner and less painful for the horse. Drainage is largely comprised of white blood cells mixed with discarded tissue fragments and blood. Commonly this is referred to as pus. As long as the odor of the drainage remains inoffensive, it is normal and desirable.

Drainage should continue for two to three weeks. If the scrotal incisions suddenly close up before two weeks or if there is a persistent bad smell, call your veterinarian immediately.

Because of surgical trauma, the gelding's sheath will swell to some degree. Accumulation of fluids in the area is normal for four to five days. If the swelling becomes extreme or is accompanied by heat, it may be advisable to notify your veterinarian. A swollen sheath may make urination uncomfortable. Be sure to encourage normal urination

Preprocedure Check

Before gelding, examine each horse thoroughly to determine what the "normals" are for that individual. Look at his sheath, his legs, his eyes, his normal facial expressions. Take his temperature, pulse, and respiration. Become familiar with each horse in an unstressed condition to help you monitor his progress during the postoperative and recovery period.

A cowboy is a man with guts and a horse.

— Will James

and bowel movements by offering your horse fresh water at all times and ensuring that he gets adequate exercise.

EXERCISE. When the new gelding is coordinated enough to navigate, he can be turned out with his usual pasture mates, providing they are not too rowdy. The best prevention and treatment for sheath swelling is a conscientious exercise program. However, because the gelding will understandably be stiff, don't expect him to exercise adequately on his own.

A combination of hand-walking, free longeing, ponying, and free exercise can be used. Hand-walking is the best method for the very stiff colt on the first day after gelding. Free exercise is the least labor-intensive exercise option but doesn't guarantee that a horse will exercise when he needs it the most. Left to his own devices, the new gelding that is very stiff might choose to stand relatively still all day. After just five minutes of forced exercise, however, the scrotal incisions usually reopen and drain, relieving the

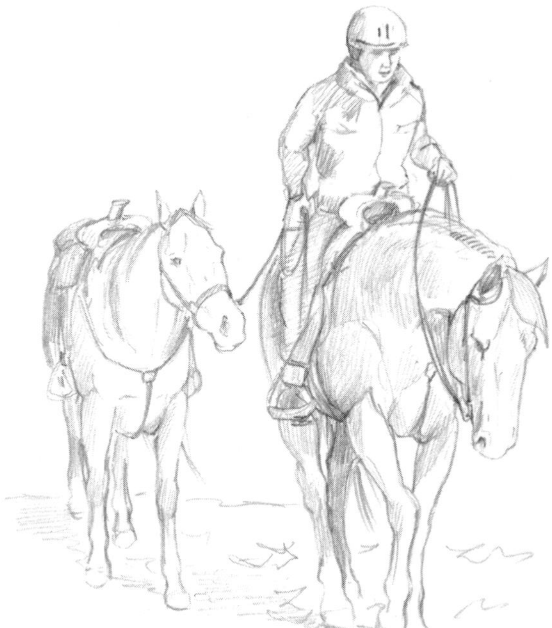

Ponying is a great way to accustom a young horse to the saddle and provide exercise during the post-gelding period.

Daily Post-Op Flushing

To minimize hair loss and skin chafing, and to decrease the chances of the horse rubbing his rear end and tail, clean the hind legs and the area under the horse's tail each day. Using warm water if possible, hose off the drainage, blot dry with a clean towel, and apply a fresh coat of petroleum jelly. During the washing, don't spray directly into the wound. Too much washing and wiping can also be irritating to a horse's skin, so strike a balance. Bath training prior to gelding will help make this daily washing just another routine. To encourage the youngster to stand still, have an assistant hold up a front foot, but be sure the young horse has had prior hoof handling.

pressure that caused the stiffness. The horse then seems more comfortable and strides out much more freely.

GELDING COMPLICATIONS. Some complications can arise even with a routine castration. Probably the most common is swelling that spreads down the hind legs. Hind-leg swelling is the body's sympathetic response to the swelling in the sheath area and, more probably, the premature closing of the incisions and inability of the area to drain. Although you can provide temporary relief to the swollen legs with cold water or massage, ultimately the incision will need to be reopened to ensure proper drainage. Until closure at about two weeks, there should be a gradual decrease in the amount of drainage: copious at first, scant toward day 14.

If drainage halts abruptly, use a warm compress on the scrotal area to soften the crusted incision area and then exercise the young horse immediately. This will usually cause the incision to burst open and release the accumulated pus. If the premature closure is persistent, your veterinarian may need to enlarge one or both of the incisions.

If the spermatic cord was not emasculated thoroughly, excess bleeding may result and the cord may need to be

Make a Schedule

It's best to approach the new gelding's exercise needs formally and follow a schedule, such as three 15-minute sessions each day for the first three days after surgery; two 30-minute sessions each day for the next week; then one 60-minute session each day until healing is complete, which is usually about two to three weeks after surgery.

NOT ALWAYS TRUE

Historical Horsekeeping

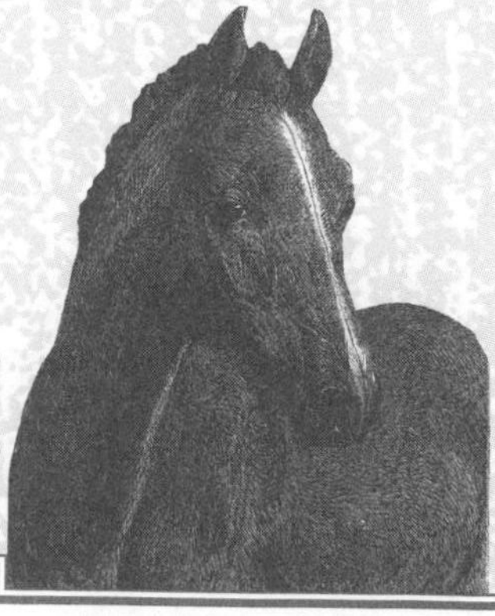

"Colts should be castrated in April, or at the end of May, after which operation they should have one hours' walking exercise every day, to prevent swelling and inflammation, and not heating food given them — bran mashes and hay will be best — and as soon as they are all right, they may be put to grass again. Colts castrated in the cold season of the year are likely to have permanently a rough coat."

— The Book of the Horse *by Samuel Sidney, 1880*

clamped. In other cases, if too much spermatic cord was pulled out of the abdominal cavity during the surgery, after emasculation the stump may retract into the abdomen. The subsequent bleeding and infection that would likely follow might require major abdominal surgery.

Sometimes after recumbent surgery, horses exhibit temporary facial paralysis, but it is uncommon. It can be caused by the halter's hardware pressing on a facial nerve when the horse's head is on the ground during the castration. That is why is best to adequately pad the horse's head and face with a soft blanket, especially in the area of the noseband hardware and side buckles of the halter. Temporary paralysis may manifest as a drooping lip, a flaccid nostril on one side, or a floppy ear. Sometimes the horse's eye will water continually. It is possible that a horse could have difficulty eating if the paralysis affects both sides of the face. Generally the side that he was lying on is the one that is affected. Recovery takes about 10 days.

No Problems

Most gelding procedures occur without incidents. Preparation, observation, and daily care will help the young horse recover quickly.

Gelding and Physique

Although a gelding and stallion may have similar muscle bulk, a stallion's muscles exhibit more definition because a gelding's muscles tend to be covered with a layer of fat, giving him a rounder appearance.

Horses gelded before puberty usually grow taller than if they were left stallions. The testosterone rush at puberty triggers the closure of the epiphyseal plates (where bone growth takes place), so the stallion essentially quits adding height at puberty. The horse gelded at one year of age has a gradual, delayed puberty and the additional time may allow him to add extra height.

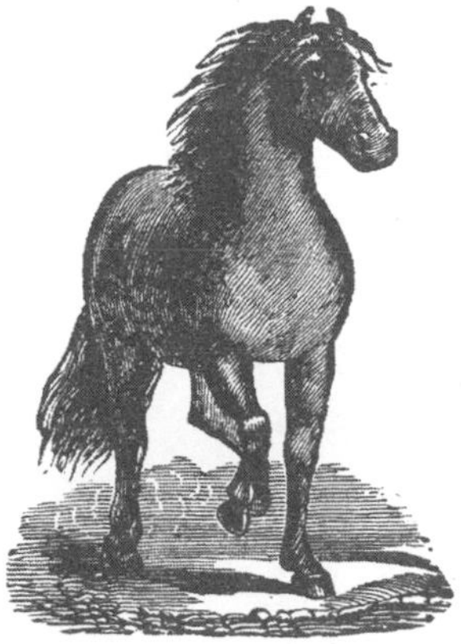

> *Depending on what age he was gelded, the horse may need as long as four to six months to mentally and physically forget he was a stallion.*

AFTEREFFECTS OF GELDING. Two weeks after the horse's surgery, from outward appearances, he is a gelding. However, past behavior patterns and a low level of androgens make the yearling continue to act somewhat like a stud colt. Use caution in turning the new gelding out with a group of mares, for example. He may learn a lesson the hard way. Depending on what age he was gelded, the horse may need as long as four to six months to mentally and physically forget he was a stallion.

After castration, the gelding's metabolism is likely to slow down. Therefore, to maintain optimal condition, a gelding usually requires less feed and more exercise than his stallion counterpart.

Fine Facilities

Facilities Maintenance Checklist

- ❑ Repair any roof damage, loose fasteners, or cracked shingles
- ❑ Check gutter and clean out
- ❑ Repair walls, inside and out, from kicking, rubbing, chewing
- ❑ Paint or otherwise treat wood inside and out
- ❑ Replace any chewed wood and use protective metal edging
- ❑ Closely monitor insects such as termites or cockroaches and rid the building of them at first sign
- ❑ Adhere to a stringent rodent control program
- ❑ Schedule an annual barn cleaning (see January Fine Facilities)
- ❑ Replace or update latches and locks as needed
- ❑ Make sure all light bulbs and fixtures are in good working order
- ❑ Clean all windows and be sure they are in good working order
- ❑ Repair leaky hoses, hydrants, and faucets
- ❑ As needed, perform stall floor renovation; even matted stalls can use a breather, freshener, or re-laying over time
- ❑ Replenish tool room with needed hand tools and supplies
- ❑ Perform regular fence checks but plan for an annual fence overhaul (see February Pasture Perfect)
- ❑ Schedule and adhere to annual (or more frequent) vehicle maintenance (see January and April RPMs & PTOs)

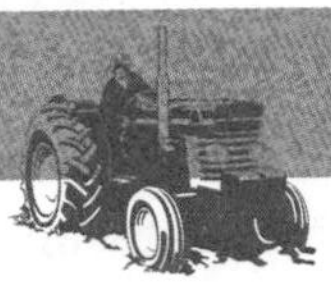

PASTURE HARROWS

Pastures that are going to be rested for the winter can be harrowed after the final mow. The best type of harrow for this job is either the English harrow or the spike tooth harrow.

The English harrow is made of heavy wire stock (7/16-inch to 1/2-inch) that criss-crosses in a diamond-shaped configuration and may or may not have protrusions called teeth (tines) on the bottom side. The teeth, which make the harrow more aggressive, range from 7/16 inch to 5/8 inch in diameter and are from 3½ to 4 inches long. A good English harrow is usually heavy and costly, but does a wonderful job of smoothing rough spots. They are excellent for leveling gravel driveways, spreading manure in a pasture, and aerating the soil without ripping it up. Homemade drags made of chain-link fence attempt to simulate the English style, but they lack teeth, and their light weight makes them bounce on top of the soil rather than doing much smoothing or leveling.

Like pull-type discs, some English harrows can be difficult to load, and when you move them by dragging them behind the tractor, they harrow everything behind you. Others attach to the three-point hitch and can be lifted for transporting. Some can be rolled or hung up for convenient storage. An English harrow connects to the tractor's drawbar by means of its own drawbar. The harrow's drawbar is a long horizontal bar or pipe that attaches along the entire front of the harrow. You can use a 6-foot drawbar for a 6-foot harrow; a 12-foot drawbar for two 6-foot harrows set side by side; or even a 24-foot drawbar for four 6-foot harrows.

Some harrows have adjustable tines. You can set them straight down for maximum penetration or angle them backward to break up surface clumps. The harrow can also be flipped upside down with the tines pointing upward for

TIPS & TECHNIQUES

Oil All Latches

When the cold, wet weather hits, many panel gate latches freeze. To prevent this, prior to winter weather, oil all latches with WD-40 or light machine oil. If a latch does freeze, use a small propane torch to thaw it out.

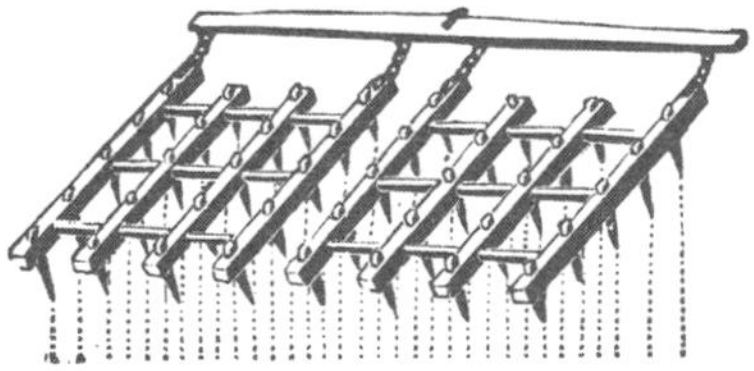

A spike-tooth harrow has a rigid frame with teeth that look something like old railroad spikes sitting on rotating bars that can be adjusted for work or transport.

use as a drag mat. Harrows can be ganged, with one following the other to perform two chores at once. For example, the first one can be set with the tines straight down to dig up the soil and the second one with the tines backward to break up the clumps, or the first one could break up clumps with backward tines while the second one is flipped over to smooth out the surface.

A spike-tooth harrow has a more rigid frame with teeth that look something like old railroad spikes sitting on rotating bars that can be adjusted for work or transport. With the teeth in full upright position, you can rip up pastures in the spring; with them set at an angle, the harrow works more as a leveler and smoother. Most spike-tooth harrows have replaceable teeth, as the teeth become blunted after long or hard use.

> *To turn and* **wind a fiery Pegasus And witch the world with noble horsemanship.**
> — William Shakespeare, *Henry IV*, Part 1

MORE IN DEPTH

TO BLANKET OR NOT TO BLANKET

I define a stabled horse as a horse with a short coat that is kept in an unheated barn with no direct sunlight. If a stabled horse is not short-coated or clipped, if the stall of the horse has direct sunlight, or if the barn is heated, adjust the recommendations in the accompanying chart accordingly. A turned-out horse is one that is allowed free exercise, has a natural winter coat, lives outdoors but has shelter from wind, and benefits from solar gain during the day. If the turned-out horse has a short coat, does not have shelter from the wind, or does not have access to shade, take that into consideration when referring to the chart. A blanketed horse should always be clean and dry.

Temperatures listed do not take into consideration the effects of the wind. During very hot weather, a wind can cool by evaporative cooling. During cold weather, wind creates a chill factor. When blanketing during cold, windy weather, figure that for every mile per hour the wind blows, it lowers the temperature 1°F. During fly season, substitute fly sheets

Choosing the Right Blanket

Temperature	Stable Horse	Turnout Horse
100° F	antisweat sheet, fly sheet, or nothing	antisweat sheet, turnout fly sheet, or nothing
90° F	antisweat sheet, fly sheet, or nothing	antisweat sheet, turnout fly sheet, or nothing
80° F	antisweat sheet, fly sheet, lightweight stable sheet, or nothing	turnout fly sheet, lightweight turnout sheet, or nothing
70° F	stable sheet, fly sheet, or nothing	turnout sheet, turnout fly sheet, or nothing
60° F	stable sheet	turnout sheet or nothing
50° F	heavy stable sheet, or lightweight blanket	turnout sheet or nothing
40° F	midweight blanket	lightweight turnout blanket or nothing
30° F	midweight blanket	lightweight turnout blanket or nothing
20° F	heavyweight blanket	midweight turnout blanket or nothing
10° F	heavyweight blanket and hood	midweight or heavyweight turnout blanket or nothing
0° F	heavyweight blanket and hood	heavyweight turnout blanket and hood
-10° F	double blanket and hood	heavyweight turnout blanket and hood
-20° F	double blanket and hood	turnout blanket and hood
-30° F	double blanket and hood	turnout blanket and hood

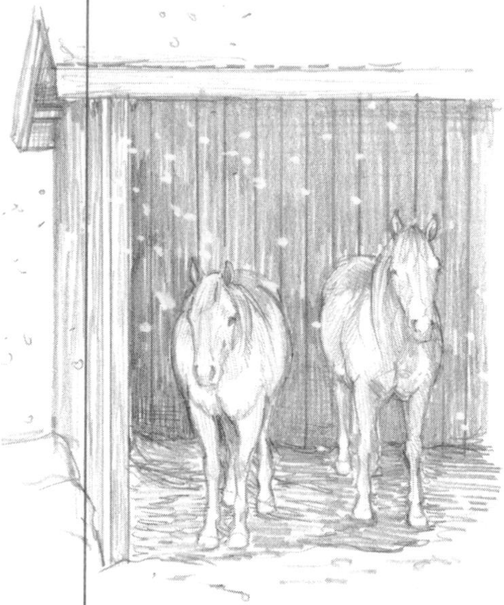

Horses allowed to grow a long winter coat do well with adequate shelter.

whenever possible, taking care to choose a durable one for turnout. During the rainy season, substitute a waterproof, breathable rain sheet for the turnout sheet. During snow season, substitute a waterproof, breathable winter turnout blanket for the turnout blanket.

Cleaning a Winter Blanket

While the blanket is still on the horse, brush the outside of the fabric to remove any mud or other debris. If the outside is fairly clean except for a few manure or grass stains, you can spray the spots with a solution of your regular blanket wash product. Let it set for 30 seconds and then scrub with a textured sponge. This is easiest to do on the horse.

Now remove the blanket from the horse and lay it out in a clean area, such as on the rubber mats of the grooming area. Brush the wither fleece to remove any hair or debris and to fluff it so it will wash more thoroughly. Brush the inside of the blanket with a stiff-bristled brush to loosen patches of hair. Hair can damage your washing machine, and it will just spread in the wash water and distribute itself over the whole blanket. The more hair you can loosen and

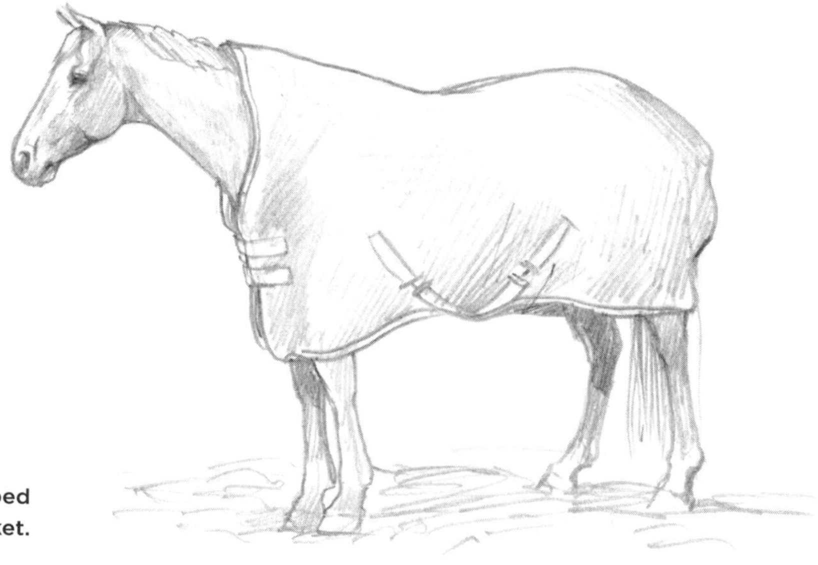

A short-haired or clipped horse needs a storm blanket.

remove, therefore, the better your blanket will look coming out of the washer and the longer your washing machine will last. Vacuuming will remove the hair from the blanket lining more easily and thoroughly.

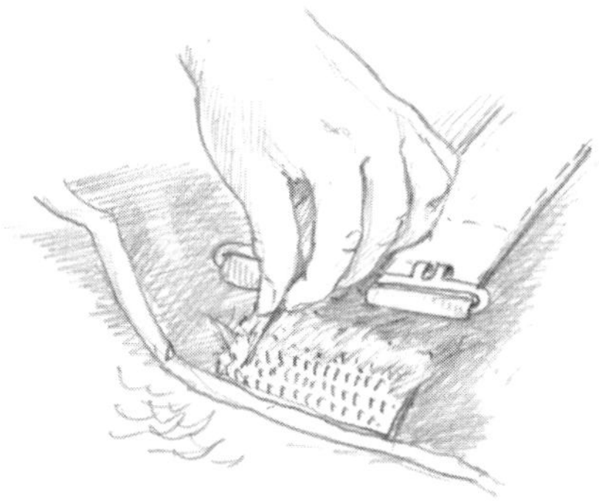

Use a darning needle to pick hair out of Velcro, and use duct tape to capture the last bits.

Unbuckle all leg straps and chest buckles, and untie tail cords. Clean the Velcro if necessary by using a darning needle to lift the hair pads and duct tape to remove stragglers. Then seal the Velcro with separate pieces of Velcro kept on hand specifically for wash day. You can buy Velcro by the foot off the roll in varying widths at any large fabric store. Cover all buckles with socks to protect the inside of the washer tub from chipping. Tie or rubber-band the socks onto the buckles.

Always read and follow the blanket manufacturer's washing instructions. Add the laundry products to the wash water. Then load the blanket into the machine according to its specific washing requirements. If the outer shell is water resistant or waterproof, it is best to fold the blanket inside out. Otherwise, the waterproof shell will prevent water from flushing through the blanket and washing will be uneven: dry spots, dirty spots, unrinsed areas, and places that are soaking wet at the end of the cycle. If the outer shell is not waterproof, load the blanket with the dirtiest side facing outward.

Use a front-loading machine without an agitator whenever possible. If you must use a top-load machine, carefully lay the blanket around the agitator in a circle, trying to keep all of the straps inside the blanket.

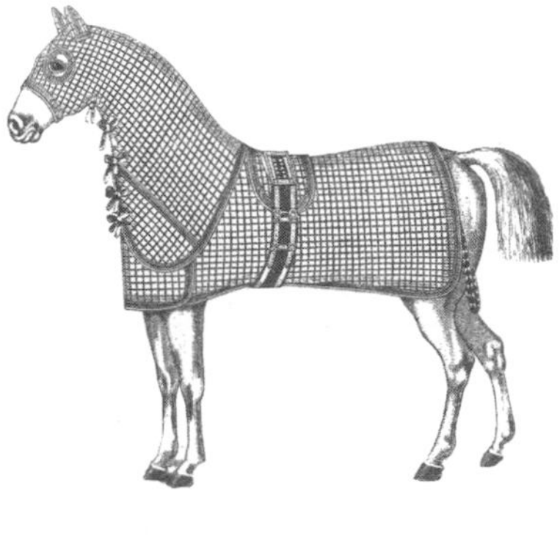

Blanket Construction

The outer layer of well-made domestic blankets usually consists of high-quality, tightly woven, durable materials such as Cordura, nylon pack cloth, duck canvas, or, in the case of coolers, 100 percent wool. Blankets made of acrylic, other fleeces, acetate, or fibers with loose, open, or uneven

Overheating

Overheating can be a real problem with blanketed horses. Often horses are turned out to exercise in the same blankets they wore all night. What is appropriate for low nighttime temperatures in a barn, however, is not necessarily desirable for a sunny paddock, even though there may still be snow on the ground. In particular, an unblanketed dark horse has the capacity to absorb much of the sun's energy.

Some waterproof blankets do not allow heat to escape from normal body respiration. Blanketing a horse too warmly can cause the horse to sweat, then chill, which lowers his resistance by sapping his energy. This is an open invitation for respiratory infections.

Overheating and sweating also encourage a horse to roll in his blanket, which is hard on the blanket and can be dangerous for the horse. Check to see if your horse is a comfortable temperature by slipping your hand under his blanket at the heart girth area.

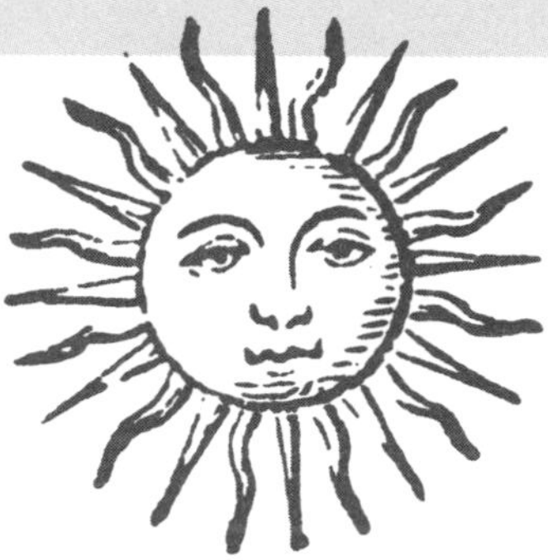

weaves are easily shredded, shrink unevenly, or may be impossible to thoroughly clean.

Most nylon products are tough, resist tearing, and provide a smooth, dense surface. Nylon-lined blankets keep the coat slick and don't easily pick up hair and dirt, so they don't require frequent washing. Fleece- and blanket-lined blankets accumulate a lot of debris so are very difficult to keep clean and difficult to repair well. In addition, fleece and blanket linings compress over pressure points on the horse's body such as the shoulders, hips, and withers. Often such blankets are also heavy, so they result in bare or raw spots on the horse. Nylon-lined blankets are less likely to cause hair loss. In the case of a horse that is very sensitive, even with a well-fitted blanket, a pure silk lining can increase comfort.

For more on horse clothing, see page 455.

Polyester insulation is light, warm, and comfortable for the horse. It is easy to wash and dry, and allows air to circulate more freely through the blanket. Whether a horse might get wet from external moisture or from his own body heat and sweat, it is important for the moisture to be able to escape from the blanket. Foam-stuffed blankets, unless they are of a very light foam, are not as breathable as polyester, are generally heavier, and are stiffer when dirty.

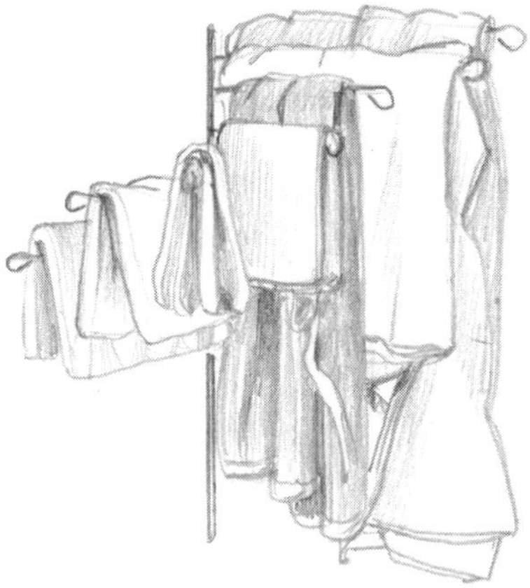

My husband, Richard Klimesh, designed and hand-forged this swinging blanket rod system.

PREVENTING DAMAGE TO BLANKETS

To prevent costly repairs or the need to replace blankets, follow these rules of blanket management.

CLEANLINESS. Never put a dirty blanket on a clean horse, or any blanket on a dirty horse. This would be an open invitation to rubbing and rolling. Dirt, manure, urine, and sunlight can be fatiguing to the blanket's fibers. A dirty blanket is not only unhealthy and uncomfortable for a horse, but the blanket can even rot if it is wet or dirty for prolonged periods of time. Ideally, a blanket should be removed from the horse daily. The underside of the blanket should be checked for debris and lightly brushed or wiped. The horse should be exercised, groomed, and then reblanketed.

BLANKET FIT. Blankets last longer and are more comfortable for the horse if they fit properly. Blankets that are too small can cause rub marks and sore spots on the withers, shoulder, chest, and hips. Too-large blankets can slip sideways and end up almost upside down, which can cause the horse to become dangerously tangled, to say nothing of the almost certain demise of the blanket.

It is usually possible to find a ready-made blanket to fit almost any size and shape of horse. If you have a hard-to-fit horse, however, or are trying to utilize a blanket that you already have, customizing can make a blanket fit better. Some of the customizing most commonly done includes cutting back the blanket at the withers or shoulder, adding fleece at the withers, adding a tail piece, cutting up higher

Car Wash to the Rescue

As with saddle pads, you can also do a fairly good job washing a heavy winter blanket at a car wash with a high-pressure sprayer. Clean the bay very well first and then lay the blanket out on the concrete floor and spray it. Don't use the car wash detergent, however; bring your own. Once you feel you have rinsed all the soap out, put in a few more quarters and make sure.

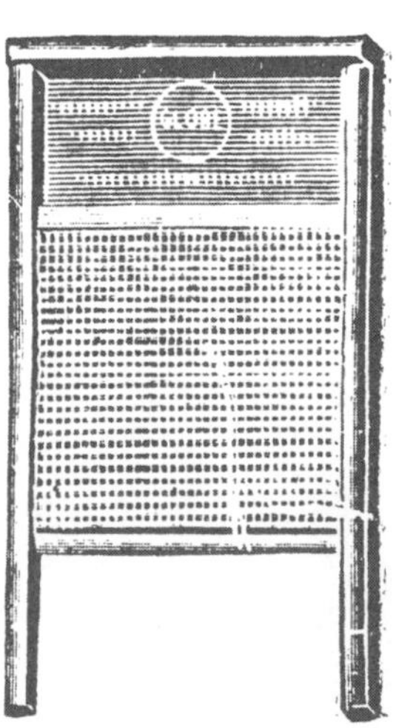

at the tail, moving the front buckles, or making an open front a solid front. Hoods can also be customized to make the ear holes more comfortable or to adjust the eyeholes.

Sometimes even a properly fitted blanket shifts around a lot on a particular horse, even with the surcingle straps snug. For these instances, use an elastic or cotton web surcingle (roller) over the blanket to hold it in place. Because coolers are not designed to be securely fitted, never turn out a horse wearing a cooler or he will most certainly step on the cooler and damage it.

WASHING BLANKETS

If a horse is blanketed daily, his blanket should be washed twice a month. Most winter blankets will not fit in a home machine and many Laundromats frown on horse laundry. You probably have a custom blanket laundering and repair service in your area.

If you do the washing yourself, use a moderate amount of mild laundry detergent and no bleach, as some horses are very sensitive to chlorine. You may also wish to add an odor eliminator to the wash cycle. Industrial cleaning supply companies carry commercial brands; washing soda is available at the grocery store.

Most blankets can be washed in warm water. Exceptions are 100 percent wool coolers (which often must be dry-cleaned), blanket-lined blankets, and those with specific cold-water instructions, such as waterproof blankets or those with leather straps.

Be sure all of the soap gets rinsed out. If you use the proper amount of detergent, most commercial machines (front-loading heavy-duty) do a good job of rinsing and spinning "dry."

DRYING. The best way to get the water out of the blanket is to roll it tightly and squeeze several times each way. It is best to line-dry all horse blankets except light sheets. Most blankets don't require reshaping. However, the lining of blanket-lined blankets often stretches, while the covering, frequently of cotton duck, shrinks just a little bit. These blankets may have to be stretched back into shape. As the blanket is drying, oil the leather straps with pure neat's-foot oil or rub Murphy's oil soap paste into the leather to soften and preserve it.

BLANKET REPAIR

The most frequent blanket repair needs are ripped surcingle straps, broken hardware, ripped-out leg-strap holes, and miscellaneous tear holes.

Torn stitching of surcingle straps can result from poor workmanship, fatigued thread, or the horse catching the blanket on something in the stall or trailer. If surcingle straps are left too loose, they are an open invitation for damage to the blanket.

Bent or broken buckles, especially the T-shaped hooks, often need to be replaced. To avoid such a repair, buy blankets with high-quality hardware of stainless steel or brass. A new type of nylon and polypropylene low-profile side-release buckle is also now available. This hardware is lighter than metal and won't rust or corrode; however, the side prongs of the buckle have been known to break.

The rectangular loops where the leg straps slide through may rip out if they are not reinforced by a durable material. Often they are surrounded by vinyl, but the vinyl can crack.

Holes in blankets come in all shapes and sizes and are caused by the horse chewing his blanket, catching it on something in the stall, or rubbing or rolling excessively while wearing it, or by another horse grabbing it.

Rubbing can also damage hoods, especially around the eyes and ears. Keeping the horse scrupulously clean can

Blanket First Aid

Frequently check the stress points on blankets: around the surcingles, leg straps, and front buckles. Take care of minor damage before it becomes a major problem.

Some tips:

- ❑ Use your mane-braiding thread and needle to whip a few stitches across the tear until you can have it repaired.
- ❑ Use duct tape or another adhesive tape as a quick and handy first aid for rips.
- ❑ Nylon patch kits made for tents also work well as first aid for tears. In some cases, such a patch may be good enough to be stitched down and serve as the permanent repair.

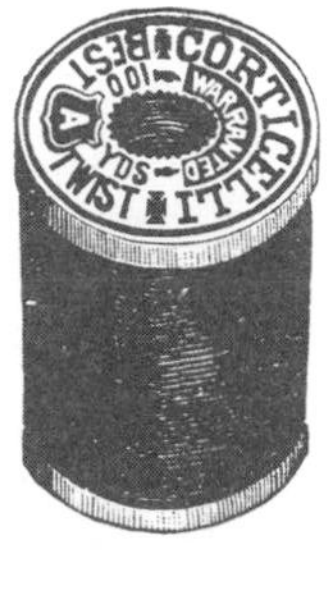

prevent much of this rubbing. If a hood is damaging the mane, it can be lined with silk.

Finally, if you are putting an expensive blanket on a horse that hasn't been blanketed before, put a sheet over the blanket to protect it until you can assess his tolerance and habits.

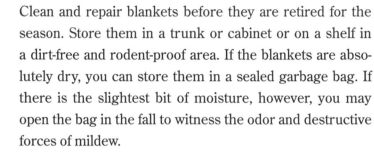

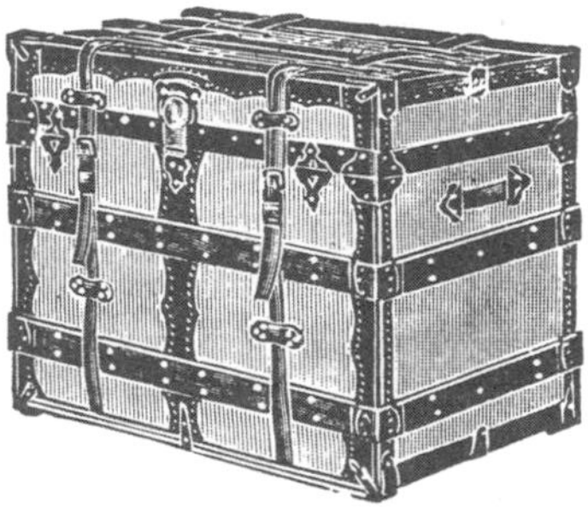

BLANKET STORAGE

Clean and repair blankets before they are retired for the season. Store them in a trunk or cabinet or on a shelf in a dirt-free and rodent-proof area. If the blankets are absolutely dry, you can store them in a sealed garbage bag. If there is the slightest bit of moisture, however, you may open the bag in the fall to witness the odor and destructive forces of mildew.

Blankets, and especially their insulation, provide irresistible nesting materials for mice, and dirty, sweaty, or manure-covered stored blankets attract insects as well as mice. If you have a moth problem, put a few mothballs between the layers of each stored blanket.

HORSEKEEPING ACROSS AMERICA

THE COLD ZONES: CANADA AND THE NORTHERN UNITED STATES

In cold winter climates, several factors affect a horse's warmth.

HAIR COAT. Usually a natural winter coat is all a horse needs to stay warm, provided that he is healthy and in good flesh, he has shelter from wind and precipitation, and he is fed adequately. If a horse has a short coat or a clip (see

December Beauty Shop) he will chill more easily than a horse with a long winter coat.

BLANKET. A blanket can be used to provide added warmth if a horse is old, ill, or thin, or if he has a short coat or doesn't use his shelter. Blankets can also be used to keep a horse's coat cleaner. See more about blankets elsewhere this month and in September and November Clothes Horse.

SHELTER. Not only do horses not need a heated barn, but their respiratory tracts also remain healthier in the fresh air of unheated barns or run-in sheds during cold weather.

WIND. To avoid loss of body heat (see February Wacky Wonderful Weather), provide shelter to block the prevailing winds.

DAMPNESS AND PRECIPITATION. A wet horse will become chilled more quickly than a dry horse will because the moisture flattens the long winter coat, thereby taking away its fluffy insulating quality.

ILLNESS. An ill horse may not move around much and consequently has decreased circulation. Provide the ill horse with maximum protection, therefore, in order to ward off chills.

WEIGHT. A thin horse will become chilled more quickly than a fat horse will, but fat is not healthy either. See the winter weight gain rule in September Feed Bag.

NUTRITION. A horse's ration should be adjusted according to the temperature. See September Feed Bag for the cold-weather feeding rule.

The horse loves his oats more than his saddle.

— Russian proverb

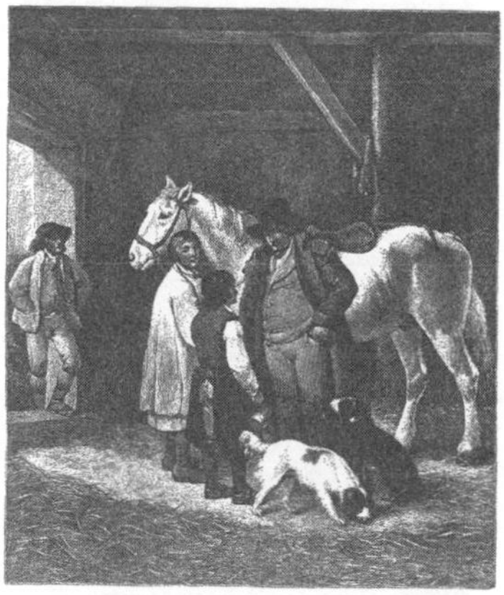

Cryptorchid

Q

Can a cryptorchid be used as a stud? I just found out today that the seven-year-old Paint I bought this year is a unilateral or bilateral cryptorchid [one or both of his testes failed to descend normally as he developed]. While he has been at a barn with 11 other horses (four geldings and seven mares), he has been no problem, but he displayed stud behavior when turned out in the arena. That's when we had him tested.

Our vet tends to be on the cautious side and encouraged me to sell him. We really like him and he is a beautiful animal. I wish he could stand as a stud because people have already asked if he was a stallion, wanting to have him cover their mares.

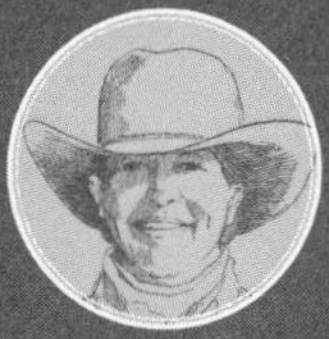

Ask Cherry

A

It's tough when there are things about a horse that you like but there is one big issue that stops you in your tracks. The bottom line is this: Your horse is not suitable to be a breeding animal. The testes cannot be dropped into proper position surgically. Researchers are experimenting with hormonal treatment for certain cases of cryptorchidism, but it would be an option only if you have access to a veterinarian or clinic that is using this technique and your veterinarian feels your horse would be a candidate.

It's possible that your horse was a unilateral cryptorchid and the previous owner had the one descended testicle removed, hoping the horse would act like a gelding. If only the visible testicle is removed during gelding, then the cryptorchid horse may appear to be a gelding but will likely display varying degrees of stallion behavior — chasing or herding mares in the paddock, mounting mares, or acting aggressive toward other male horses.

If a veterinarian's examination reveals that this horse has one or two testicles in the inguinal canal and gelding can be performed through the flank with the horse standing, this would be a good solution. If the exam reveals that there are one or two testicles in the abdomen, weigh the cost and risk of abdominal surgery against your attachment to the horse.

If you decide to sell the horse, be sure to let the new owners know about his condition. If you don't, they could be hurt when his stallion behavior emerges.

EARLY WINTER

NOVEMBER TO DECEMBER

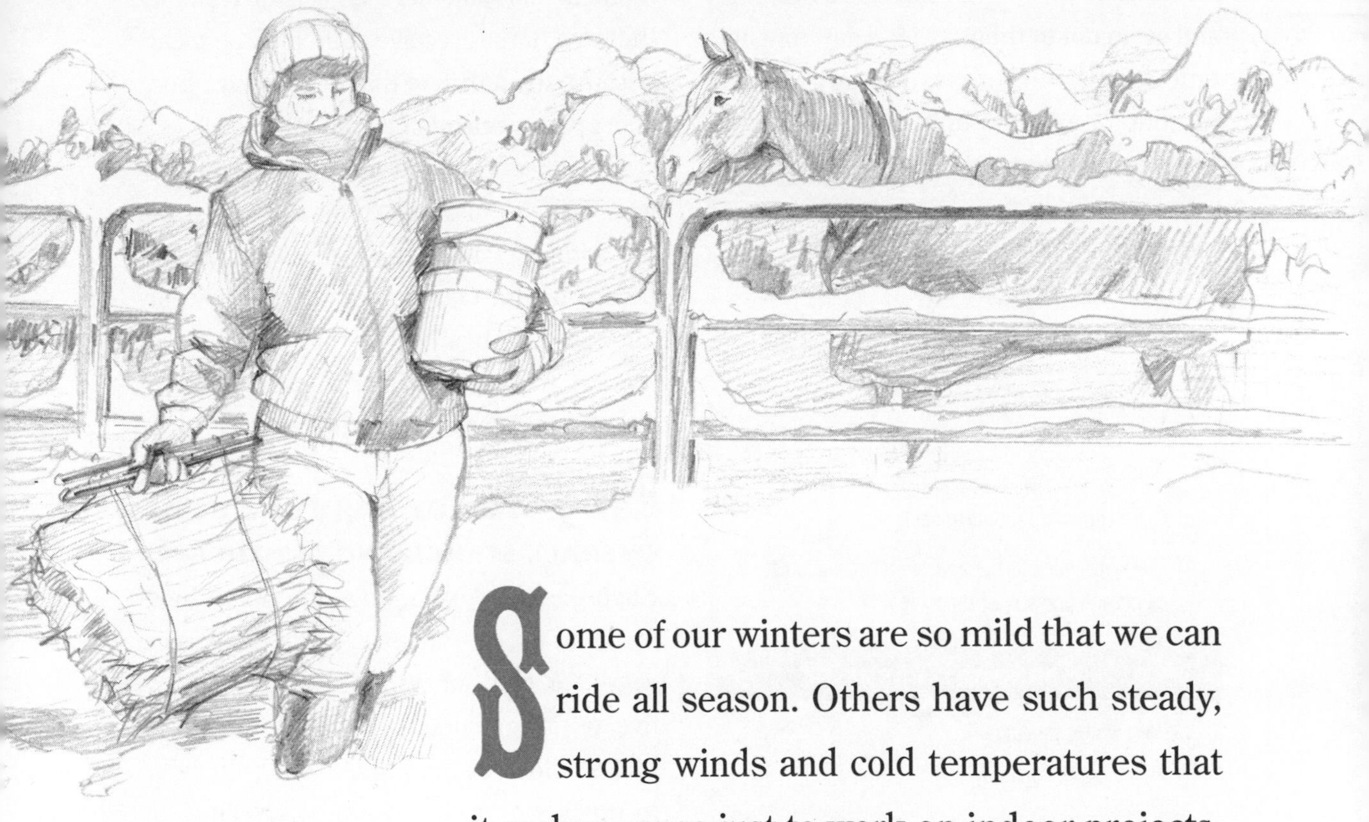

Some of our winters are so mild that we can ride all season. Others have such steady, strong winds and cold temperatures that it makes sense just to work on indoor projects. Often, therefore, at this time of year we are simply horsekeepers — feeding, scooping, and providing veterinary and farrier care. These tasks are not only necessary but, to me, they are also deeply satisfying.

This season usually marks the beginning of a slow-down. Even though the cold days and long nights might allow us a bit more R&R, our horses need as much care, if not more, during the winter. Although some horses might still be out on pasture full time (depending on the year and pasture condition), we have been carrying hay and grain out to them, twice a day, for some time now. Some horses are in pens with turnout for exercise only.

Weekly Tasks

- ❑ Restock the hay supply in horse barns
- ❑ Check grain supply
- ❑ Check bedding supply
- ❑ Dump and scrub all waterers, troughs, tanks, tubs, and buckets
- ❑ Scrub feed dishes
- ❑ Check veterinary supply needs
- ❑ Check upcoming farrier and veterinarian appointments and prepare for them

Seasonal Tasks

- ❑ Make winter shoeing plans
- ❑ Monitor winter water intake
- ❑ Increase roughage when below freezing
- ❑ Keep winter feeding areas clean of old feed
- ❑ Spread manure
- ❑ Clean tack and get ready for spring!
- ❑ Monitor pastures daily
- ❑ Remove horses from pasture while there is still vegetation in the field

During the winter it is necessary to keep a close eye out for signs of wood chewing, because horses that have been used to unlimited pasture turnout and are confined during wet, cold weather are the most likely candidates for this vice. An anti-chew kit is kept at the ready to treat freshly chewed wood the moment it is spotted. I increase the feed that the barn horses receive at their three meals because the nutrition that they receive from short pasture turnout is minimal.

Because there are still horses on pasture, I go out to check them at least once a day with my Pasture Kit. I often do this just before lunch. Our horses might be wearing sheets or blankets or they might be *au naturel*, with fluffy winter coats, depending on our plans for them for the winter.

Early Winter Visual Exam

OVERALL STANCE AND ATTITUDE. As I approach the barn, does the horse have his head up, are his eyes bright, and is he eager for feed, or is he lethargic, inattentive, or pacing and shivering?

LEGS. I look at the horse from both sides to quickly spot any wounds, swelling, or puffiness. With winter hair, I might have to feel for any abnormalities.

APPETITE. Has the horse finished all of his feed from the previous feeding? I keep track of winter weight with a rib check (see November Feed Bag).

WATER. Is there evidence that he has taken in a sufficient amount of water?

MANURE. Is the fecal material well formed, or hard and dry, loose and sloppy, covered with mucus or parasites, or filled with whole grains? Are there at least three manure piles since I last fed the horse?

PEN, SHELTER, OR STALL. Are there signs of pawing, rubbing, rolling, thrashing, or wood chewing?

BLANKET. If the horse is wearing a blanket, I check underneath for heat or signs of past sweating and check that all straps are fastened and the blanket is properly positioned. I also feel his ribs and check if the blanket has been rubbing off any hair, especially at the shoulders and withers.

✳	My Day	A Horse's Day
6:30 AM	Rise.	
7:00 AM	Chores, visual exam, feed barn horses.	Eat.
7:30 AM	Breakfast.	
8:00 AM	Work in office, domestic duties.	
9:00 AM		Walk over to the water tub for a drink.
9:15 AM		Return to the feed area or back out to pasture.
10:00 AM		Doze or lie down.
11:30 AM	Walk out to pasture horses and give visual exam.	
12:00 PM	Chores, then lunch.	Eat.
1:00 PM	Work in office or barn, ride.	
2:00 PM		Drink.
3:30 PM	Turnout.	Doze, lie down, or turnout.
5:30 PM	Bring horses in.	Return to pen.
6:00 PM	Chores.	Eat, drink, mosey until dawn, keeping alert for unusual sights or sounds.
6:30 PM	Supper for horsekeepers.	
8:30 PM	Nightly movie.	
10:30 PM	Go to bed.	

NOVEMBER

As if trying to hold onto the last strands of autumn, I find myself stretching out chores, taking more time than necessary to work each horse, sometimes just dismounting and strolling back to the barn, taking it all in. In the evening, Richard and I often stand up at our barn, overlooking the valley. Sometimes we're treated to the swooping of bats just as the stars begin to appear. And some years, our November is an extension of fall and becomes an extra bonus for us to enjoy.

Day Length in Hours

Latitude	Jan 1	Jan 16	Feb 1
60°N	8.31	7.09	6.1
55°N	9	8.05	7.32
50°N	9.52	8.75	8.18
45°N	9.93	9.3	8.83
40°N	10.27	9.75	9.37
35°N	10.56	10.13	9.82
30°N	10.81	10.46	10.21

See page 22 to find your latitude.

WACKY WONDERFUL WEATHER

STANDARD TIME

"Spring forward, fall back." During the change back to Standard Time, we turn our clocks back an hour, effectively moving an hour of daylight from the evening to the morning. In the United States, this change occurs at 2:00 a.m. local time; thus, in the fall, clocks fall back from 1:59 a.m. to 1:00 a.m.

The Energy Policy Act of 2005 amended the time change dates for Daylight Saving Time in the United States. Beginning in 2007, DST will begin on the second Sunday of March and end the first Sunday of November.

Daylight Saving Time is not observed in Hawaii, American Samoa, Guam, Puerto Rico, the Virgin Islands, and Arizona.

PREPARING FOR HIGH WINDS

In advance of any winter storm, secure your property. Remove dead trees or overhanging branches near structures, loose roofing materials, and objects in yards or on patios, roofs, or balconies that could blow away. If a wind advisory or high wind warning is issued:

- Take shelter. Decide whether your horses are safest indoors or on pasture.

To Do

- ❑ Deworm
- ❑ Rhino #1 for broodmares
- ❑ Hoof trim and shoe
- ❑ Work arena
- ❑ Scrub feed tubs and buckets
- ❑ Move hay to barns
- ❑ Rib check
- ❑ Dry baths

To Buy

- ❑ Beet pulp pellets
- ❑ Senior feed
- ❑ Corn oil
- ❑ Light bulbs

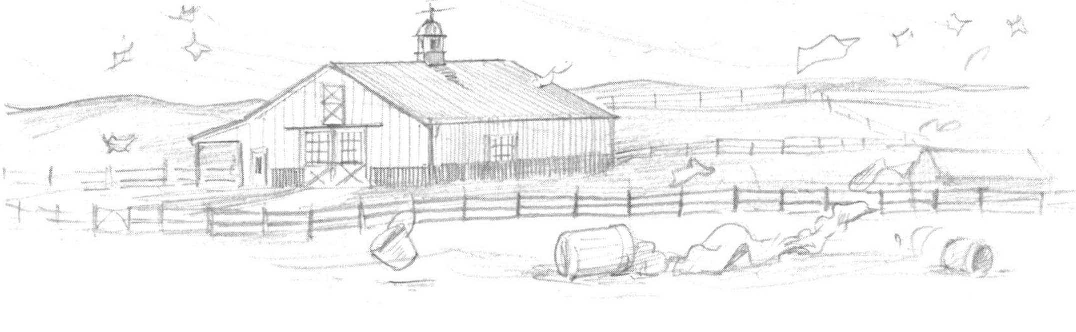

If you live in a high-wind area, routinely keep things picked up and battened down.

High Winds

If you and your horse are caught outside during high winds:

★ Take cover next to a building or under a shelter, clear of roadways or train tracks.

★ Watch for flying debris. Tree limbs may break and street signs may become loose during strong wind gusts.

- Tune in to local weather forecasts and bulletins issued by the National Weather Service on local TV and radio stations.
- Shutter windows securely and brace outside doors.
- Bring in unsecured objects from arenas, barnyards, patios, and balconies and secure outdoor objects that could blow away and cause damage or injury.

In the event of a downed power line, immediately call to report the situation to your local utility emergency center and to the police. Do not try to free lines or to remove debris yourself. Avoid touching anything that may be contacting the downed lines, including vehicles, tree branches, horses, or people, or you may become a victim. Puddles and even wet or snow-covered ground can conduct electricity in some cases. Warn others to stay away (see map, page 516).

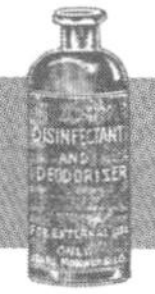

VET CLINIC

FYI

Slow Drinkers

A horse drinks by closing his lips and creating suction with his tongue, so it can take quite a bit of time for a horse to get his fill of water. Horses drink about a third of a pint per swallow, or 1 gallon in about 30 seconds, coming up for air after about 10 swallows.

WINTER WATER ISSUES

As the weather gets colder, be sure your horses are drinking enough water. They require between 4 and 20 gallons of drinking water a day. Water should always be available, clean, and of good quality. A horse's water intake will increase with environmental heat, exertion, lactation, increased hay ingestion, some illnesses, and increased salt intake, and it will decrease in extremely cold weather and during some illnesses. If a horse doesn't get the water he needs on a regular basis, he could suffer impaction colic, in which the contents of his intestines aren't moist enough to move properly through his digestive system.

To determine if a horse is dehydrated, perform the pinch test (see January Vet Clinic). Pick up a fold of skin on the horse's neck between your thumb and index finger.

Release the skin. It should return to its normal, flat position in one second. If a ridge remains, the horse is slightly dehydrated. If the skin remains peaked in what is called a "standing tent," the horse is dehydrated and could require immediate veterinary attention.

WATER IN WINTER. In very cold weather, providing freshly drawn water might encourage a horse to drink more water than if he has to eat snow or drink from an icy pond or trough. However, many horses will not drink artificially warmed or too-hot water. If you are in a cold climate and do not have heated watering devices, draw fresh buckets from the tap or hydrant several times a day to offer each horse. Horses prefer freshly aerated water at 35 to 40°F.

ADJUSTING TO UNFAMILIAR WATER. Because horses have such an exquisite sense of smell and taste, they often refuse to drink foreign water when they are away from home, even though it may be perfectly safe. To prevent a horse from going "off water" when traveling or when you move to a new location, you can flavor his home water for a while before leaving. Then flavor the new water with the same substance so it will smell and taste the same as what he was used to at home. Try a few drops of oil of peppermint, oil of wintergreen, molasses, apple juice, or soda. Use the additive sparingly and test each horse ahead of time so you know what will work before you move him.

COLIC

Colic is a pain in the abdomen, which can be mild and temporary or complicated and fatal. There are several types of colic in the horse:

- **Impaction** colic occurs when the intestines are blocked by a mass, which is usually food but could be a large batch of worms purged after deworming.

Enteroliths

Intestinal stones, or enteroliths, can become quite large and can cause colic, requiring surgery for removal. Enterolith formation has been linked to digesting alfalfa. Other contributing factors include lack of pasture, hard water, middle age (11.4 is the mean age), and certain breeds (including Arabians, Arabian crosses, Morgans, Saddlebreds, and Miniatures). California has the highest incidence of enteroliths followed (in no order) by New Mexico, Texas, and Utah.

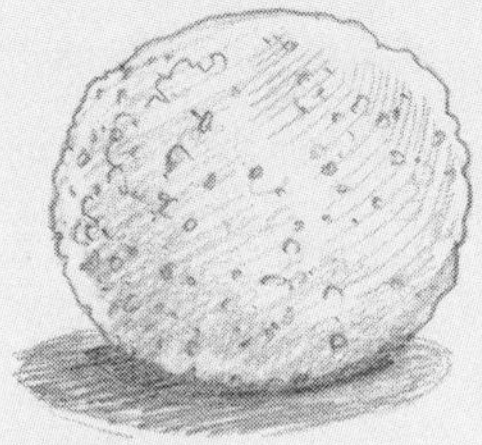

Enterolith

Signs of Colic

- ★ Pawing
- ★ Looking or biting at the side
- ★ Kicking at the abdomen with the hind legs
- ★ Lying down and getting up
- ★ Rolling
- ★ Standing stretched out
- ★ Attempting to urinate

Colic Prevention

- ★ Provide adequate water, salt, and minerals
- ★ Provide adequate exercise
- ★ Deworm regularly
- ★ Feed regularly, offering hay before grain
- ★ Use medications with caution
- ★ Don't feed on sand or gravel
- ★ Provide annual dental care
- ★ Minimize grain (use horse-proof locks on grain room)
- ★ Make feed changes gradually
- ★ Feed high-quality hay

- **Flatulent** (gas) colic often occurs from something the horse ate that produces gas, and since horses don't burp, the gas builds up until it can be released rectally.
- **Spasmodic** colic occurs from violent intestinal contractions.
- **Torsion** colic refers to the displacement of a portion of the intestine. When this occurs, the intestine has usually twisted, causing an absolute blockage that requires surgery.
- **Inflammatory** colic refers to cases in which the small or large intestine is inflamed from a feed, chemical, or illness.

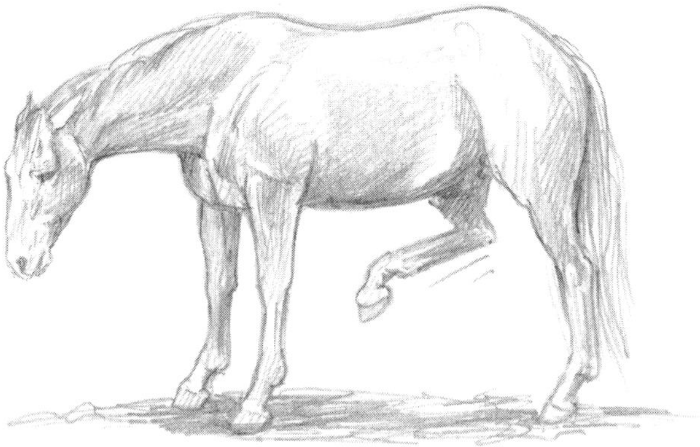

Kicking at abdomen

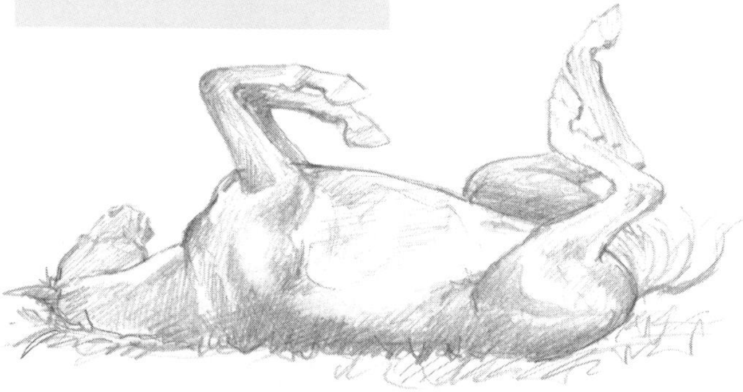

Rolling

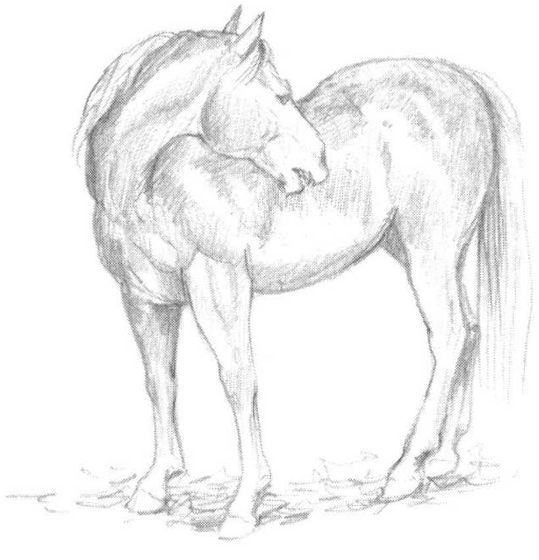

Biting side

FOOT NOTES

BAREFOOT IN THE WINTER

You may have heard the advice, "Pull his shoes and turn him out for the winter." Although this suggestion has merit in certain situations, for some horses such a plan would lead to chronic hoof problems.

The practice gained popularity during the era of horse-powered agriculture in areas with long, hard winters when most of the driving teams were not kept in full work. Turning a shod horse out in a snow-covered cornfield, plowed field, or winter pasture would have been an open invitation for lost shoes. Also, a horse shod with plain shoes usually has poorer traction in many footings than a barefoot horse. What's more, shod horses turned out and fed in a group are more likely to injure one another if they kick. So, to the turn-of-the-century Midwest draft-horse manager, pulling the shoes for the winter made sense.

Today's horse management is characterized by year-round use, increased confinement, and individualized

Over the river
and through the wood,
To Grandfather's
house we go;
The horse knows the way
To carry the sleigh,
Through the white and
drifted snow.
— Mrs. Lydia Maria Child

Evaluating Hoof Conformation

Barefoot candidates should have all of the following:

- ★ An upright hoof and pastern axis of 54 degrees or greater
- ★ A heel angle parallel to the toe angle, with minimal tendency to under-run heels
- ★ A hoof free of dishes or flares
- ★ The wall straight from the coronary band to the ground
- ★ The hoof horn of high quality material: thick, dense, hard, and solid, yet resilient because of a proper balance between internal and external moisture
- ★ A thick hoof wall through the quarters and into the heel
- ★ A well-cupped, durable yet resilient, concave sole

For Want of a Nail

If thin, well-designed horseshoe nails are used properly, and old nail holes in the hoof are filled, nails pose no real threat to the health of the hoof. However, when large nails are driven indiscriminately, and old nail holes are left open to invasion by moisture, soil, and manure, the strength of the hoof wall suffers. Compared to an instance of poor shoeing, therefore, the barefoot horse may be better off. Bad shoeing is often worse than none at all.

feeding. Yet for some reason, many horse owners still feel they should adhere to the age-old practice to ensure hoof health. The common belief is that pulling the shoes allows the hooves to "spread out and breathe." In fact, what often happens is that the hooves flatten out and break.

To determine whether going barefoot is a viable option for your horse, evaluate his hoof conformation to see if it resembles the "ideal" hoof that can go barefoot or the "problem" hoof that should not.

PROS AND CONS. The primary advantage to letting a horse go barefoot is that it costs less in the short term. A hoof trim costs approximately one-third or less of the price of a standard shoeing. To determine the overall savings, however, take into account the extra farrier and/or vet costs incurred the following spring, summer, and fall, which result from damage that occurred during the barefoot winter months.

A properly trimmed unshod hoof is easier to maintain, as it more easily self-cleans than a shod hoof. A bare hoof wall can more readily release excess moisture and can better maintain an optimal moisture equilibrium. A barefoot horse has quite good traction in a variety of low-demand situations, especially if the hooves are naturally balanced, with dense hoof horn and a well-cupped sole.

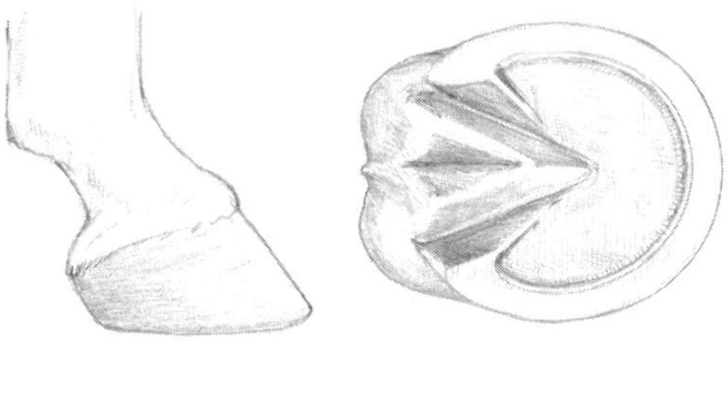

Hoof that could go barefoot.

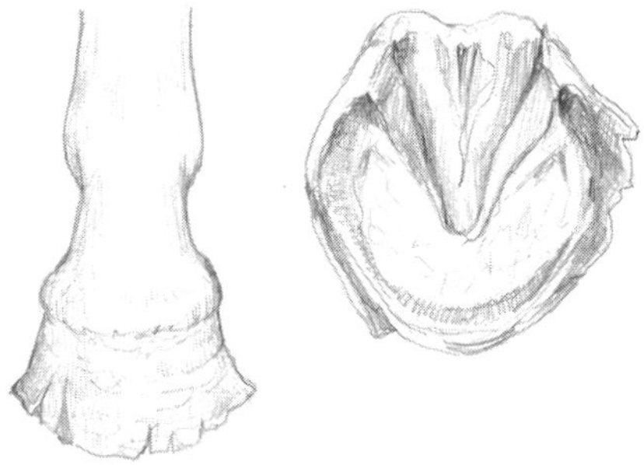

Hoof that should not go barefoot.

In some situations, such as on rocks, concrete, and hard ice, the barefoot horse has better traction than the conventionally shod horse does. However, such footing can cause excess wear of the bare hoof. Conventional shoeing decreases hoof wear, and specialized shoeing is available to increase traction.

Shod horses, especially those shod with borium, ice nails, or caulks, are potentially more dangerous to other horses and humans who are kicked or stepped on. Barefoot horses are safer to others as well as to themselves.

Unfortunately, many horses' hooves do not do well going barefoot in a domestic environment, especially with inconsistent hoof care. Such hooves have the tendency to form long toes, low heels, and under-run heels, where the heel angle is lower than the toe angle by 5 degrees or more. They often have dishes or flares, which can result in wall breakage. The hoof wall is thin and weak at the quarters and heels. The sole is flat or dropped.

When a horse's shoes are pulled, it can take a year or more, even with regular hoof care, for his hooves to adapt and be conditioned to going barefoot.

THE HOOVES OF WILD HORSES. Wild horses' hooves are characteristically steeper than those of domestic horses, ranging from 50 to 60 degrees in front and 53 to 63 behind. They exhibit a naturally rounded edge (perimeter), with the front hooves rounder in shape and the hinds more pointed. The hooves are even, well proportioned, balanced, and symmetric.

Wild Hooves

Wild horses are not a breed but a mix of domestic horses living in a natural environment. Their freedom of movement over a dry, rugged terrain has much to do with their solid hoof qualities. It has been found that neither sex nor color of hoof has any obvious effect on hoof measurements or shape.

The basest horn **of his hoof is more musical than the pipe of Hermes.**

— William Shakespeare, *Henry V*

FEED BAG

An old horse does not forget his path.
— Japanese proverb

COLD WEATHER FEEDING RULE REMINDER

For every 10°F below freezing (32°F), increase the hay portion of your horses' ration by 10 percent.

DO A RIB CHECK

This is the time of year when it can be difficult to see your horse's weight and condition, so you will need to feel his ribs. Refer to the Horse Body Condition Criteria in May More In Depth.

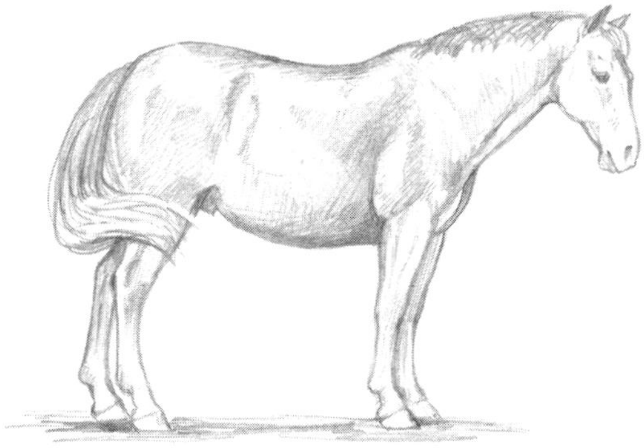

Too fat

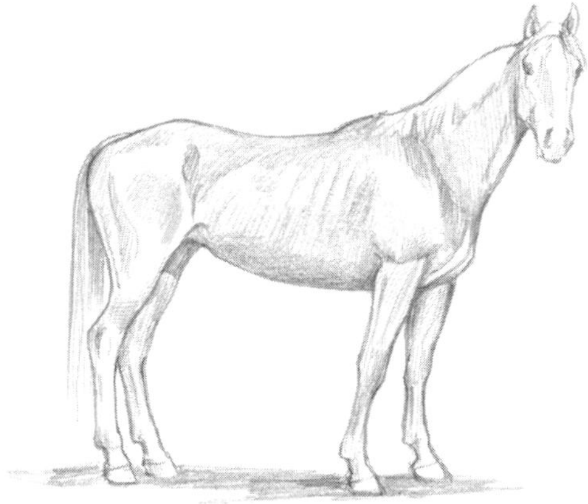

Too thin

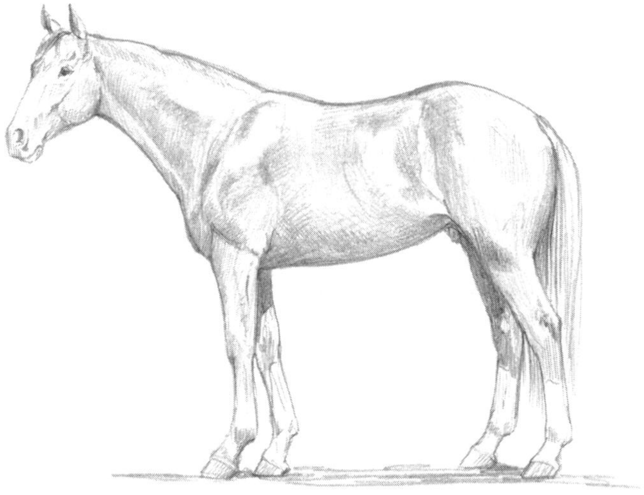

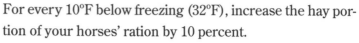

Just right

A horse's weight is considered about right when he scores in the middle of a horse condition scale. Using a scale from 1 to 9, 1 represents emaciated and 9 represents extremely obese. As an overview:

- A horse with a body condition score of less than 4 has less energy and lower resistance to disease and cold, and may have trouble breeding.
- A horse at 5 to 7 is usually at the optimal weight.
- A horse with a score of 8 or 9 is just a step away from colic or laminitis. Obese horses also have low energy and reproductive problems.

To determine your horse's score, stand about 20 feet away and inspect him from each side, the front, and the rear. Is your overall impression that he is too fat, too thin, or just about right? If you can see a horse's ribs or feel them very easily, he will score 4 or lower. If you can't see the ribs, but you can feel that they are there under a slight covering, he will score 5 or higher. At 7 the spaces start to fill in with fat between the ribs and will feel spongy.

Aim to keep your horse at optimal weight year-round. The exception to the rule: if you live in an area with very cold winters, allow your horse to gain a little fat in the fall to help insulate him when temperatures drop. For example, if he normally scores a 6, let him move up to a 7 in October and maintain that weight until spring, when increased work will bring him back to his normal working condition of 6.

BRAN MASH

During chilly winter days, when you might look forward to that steaming bowl of oatmeal, your horse would probably welcome a properly prepared mash. Read about beet pulp mash in January Ranch Recipes and March Feed Bag.

Before making a bran mash, know that wheat bran mash has its pros and cons. Wheat bran is lower in energy than grains but much higher in phosphorus. It is a good source

Ranch Recipes

Bran Mash

For one horse:

★ 3 cups hot water

★ 3 cups wheat bran

★ Cover and let steam for one hour.

Optional: Add up to 1 cup of molasses, sweet feed (grain), chopped apples, or carrots before serving.

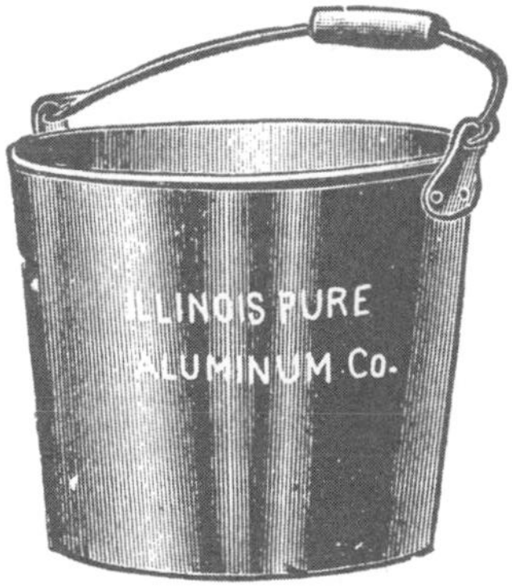

One problem with wheat bran is that the excess phosphorus interferes with calcium absorption.

of roughage and hydration and it is palatable, but it is expensive. It might best be an occasional treat or to improve bowel motility, for example, in older horses.

> *Look back at*
> our struggle for freedom,
> Trace our present day's strength to its source;
> And you'll find that man's pathway to glory
> Is strewn with the bones of the horse.
> — Author Unknown

One problem with wheat bran is that the excess phosphorus interferes with calcium absorption. The deficiency can lead to calcium being metabolized from the bones (usually of the face, legs, and ribs) and a condition called big head (nutritional secondary hyperparathyroidism), in which fibrous growths replace the decalcified (less dense) bone. One solution is to mix alfalfa pellets (a source high in calcium) in with the mash.

Another problem is that the intestinal bacteria needed to digest hay and grain might be destroyed by a long-term diet of bran mash. When normal fermentation patterns are interrupted, colic can result. Beet pulp is a more economical and more nutritious source of fiber and doesn't have the risks associated with feeding too much wheat bran.

WILD LIFE

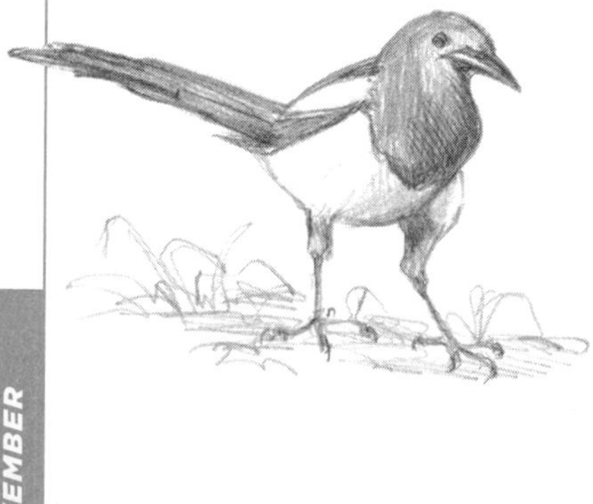

MOUNTAIN PENGUINS (MAGPIES)

We love 'em. We hate 'em. Magpies sail in gracefully, looking so elegant and even exotic in their iridescent black tuxedos, tails, and crisp white shirts. But that's where the romance often ends. Also known as camp robbers, these noisy, squawking, boisterous bullies of the bird world can take over a bird feeder so no other birds can visit. And they can swarm in cackling bunches right outside your bedroom window.

Magpie is the common name for the black-billed, long-tailed *Pica pica*, which is abundant throughout western North America, Europe, Asia, and North Africa. Magpies belong to the family Corvidae (see West Nile Virus in June Vet Clinic) and are related to jays and crows (who are also noisy and bold). They average 20 inches long, their tails accounting for more than half their length. Magpies are often found near livestock, where they feed on dung- and carrion-associated insects, and forage for ticks and other insects on the backs of domestic animals. I've often seen magpies on the backs of my horses at pasture.

Perhaps their most notorious behavior is picking wounds and scabs on the backs of livestock. If they find an open wound, such as that from a new brand, they may pick at it until they create a much larger sore. The wound may eventually become infected, which, in some instances, may kill the animal. In addition, magpies, like ravens, may peck the eyes out of newborn or sick livestock.

Joy or Vanity?

The magpie is symbolic in some cultures:

Chinese. The "Bird of Joy"; good fortune. A chattering magpie signifies good news, the arrival of guests. Under the Manchu dynasty it also represented imperial rule.

Christian. The Devil; dissipation; vanity.

CLEAN-UP CREW

STALL FRESHENERS

Barn lime (calcium hydroxide, slaked lime, or hydrated lime) was once the old standby for deodorizing and drying out stall floors. It lowers the acidity of the urine and causes dirt particles to clump, thereby allowing air to dry them out. Although cheap and readily available, barn lime is not especially safe or effective; in fact, it is highly alkaline and can irritate your skin or your horse's, especially when damp. Horses that eat from heavily limed floors can suffer mouth, throat, and lung damage.

Products containing zeolitesare are safer, far more absorbent than lime, and better at reducing ammonia odors. They are nontoxic to people and animals, nonflammable, and environmentally friendly.

Zeolites are a group of naturally occurring minerals, hydrous silicates, which were deposited as a result of volcanic activity millions of years ago. Their honeycomb-like

NOVEMBER Manure Pile Maintenance

PILE A
Sell, store, or spread.

PILE B
Quit adding, turn once.

PILE C
Start pile.

Odd Word

cast. When a horse lies and rolls next to a stall wall, becoming trapped and unable to get up.

Pasture Perfect

Winter Water

Sometimes in a period of snow and bitter cold, the creek freezes thick and seems to go dry. Even if we can break all the way through the ice, we find bare ground below. The water flow has gone underground. One 8°F morning, it looked as though we would have to bring the horses in from the pastures or set up water troughs for each pasture. The next morning, however, we had a warm-up to 41°F and the water started flowing above ground again.

structure gives them a very large surface area, which enables them to absorb tremendous amounts of odors.

Foul-smelling gases latch on to dust particles that have a positive molecular charge. Zeolite molecules have a negative molecular charge, so they act like magnets to attract dust particles, thus helping clear the air of odors as well as dust. In a similar manner, zeolites trap positive ammonium ions directly from urine, which makes them especially effective at reducing ammonia odors.

The honeycomb structure of zeolites, with millions of tiny micropores, also enables them to absorb more than 25 percent of their weight in water. Furthermore, zeolites do not become dangerously slippery when wet, which is important if your stall flooring consists of wood or solid rubber mats.

There's no need to let the stall dry out completely when using zeolites. Remove wet bedding, cover damp areas with 1⁄16 inch to 1⁄8 inch of zeolite product, plus a layer of dry bedding, and return the horse to the stall. The zeolites will absorb moisture and odors and hold them until the next stall cleaning. If odors are mounting but you don't have time to clean stalls, sprinkle a zeolite on the wet spots or place an open-topped container near the stalls to absorb odors.

One would think that a material that worked so well must carry some precautions, but studies have demonstrated that zeolites are essentially nontoxic to people and animals, whether ingested, on the skin, breathed, or in the eyes. They are nonflammable, environmentally friendly, and can be safely handled around horses' water and feed with bare hands, which is especially nice for those suffering from chemical sensitivity. They have a neutral pH of 6 to 8 and, as an added benefit, used zeolites are loaded with ammonium ions, which makes them an excellent slow-release fertilizer for gardens, flower beds, yards, fields, potting soil, and plant beds.

Pest Patrol

Fire Ants

Red fire ants first entered the United States from Brazil by way of Mobile, Alabama, in the 1930s. They now infest much of Texas and have spread into California. When you or your horse disturbs a fire ant mound, the ants swarm up your or your horse's leg and inject venom, often in multiple sites. The bite burns, swells, forms a blister, and itches for days.

Fire ants cost farmers and ranchers 6 billion dollars in lost production annually. This can include damaged equipment, loss of livestock (such as baby calves), and loss of time when harvesting, because ants can jam balers and combines, and the farmer must slow down due to rough ground from the sizable ant mounds. Electrical systems are attractive to fire ants, so they often swarm and short out air conditioners, water pumps, relay switches, and transformers.

Yards and grazing and haying land are often treated in November to decrease fire ant populations. You can broadcast pesticides at this time of year, or you can treat the mounds in late August to October.

Droughts naturally suppress water-loving fire ants. During their decline, however, ticks, chiggers, fleas, and cockroaches dramatically increase, because fire ants normally eat the eggs and larvae of these insects, as well as devouring boll weevils and sugar cane borers. Consequently, even though fire ants are pests to be watched out for and reckoned with if they run rampant, some stockmen have recently missed the valuable service they perform.

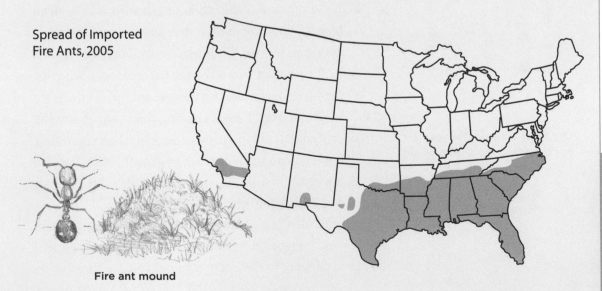

Spread of Imported Fire Ants, 2005

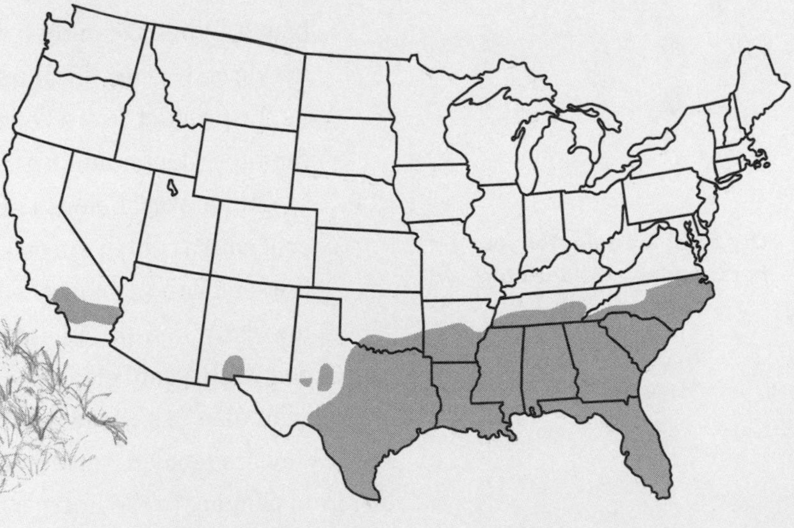

Fire ant mound

BEAUTY SHOP

Always smile
when you are riding
because it changes
your intent.
— James Shaw

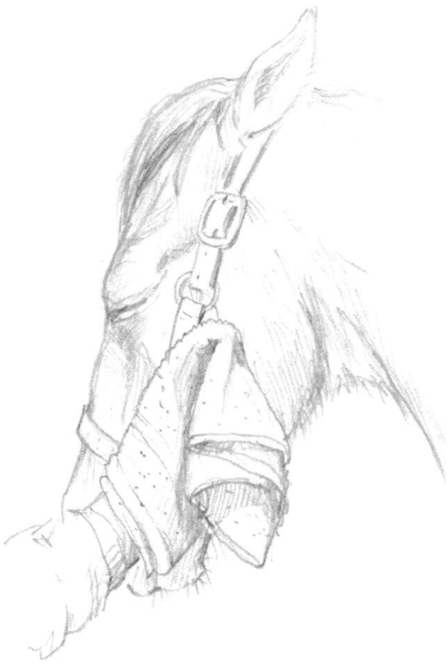

Dry baths are safer for your horse during a cold winter.

DRY SHAMPOO

This time of year, it is often too cold to give a horse a wet bath, and sometimes when you need to clean up a horse, there isn't easy access to water. That's when dry shampoo comes in handy. It works on horses that are dusty, dingy, or scurfy, or have dry sweat marks or green manure stains. (The term "dry shampoo" is a misnomer because many of the products for horses are liquids in a spray bottle.)

For spot cleaning, removing sweat marks, or cleaning the head, here are some tips.

1. Mist (don't soak) a clean terry cloth or a terry-lined sock turned inside out and fitted onto your hand like a mitten.
2. Rub against the direction of hair growth. This is especially important with long winter hair.
3. Find a clean spot on the cloth or sock, add more spray, and repeat the rubbing.
4. Continue misting until the cloth or sock no longer removes dirt.
5. Let the hair dry and then brush with a soft, clean brush. When cleaning larger areas, spray the product directly onto the horse's coat. For best results, let the product "work" on the hair coat for one to five minutes, depending on the product and how dirty the horse was, before rubbing the product into the coat with a rubber curry or fingers. Then vigorously buff and rub (against the hair growth) with Turkish towels. When the horse is nearly dry, set the hair coat with a soft, clean brush.

You can also use these products in a preventive manner. If they are labeled "antistatic", they will keep dust and dirt from clinging to the horse's hair. If you use them while

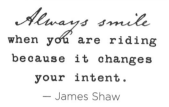

grooming the horse before work, sweat and dirt don't tend to stick to the hair, making after-work grooming much easier. However, if you use a waterless cleaner too often without a bona-fide bath in between, the horse's hair and skin tend to dry out or develop a buildup.

Although most products say that they are safe to use in the saddle area, many of them make the hair quite slick, so I'd suggest cleaning the saddle area with vigorous grooming, vacuuming, and a damp cloth.

> *en español*
>
> **rodeo.** Comes from *el rodeo,* 'a cattle roundup'; a public display of cowboy skills.

TACK ROOM

WINTER RIDING CLOTHING

Choose fabrics carefully. You'll find that certain garments make you feel so toasty and comfortable that you'll want to wear them for more than riding. Other items may not allow you to cool properly, may cause itching, or may generally be uncomfortable.

Design your winter riding wear so that perspiration has a place to go. Fibers and clothing materials will transmit, repel, or absorb moisture. Wicking is a process whereby perspiration is transported from the body's skin to the underclothing, and then to outer layers of clothing or to the air. This can happen in several ways.

- Some fabrics with close-together fibers, such as silk, allow sweat to climb the fibers by capillary action to the outerwear.
- Open-weave, nonabsorbing fabrics, such as polypropylene, remove sweat from the body by allowing body vapors to be transmitted outward.
- In a type of wicking called spreading action, water molecules are attracted to certain types of dry fibers, such as the treated polyester called Capilene, more

> **FYI**
>
> **Winter Layers**
>
> The layers necessary for winter riding usually consist of:
>
> ★ An inner layer to handle perspiration
>
> ★ A middle layer to provide insulation
>
> ★ An outer layer to cut the wind and provide protection from precipitation, if necessary.

Riding in the Cold

If you are cold, you can warm up by increasing your activity level. Move from a walk into a posting trot, or get off and lead your horse to restore the blood flow in your legs and arms. If you are too warm, temporarily decrease your activity level and gradually vent your body heat. A too-rapid evaporation of body moisture and heat can lead to chilling, so adjust your clothing in small stages rather than all at once.

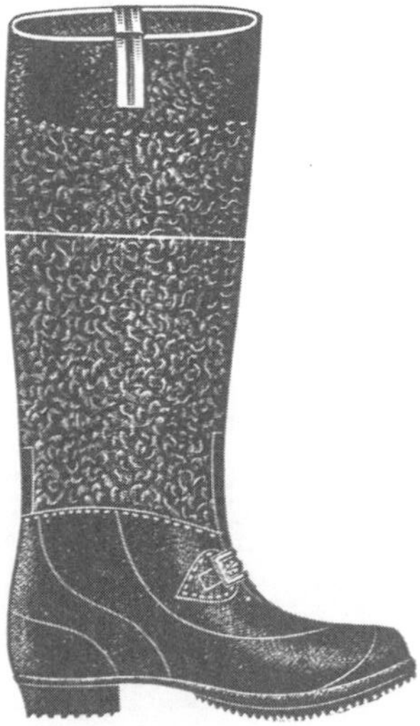

than they are to other water molecules. The moisture migrates through the clothing, always seeking the driest fibers, thereby moving to the outer layers and eventually dissipating.

Dress yourself in layers in order to trap air, which helps to keep cold out and body heat in. Proper layering prevents overheating, soggy clothes, and subsequent chill. It allows you to peel off layers to accommodate the various activity levels during a riding session.

Dress according to your proposed activity level. Rate your upcoming ride as passive, active, or very active. Pleasure riding or hacking at the walk is quiet and passive, so the extremities (fingers and toes especially) may get cold from decreased circulation. Cross-country galloping, however, is very active for the rider and rarely results in coldness during reasonable environmental conditions.

Avoid tight clothing. Pressure on surface capillaries from tight garments tends to slow circulation and decrease body warmth. Loose clothing traps fluffy layers of air that act as insulation.

Dressing for a Winter Ride

Routinely carry compact, lightweight accessories that will provide added warmth in the event of a weather change. Whether you are heading out for a road ride or just out to your arena, be prepared with a neck gaiter, scarf, or extra gloves. These items often take up little space in your pockets or in a saddle pouch, but can make a real difference in your comfort and well-being. If you will be more than 10 minutes away from shelter, tie a storm coat on your saddle.

FEET. The secret to warm feet starts with sock liners and well-designed, roomy, insulated boots. A thin sock liner used in conjunction with a medium-weight outer sock provides wicking, insulation, and cushion. The thickness of your outer sock will be determined by your activity level, the insulating quality of your boots, and the boots' fit. Be sure to choose boots that fit well but are not the least bit tight. Even a slight pressure at the toe or instep will cut off circulation and result in cold feet, no matter how high-tech your socks are.

Good-quality insulated boots have an inner layer (often with a removable sole) made of perspiration-wicking material, a middle layer of selectively permeable material to act as a mediator between the foot's perspiration and the moisture in the environment, and an outer durable, yet porous, covering, such as leather or nylon. Although canvas or nylon snowpack-type boots with felt liners are warm and roomy and conform to layering recommendations, they are often too wide and loose to use safely in a stirrup iron, and they prevent the use of spurs.

TIPS & TECHNIQUES

For Warmer Feet

Outfit your stirrup irons with a rubber tread pad to further insulate your foot from the cold metal.

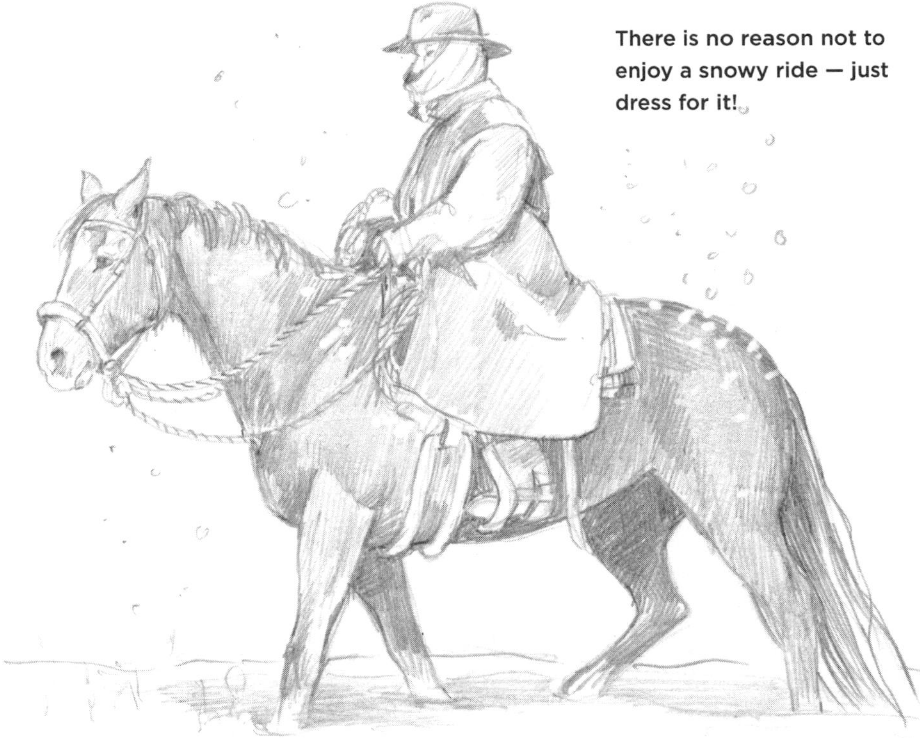

There is no reason not to enjoy a snowy ride — just dress for it!

Horse Sense and Safety

Guiding a Horse

★ When leading, if necessary use your right elbow against the horse's neck to keep him straight and to prevent him from crowding you.

★ If a horse resists or balks when you try to lead him, do not get in front and try to pull. Instead, stay in the proper position at the shoulder and urge the horse forward with a light tap from a long whip held in your left hand.

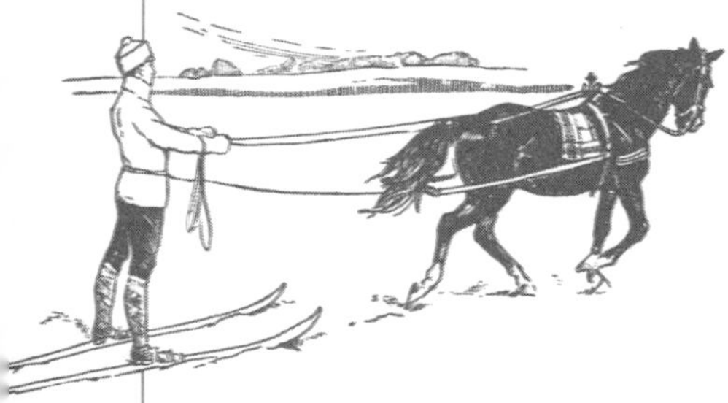

HANDS. If it's not necessary for you to have a very close feel of your rein action, consider a pair of puffy but lightweight and incredibly warm Thinsulate gloves. If you ride with close contact, on the other hand, use a pair of glove liners under a slightly oversized pair of thin leather riding gloves. When temperatures are moderate, you may find a pair of cross-country ski gloves, usually a blend of warm fabrics and leather, just perfect.

HEAD. Since your body can lose a great deal of heat through your head, don't be casual in your selection of headgear. During the coldest weather, and especially those days with wind, use a hat with an adequate insulation layer as well as a tight outer cover to deter heat loss from convection by the wind. A sheepskin hat with ear and forehead flaps keeps the most severe winter winds from chilling the head. Some Thinsulate ski hats with tightly woven outer shells of polyester or nylon also work well.

During storms, hats with brims offer some shelter from driving snow, but often no protection for the ears. If you have a brimmed hat that is slightly too big, you can wear a lightweight headpiece such as a hood, neck gaiter, or ski balaclava under it. Hats with brims also provide some protection from the glare of the winter sun, which is especially intense when there is snow on the ground.

Good-quality sunglasses, however, should be an integral part of your winter outfit, too. Use those with at least 98 percent protection from ultraviolet (UV) rays. Tinted lenses that provide less protection are worse than no sunglasses at all, because the dark lenses encourage the pupils to dilate, thus letting in more harmful glare.

NECK. To keep your neck warm, choose articles that can be removed or loosened to vent body heat and perspiration.

Neck gaiters easily slip off when they are no longer needed. Jackets with high zip collars and protective plackets allow you to choose how much protection your neck gets, and the plackets prevent zipper rub. A zippered turtleneck allows you to vent body heat all the way down to your under layer, which is essential during high-activity riding.

LEGS. The best bet for very cold weather and passive to moderately active riding are insulated pants specifically designed for riding. Such winter riding pants are designed to insulate and resist the wind as well as to provide comfortable, secure riding without bulk. Depending on your body thermostat and the weather, you may wish to wear long underwear with these pants, but the most that would be required would be a pair of silk liners. If you wear jeans or breeches, choose a roomy pair and use them in conjunction with light-, middle-, or heavyweight drawers. Sheepskin saddle-seat covers will also add to your warmth. If you

STILL TRUE TODAY

Historical Horsekeeping

"One of the most serious objections to stables as they are usually constructed throughout the country is the lack of proper ventilation. Usually they are nothing but close boxes, and entirely too small for the number of horses kept in them. The doors and windows are closed, and the bedding, saturated with ammonia, is tucked away under the manger. Anyone going into such a stable, especially during warm weather, will have the eyes immediately affected by the escape of ammonia, which, with the contamination of the air, caused by being breathed over and over, makes it even sickening to breathe any length of time." — Magner's Standard Horse and Stock Book *by D. Magner, 1916*

Winter Wear Questions

When choosing your clothing for winter riding, consider the following:

★ Is the garment comfortable and warm?

★ Is it designed to allow you to move freely?

★ When you are mounted, are the legs of the drawers or pants long enough to cover your ankles?

★ Does the jacket unzip from both the top and the bottom?

★ Are the boots safe in stirrups and can spurs be used with them?

★ Does the garment allow the feel necessary for riding?

★ Is it so bulky and heavy that it will impede riding?

★ Does hay stick to the fabric?

★ Is it washable?

★ Is it durable and well made?

Upper-Body Clothing Options

Because your upper body benefits from the heat of body metabolism (circulation, respiration, and digestion), it rarely gets cold if properly covered. Here is where you need to give some thought to removable layers. Choose a long-underwear top to suit your activity level and cover it with an insulating layer (wool, down, or Thinsulate), followed by a wind-resistant yet breathable layer (nylon or densely woven cotton). Some jackets and riding coats are both insulating and wind-resistant. During weather in the 30s and 40s, when a jacket might not be necessary, a good combination is a silk turtleneck, heavy wool sweater, and riding vest.

Outer garments that unzip or unsnap from both the top and the bottom are most appropriate for riding. Riding jackets must have freedom of movement in the shoulder and arm area. Longer coats must have flaps or gussets that conform to the cantle.

For protection during a storm, choose clothing with a tightly woven, waterproof outer layer. A flannel-lined New Zealand storm coat used in combination with long underwear, a wool shirt or sweater, and a down vest if necessary, keeps the worst storms from chilling you or damaging your saddle. Pants, jacket, and vest give you more freedom of movement than a long coat and offer the same good protection for the rider, but not for the saddle.

plan to get off your horse to lead, you can keep your lower pant legs warm and dry and prevent snow from sneaking into your boots by using gaiters.

Rather than looking at winter as a dormant time, if you dress properly for the weather, you will find that cold-weather riding can be enjoyable and beneficial for both you and your horse.

FARM OFFICE

HORSE INSURANCE

If you have valuable horses or board horses, consider horse mortality and/or horse health insurance. Look for an agent that specializes in equine insurance and writes with companies that have an A or A+ rating. Insurance companies are rated from AAA to C- by independent sources that evaluate their financial strength, or ability to pay a claim. Some sources of insurance ratings include A. M. Best, Standard & Poor's, and Moody's.

Mortality insurance is a form of term life insurance for your horse. It pays the value of the policy if the horse dies of natural or accidental causes (with certain exclusions). It might also pay if the insurance company agrees that a severely sick or injured horse should be euthanized. Full mortality insurance covers all causes of death, including illness and injury, and may include proven theft. A thorough physical examination is usually required before a full mortality policy is issued and, even if the horse passes the examination, the insurance company may have standard exclusions for certain causes of death.

The policy amount is the value of the horse. Mortality insurance rates are based on the type of policy and the value of the horse. Rates vary according to the breed, age, and use of the animal. The value is usually the purchase price of the horse, or if homebred, twice the stud fee. Sentiment or replacement costs are not a part of the value. A horse's policy value can be increased by factors such as winnings or sale of offspring, which must be proved and submitted to the insurance company. Generally, insurance underwriters take care in establishing the true value of the horse at the time the policy is written so that there aren't problems at the time of loss. If an insured horse dies or is seriously ill or injured, notify the insurance company immediately and according to the specific instructions outlined in the policy in order to avoid difficulties with your claim. A mortality insurance policy might be a good idea if you can't stand the financial risk of losing your investment in the event of a horse's death or serious injury.

Horse health insurance includes surgical-only, major medical, and unborn or prospective foal coverage. Health

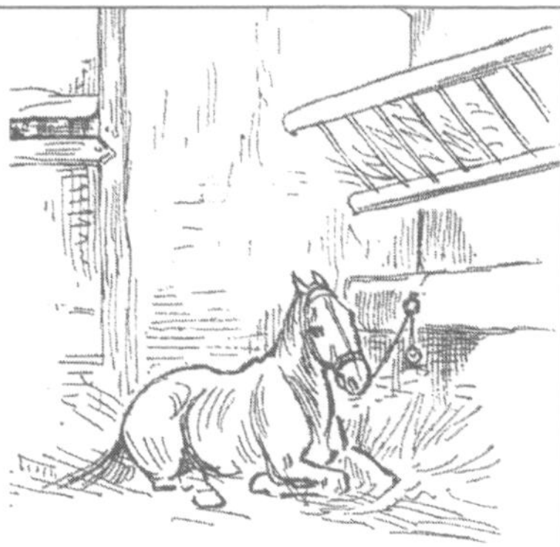

"Go anywhere in England where there are natural, wholesome, contented and really nice English people; and what do you always find? That the stables are the real center of the household."

— George Bernard Shaw, *Heartbreak House*

insurance is usually only available for horses already covered by a full mortality policy. Surgical-only insurance customarily pays for the veterinarian's surgery bill in nonelective surgery such as colic. In addition, some associated costs such as portions of X-rays and drugs might be paid. But anesthesia and board at the clinic might not be covered, resulting in a net coverage of the total expenses of only about 50 percent. Often, elective surgeries such as castration are not covered.

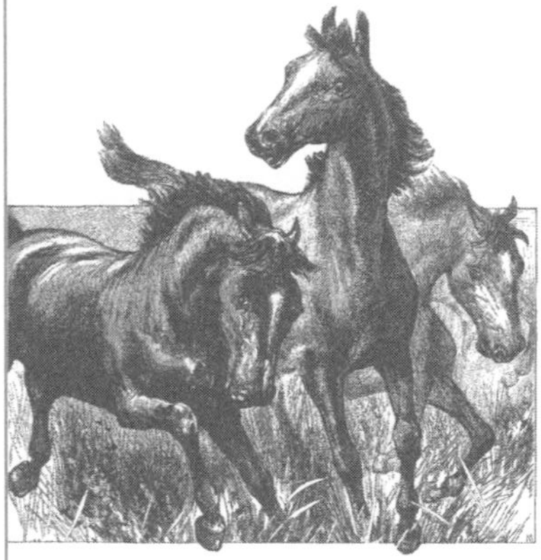

Policy costs are a flat fee per horse per year. There is usually a small deductible and a maximum claim amount. Major medical insurance usually pays surgical and nonsurgical expenses. Although these policies have a larger deductible and higher premiums than surgical-only endorsements, most major medical policies pay the entire cost of the treatment (over the deductible) up to the policy amount. Medical insurance requires an application and a completed and signed veterinary exam form.

Clothes Horse

Outdoor Horse Clothing

During the winter, when a horse lives outdoors or when a stabled horse is turned out for the day, he would benefit from a waterproof, breathable turnout blanket. When it is muddy or snowy outside, a long, lower hemline protects the legs and keeps them cleaner when the horse lies down. (See more on blankets in July and October Clothes Horse and September More in Depth.)

Don't put a blanket on your horse and then just forget about it. At least once a day, put your hand under his blanket. If it feels hot or sweaty underneath, your horse will get chilled. Also, every day, be sure the surcingles and leg straps are securely fastened, and look for signs of blanket rubs, especially in the shoulder area.

Insurance Applications

The **owner application** asks such questions as these:

- ★ What type of fencing do you have?
- ★ How often do you deworm and what type of dewormer do you use?
- ★ Has there been infection or contagious disease on the premises in the last 12 months?
- ★ How many of your horses have died or been destroyed in the last three years?
- ★ Are there any liens on this horse?
- ★ Is there any indebtedness due because of the change of ownership on this horse?
- ★ Has your insurance ever been canceled or refused?
- ★ Is this horse insured now? Has he ever been insured? With whom?
- ★ Who will be providing care for this horse?

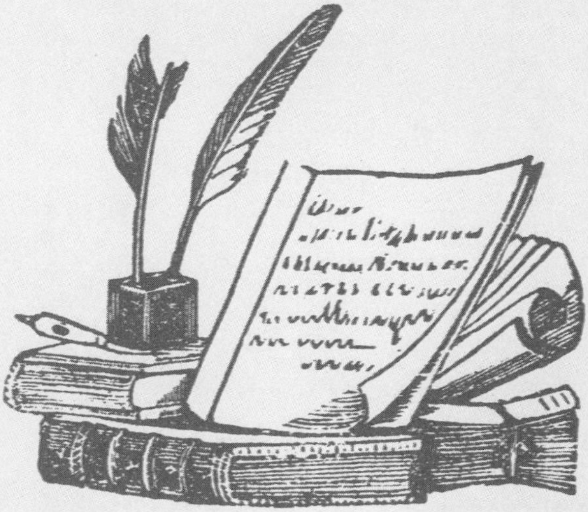

The **veterinary exam** for insurance varies depending on whether the policy will contain riders for surgical or major medical. Some of the things the veterinarian will check include:

- ★ Temperature, pulse, and respiration
- ★ Condition of eyes
- ★ Evidence that the horse is a "bleeder"
- ★ Evidence of nerving
- ★ Evidence of laminitis
- ★ Evidence of blistering or firing
- ★ Past lameness
- ★ Past surgeries
- ★ Fecal exam results
- ★ Scars
- ★ Male: castrated or both testicles evident
- ★ Female: mare in foal; past breeding or foaling problems; reproductive exam
- ★ Any vices or bad habits
- ★ Deworming program, parasite problems, colic problems
- ★ Any congenital abnormality or deformity
- ★ Results of Coggins test
- ★ Any other medical facts that should be brought to the attention of the company

PRE-RIDE WINTER WARM-UP

For your horse, keep the saddle and pad in a heated tack room if possible to avoid contributing to a "cold back": he humps and bucks when first saddled or ridden. Fasten cinches so they are secure enough but not excessively tight, and let the space between the horse's back, pad, and saddle warm up gradually. Keep the bridle in the tack room too, and further warm the bit by holding it in your gloved hand before putting it in his mouth.

When you lead, be ready for a hop. Before you mount, untrack your horse to the left and right, then finish tightening the cinch. You could prepare your horse further by doing a few in-hand exercises or longeing him if he is particularly frisky. When you mount, sit for a moment, even as long as a minute, before you move off, and then work on long, slow, steady work, such as a walk on a loose rein followed by a posting trot.

TIPS & TECHNIQUES

Before You Mount

Grooming and tacking should warm you up sufficiently. If not, a few overhead arm exercises and a short jog should get the blood flowing.

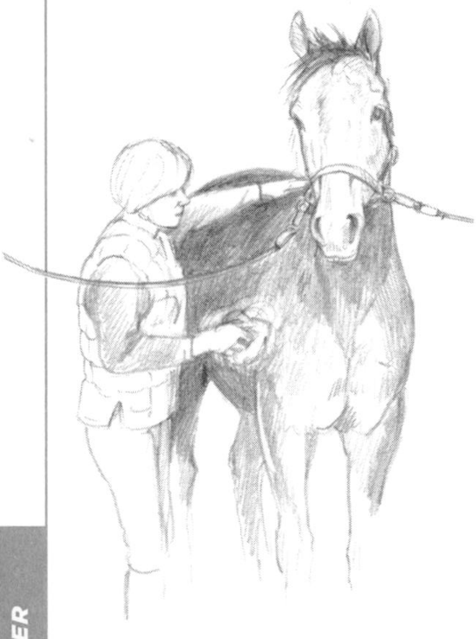

Grooming will help you warm up before a ride.

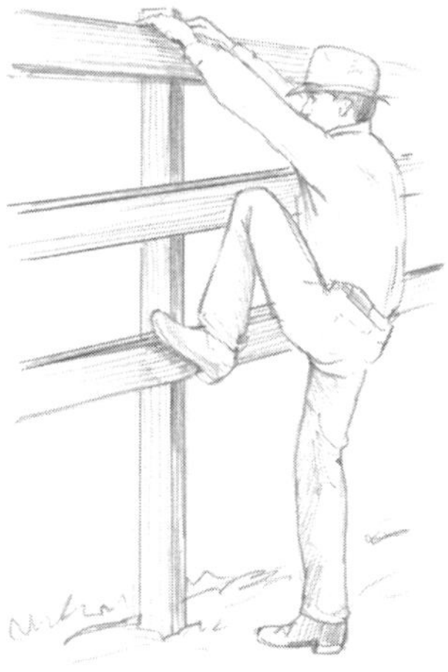

Stirrup stretch: Before mounting up, stretch the muscles of your legs and arms.

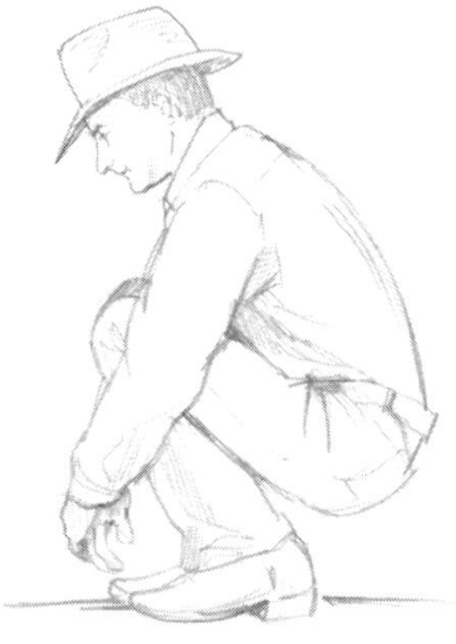

To give your back a good stretch, assume the campfire pose.

REPRODUCTION ROUNDUP

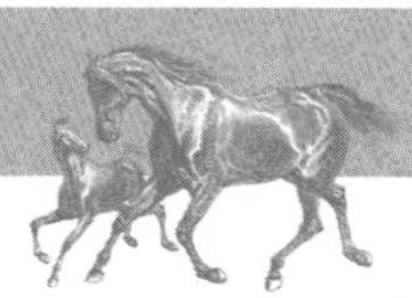

BEHAVIOR DURING ANESTRUS

Now that it is winter, make note of your mare's anestrus behavior. "Anestrus" refers to the time period when her reproductive system is quiet or shut down for the winter, and she is not cycling. Get to know your horses' "winter mare" personalities. Some mares during the winter, like geldings, are very neutral and predictable. Others may seem sluggish while some are always aware of "where the boys are." It will vary greatly among mares.

EARLY CYCLING

Increased day length starts mares cycling, and 16 hours seems to be the magic number. If you want to breed your mare earlier than May, begin using lights to artificially create a longer day. Adding light in late afternoon so that the horse's "day" is 16 hours results in her cycling within 60 to 90 days. Therefore, if you want to breed your mare early, start this program at the end of November. The mare must have the extended light period every day or the effort will not work, and the longer light period must last until at least May 1 or cycling will stop.

BROODMARES' RHINO #1

Pregnant mares should receive vaccinations against rhinopneumonitis virus (equine herpes virus 1p and 1b) to help prevent abortion due to viral infection. Vaccinations should be given at the fifth, seventh, and ninth months of pregnancy. Other horses on your premises might also require rhinopneumonitis vaccines. Ask your veterinarian to recommend which rhino vaccine to use for your situation.

The rhinopneumonitis vaccine must be administered IM, deep in heavy muscle. Your horse must exercise following

Early Cycling How-to

Research has shown that 24-hour light has the same effect as no light, so your goal for an early foal is 16 hours of light, no more, no less, every day until at least May 1.

To get 16 hours of light, use timers to turn barn lights on and off (for example, on at 5:00 p.m., off at 10:00 p.m.), and check them daily to be sure they are working. A 200-watt incandescent light bulb (or two 40-watt fluorescent bulbs) in each stall is sufficient. As noted in February Beauty Shop, this program will cause the horse to shed earlier too, so in a cold climate, the mare may require more feed and/or blanketing.

the injection to promote absorption and to prevent muscle soreness. For mares heavy in foal, hand-walk 15 to 30 minutes per day for three or four days after the injection.

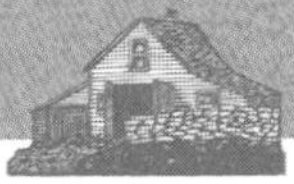

FINE FACILITIES

KEEPING A HORSE IN A STALL

The smaller your acreage and the closer you live to an urban area, the more likely it is that your horse will spend part of his time in a stall. Although it is a space-efficient way to keep a horse, a stall requires a large investment of capital and time. You must have a well-designed barn, feed at least twice a day, clean the stall morning and evening, and exercise the horse every day by riding, longeing, driving, ponying, or providing active turnout. Even with all that, stall life doesn't suit every horse.

For the best chance of success, start with a good stall. A good stall environment begins with a minimum space of 12 feet by 12 feet with an 8-foot-tall by 4-foot-wide door. Many horses over 1,100 pounds or 15 hands are much neater and more content in a 12-by-14-foot or 12-by-16-foot stall.

For hoof and respiratory health, locate the barn on a well-draining site. The base of the floor should be of porous material, such as 10 to 12 inches of gravel. The flooring, which goes on top of the base, should be comfortable and safe, such as rubber mats. The bedding must be nontoxic, clean, dust-free, comfortable, and unpalatable.

The stall walls and doors should discourage rubbing, be able to withstand damage from kicking or chewing, allow ventilation to flow through the stall, and let the horse look out. There should be a clean place for the horse to eat hay (preferably at ground level), a grain feeder, and a large water pail or automatic waterer.

TIPS & TECHNIQUES

IM Injections

Administer injections yourself only if you are fully capable of giving an aseptic IM (intramuscular) injection. If you would like to be able to vaccinate your horses in the future by yourself, see *Horse Health Care* (in Recommended Reading) and then ask your veterinarian to demonstrate and coach you so you can learn.

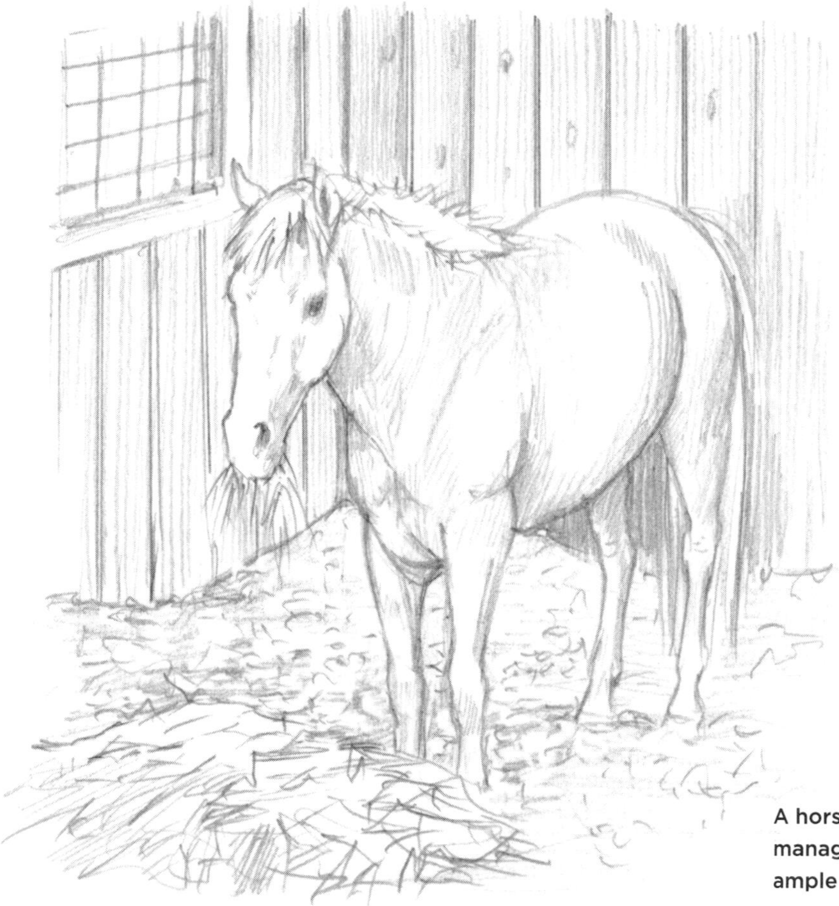

A horse can be happy in a well-managed stall providing he gets ample exercise.

The stall should be located where there is not a lot of noise or bright lights. The barn environment overall should be healthy, with plenty of ventilation (from windows, doors, vents, or fans) that keeps the temperature in the range of 30 to 80°F and humidity in the range of 35 to 60 percent.

NOT ALWAYS TRUE

Historical Horsekeeping

"Carrots are a good laxative and alterative before frost, but are too cold and constipating during cold weather. They may be fed in October, November, and December but in the Northern States not later."

— Magner's Standard Horse and Stock Book *by D. Magner, 1916*

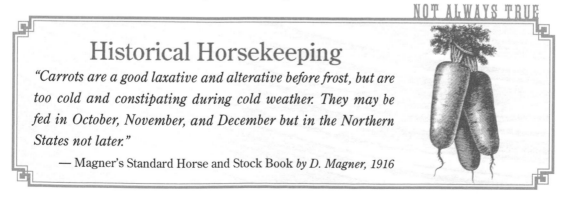

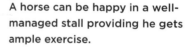

STALL KICKING

Few vices can be as destructive to your horse, your facilities, and your peace of mind as stall kicking. Capped hocks and curbs are often associated with chronic stall kickers. Loose, lost, or shifted shoes are common with stall kickers.

> **Movie of the Month**
>
> ***DANCES WITH WOLVES* (1990)**
>
> Kevin Costner's masterpiece about Lt. John Dunbar, a soldier assigned in the 1860s to a remote post in Sioux Indian country along with his buckskin horse, Cisco. He befriended Kicking Bird, played impeccably by Graham Greene, adopted the Indian lifestyle, and became "Dances with Wolves." Much excellent bareback riding, including an action-packed buffalo hunt. Some very sad realities in this movie however, but with each viewing, it never fails to inspire.

CAUSES OF STALL KICKING. Kicking is part of socially acceptable play among horses, so stall kicking may begin as a natural behavior but may quickly become an exaggerated and obsessive habit. Like many stable vices, it may be contagious between neighboring horses.

In some cases kicking occurs between neighbors who don't get along. A mare that has gone out of estrus (and in some instances, one that is in estrus) may kick at the horse in the next stall, whether it is a stallion, a gelding, or another mare. Others may have a personality or pecking-order conflict. And other horses that are protective of their feed and personal space may use kicking as a territorial protection measure.

Some horses have learned that a great way to elicit attention from humans, and perhaps even get an extra measure of feed, is to kick. The noise brings someone to the

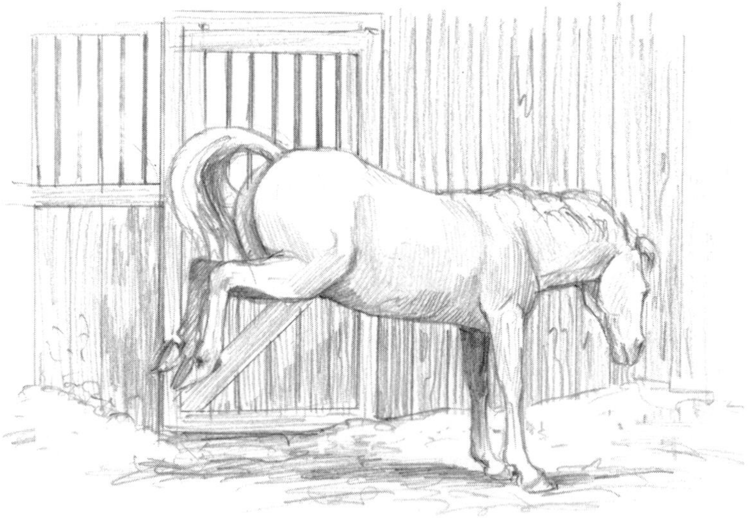

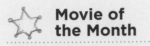

Stall kicking can be damaging to the facilities and injurious to the horse.

stall, often with a diversionary flake of hay or a handful of wafers. The kicking horse has not only received what he wanted but has even been rewarded for kicking.

CURING STALL KICKING. Before trying any corrective measures, be absolutely sure that the horse is receiving regular adequate exercise and appropriate feed and has reasonable neighbors. For the pros and cons of stall life, see *Horsekeeping on a Small Acreage* (in Recommended Reading).

A horse's ration should be tailored to meet his energy needs. An overfed, underexercised horse is a prime candidate for becoming a stall kicker.

If stall kicking is obviously due to boredom or confinement, the horse can be given additional work sessions or turnout time in a pasture or run. If this is not possible, a stall toy may offer a diversion. When kicking is due to an incompatible neighbor, shifting the horse's position in the barn may help. If kicking is a means of begging for a treat, tying the horse in his stall so that he cannot reach a wall often prevents kicking but may precipitate pawing.

TIPS & TECHNIQUES

Put Him to Work

Any horse, and especially an energetic, inquisitive horse, should have active, sustained exercise at least five times a week.

STILL TRUE TODAY

Historical Horsekeeping

"It may be well to reiterate: the best average heat for a stable should be from sixty to not to exceed sixty-five degrees; that the air should be normally dry, for if there be any moisture about the stables, it will hang about the horses in the shape of a mist, and the animals when they are brought into the open air, although their skin will be as fine as can be imagined, will shiver as if they had just made their exit from a warm bath."

— Prairie Farmer Horse Book, *Jonathan Periam, 1891*

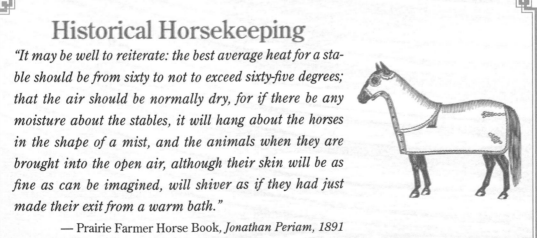

RPMS & PTOS

WISH LISTS

This is a good time to write up your wish list — things you'd like to have and need to work into your or Santa's budget. Some examples:

- An upgrade to a ¾- or one-ton truck so you can haul a bigger horse or hay trailer.
- A horse trailer with a dressing room that's large enough to sleep in on an overnight trail ride.
- A larger, more powerful tractor.
- A generator for those power outages that seem to be becoming more frequent.
- A hay elevator to make hubby's work a little easier.
- A garden tractor with a belly mower for those tight spots.
- A utility vehicle for those pasture chores and guest tours.

> *The best horse* doesn't always win the race.
>
> — Irish proverb

MORE IN DEPTH

HORSEKEEPING IN THE SUBURBS

As urban corridors are subdivided into small acreages, you may find yourself setting up horsekeeping in or near a residential neighborhood. Such a location involves some special considerations to maintain good neighborly relations and satisfy legal requirements.

- **Manure management.** Your sanitation plan must be impeccable. Manure piles must be concealed and well managed to control odor and flies.
- **Noise control.** Whinnying horses, a blasting barn radio, a megaphone used during lessons: all of these

seem perfectly normal to a horse owner, but may not be to a neighbor who cherishes peace and quiet.

- **Aesthetics.** Where you see a beautiful pasture, your neighbor might see a field of weeds and manure. Appearances matter when neighbors are close, so mow, paint, and repair as needed.
- **Security.** It is imperative that your horses stay on your property and not be able to access your neighbors' garden, lawn, trees, or buildings by leaning, reaching, or escaping. If your neighbors also have horses, consider instituting a 20-foot buffer zone (double fence) between properties so the horses can't contact each other.
- **Boundaries.** Buildings and other facilities must be placed a certain distance from property boundaries, street rights-of-way, and your home.
- **Traffic.** The coming and going of your truck and trailer, manure removal services, feed trucks, and the like may be a source of consternation for neighbors.
- **Dust.** Some properties are subject to a permit and fees for dust raised ("fugitive dust"). Any bare or disturbed surfaces, such as arenas, round pens, paddocks, runs, and driveways, could qualify. (See July Clean-up Crew for more on fugitive dust.)

FYI

Be a Good Neighbor

Stay in touch with neighbors so you can work out small problems before they become big ones. Stay informed. Be active in your local government so you can defend challenges to your rights as a land and horse owner.

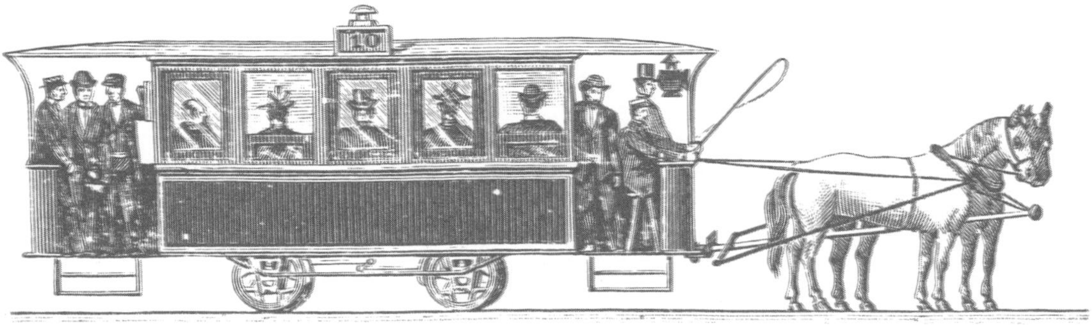

WIND TUNNEL IN THE WEST

While high winds are commonly associated with severe thunderstorms, hurricanes, and nor'easters, they may also occur as a result of differences in air pressure, such as when a cold front passes across the area from the Pacific Northwest or Canada. High winds are common during the winter in the western United States and can cause downed trees and power lines, flying debris, and collapsed buildings. These in turn lead to power outages, transportation disruptions, damage to buildings and vehicles, and injury or death.

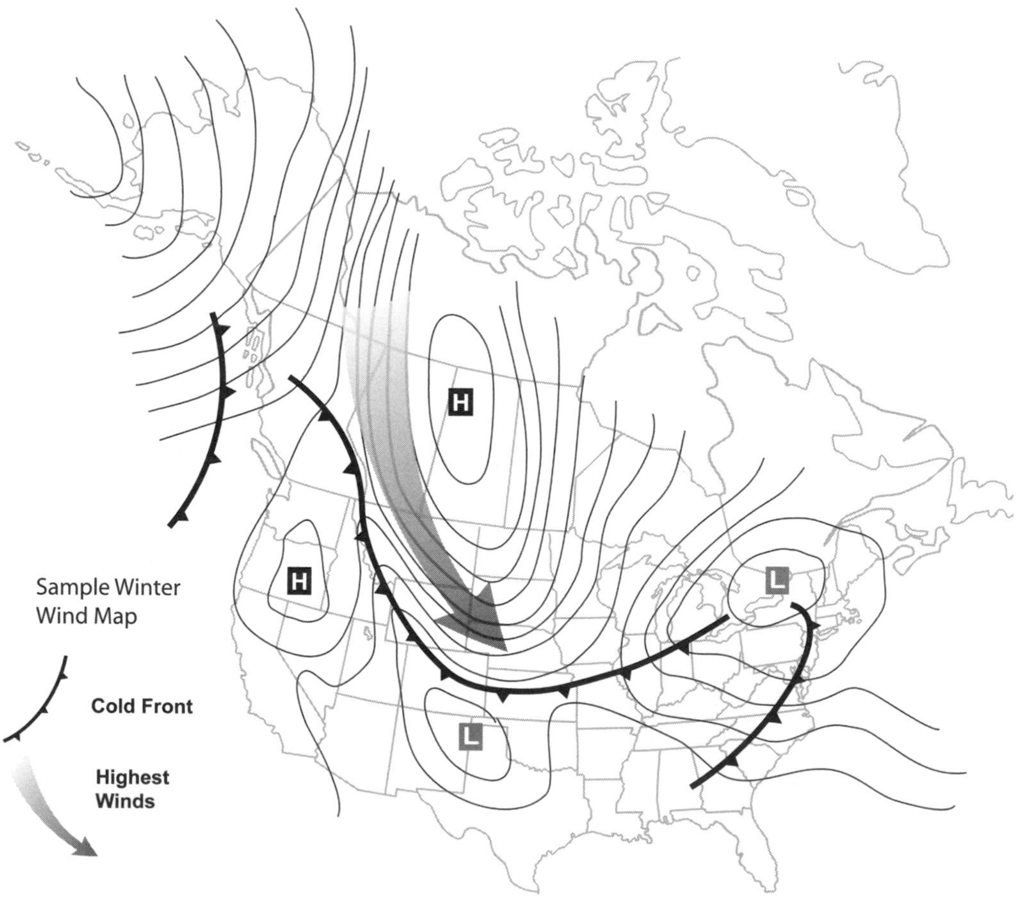

National Weather Service Terms

Wind Advisory. Sustained winds of at least 30 miles per hour (mph) for one hour, with 45–57 mph gusts.

High Wind Warning. Sustained winds of at least 40 mph for one hour or more, or gusts to 58 mph or more. Issued when high winds affect the forecast area and threaten life and property.

Beaufort Wind Scale. A simplified scale developed to aid in the estimation of wind speed and typical effects:

★ **25–31 mph: Strong Breeze.** Large branches blow; telephone wires whistle; umbrellas unwieldy.

★ **32–38 mph: Near Gale.** Whole trees in motion; resistance felt while walking against the wind.

★ **39–46 mph: Gale.** Twigs break off tree branches; wind impedes walking.

★ **47–54 mph: Strong Gale.** Slight structural damage.

★ **55–63 mph: Storm.** Rare inland; trees uprooted; considerable structural damage.

★ **64–72 mph: Violent Storm.** Very rare; widespread structural damage; roofing peels off buildings; windows broken; mobile homes overturned.

★ **73 + mph: Hurricane.** Widespread structural damage; roofs torn off homes; weak buildings and mobile homes destroyed; large trees uprooted.

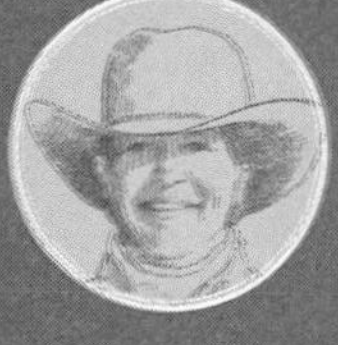

Ask Cherry

Stall Flooring

Q What is the best kind of flooring to have in a stall? We are building a new horse barn and want to know about the stall floor to make it as easy to keep clean as possible. The stalls will be 10 feet by 16 feet. The stalls will be used to feed and hold a horse for foaling. Thanks for your time.

A I prefer interlocking rubber mats over decomposed granite or another well-draining, well-packed base. I normally bed with shavings, but use straw for foaling.

DECEMBER

Some of my most memorable and beautiful rides have been in deep winter snow. Plowing through the drifts, however, can be a lot of hard, sweaty work for a horse. So if I plan to do a lot of winter riding, now is the time of year to body-clip.

I appreciate my horses so much that every year I think hard about what I could do to show my appreciation for another wonderful year. And here it is, straight from the horse's mouth: Be the best horsekeeper I can be.

Day Length in Hours

		Date		
		Dec 1	Dec 1	Dec 1
Latitude	60°N	6.1	5.56	5.66
	55°N	7.32	6.93	7
	50°N	8.18	7.88	7.93
	45°N	8.83	8.6	8.64
	40°N	9.37	9.17	9.21
	35°N	9.82	9.66	9.69
	30°N	10.21	10.08	10.1

See page 22 to find your latitude.

WACKY WONDERFUL WEATHER

While it can be a month of extreme cold in many parts of the United States and Canada, December means perfect riding weather in the South and Southwest. If your area experiences an annual deep freeze, provide shelter in the form of a stall, shed, overhang, trees, and/or blankets. Make sure all horses can find protection from wind and moisture.

To Do

- ❑ Hoof trim and shoe
- ❑ Scrub feed tubs and buckets
- ❑ Move hay to barns
- ❑ Winter clip

To Buy

- ❑ Complete feed wafers
- ❑ Grain
- ❑ Dewormer
- ❑ Carrots

WINTER SOLSTICE

In astronomy, the winter solstice is when a hemisphere is most inclined away from the sun, resulting in the shortest day and the longest night of the year. In the northern hemisphere, the winter solstice usually falls on December 21 or 22; in the southern hemisphere, on June 21 or 22.

VET CLINIC

VET FACILITIES

Here are some things you can do to make life easier for your veterinarian.

- A veterinarian, like a farrier, should be able to get his or her truck close to the sheltered work space in the barn.
- Access to hot and cold water is a big plus, because many veterinary procedures involve washing various parts of the horse.
- The footing should be solid with good traction, and sloped to drain water away from the work area, so the vet doesn't have to stand in water.
- Good lighting is especially important for vet work. Besides ample permanent lights, portable lights

O, Wind,
If Winter comes, can Spring be far behind?
— Percy Bysshe Shelley, *Ode to the West Wind*

TIPS & TECHNIQUES

A Handy Extra Stall

Having an extra stall in your barn, and rotating horses so one stall can dry out thoroughly, will minimize floor maintenance.

should be available to spotlight certain areas on the horse. Plenty of outlets installed in convenient locations will make it easier for the vet to use clippers, ultrasound, and other equipment.

- A rubber mat over the textured concrete prevents excess hoof wear, as from pawing.
- A counter or table close to where the vet is working is very useful for setting down tools and keeping supplies at hand without having to place them on the floor.

Note that a wash rack can also double as a vet area.

STOCKS. A professional palpation chute (stocks) is designed to safely contain a horse while allowing a veterinarian to work on him. The solid doors on the front and rear of stocks protect a person from being kicked or struck. The floor slopes to a drain located between the two stocks. With doors on both ends, the horse can be led in and then out of stocks without having to back up.

"Loose stocks" are roomier and multipurpose. Located next to a barn under a roof overhang, they are designed as a place to train young horses to stand quietly and to let a horse dry after a workout or a bath. They can also be used for vet work. The cross-ties and pipe rails allow some movement, but keep the horse from swinging too far sideways. There's enough room in loose stocks for a farrier, vet, or groom to work on a horse.

Odd Word

stare. When a horse's hair coat sticks straight out, it is "staring" rather than lying flat and gleaming.

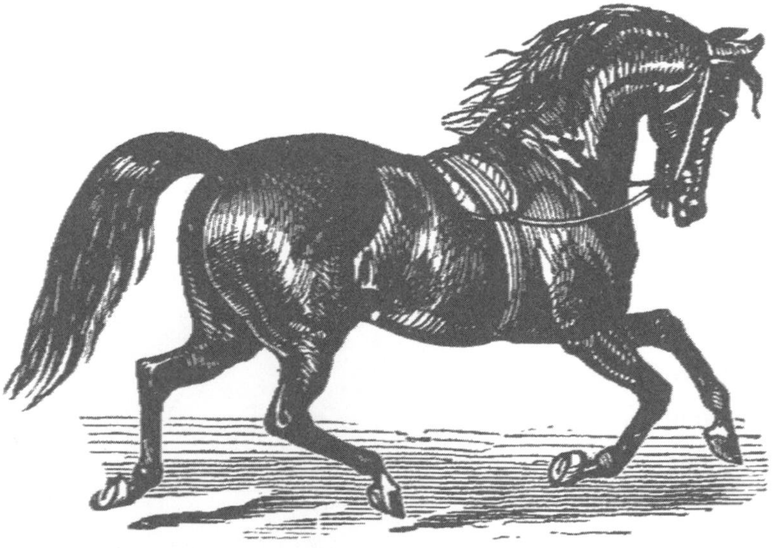

FOOT NOTES

A FOUNDATION FOR HEALTHY HOOVES

Your horse's living quarters, whether stall, pasture, or paddock, should have well-drained footing. The site for your barn should be properly prepared so that the soil and other materials beneath the floor percolate well. Ideally, the finished level of the barn site should be 8 to 12 inches above ground level. If the existing soil is well drained, the site can be prepared by the addition of 6 inches of crushed rock covered by soil. Pure clay (a traditional favorite) packs firmly but does not percolate well. Soil blends or synthetic materials (depending on locale) might work better than clay for site preparation.

A site with poorly drained soils requires excavation to between 3 and 10 feet. Several feet of large rock should be laid at the base of the excavation. Crushed rock of decreasing sizes should follow in layers, leaving about 1 foot for the site's topsoil. A mixture of clay, sand, or other materials (such as road base or small gravel) usually works well.

Five Keys to Healthy Feet

Hoof health depends on:

★ good facilities

★ sanitation

★ exercise

★ good nutrition

★ competent farrier care

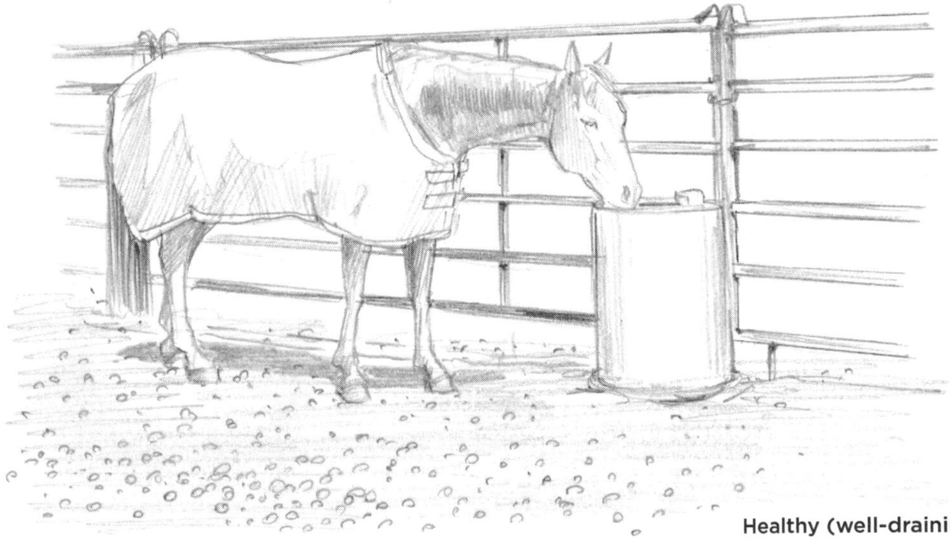

Healthy (well-draining) pen footing.

Choosing Flooring

Factors to consider when choosing flooring include:

- ★ Initial cost
- ★ Longevity
- ★ Maintenance
- ★ Cushion
- ★ Drainage
- ★ Odor retention
- ★ Ease of cleaning and sanitizing
- ★ Traction

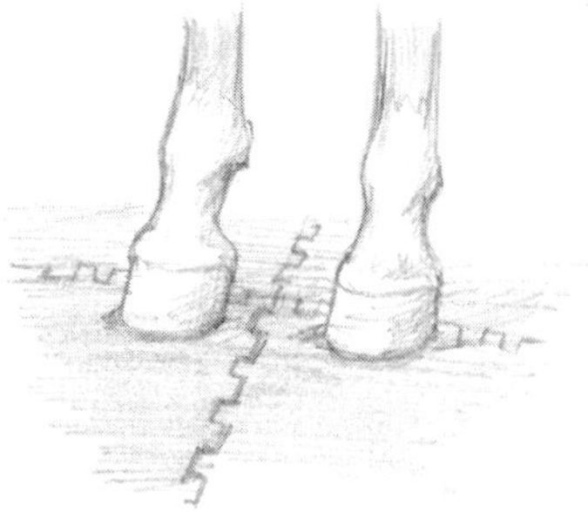

Good stall flooring

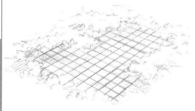

Grids are suitable for outdoor application in high-traffic areas.

Stall Flooring

The stall flooring is the layer added on top of the prepared site. Be sure to consider the type of bedding you plan to use, as some flooring/bedding combinations are undesirable.

TAMPED CLAY. For box stalls, the tamped clay floor has been a traditional favorite because it provides cushion and good traction and is warm and quiet. Tamped clay does not drain well, however, so clay stalls must be sloped to allow drainage. In addition, urine pools can create large potholes, requiring the clay floor to be leveled routinely and overhauled annually.

MIXTURES. Mixtures of clay and sand or clay and crushed rock are usually readily available and have improved drainage over pure clay, while retaining most of the desirable features of the clay floor. Road base is often such a mixture — a blend of crushed limestone and clay. While a road base blend may result in better sanitation, however, it can be more unstable under a horse's movement so can become mixed in with the bedding, be ingested with the feed, and turn into a pawing horse's delight.

CONCRETE. Although it makes a low-maintenance, permanent floor that is fairly easy to sanitize, concrete requires very deep bedding because it can be hard, cold, and abrasive. A pawing barefoot horse can severely damage his hooves on a concrete floor. Concrete floors must be designed with a drain or a slope and should have a textured surface to ensure good traction.

"RUBBER" STALL MATS. Usually a combination of rubber, clay, nylon, and rayon, these mats act as an intermediary between the soil and the bedding. They have superior cushioning, so they are comfortable, can be easily sanitized, make stall cleaning easy, decrease dust so horses stay cleaner, and decrease the amount of bedding required by up to 50 percent. They also prevent a pawing horse from digging holes in the stall. Stall mats are initially expensive, however, and if they are not properly texturized, they can be slippery.

STALL MATTRESSES. A stall mattress system consists of two parts: a mattress and a cover. The mattress is a thick rubber-filled cushion. The cover is a Latex or rubber sheet fastened to the sides of the stall. Plenty of absorbent bedding must be used to soak up urine.

INTERLOCKING PLASTIC STALL GRIDS. The large holes and spaces in the grids are filled with sand or road base, providing a tough floor with good drainage. If properly installed, such a floor is impervious to a pawing horse; however, the sand may be ingested along with the feed.

WOOD. An old-time favorite for tie stalls, wood is really not appropriate for box stalls. Although it is warmer than concrete and fairly durable if treated, it can be slippery, is difficult to sanitize and deodorize, and can be noisy under a nervous horse.

EXERCISE FOR HEALTHY HOOVES

Exercise is essential for maintaining overall health and for the development of dense, tough hooves. All horses of all ages need exercise every day — either a ride or a minimum of two hours of turnout in a large pen or pasture. The many benefits of exercise include assistance in the development and repair of tissue. It can improve the quality and strength of bones, tendons, ligaments, and hooves. Regular, moderate stress creates dense, stress-resistant bones and hooves. Exercise also conditions and stretches muscles and tendons, resulting in less chance of injury and lameness.

Exercise Options

- ★ Riding
- ★ Turnout
- ★ Ponying
- ★ Longeing and long lining
- ★ Electric horse walker
- ★ Treadmill
- ★ Swimming

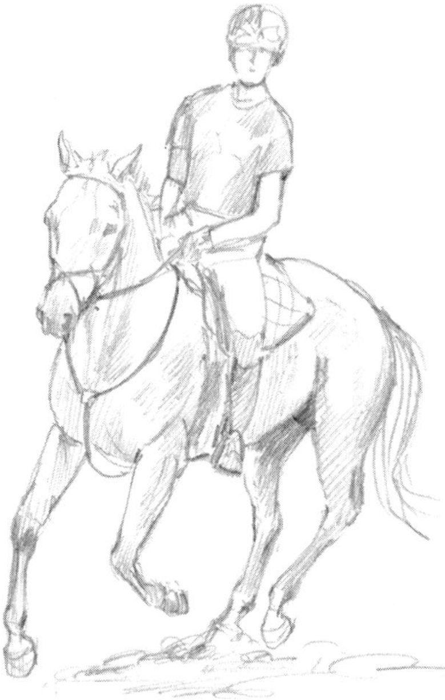

Riding is an ideal way to provide and get exercise.

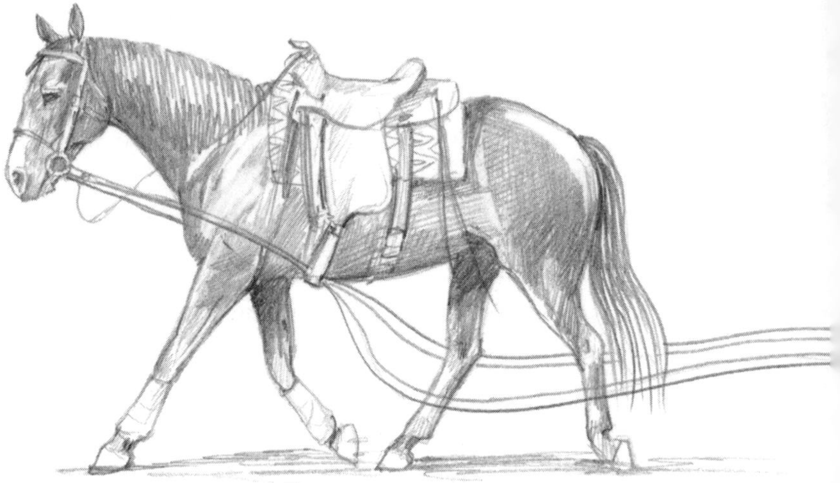

Ground driving is another great training and exercise tool.

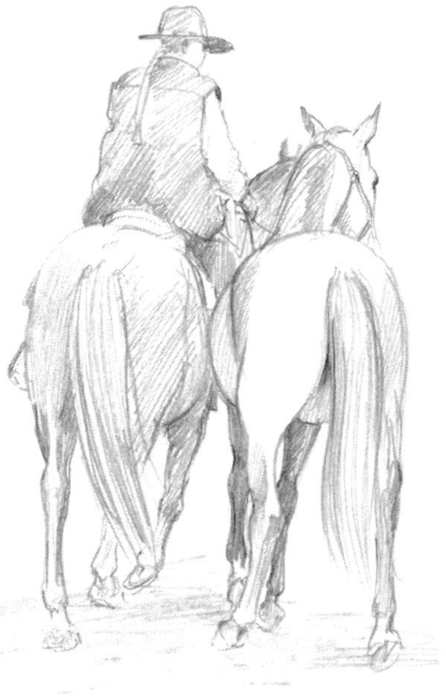

Ponying is an excellent way to exercise two horses.

It is important that any exercise area be safely fenced and free from hazardous objects. Footing should not be excessively deep. Hyperextension of the fetlock in deep sand can do permanent damage to tendons. Rocky footing can encourage the development of dense, tough hooves but can also cause hoof damage, especially if the horse's hooves are weak and vulnerable when he is first turned out in a rocky pasture. (See June Training Pen for more details.)

DAILY HOOF INSPECTION

Your routine examination (which can occur at each feeding) should include noting your horse's overall stance and attitude, the condition of his legs, how he moves, and clues in his living area. If you notice a discrepancy in his legs or hooves, halter your horse and bring him to an area where you can give him a thorough visual check, clean his hooves, and palpate his legs. So that you have a baseline for comparison in relation to texture, temperature, and sensitivity of your horse's legs and hooves, be sure to carry out a preliminary examination when everything appears normal.

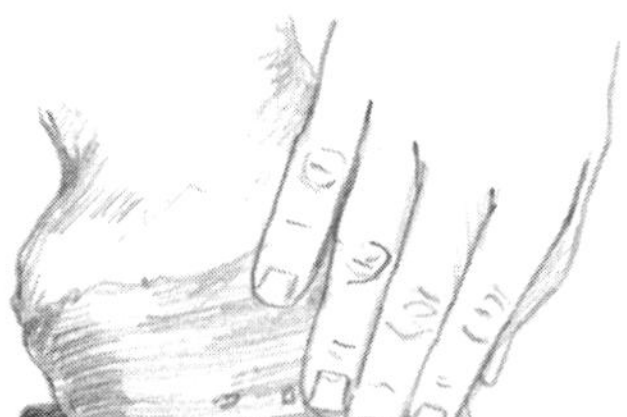

Feel the hoof for loose or rough clinches.

How to Examine Hooves

1. Notice which leg he is resting.

2. Notice if his front legs are both ahead of or behind their normal (vertical) configuration.

3. Notice if his hind legs are ahead of or behind their normal configuration.

4. Notice if he is reluctant to walk to the examination area.

5. Wipe any mud or manure off the hoof wall and coronet.

6. Pick out all of his hooves.

7. Note any sensitivity in the clefts of frog (including the central cleft) when using a hoof pick to clean them.

8. Look for embedded rocks, splinters, nails, or other objects in any part of the hoof, including the coronet.

9. Test each branch of the shoe to see if it is loose.

10. Sight down the bottom surface of the shoe to see if it is still flat. Sometimes the heel of a shoe will be stepped on and bent down and go unnoticed because it is still tight.

11. Note if the shoe has slipped or twisted off to one side.

12. Note if the shoe has slipped backward. (Be careful not to confuse this with a shoe that has purposely been set back by your farrier.)

13. Check the clinches to see they are tight or if they have opened up and started to pull through the hoof.

14. Look for signs of injury on the coronary band, bulbs, or lower leg.

CLEANING A HOOF

Here's how I clean a hoof. First I use the side of the hoof pick to scrape mud off the outside of the hoof wall. A stiff brush will further clean the hoof wall and make it less messy for you or your farrier to handle. Then I pick up the foot. I hold the hoof pick with the blade facing away from me. I remove the debris from the sole and the clefts of the frog (the V-shaped rubbery cushion located between the heels on the bottom of the hoof). Then I turn the pick toward me and clean around the inside edge of the shoe if the horse is shod. I remove any remaining debris from the frog.

There is a great variety in hoof picks. Choose one that is comfortable in your hand so you will use it often!

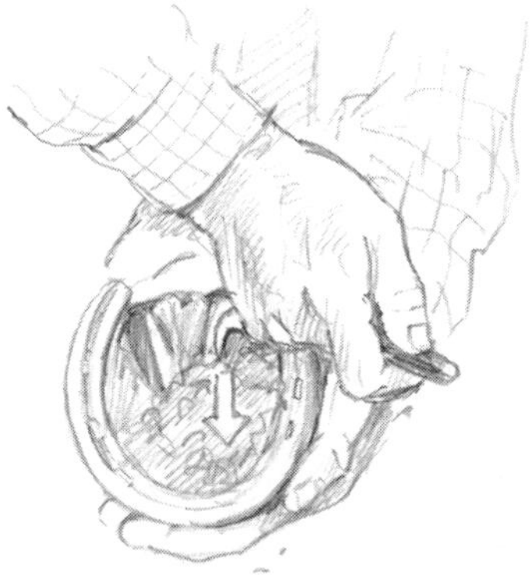

Clean hooves daily.

Cold Weather Feeding Rules

- ★ Increase roughage by 10 percent for every 10°F below freezing.
- ★ Make sure there is free-choice open water to drink. Provide water using tank heaters or automatic waterers, or break the ice in creeks, ponds, or troughs. Do not expect your horse to get his needed moisture from snow.

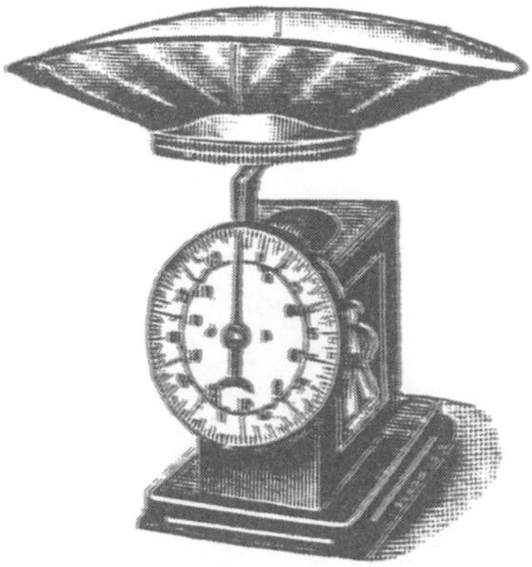

FEEDING FOR HEALTHY HOOVES

Feeding horses can be a complex topic. The following nutrition guidelines relate specifically to hoof health. In short, supply required nutrients and do not overfeed, which can lead to laminitis, a debilitating condition of the hooves.

- **Know each horse's feed requirements.** Commercial feeds or hays may not provide all a horse needs. Several important nutrients, such as biotin and methionine, that are necessary for high-quality hooves are often deficient in horses' rations.
- **Know exactly what you are feeding.** Read and understand the feed tags of commercially prepared feed. If you buy large batches of hay, have it tested for its nutrient content.
- **Monitor your horse's weight** routinely to determine the amount of feed required, to prevent obesity, and to minimize the chance of laminitis. A hundred extra pounds of body weight plus 200 pounds of tack and rider can be very harmful to your horse's feet and limbs.
- **Know exactly how much** you are feeding. Weigh feed to prevent obesity.
- **Feed grain only if a horse requires it:** young, growing horses, horses in hard work, and lactating broodmares are in this category.
- **When turning a horse out to pasture** for the first time, be sure the horse has had a full feed of hay. Limit grazing to one half hour for the first two days. Then one half hour twice a day for two days, then one hour twice a day, and so on.

  Monitor horses that are on pasture; they can quickly become overweight or suffer laminitis.

- **Be sure it is impossible** for a horse to get into the feed room. Horses do not know when to stop eating and can literally "eat themselves to death." An excess amount of grain can cause colic or laminitis.
- **Do not feed a horse immediately** after hard work and do not work a horse until at least one hour after a full feeding. The horse is a digestively sensitive creature and requires consideration in work requirements surrounding meals.
- **Feed the highest-quality hay** you can find.
- **Provide free-choice salt,** minerals, and water.
- After formulating the hay and grain portion of your horse's ration, **choose a hoof supplement** that provides any missing nutrients. Frequently hooves (and hair coat) benefit from the addition of DL-methionine, lysine, calcium, biotin, and other substances to the ration.

He doth **nothing but talk of his horse.**

— William Shakespeare, *The Merchant of Venice*

PASTURE PERFECT

SNOW RULE FOR TURNOUT

As long as there is at least a 4-inch snow cover on the pastures, the horses can be turned out to enjoy free exercise and a good roll. If the weather is mild, we often feed the pasture horses on the snow, which is a great, clean place to lay out the hay rations.

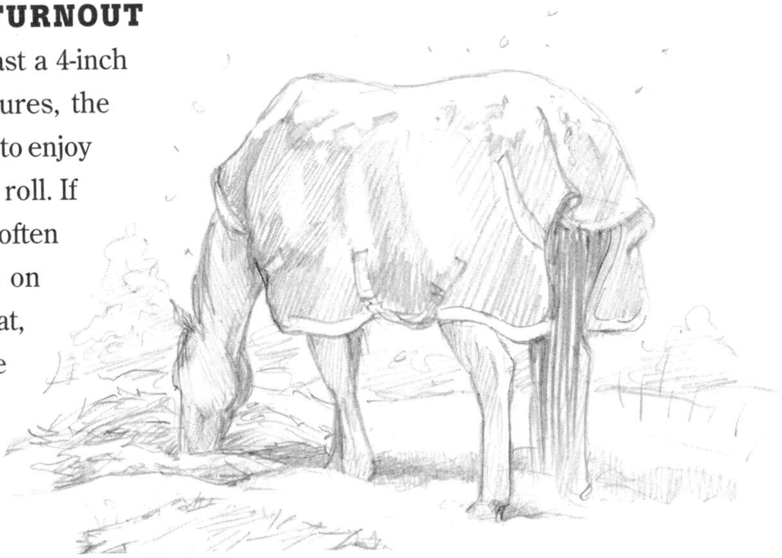

WINTER: *DECEMBER*

Pest Patrol

Killer Bees

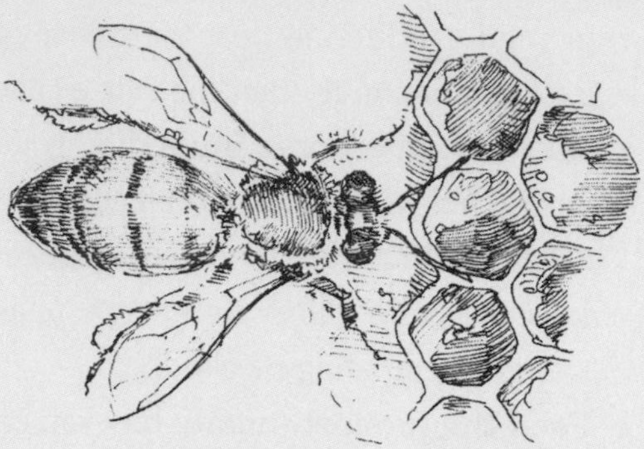

Killer bees, or Africanized honeybees (AHB), are a cross between Brazilian honeybees and aggressive African bees. Decades ago, the African bees were imported to Brazil for laboratory work. Some escaped, crossbreeding with native bees. They began moving north at a rate of about 200 miles per year. They entered Texas in 1990 and have spread through Nevada, Arizona, New Mexico, California, and other parts of the southeast United States.

They are very defensive and aggressive. If a hive is disturbed, a person or animal can be stung up to 100 times. Although their venom isn't any more potent than that of regular honeybees, they can cause serious injury or death because they attack in great numbers and pursue victims for great distances. Once disturbed, a colony can remain agitated for 24 hours, attacking people and animals within a quarter mile of the hive for no reason. In South America, there have been more than 1,000 fatalities; fewer than 10 deaths have occurred in the United States so far.

Be alert for the sight of bees coming into and out of an opening, such as a crack in a tree, cactus, or wall; a hole in the ground; or a vacant building. Check the box opposite for some tips.

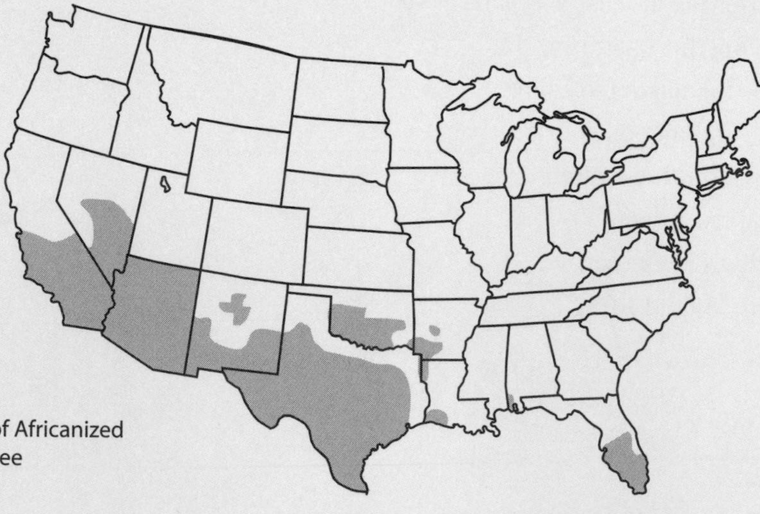

Range of Africanized Honeybee

WILD LIFE

OUR CHRISTMAS EAGLE

A few feet from our kitchen sink window is a huge, flat granite rock where we put extra treats for our cats — if they can beat the magpies to them! One day Richard and I were skinning and sectioning a huge turkey that I was going to use for a Christmas curry. As you may know, a raw turkey yields a huge bowl of fat and skin, so halfway through our task, I took the first of the orts out to the feeding rock.

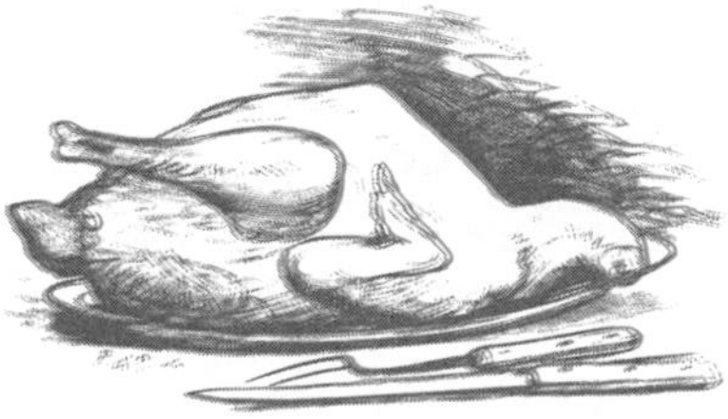

Bee Safe

When working on your farm or ranch or riding your horse:

- ★ Listen for the sound of bee activity.
- ★ Wear light-colored clothing. Bees tend to attack dark things. Dark clothing, dark hair, or anything dark in color could draw the animus of the AHB.
- ★ Bees are sensitive to odors, both pleasant and unpleasant. The smell of newly cut grass has been shown to disturb honeybees. Avoid wearing floral or citrus aftershaves or perfume.

If you come upon bees when riding, whether killer bees or not, depending on the situation, it might be best to quickly escape. If you can control your horse at a gallop, that would be the best plan. If think your horse might panic, however, you could consider dismounting and leading him quickly but calmly away from the area. If possible, put a bandana over your face and a shirt over your horse's head as you escape, because bees usually go for the head on both humans and animals.

When you are away from the threat, examine yourself and your horse. Removing the stingers soon after attack will lessen the amount of venom entering the body. Scrape the stingers off the skin with a blunt instrument or credit card. Don't remove bee stingers with your fingers or tweezers, because the pinching action forces more toxin into your body or your horse's.

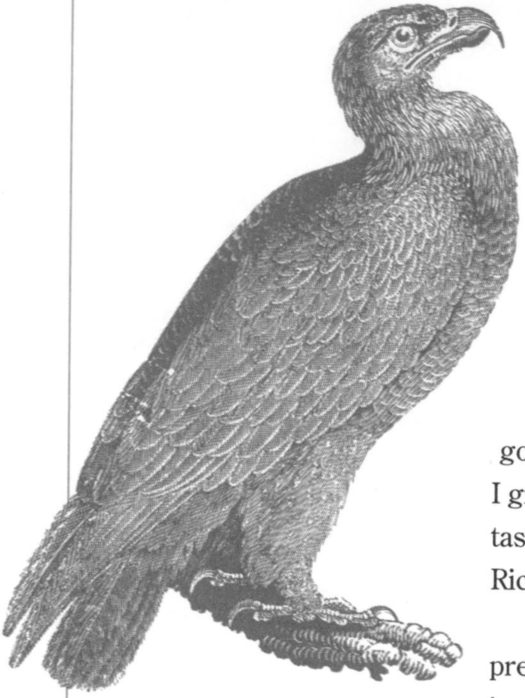

It was less than a minute before the "mountain penguins," as we call the magpies, showed up to feast. They would stand on a piece of skin with one foot and tear into it with their heavy black bills. We stood next to each other working and intermittently looking up to glance out the window and watch the penguins get a good meal.

Once, when I was looking up and Richard was looking down, I saw a huge shadow pass over the rock. Before I could speak, it materialized into an enormous golden eagle who landed there — just a few feet from us. I grabbed a breath, and to be sure my pal also saw this fantastic site, without moving, I whispered intently, "Richard, Richard. Look, look."

I had seen live eagles in raptor exhibits, but nothing prepared me for this wild eagle, so big, so close, so amazingly powerful. In a few seconds, he gulped what would have been a week's meal for a family of magpies. And then he was gone.

We both said "Wow" about ten times, and before we could form any more coherent words, he graced us with another landing! This time he stayed much longer, allowing us to admire his wonderful leg feathers that went all the way down to his toes, his strong talons, and powerful hooked bill. He was truly majestic and a special Christmas present indeed. (See more about eagles in April Wild Life.)

I will not change my horse
with any that treads but on four pasterns.
When I bestride him, I soar, I am a hawk: he
trots the air; the earth sings
when he touches it.

— William Shakespeare, *Henry V*

SANITATION FOR BETTER HOOF HEALTH

Sanitation practices are essential for your horse's hoof health. Urine breaks down into products that contain ammonia, with a pungent vapor that is injurious to the eyes and lungs. The combination of dung and urine is a perfect medium for the proliferation of bacteria, which can begin destructive processes on hoof horn. When certain fecal bacteria ferment, their secretions can dissolve the intertubular "hoof cement." Moist manure softens, loosens, and encourages the breakdown of hoof horn cells.

MOISTURE CONTROL. By now you know that making a horse stand in mud is often the worst thing you can do — and that hoof dressing should not be indiscriminately slathered on your horse's hooves to "moisturize" them. Since the modern riding horse evolved on semiarid plains, the healthy hoof is designed to be dry and hard. Your role as manager of your horse in confinement is to provide an environment that allows the hoof to be dry, hard, and healthy.

The effects of repeated wet/dry conditions can be devastating to hooves. Hoof conditions worsen during hot, humid weather, especially when horses are turned out at night in dew-laden pastures and then are either left out where the sun will dry the hooves or put in a stall where the bedding dries the hooves. Horses that receive daily baths or rinses or those that repeatedly walk through mud and then stand in the sun experience a similar decay in hoof quality. In both cases, the hoof is going through a stressful moisture expansion and contraction cycle, which is damaging to the hoof structures. In the process of drying out, the hoof develops cracks, and the cracks are packed with mud so they continue getting larger and spreading. In addition, the

A Healthy Balance

If your horse is getting adequate exercise and the footing of his stall, pen, or pasture is well drained, the moisture balance between the inner and outer layers of his hooves probably remains at a relatively constant, healthy level. If your horse stands inactive for long periods of time, however, sufficient moisture may not be delivered via the blood to the hoof, and his hoof walls may tend to contract.

On the other hand, if his hooves contain too much moisture from water, mud, frequent baths, or excessive hoof dressing, they become soft, the hoof spreads, and the layers separate.

Six-Step Hoof Plan

Follow these guidelines to maintain your horse's hooves at an optimal, constant moisture level:

1. Keep stalls dry.
2. Provide turnout areas that are not muddy.
3. Minimize bathing.
4. Minimize wet/dry episodes, such as hosing legs and then putting the horse in a stall with dry sawdust bedding.
5. Use hoof dressing discriminately.
6. Use a hoof sealer when appropriate, such as during the wet seasons, if the horse must be bathed frequently, if the hooves show signs of surface cracks, or if your farrier has rasped the wall of the hoof to shape it during trimming.

cellular cement that holds the hoof horn together breaks down. The result is a frayed, pulpy mass of fibrous tubules. Drying mud and water also leach out essential nutrients and oils that are responsible for maintaining hoof flexibility.

(See July Foot Notes for information on hoof dressings and sealers.)

HOOF-HEALTHY BEDDING. Bedding should be easy to handle, absorbent, and comfortable. The bedding with the highest water-absorbing capacity, however, is not necessarily best. Extremely absorbent bedding sops up too much urine and if the bedding is not changed frequently, the horse's hooves will be subjected to constant wetness. On the other hand, a bedding with very little absorbency lets too much moisture pass through to the flooring and can result in pooling. The ideal bedding in most cases has a moderate absorbency and is free from dust, mold, and injurious substances. (See October Clean-up Crew for more on bedding.)

DECEMBER
Manure Pile Maintenance

PILE A
Sell, store, or spread.

PILE B
Turn once, water as needed.

PILE C
Turn twice, water as needed.

BEAUTY SHOP

WINTER CLIP

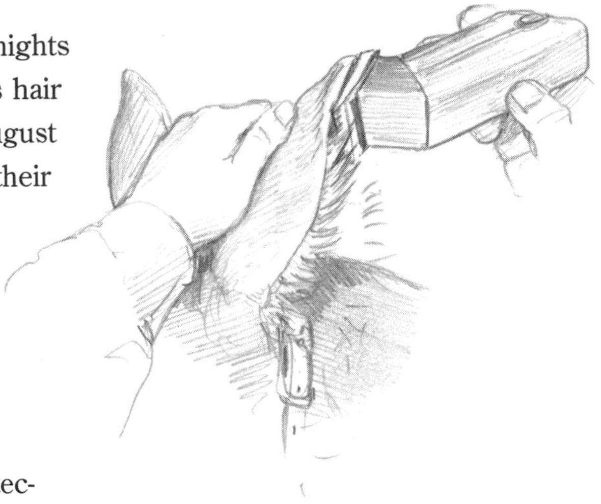

If you need to tidy up your horse's ears for the winter, just clip them flush and maybe tweak the outline.

The shorter days and longer, cooler nights of fall trigger a change in your horse's hair growth. In temperate climates, in August or September, horses begin shedding their short summer hair and replacing it with longer winter hair. The fluffy coat characteristic of horses turned out in the northern states and Canada is usually completely grown in by November. For these horses, the natural coat is an ideal form of protection, as the long hair traps a layer of warm air next to the body, which acts as insulation. During cold temperatures, piloerector muscles make the hair stand up, which increases the coat's insulating potential.

However, long winter hair can create difficulties for you if you intend to ride your horse actively during the winter. If you do plan to keep your horse in work throughout the winter, you should consider one of the following: blanketing, clipping, or a combination of clipping and blanketing.

BLANKETING. To minimize the density of the winter coat your horse grows in the fall, you can begin blanketing him in August and using lights (see November Reproduction Roundup) so that his body receives the signal that only short to medium hairs are required to replace the summer coat. Of course, once you begin blanketing, you will need to continue blanketing your horse all winter.

BODY CLIP. In areas with moderate to severe winters where horses grow a substantial winter coat, you may need

> **Ear Clip**
>
> Certain places on a horse's body have extra hair for a reason. The ears, for example, grow extra hair both inside and outside in the fall to keep them warm during the winter.

Horse Sense and Safety

Don't Wrap that Rope

Never wrap a rope or strap around your hand, arm, or other part of your body. If a horse spooks suddenly and bolts, you may be unable to free yourself from him and could be hurt badly.

TIPS & TECHNIQUES

Clipper Blades

For most body work, heavy-duty clippers with a wide head work best. Small clippers are necessary for the legs, head, and tight areas such as the elbows. The clippers for the body work should be outfitted with #10 or #15 blades, which cut hair to about a quarter inch. Never use a surgical blade (#30 or #40) for a body clip, as it would remove the hair right down to the skin.

to use a type of body clip to minimize grooming and cooling-out time. If you choose a conservative clip and your winter is mild, you may be able to turn out a clipped horse without blanketing him. In most wintry states, however, it is necessary to blanket a clipped horse.

Body clipping will allow you to work your horse vigorously during the winter. Clipped horses sweat less, and what sweat there is will be able to dry more quickly. The clipped horse can be cooled out much more effectively and safely than the unclipped horse. Also, the clipped horse is tidy in appearance and relatively easy to keep clean, an important factor in the nonbath months.

Body clipping won't appreciably improve the appearance of an unhealthy horse — such a horse will just have a bad short coat instead of a bad long coat. But the healthy horse in active work can benefit greatly from a winter clip.

CLIPPER TIPS. Before you bring your horse in the barn for his clip, be sure your clippers are in working order and that you have several sets of sharp blades on hand.

In very general terms, there are two types of clippers: heavy-duty and light-duty. The heavy-duty clippers are suitable for body and leg clipping. They are designed to be used for extended periods of time because they cool while they are being used. Light-duty clippers are suitable for small jobs, such as trimming the muzzle, throat, ears, and bridle path, and perhaps a touch up on the legs. If you use light-duty clippers for removing heavy winter hair, not only will the blades quickly become dull, but the motor may overheat and burn out as well.

Up rose the wild old winter-king
And shook his beard of snow.
— Charles Godfrey Leland

Types of Clips

There are three basic types of body clips, each with many variations and styles: the full clip, the hunter clip, and the trace clip. **The full body clip** consists of shortening the hair on the entire horse, including the head and legs. Immediately after a full body clip, most horses, especially bays and chestnuts, appear to be a lighter color.

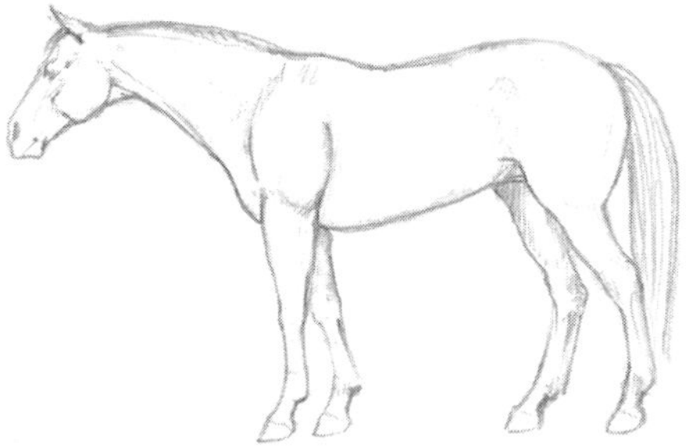

Full body clip

The (field) hunter clip. This is essentially a full body clip, except that long hair is left on the legs and saddle area. For protection when working in snowy fields, the winter hair remains on the legs from the elbows and stifles down to the coronary bands. In addition, a patch the shape of the saddle pad is also left so that the horse's back is less prone to chill after work.

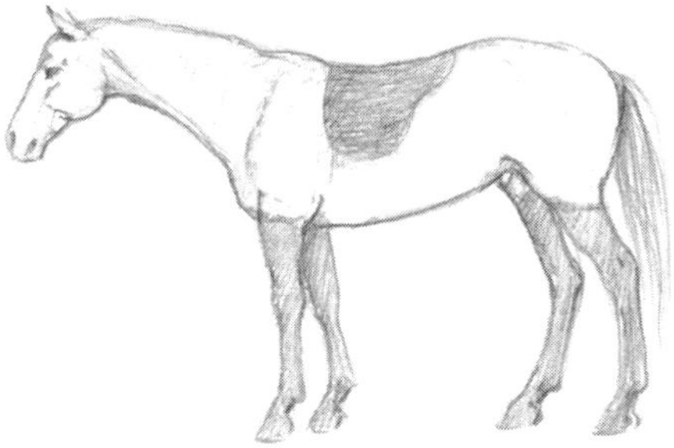

Hunter clip

The trace clip. This was originally designed for harness horses that worked in the winter. The hair is clipped in the areas where a horse sweats: the throat, chest floor, belly, inner thighs, and under the tail. A conservative trace clip may involve removing a strip of hair 8 to 10 inches wide from the throat under the belly to the anus. The basic trace clip can be embellished with sharp geometric designs and circles so it fits the needs of a more aggressive exercise program.

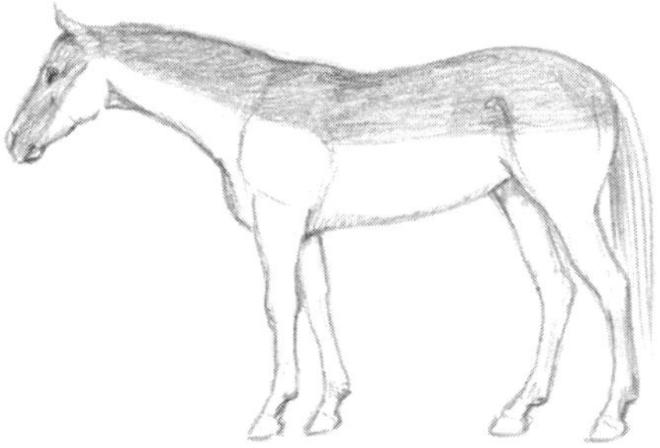

Trace clip

Clipping Procedure

- ★ Begin clipping on the shoulder or the barrel with the large-headed clippers. To get a consistent clip, hold the clippers with the blades flat against the horse's body for the entire session.
- ★ Aim the clipper head directly against the hair growth. You will probably be surprised at how many times the hair growth changes direction on the horse's body.
- ★ Using short strokes rather than long strokes results in fewer "tracks," or residual clipper lines.
- ★ As you clip, keep the blades clean and cool. With the clippers running, dip just the tips of the clipper teeth into a commercially prepared blade wash or kerosene. This will cut any oily or dirty residue that has built up on the blades. With the blades pointed toward the floor, shake the excess fluid off the blades before tipping them upright to resume.
- ★ If you notice that the sound of the motor changes, it may be that the blades need to be lubricated. Refer to your owner's manual. Some models require oiling. Others recommend a spray lubricant be used directly on the blades. The lubricant cools the blades and removes small dirt particles, thereby further reducing friction.
- ★ Keep the air intake screen clear of hair, or the motor will not cool properly. If the clippers overheat, you must stop using them until they cool. Hot clippers not only can hurt your horse, but the motor can also burn up irreparably.
- ★ Once you finish clipping the fleshy body parts such as the shoulders, chest, barrel, belly, and thighs, use small clippers on the extremities such as the legs and head.
- ★ When you are finished, thoroughly clean your clippers before putting them away. Leaving hair, sweat, and scurf on the blades can result in rusted blades that will not clip well the next time you want to use them.
- ★ Finally, curry your horse vigorously, vacuum him, and rub some oil or conditioner into his coat. Groom the clipped horse daily to restore the oil and shine to his coat.

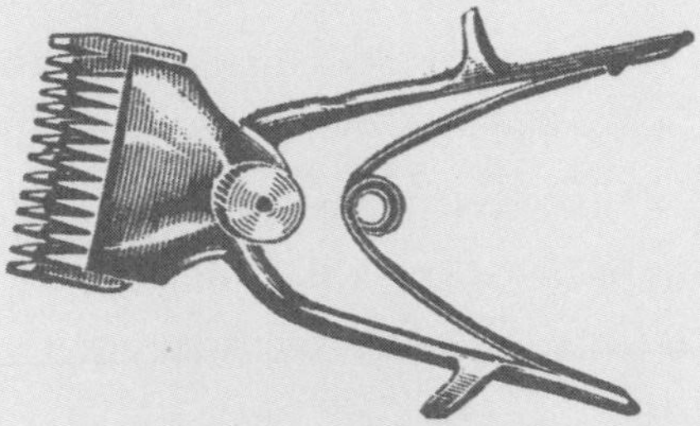

Body Clipping Basics

Here are some tips for the first time you clip a horse.

Take the time to outline a plan. Mentally go through each step of the procedure to be sure you will have everything on hand that you need. Budget enough time for the job. Figure about two to three hours to clip a horse.

Approach the task with patience. If you get frazzled or hurried, your clip will show it. If it is your first time doing a body clip, ask a knowledgeable friend to coach you through the tough spots.

Everyone stay calm. A calm, experienced horse will make your first clipping job easier. *If* you must clip a young or nervous horse, ask your veterinarian to recommend an appropriate tranquilizer.

Cleanliness is a virtue. Be sure the horse is very clean before you begin clipping. Dirt can dull clipper blades very quickly. If bathing is possible, wash the horse the day before clipping and let him dry unblanketed. If it is too cold for bathing, thoroughly groom the horse using a rubber curry and vacuum so that the clean hair stands out from the body when you are finished.

TIPS & TECHNIQUES

Clear the Deck

Braid the mane and wrap the tail to keep them out of the way while you are clipping.

Tack Room

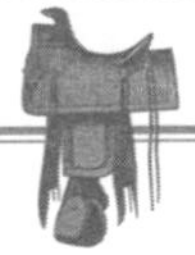

Leather-Cleaning Tools

Having the right tools and products on hand for cleaning leather will help you do a good job. Here's what I use:

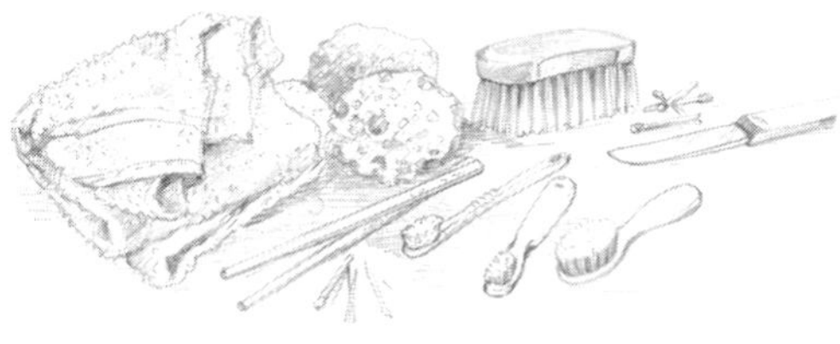

- ★ Warm water, Turkish towels, and sponges
- ★ Special leather cleaning products that don't strip oils or clog pores
- ★ Soft bristled brushes, including an old toothbrush, for lifting dirt out of tooled leather
- ★ A dull knife, wooden chopsticks, and wooden matches for removing those stubborn little "jockeys" (the dark, crusty buildup of sweat and dirt on the underside of leather)

(See more about leather care in January Tack Room.)

WINTER: *DECEMBER*

CLOTHES HORSE

Cleaning Velcro

To clean the hook surface of Velcro, you can run a large darning needle between the rows of hooks. This loosens and lifts the debris in a pad, which you can then remove with your fingers. Use a toothbrush to brush out the last bits, and make a loop of duct tape to pick up the final stragglers.

PROTECTING VELCRO

Hook-and-loop fasteners, commonly known as Velcro, are on all sorts of horse tack, from blankets to shipping boots to exercise boots. Velcro has a hook portion and a loop portion. The loop portion usually stays fairly clean, but the hook portion is a magnet for horse hair, thread, hay, lint, and other debris, which clogs the hooks and keeps them from gripping. To keep Velcro aggressive, fasten it when it is in use, when it is not in use, and when it is being laundered. However, if blankets and boots are fastened when they are put in the washer, they may not get thoroughly clean. As a remedy, I purchase some extra loop portion at my local sporting goods store, where it is sold in various widths by the yard. I cut it into the lengths I need to protect the hook portions in the washing machine.

FARM OFFICE

TIPS & TECHNIQUES

Legalities

If you are thinking of taking in boarders, be sure to read about legal issues for horse owners (see Recommended Reading) and look through the horse motel guides.

BOARDING

Boarding requires labor, patience, and a love of not only horses, but also dealing with people. Although inconsiderate owners are often part of the bargain, there are many wonderful people who appreciate a fine level of personal service.

Demand will vary greatly from region to region. You will need to spend money on facilities and advertising, and then wait until your reputation builds. And you will need to have boarding contracts, waivers, and other forms drawn up by an attorney specializing in equine law in your state.

TRAINING PEN

APPROACHING

When I approach a horse to catch him, I do not walk right at his head, which could cause him to turn and move away from me. And I do not approach him directly from the rear in one of his blind spots, because I could surprise him and make him spook or even kick. Instead, I gaze indirectly at his neck and shoulder area, and as I approach I speak to him: "Hey, boy, how are you doing?" And when I get close enough to touch him, instead of touching him on the face, I touch his neck or withers, a place a horse likes to be touched, before I halter him.

CATCHING TACTICS

Nothing can be so frustrating as a horse that refuses to be caught, and few things can be as dangerous as turning loose a horse that jerks away prematurely, often wheeling and kicking as it gallops off. The horse that keeps just enough distance between him and the approaching trainer and the horse that pulls away when being turned out have one thing in common — disrespect of the trainer and the equipment. As with most training situations, it is best to prevent such habits with regular sessions for young horses, in this case, catching, haltering, and unhaltering. Leaving a halter on a horse is dangerous and sidesteps the important lesson of haltering and unhaltering.

Once a horse has successfully avoided being caught several times, whatever the initial reason was, he may continue the behavior merely out of habit. There may no longer be an unpleasant condition to blame for the action, but the horse still shuns the handler. In other cases, avoiding the trainer may just be an enjoyable game of tag.

The Horse's Point of View

Horses are generally difficult to catch because of fear, resentment, or habit. Unhandled horses move away from the unfamiliar sight, sound, and smell of the trainer. Other horses may evade the handler because they resent the treatment they get after they are caught: excessively hard work, ill-fitting gear, painful doctoring, or tactless training.

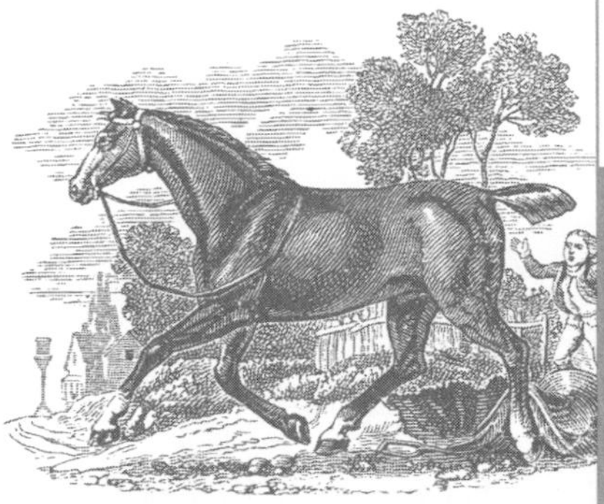

> **Movie of the Month**
>
> ***THE LORD OF THE RINGS* (2001)**
>
> This magical trilogy is full of gripping horse scenes, from the squalling, frothing, roughshod black mounts handled cruelly by the Ringwraiths to the glowing spirit of Shadowfax, the Lord of All Horses, ridden bridleless by Gandalf. Look for the sensitivity of Strider's horse Brego; the great lead changes and jumping of Arwen's grey horse Asfaloth; and the Elvin spell that creates a thundering herd of water horses to defeat the Nazgul.

THE WALK-DOWN METHOD. Whatever the reason, and whether developing good manners in a young horse or retraining a problem horse, few methods produce such long-lasting results as the "walk-down method." Because it is based on persistence, it may be time consuming at first, but it is worth the investment. Begin the lessons in a small enclosure and gradually increase the size of the area.

When approaching the horse, don't be threatening in body language. Always walk toward the horse's shoulder, never his rump or his head. Move at a smooth, slow walk. Don't look directly at the horse, but keep him in your peripheral vision. When the horse stands and allows you to approach, scratch him on the withers and then walk away. Always be the first to turn and leave. Don't catch and halter the horse each time he lets you touch him. Soon it will take just a few seconds for the horse to decide to stand still.

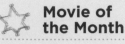

When approaching a horse, don't be threatening in body language.

CORNERING THE HORSE. If a horse must be caught more quickly, he could be run into a chute or cornered by two or three experienced people. The natural tendency of a

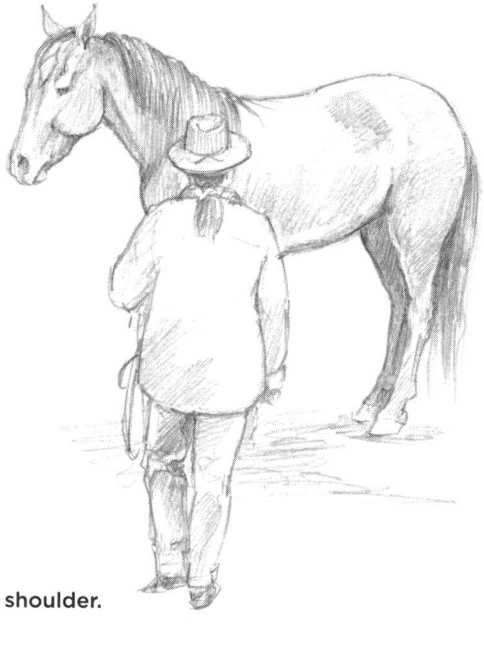

Whenever possible, approach a horse at his shoulder.

cornered horse is to turn his hindquarters toward danger. If a horse is unsure of humans, he will behave this way as a defensive measure. The object of whip-breaking a horse is to make him face the trainer. Using a whip on a horse's hocks or rump will often cause him to turn around. But a whip in the hands of the wrong person can cause a horse to jump out of the enclosure, trample the trainer, kick, or strike. Whip-breaking should be attempted only by an experienced trainer.

Because it is unsafe to go past a horse's rump to reach his head in a corner, the horse must be taught to turn around. Usually, popping the horse over the tailhead with the end of the lead rope gets his attention and he turns to see what happened. Using a reassuring voice and a scratch on the neck or withers, the trainer should let the horse know that he has behaved properly.

HALTERING. Haltering in a safe, organized fashion prevents mishaps and bad habits. Approach the horse from the near (left) side and hold the unbuckled halter and rope in

Good vs. Bad Habits

Horses can quickly develop bad habits regarding catching, haltering, and unhaltering. That's why it is necessary to follow a regular routine until good manners are established.

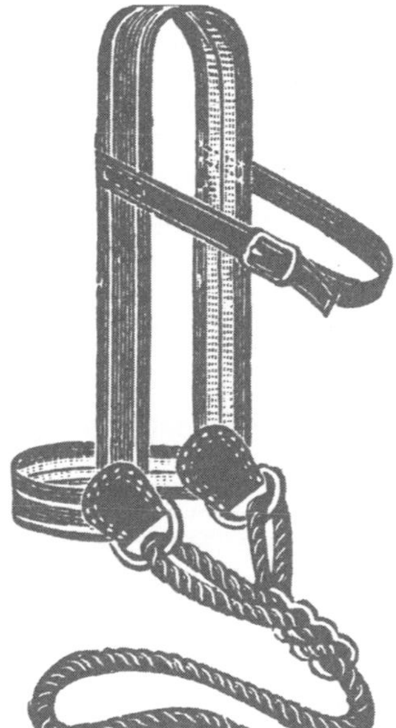

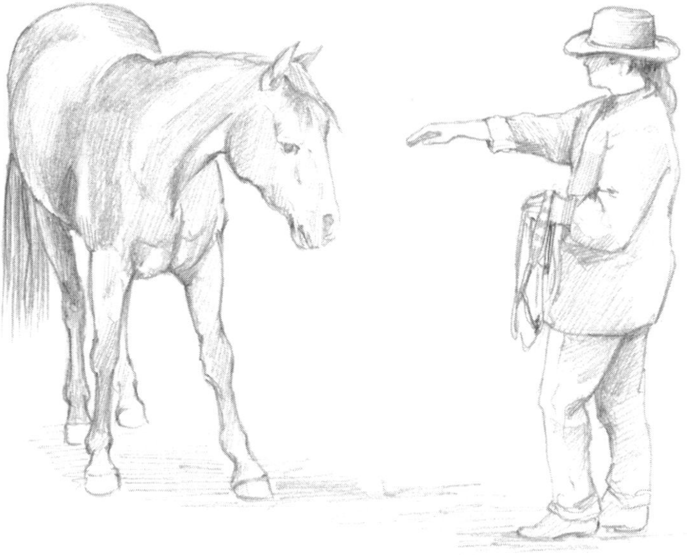

If you must approach from the front, reach out and touch his neck or shoulder, not his face.

Ranch Recipes

Braunsweiger Balls

To give a deworming pill to my cats, I cut it in fourths with a pill cutter and then hide each tiny quarter inside a ball of irresistible (to cats) braunsweiger (liverwurst or liver sausage). Over the previous few days, I prime the pump by calling the cats to a series of large tree stumps we have at our back door and tossing them blank balls.

Once they have the routine down, it is time for the loaded balls. On deworming day, they get the dosed balls and gulp each one down quickly so one of the other cats doesn't get it. With this method, I've never missed.

Haltering in a safe, organized fashion prevents mishaps and bad habits.

your left hand. With your right hand, scratch the horse on the withers and then move your right hand across the top of the neck to the right side. Pass the end of the lead rope under the horse's neck to your right hand and make a loop around the horse's throatlatch. Hold the loop with your right hand. If the horse tries to move away at this stage, you can effectively pull his head toward you while levering your right elbow into the middle of his neck.

To halter, hand the halter strap with the holes in it under the horse's neck to your right hand, which is holding the loop. With your left hand, position the noseband of the halter on the horse's face and then bring the hands together to buckle the halter.

TURNING LOOSE. Turning a horse loose follows the same procedure in reverse order. First, apply the loop around the horse's neck, and then remove the halter. Hold the horse momentarily with the loop, then release the loop and gently push the horse away with your right arm or hand. If you are dealing with a chronic bolter, try dropping a few feed wafers on the ground before you turn the horse loose. He soon will think more about inspecting the ground where he stands than about running away.

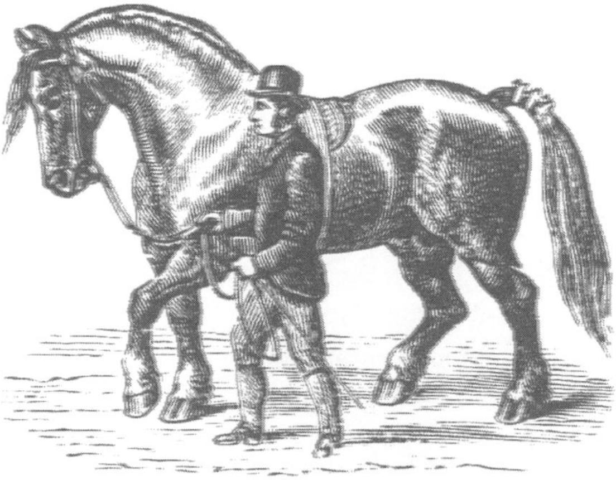

REPRODUCTION ROUNDUP

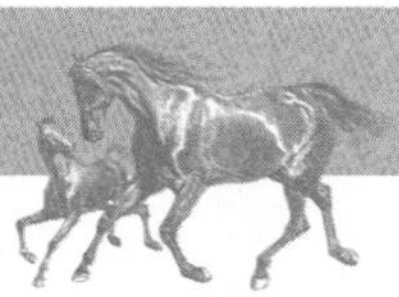

SPAYING A MARE

Although removing a mare's ovaries is not as commonly performed as gelding is, there are circumstances in which spaying a mare can be advantageous. If a mare has developed dangerous behavior as a result of hormone imbalances resulting from an ovarian tumor, removing the ovaries can redeem the mare's chance at a useful non-breeding role. Mares with granulosa tumors most often display wicked habits such as squealing, biting, kicking, and exhibiting stallionlike behavior. In 90 to 95 percent of cases, surgical removal of the tumor and/or ovaries eliminates the undesirable behavior.

Mares that have developed cresty necks and voice changes most often retain these characteristics after surgery. Less dangerous mares who have irritable, fussy, or silly periods every month may be unreliable in terms of show, race, or ranch work. If a mare is valued, but not for breeding purposes, spaying may provide the necessary alternative to produce a more solid performer.

A nonsurgical treatment for mares with undesirable estrous behavior is the administration of an oral synthetic progesterone. Progesterone is the calming female hormone responsible for maintenance of pregnancy, and its inhibiting effect on the occurrence of the estrous cycle might provide temporary help during a prospective broodmare's show or race career.

Methods of Spaying

If more permanent measures are required, the mare owner must look to surgical alteration. There are three methods of removing the ovaries: abdominal surgery, flank incision, and the vaginal approach.

en español

vamoose. Comes from *vamos,* meaning 'let's go '.

concho. Comes from *la concha,* 'a metal disk, usually of decorative silver, set on a leather rosette for decoration or for securing the saddle to the tree'.

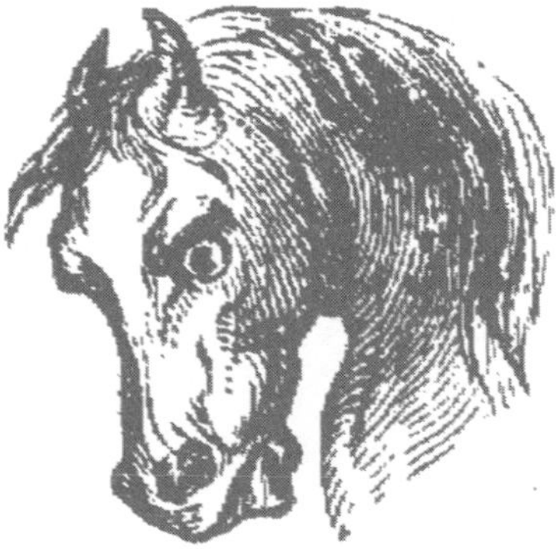

Major abdominal surgery under general anesthesia is the most expensive method and involves the longest recovery period, yet may be the only option available to horse owners in many locations. The ventral midline incision made from the umbilicus toward the udder gives the practitioner easy access to the ovaries. The surgeon has absolute hemorrhage control, which is essential when dealing with the highly vascular ovary with a tumor. Major vessels are tied. The patient usually remains in the hospital for observation for 10 to 12 days, then is restricted to box-stall or paddock confinement for an additional 30 days. It is usually 90 days from the date of surgery until the mare can return to training. As with all major abdominal surgeries, there is the risk of anesthesia and postoperative complications such as colic.

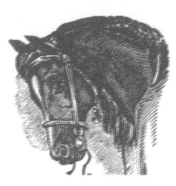

"A lovely horse is always an experience. . . . It is an emotional experience of the kind that is spoiled by words."

— Beryl Markham in *West with the Night*

Effects of Spaying

Spayed mares no longer have estrous cycles, so do not exhibit estrous behavior. Otherwise, there are no behavioral changes associated with an ovariectomy. Likewise, other than the absence of ovaries and the decrease in estrogen production, there are no physical changes. The mare's metabolism does not slow down, so she does not become an easier keeper. Spayed mares do not lose their feminine features. Your mare will look as sweet as she did before surgery. More important, she will behave more consistently.

Removing a mare's ovaries is a permanent way of altering her estrous cycle and behavior. After careful consideration of breeding potential and intended use, spaying may be the answer to one of your mare management questions.

The flank approach is usually performed with the horse standing in stocks, under the influence of a tranquilizer and local anesthetic. Often a 4-inch incision is made in each flank to allow the surgeon easier access to each ovary. Removal can be made with an emasculator, such as that used in the gelding process, or with a chain-loop ecraseur. Recovery is quicker than with abdominal surgery. Beginning with one day for observation in the hospital, the horse should spend 10 to 14 days in stall or paddock confinement and return to work 30 days from the date of surgery. Generally, the flank method has few complications but does yield minor scars.

The vaginal approach is the fastest, most inexpensive method, with a cost about a quarter that of abdominal surgery. However, the vaginal approach requires a higher level of technical expertise and may not be widely available. Mares must be free from reproductive tract infection and are routinely put on antibiotics before and after surgery. It is especially important when choosing this method to fast the mare for 24 to 36 hours prior to surgery to ensure minimal intestinal fill.

The mare is restrained in stocks, under the influence of a tranquilizer and local anesthetic. The surgeon makes entry through the vulva and a small incision is made in the vagina. The ovaries are severed from their attachments by utilizing a chain-loop ecraseur. No ligation of vessels is required and no vaginal sutures are necessary. There is little trauma or jeopardy involved in the vaginal approach. After surgery, the mare is usually kept standing in cross-ties for 24 to 48 hours, because lying down might allow protrusion of intestine through the incision. During this time she should be periodically handwalked for exercise. After three to four days in a box stall, she can be turned into a paddock for a week, and then returned to work.

LOOKING AT HORSES

Topline

The ratio of the topline's components, its curvature, the sharpness of the withers, the strength of the loin, the slope of the croup, and the length of the underline in relation to the length of back all affect a horse's movement.

A rule of thumb is that the neck should be greater than or equal to the length of the back, and that the hip should be at least two-thirds the length of the back. The neck is measured from the poll to the highest point of the withers; the back from the withers to the loin, located above the last rib and in front of the pelvis; and the hip from the loin to the point of buttock.

Be sure to look at the neck from both sides because the mane side often appears shorter than the nonmane side.

When to Spay

When to spay a mare depends somewhat on the reason for the surgery and the subsequent method of choice. Abdominal surgery would be necessary for the mare with a large ovarian tumor and could be performed at any age. It would also be appropriate for routine ovariectomy of the yearling, as the longer recovery time would not interfere with a performance schedule. From a technical standpoint, both the vaginal and flank methods are best suited for a mare of two to three years of age whose mature proportions allow the surgeon room to operate.

FINE FACILITIES

FARRIER WORK AREA

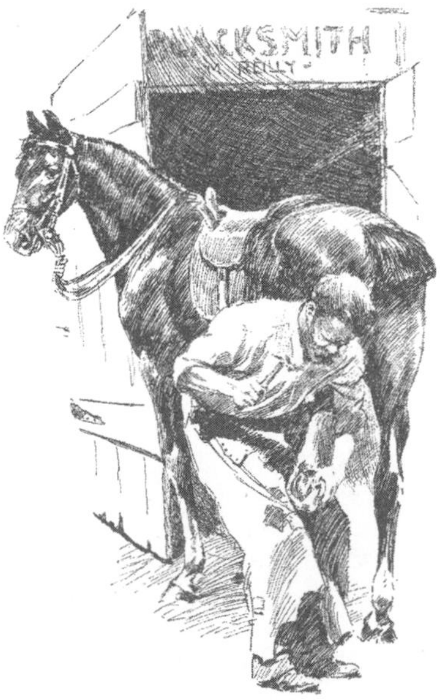

An important part of your facilities is an all-weather, level, well-lighted work area for your farrier so he can do his best work. Your farrier may have personal opinions about the type of floor he prefers or whether he likes to work in a small enclosure or a large, open area. However, certain amenities help any shoeing to proceed safely and efficiently, such as:

- The shoeing area should be well lighted, uncluttered, and level.
- The flooring can be concrete, rubber, wood, or asphalt. Tile, very smooth concrete, and some rubber mats can be slippery when wet.

Your farrier should not be expected to shoe in a driveway, in the snow, out in the middle of a pasture, in a muddy or rocky paddock, or in a dusty barn aisle. Gravel can damage a freshly trimmed hoof in a matter of seconds while the farrier is preparing the shoe. Shoeing in a barn aisle full of potholes makes it very difficult for the farrier to assess limb balance accurately, not to mention for the horse to stand squarely.

In temperate climates, there should be a well-lighted indoor shoeing area that is out of the snow and wind. During the summer and in the southern states, some farriers prefer to work in a shaded outdoor area where the breeze can keep the farrier and the horse cool. Since most farriers use electric tools for shoe preparation, the shoeing area should have access to 110-volt electrical outlets.

Snow Day

During very deep snow periods, keep horses indoors. Monitor fence lines so that pasture horses do not inadvertently step over a fence and become entangled.

Tying Options

Some farriers prefer to have horses held by an experienced horseman for shoeing. It is best if the handler stands on the opposite side from the shoer to keep the horse from moving away from him. Other farriers would rather work with the horse tied at a hitching post or in cross-ties. The tie area should be strong and safe.

When tied at a hitching post, the horse should be tied at or above the level of the withers with approximately 2 to 3 feet of rope between the halter and the post. A shorter rope prevents the horse from attaining a comfortable head position and makes it difficult for him to move freely when asked by the farrier. A longer rope often allows the horse to lower his head too much and move his body around.

The height of cross-ties will vary according to the width of the alley spanned. Very wide alleys require long cross-ties that must be mounted high; cross-ties in narrow alleys are shorter and can be mounted so that the ties aim almost horizontally at the cheekpieces of the horse's halter.

If your horses have come out of muddy lots, be sure to clean them, especially their shoulders, hindquarters, and legs, which the farrier will be contacting. Also, scrape and then wipe the mud off the hooves rather than hosing them off. Clean, dry hooves are much safer and more pleasant for the farrier to work on than slippery, wet hooves.

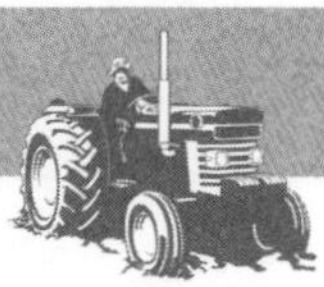

RPMS & PTOS

FRONT-END LOADERS

A front-end loader is a large bucket mounted on the front of the tractor and used for scooping up and moving quantities of material. On a horse farm, that material is most often manure, but a front-end loader can also move gravel, dirt, bedding, and even snow. If your tractor didn't come with a loader, you can add one (made by the same manufacturer or a third party) along with an auxiliary hydraulic system, as long as the loader is specifically designed to work on your tractor.

When choosing a tractor and loader to perform the tasks you plan on doing, consider breakout force (a loader's capacity to break through and lift hard-packed earth), which can range from 900 pounds to 9,000 pounds, and maximum load lift capacity, which can range from 515 pounds to 5,140 pounds.

Consider also maximum lift height, which can range from 75 inches to 169 inches clearance with the bucket in the dumped position, and the reach of the arms at maximum lift height. All of these figures will help you determine if a tractor has the power and scope to reach where necessary, such as over fences, panels, or walls, or deep into sheds.

A mid-mount loader frame, which attaches just ahead of the operator, is best, as it eliminates the need for bulky bracing at the front of the tractor. Valves and hoses mounted at the midsection instead of the rear of the tractor make hookup easier. Pay special attention to the mounting dimensions, size of the loader in relation to tractor horsepower, and operating clearance. As you shop, check to see what different-size buckets and other attachments are available that can interchange with your standard bucket.

TIPS & TECHNIQUES

The Time Factor

Other factors are bucket dump time, rollback time, dump angle, and rollback angle, all of which contribute to the time required to cycle through a repetitive task such as loading manure onto a spreader. If working rapidly is important, you might want to consider a self-leveling loader, as it will decrease spilling and allow you to keep a quick work pace.

A pipe frame trip-bucket loader, usually found on older tractors, can be raised and lowered hydraulically, but the tipping of the bucket itself is an all-or-nothing situation. With their limited control, trip buckets are notorious for either skipping over the top of your intended load, or digging in too deep and tearing up the earth underneath.

Double-action hydraulic buckets are much more versatile than trip buckets because you can control the position of the bucket with a much finer degree of movement. This allows you to sprinkle the material you are unloading rather than just dumping it in a pile, as is the case with a trip bucket. You operate the bucket with a single joystick hydraulic control that is intuitive for many novice operators. All four movements (lifting bucket, lowering bucket, tilting bucket forward, and tilting bucket backward) are performed with one hand on one lever.

If you plan to use several sizes of buckets, perhaps a large one for sawdust and a smaller, heavier one for gravel, a quick-attach option for the entire loader and/or the bucket is handy. It makes it simple to remove the bucket if

Snow Removal

If a tractor and equipment have been properly maintained all year, they will be ready to go to work when you need them for snow removal.

In order **to go fast, one must go slow.**

— Old horseman's proverb

Often the **slower you go, the faster you get there.**

— Cherry Hill

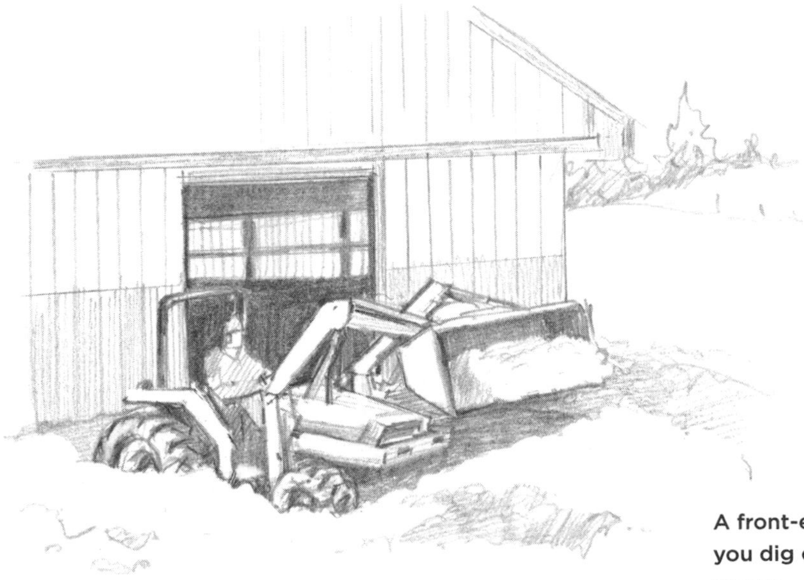

A front-end loader will help you dig out from those big snows.

> TIPS & TECHNIQUES
>
> **Loading Up**
>
> You may have to weight your tractor's tires or add ballast elsewhere (on the frame or at the rear) to properly balance your tractor for loader operation. This is important, especially if you plan to attach other implements to your loader or carry heavy material in the bucket, which positions the weight much farther ahead, out in front of your tractor.

it obscures your view and you want to remove it when not in use, or if you want to replace the bucket with another implement. Some quick-attach designs require tools and aren't as convenient as the ones that only require the flip of a handle. Some implements can be added right to the bucket using bolts or chains, including such things as a manure fork, bale spear, or pallet fork. Some loaders even offer a skid steer loader-compatible quick-attach device, which enables you to use backhoe or posthole digger attachments designed for skid steers.

A tractor with a loader should have a grill guard to protect the front of the tractor from material or items falling out of the bucket. If shopping for a used loader, look for signs of stress: bowed arms, a bent bucket, welded repair spots, worn-out pins and bushings, and leaking hydraulic cylinders.

A BLADE FOR ALL SEASONS

A blade is a moldboard with a cutting edge that is used for pulling or rearranging dirt, manure, bedding, or snow. The moldboard is curved to minimize drag and to roll dirt or snow off the blade. A blade can be rear mounted (most common), belly mounted (in the middle of the tractor) or front mounted, although a front-mounted blade is more commonly called a plow. A hydraulically operated front-mounted plow comes in handy in areas with high snowfall, especially if you have long lanes or roadways to barns and other buildings to keep clear. Most plows have adjustable skid shoes at the bottom edge to keep from digging into the road.

A blade can be used annually to level the footing in pens as well as to remove snow from driveways.

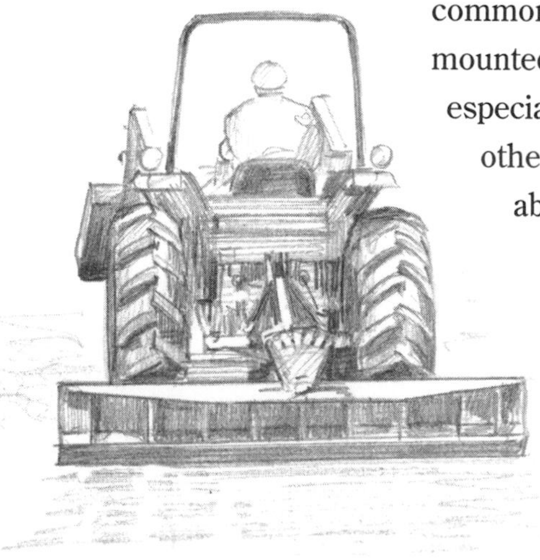

The typical horse farm blade is a 5- to 8-foot-wide, rear-mounted, three-point blade, although blades are available up to 14 feet wide. A blade can be used straight, at an angle, or swiveled completely around (by removing a pin) so that it can push backward. The three-point adjustment can keep the blade level or tilt it to one side or the other. Smaller blades have all manual adjustments; some larger blades have hydraulic adjustments. Depending on the setup, adjustment is done either manually — by a rope attachment from your seat or by getting off the vehicle and moving the blade by hand — or hydraulically from the driver's seat.

A blade is handy for scraping pens, leveling driveways, and moving light snow. For moving heavy snow, a loader or plow works better. A V-plow will enable you to make an initial path through deep snow more easily than a straight plow. Another snow removal option is a snow blower/thrower that mounts like a plow at the front of the tractor to gather snow and blow it into a specified direction as dictated by the discharge chute.

A belly blade (usually 6 to 8 feet wide) is mounted just below the operator at the midpoint of the tractor where the operator can easily see what he or she is doing. There is no need to constantly turn around (which is hard on the back) or stand up (which is unsafe) to view your work. Belly blades are usually powered by hydraulics that raise, lower, or change the angle, tilt, and pitch of the blade and can shift the entire blade sideways. If you are a serious grader, you can even add an optional laser system for leveling. It is important to check on the compatibility of a belly blade with your tractor and loader. Most belly blades will not work with cab-model tractors.

Skid shoes are an optional bolt-on attachment that holds the blade off the ground a few inches to allow removal of snow or manure without digging into the road or pen surface. Another feature is that the cutting edge of many blades is either reversible or replaceable by removing bolts. Some blades have optional end plates that convert the blade into a box blade, a great help in moving or leveling material.

FYI

A Box Blade

You can buy a separate box blade, a combination ripper and blade with endplates. The box blade has adjustable teeth (scarifier shanks) at the front of the box that dig into the soil up to 4 inches and a blade, or tailgate, at the rear that can be adjusted to float or grade. A box blade is most useful for landscaping, road maintenance, loafing shed cleanup, or ditch digging.

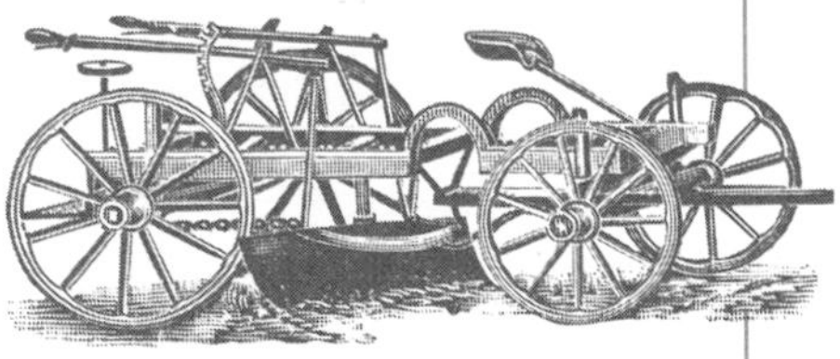

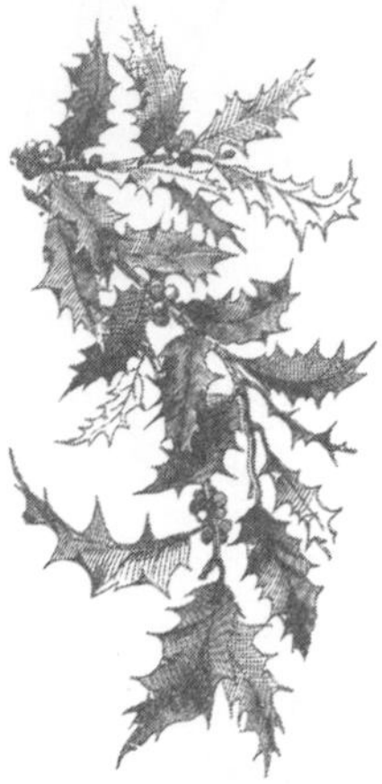

YOUR HORSE'S HOLIDAY WISH LIST

Is there is a special horse on your Christmas list that you would like to thank in some way for his enjoyable partnership and devotion to duty? If so, show that you really appreciate him by choosing something that a horse would enjoy. Pass up the reindeer antlers and choose something from this horse's Christmas wish list. As you might suspect, with horses, food items top the list.

Carrots Count

Carrots are an excellent source of carotene, the precursor to vitamin A. Vitamin A is usually the only vitamin that ever needs to be supplemented in a horse's diet. If a horse is not receiving green, sun-cured hay, he may not be getting adequate carotene.

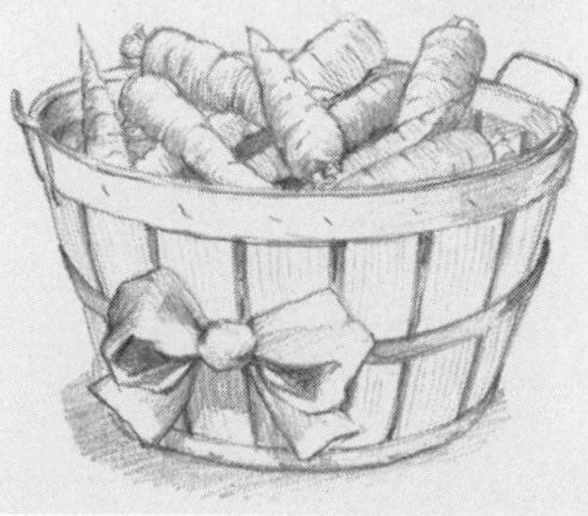

Gifts for the Equine Gourmet

A TRUCKLOAD OF CARROTS. If you have several horses, you can wish them all happy holidays with a truckload of carrots. Some farms sell a pickup load for $100 or so, delivered. If you have a cool, shady place to store them, they will likely keep until the last one is fed. Carrots provide a welcome diversion to the horse's normal ration and can be a healthy reward for good behavior.

If a truckload is not an option, then set aside the money to buy large bags of carrots or apples, especially affordable if you belong to a warehouse club. If you're on a tight budget, you'd be surprised at how many perfectly good (for horses) carrots and apples are thrown away by grocery stores every day. Befriend your local produce manager and arrange to pick up equine goodies regularly.

HOT MASH. When the temperature dips, oatmeal makes a healthy and warming breakfast for you. Likewise, at the barn, during cold weather, your horse might relish a hot grain mash. It takes a little practice and some testing to see what grains and mash consistency appeal to each horse. Don't think of wheat bran as the only choice for a mash (see January and November Ranch Recipes). Also experiment with mashes made from rolled oats, sweet feed, cracked corn, barley, shredded beet pulp, a handful of molasses or a pinch of salt, some oil, or chopped apples or carrots and you are on your way to satisfying your horse's culinary pleasures (or at least enjoying the benevolent feeling you get from trying!).

Measure and mix the dry ingredients the night before and bring them to the house in a pail. When you put the water on for your tea the next morning, boil some extra water for the mash. Usually, a 4:1 ratio of grains to boiling water is satisfactory for most horses. It is best to err on the dry side rather than the mushy side. Stir as you pour the water. Let the mash steep in a warm place for about 30 minutes, preferably covered so it can steam. Check the temperature and serve.

Take a mug of hot tea out to the barn for yourself, find a warm corner to sit, and then listen to the contented slurpings of your appreciative buddies. And know that besides the nutritional benefits, a mash during cold weather can provide your horse with the needed moisture he might be reluctant to sip from a cold bucket.

GRAIN BLOCK. A tasty treat that doubles as a pacifier for a horse that is stalled during cold weather is a molasses grain block. Sold across the country under hundreds of local feed mill labels, these blocks should be considered as an occasional supplement to the horse's normal diet. Under most feeding circumstances, they are unnecessary, but horses dearly love them. Comprised of grain products, molasses, and minerals, the 40- to 50-pound cubes have a wonderful smell and a texture that entices horses to both lick and chew them. Similar products are made for sheep and cattle, but contain a synthetic source of protein called urea, which horses can't utilize.

For horses, it is important to purchase the "premium"

Peppermint Water

Swirl a candy cane in your horse's water pail? This is not just a frivolous holiday act but can have a practical application. Peppermint oil is one substance that can be used to disguise water for the horse that is often "on the road" and will be offered different types of water to drink. Using an aromatic and tasty substance in his water, while he is both at home and away, may be the best gift you give a reluctant drinker.

Being a Horse

Probably the next most popular request on a horse's wish list is his desire to be allowed to be a horse.

Horse History Timeline

Now that it is near the end of the year, it is a good time to look back at what you and your horse have accomplished over the year. I thought it would a be perfect time to look at the big picture, too: where horses have come from and their marks in history, with special emphasis on current statistics related to North America.

BC

- **55,000,000** Appearance of Eohippus, or the dawn horse.
- **4000–3000** Domestication of horses for warfare in chariots.
- **900** First recorded use of horses being ridden as cavalry.
- **365** Xenophon, horseman and prolific author, writes *Treatise on Horsemanship*.
- **338** Alexander, son of Philip of Macedonia, riding Bucephalus, conquers the Greeks.

AD

- **610–625** Mohammed writes the Koran and forms a horse army that is devastatingly effective.
- **1494** Columbus brings horses to the Americas (West Indies); 24 stallions and 10 mares.
- **1519** Cortez brings Spanish horses to Mexico.
- **1500s** Horses are brought into Florida and the Midwest.
- **1521** Cortez and a small number of Spaniards conquer the Aztec empire (in Mexico), mainly due to their use of horses.
- **1572** Spanish Riding School established.
- **1718** First stagecoach in United States.
- **1730** Importation of English racehorses to the United States; they later became known as Thoroughbreds.
- **1777** U.S. Cavalry established.
- **1860–1862** Mail service provided by the Pony Express in United States.

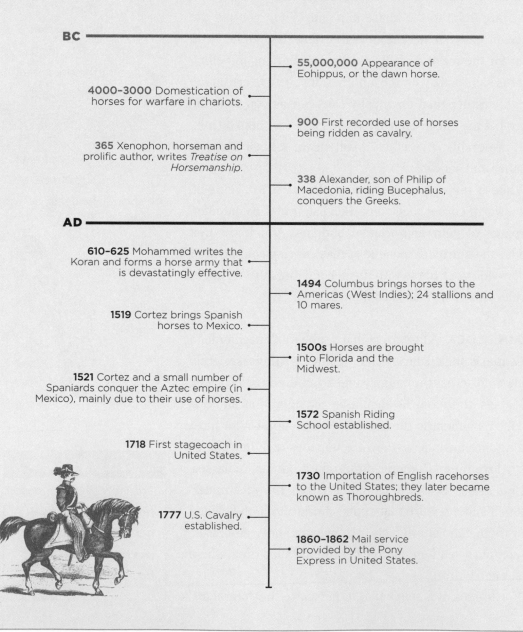

1885 First automobile in United States.

1893 Jockey Club (Thoroughbred breed organization) established in United States.

1904 First tractor invented in United States.

1912 Equestrian events now part of the Olympics.

1914 World War I uses U.S. Cavalry; Henry Ford opens the first automobile assembly line in United States.

1915 United States horse population peeks at an estimated 21,431,000.

1917 American Horse Shows Association established.

1924 U.S. farming shifts over to tractors instead of horses as farm tractors become available.

1940 The American Quarter Horse Association is established.

1941–1945 U.S. Cavalry horses function as draft and pack animals in World War II.

1949 U.S. Cavalry is liquidated.

1950 U.S. horse population reaches modern-day low of an estimated 2,000,000.

1987 U.S. horse population estimated at 5,200,000 by the American Horse Council.

1991 U.S. horse population estimated at 5,000,000 by American Veterinary Medical Association.

1992 U.S. Farm Census reported 2,049,522 horses on farms; 18 percent of farms have horses. This does not include horses that are not on farms (U. S. Department of Agriculture).

1999 U.S. horse population estimated at 5,320,000 (National Agricultural Statistics Service [NASS], Agricultural Statistics Board, U.S. Department of Agriculture).

2002 U.S. horse population estimated at 6,900,000 by the American Horse Council.

2005 U.S. horse population estimated at 9,200,000 with 2,000,000 horse owners and 4,600,000 people involved in the horse industry (American Horse Council)

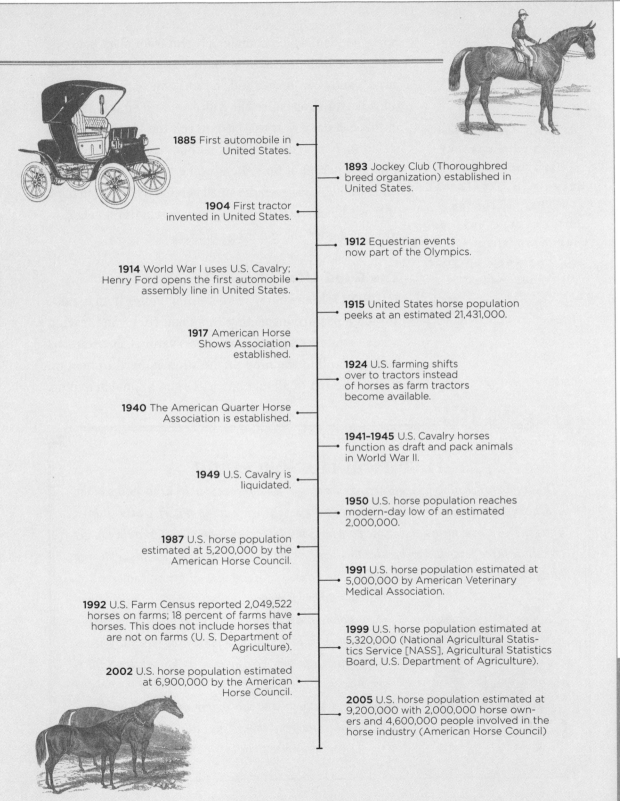

A horse never knows who may buy him, or who may drive him; it is all a chance for us, but still I say, do your best wherever it is, and keep up your good name.

— Anna Sewell, *Black Beauty*

horse version, which contains protein from plant sources, such as soybean meal. Most horses appear to enjoy these large "candy bar" blocks and, in fact, some horses are determined to finish an entire block all at once. If your horse falls in this category, you will have to roll the block out of his stall or pen each day and only let him have access to it for a limited period of time. Be sure he always has adequate water available, as even the small percentage of salt in most of these blocks will increase your horse's thirst reflex — which is a good thing during cold weather.

The Good Life

TURNOUT. Many horses like nothing better than to nose around a pasture inspecting roots and sticks and tracing recent equine history. From observations, it seems as though a roll in the mud or the snow is hard to beat on the equine list of all-time favorite recreational activities.

STILL TRUE TODAY

Historical Horsekeeping

"The importance of strict regularity in feeding is underestimated by nine-tenths of the ordinary feeders, and by fully one-half of the stablemen having the care of well bred horses. The horse, for whatever purpose he is used, if actively employed, should not get less than three feeds a day, besides the hay he eats during the night. All fast working horses should have four feeds a day. The hours of feeding are of prime importance. These should be, as closely as possible, at six in the morning, at noon, and at six at night, except at those pressing seasons of extra labor when the morning feed may be an hour earlier and the evening feed an hour later. In this case, however, nose bags should be carried to the field or they should be turned to the wagon at 10 a.m. and at 4 p.m. to take one-third their usual allowance."

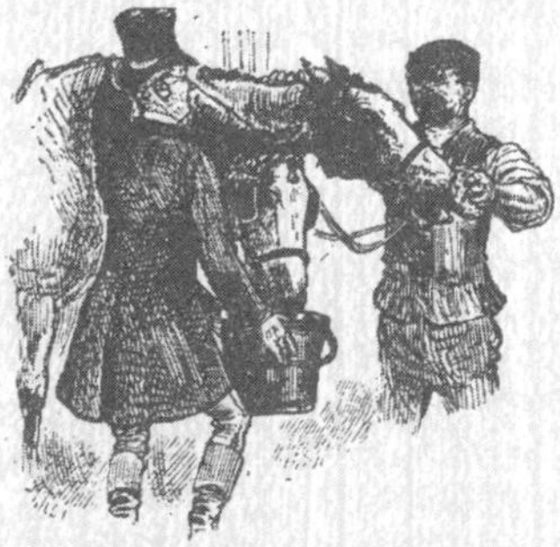

— Gleason's Horse Book *by Prof. Oscar R. Gleason, 1892*

Stall Toys

If you feel you must give an actual present to your horse, perhaps an innovative stall toy is the answer. Designed to while away the hours and discourage wood-chewing and other vices, stall toys can channel pent-up energies toward non-destructive play. Commercial models are often huge rubber balls, but a gallon milk container can work, too. Experiment with hanging the toy from various heights. Note that if your horse becomes obsessed with playing with a toy, you may see some undesirable changes in the curvature of his neck, so monitor how he plays and what height is optimal. A variation on this idea is to give a horse a sturdy beach ball to play with in a small paddock or indoor arena.

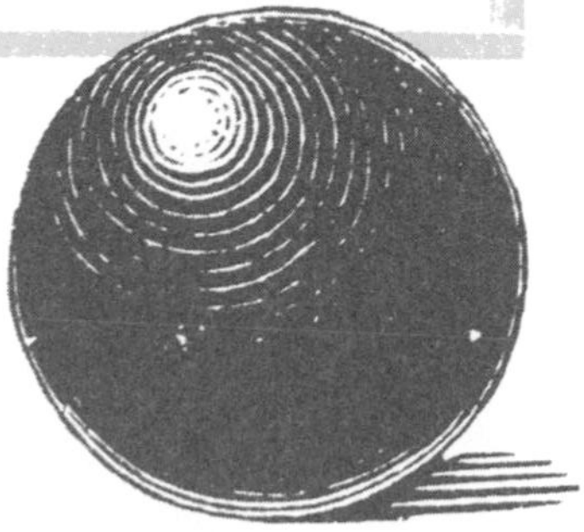

Contrary to our guidelines, horses see absolutely nothing wrong with being dirty or having their manes flop over to both sides of their necks.

TO GROOM OR NOT TO GROOM. Depending on the type of winter management that you follow, you may wish to groom, or not. A pasture horse, left to his natural devices, grows a thick, protective coat and further seals his skin from wind and moisture by accumulating a heavy, waxy sebum at the base of his hairs. Horses that are turned out for the winter should not be extensively groomed, lest you inadvertently remove your horse's valuable oily protection. The best gift for the pastured horse is to let his waxy layer stay intact (without vigorous currying), let his coat be fluffy (not smoothed down by brushing), and to offer him shelter from wet weather or piercing winter winds.

BLANKETS. If your horse would be more comfortable with a winter blanket, be sure to choose a waterproof, breathable one that can be easily laundered so you'll perform that task when necessary.

BODY STROPPING. The stalled horse that is in work not only appreciates but also requires vigorous grooming. A special Christmas session might include body stropping, which is an isotonic muscle exercise. You can use a cactus cloth or a wisp for the stropping. It's a vigorous exercise that includes pounding the large muscle masses of the neck, shoulders, and hindquarters with moderate pressure, which stimulates circulation, and then casting off waste products with a sweeping motion. Massage your horse's legs with your hands using a circular motion toward the heart. Massage your horse's head, with an ear rub for the finale — inside and out, ending with a slight pulling as you slide your fingers off the tips of your horse's ears. Be forewarned: Horses given such a body rub are likely to melt in a puddle! And ask for more.

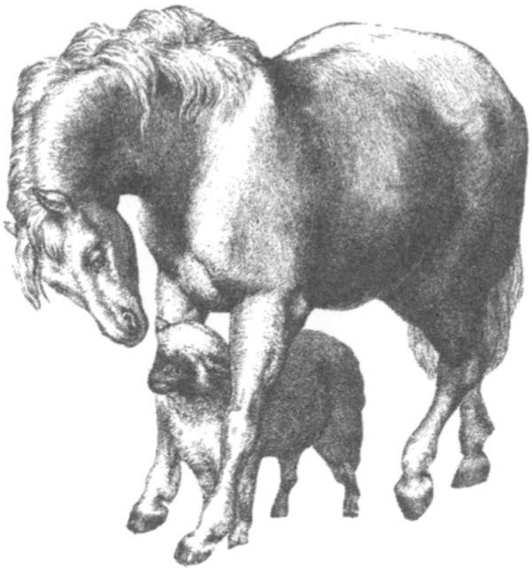

COMPANIONSHIP. If the cold weather has kept your horse in and he is lonely, he might appreciate a stall companion. Some friendships just happen and do not have to be arranged. Cats, chickens, lambs, and dogs have been known to voluntarily take up quarters with a compatible horse. The daily treks and routines of both horse and companion provide interest and comfort for each other. Pygmy goats and other pets or small livestock can sometimes be successfully transplanted in a lonely horse's stall.

As we know, the holiday season is not complete without family and friends. And so it is with equines. A real treat, especially for a stalled horse, is to be turned out with a favorite (compatible) companion. There is nothing quite so joyous as two buddies ripping and tearing in the paddock, playing all the bucking and twisting games that are so important in the horse world. Even though mutual grooming can mess up a lovely mane, it provides unequaled satisfaction and contentment for a horse that is starved for socialization.

I pray that gentle hands
May guide my feet;
I ask for kind commands
From voices sweet;
At night a stable warm
With scented hay,
Where, safe from every harm,
I'll sleep till day.

— Pony's Prayer

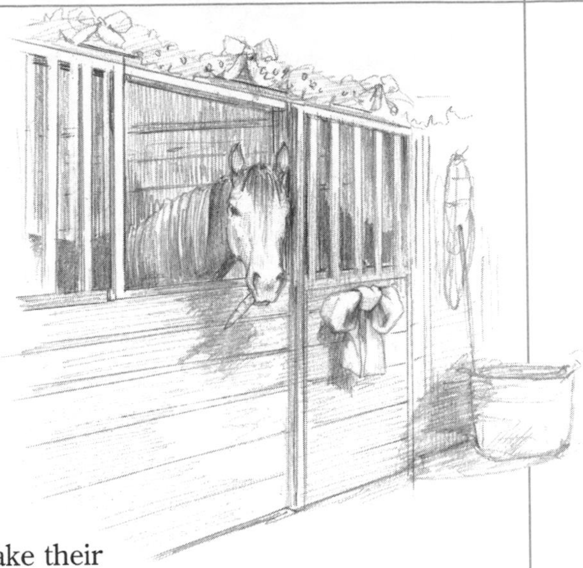

Making a Horse's Work Easier

SHOEING. Horses are appreciative when we make their work easier and more comfortable. One way to do this is to make sure your horse is shod for balance, comfort, and safety year-round. A consultation with an equine veterinary specialist or a master farrier may turn up some helpful ideas regarding your horse's shoeing. Besides checking for proper breakover and flat landing, you may be introduced to new ways to provide safe footing for winter riding.

RIDING WELL. Another way to make a horse's work easier is to become a more physically fit and athletic rider. Give your horse the gift of becoming a more effective rider. Promise to stick with the suppling exercises that help you to mount smoothly and ride more fluidly. Lose a few pounds to ease his burden. Strengthen your body and become a working member of the team, not just a passenger. Make a New Year's resolution to take some riding lessons to improve yourself so that you are a better partner with your horse.

PEACE AND QUIET. Finally, let your horse luxuriate in some peace and quiet. Offer him a comfortable place where he can doze or lie down without distracting lights and noises. Let him sigh and whinny in his sleep and wake when he's ready. Peace.

Winter Fitness

Q Do you have tips for the horse to stay fit during the winter months?

A In many ways, winter is my favorite time to ride — there are no bugs, and it's invigorating for both of us. But winter riding can pose its problems, such as early darkness if you don't have a lighted indoor arena to ride in after work. Also, the temperature here really plummets at about 4:00 p.m. and makes proper cooling-out difficult.

If you are going to keep your horses in active work, consider a combination of body clipping and blanketing. Clipping will reduce sweating during a vigorous workout and will allow you to cool your horses out more quickly and safely. Be sure to use a cooler on your horse as soon as you return after a work session. Consider using a quarter sheet when you ride. Also, winter riding might require specialized shoes for your horse. Maybe I'll see you on the trail this winter!

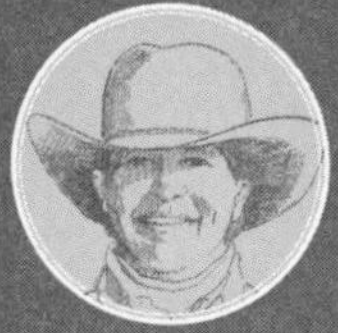

Ask Cherry

Blanket/Unblanket

Q When do I blanket my horse? Is it okay to blanket him when it's below 0°F and then remove it once the temperatures are around 20°F or warmer? Or am I better off not to blanket at all if I don't keep it on all the time?

A It depends on your horse's winter coat and his type of shelter. If he has a good winter coat, you don't do a lot of grooming or bathing in the winter, and he has shelter to get out of the wind and wet, he doesn't need a blanket. If he has a thin hair coat, if you groom or bathe him, or if he has to stand out in the wind and wet, then by all means, yes, use a winter blanket in temperatures below 15°F.

Choose a blanket that is lightweight but warm. Heavy blankets flatten the hair, so when you remove them there is no natural loft to provide air insulation. If you are blanketing your horse in cold temperatures for weeks rather than just days, then you might need to "wean" him off the blanket when the weather warms up. When days are in the 30s but the nights are in the teens, you still might want to blanket your horse at night or at least put a waterproof, windproof, breathable sheet on him as a "transition" blanket. There is no absolute or easy answer, as all horses, shelters, management, and weather patterns are so different.

APPENDIX

WEB SITE RESOURCES

Horsekeeping, Horse Training, and Horse Care Information

Cherry Hill's Horsekeeping *www.horsekeeping.com*

Weather, Climate, Natural Science

Canada Environment *www.ec.gc.ca*

Canada Weather Office *www.weatheroffice.gc.ca/canada_e.html*

Day length by latitude *www.orchidculture.com/COD/daylength.html*

Drought Monitor *www.drought.unl.edu/dm/archive.html*

Latitude map *http://geography.fullerton.edu/332/climate/latlong.gif*

National Fire Maps *www.nifc.gov/firemaps.html*

National Oceanic and Atmospheric Administration *www.noaa.gov*

NOAA wind chill chart *www.nws.noaa.gov/om/windchill*

National Weather Service Weather Maps *www.weather.gov*

National Weather Service Fire Forecast Map *http://fire.boi.noaa.gov*

USGS earthquake information *http://earthquake.usgs.gov/regional/states/seismicity*

Wind maps, National Weather Service *http://adds.aviationweather.noaa.gov/winds*

Wind maps, U.S. Department of Energy *http://www.eere.energy.gov/windandhydro/windpoweringamerica/wind_maps.asp*

Equine Health

American Association of Equine Practitioners (AAEP) horseowner's site *www.myhorsematters.com*

American Farrier's Association (AFA): *www.americanfarriers.org*

Centers for Disease Control and Prevention *www.cdc.gov*

EPA mold information *www.epa.gov/mold/moldresources.html*

The Farrier and Hoofcare Resource Center *www.horseshoes.com*

Humane ending of a horse's life: *www.agric.nsw.gov.au/reader/aw-companion/humane-destruction-stock.htm*

The Horse *www.thehorse.com*

Lyme disease map *www.cdc.gov/ncidod/dvbid/lyme/tickmap.htm*

Pasture-related laminitis in horses *www.safergrass.org*

Poisonous plants informational database *www.ansci.cornell.edu/plants/comlist.html*

Horse Information

American Horse Council *www.horsecouncil.org*

American Riding Instructors Association *www.riding-instructor.com/*

National Animal Identification System *animalid.aphis.usda.gov/nais/index.shtml*

Wild horses and burros *www.wildhorseandburro.blm.gov/index.php*

Horse ID and Security

Home Again Pet Recovery Service *www.homeagainid.com*

HorseTrac Protection Network for Microchipped Horses *www.horsetracusa.com*

Liability signs *www.kyhorse.com/store/equipment/statesigns.htm*

United Animal Nations (emergency animal sheltering and disaster relief services) *www.uan.org*

Emergency Information

Federal Emergency Management Agency (FEMA) *www.fema.gov*

RECOMMENDED READING

Anthony, Stan. *Farm and Ranch Safety Management.* Albany, NY: Delmar Publishers, 1995.

Damerow, Gail. *Fences for Pasture and Garden.* Pownal, VT: Garden Way Publishing, 1992.

Ewing, Rex A. *Beyond the Hay Days: A Refreshingly Simple Guide to Effective Horse Nutrition.* LaSalle, CO: Pixyjack Press, 1997.

Fershtman, Julie I. *Equine Law and Horse Sense.* Franklin, MI: Horses and the Law Publishing, 1996.

Fershtman, Julie I. *More Equine Law and Horse Sense.* Franklin, MI: Horses and the Law Publishing, 2000.

Hill, Cherry. *Equipping Your Horse Farm.* North Adams, MA: Storey Books, 2006.

Hill, Cherry. *The Formative Years: Raising and Training the Young Horse from Birth to Two Years.* Ossining, NY: Breakthrough, 1988.

Hill, Cherry. *Horse for Sale: How to Buy a Horse or Sell the One You Have.* New York, NY: Howell Book House, 1995.

Hill, Cherry. *Horsekeeping on a Small Acreage.* 2nd edition. North Adams, MA: Storey Books, 2005.

Hill, Cherry, *Horse Handling and Grooming.* North Adams, MA: Storey Books, 1990.

Hill, Cherry. *Horse Health Care.* North Adams, MA: Storey Books, 1997.

Hill, Cherry. *How to Think Like a Horse.* North Adams, MA: Storey Books, 2006.

Hill, Cherry, and Richard Klimesh. *Maximum Hoof Power, A Horse Owner's Guide to Shoeing and Soundness.* N. Pomfret, VT: Trafalgar Square, 2000.

Hill, Cherry. *Horse Care for Kids.* North Adams, MA: Storey Books, 2002.

Hill, Cherry. *Stablekeeping: A Visual Guide to Safe and Healthy Horsekeeping.* North Adams, MA: Storey Books, 2000.

Hill, Cherry. *Trailering Your Horse: A Visual Guide to Safe Training and Traveling.* North Adams, MA: Storey Books, 2000.

Klimesh, Richard and Cherry Hill. *Horse Housing: How to Plan, Build, and Remodel Barns and Sheds.* N. Pomfret, VT: Trafalgar Square, 2002

Knight, Dr. Tony. *A Guide to Plant Poisoning of Animals in North America.* Jackson, WY: Teton New Media, 2001.

Lewis, Lon. *Feeding & Care of the Horse.* 2nd edition. Media, PA: Williams & Wilkins, 1997.

Lodge, Ray and Susan Shanks. *All-Weather Surfaces for Horses.* London: J.A. Allen, 1999.

Malmgren, Robert. *The Equine Arena Handbook: Developing A User-Friendly Facility.* Loveland, CO: Alpine Publications, 1999.

McFarland, Cynthia, *The Foaling Primer.* North Adams, MA: Storey Books, 2005.

United States Department of Agriculture. *Plants Poisonous to Livestock in the Western States,* Agriculture Information Bulletin 415. Washington, DC: US Government Printing Office.

United States Dressage Federation. *Under Foot: Guide to Arena Construction, Maintenance & Repair.* 3rd edition. Lexington, KY: 2007.

INDEX

Page numbers in *italic* indicate illustrations, photos, or maps; those in **bold** indicate tables or charts.

C

I